Outline of Periodontics

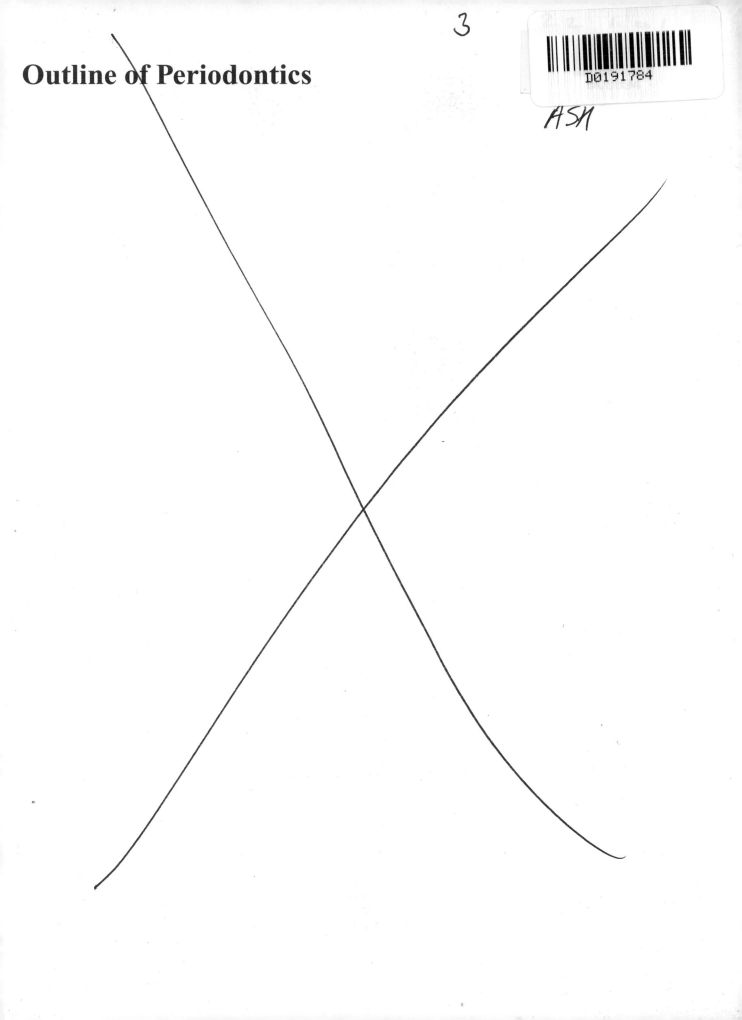

Outline of Periodontics

Fourth edition

J.D. Manson MChD, PhD, FDSRCS
Formerly Visiting Lecturer, King's College Hospital and Dental School;
Senior Lecturer in Periodontology, Institute of Dental Surgery;
Honorary Consultant, Eastman Dental Institute, London, UK

and

B.M. Eley BDS, FDSRCS, PhD
Head of Division of Periodontology and Preventive Dentistry,
Guy's, King's and St Thomas' Dental Institute, London, UK;
Honorary Consultant to King's Healthcare NHS Trust and
Guy's and St Thomas' Hospital NHS Trust

OXFORD • AUCKLAND • BOSTON • JOHANNESBURG • MELBOURNE • NEW DELHI

wright
W

Wright
An imprint of Butterworth-Heinemann
Linacre House, Jordan Hill, Oxford OX2 8DP
225 Wildwood Avenue, Woburn, MA 01801-2041
A division of Reed Educational and Professional Publishing Ltd

℞ A member of the Reed Elsevier plc group

First published 1983
Second edition 1989
Reprinted 1991, 1993
Third edition 1995
Reprinted 1996
Fourth edition 2000

© J.D. Manson and B.M. Eley 2000

British Library Cataloguing in Publication Data
Manson, J. D.
  Outline of periodontics. - 4th ed.
  1. Periodontics
  I. Title   II. Eley, B. M. (Barry M.)
  617.6'32

ISBN 0 7236 1070 3

Library of Congress Cataloguing in Publication Data
Manson, J. D. (Julius David)
  Outline of periodontics/J.D. Manson and B.M. Eley.–4th ed.
    p. ; cm.
  Includes bibliographical references and index.
  ISBN 0 7236 1070 3
  1. Periodontics.   I. Eley, B. M. (Barry M.)   II. Title.
  [DNLM: 1. Periodontal Diseases.   2. Periodontal Diseases–therapy. WU 240 M289o 1999]
  RK361 .M349
  617.6'32–dc21   99–045299

ISBN 0 7236 1070 3

Typeset by Keytec Typesetting Ltd., Dorset
Printed and bound in Great Britain by the Bath Press, Somerset

Contents

Preface to the fourth edition

'Knowledge advances by steps, and not by leaps' said Lord Macauly, nineteenth century English historian, and the history of our exploration into the aetiology and pathogenesis of periodontal disease exemplifies this slow and, more often than not, uncertain process.

The relationship between periodontal disease and oral bacteria has been suspected for hundreds of years, but it was only with the elegant experiments of Waerhaug over 40 years ago, and then of Löe, Theilade and Jensen a decade later that this connection was established on a scientific footing. Since then, the mechanisms of disease production have been clarified and the techniques of dealing with disease of the tooth-supporting tissues and its sequelae have become increasingly sophisticated and effective. In this edition we have tried to spell out clearly the most recent thinking, and to give a straightforward account of current practice. However, the mundane role of good oral hygiene remains the central pivot of sound oral health and the prevention of periodontal disease for the vast majority of our patients, and the efforts of the dental profession must be bent towards the application of our knowledge to health education. However, we should not forget the role of genetics in determining susceptibility to periodontal disease, and recent significant advances in this area have been included.

We would like to thank a number of people for their invaluable help in updating material for this new edition, including Dr M. Soory for her help with the sections on 'Gingival hyperplasia' and 'Dental implants', Mr C.A. Waterman for his help with the chapter on 'Mucogingival problems and their treatment' and Professor R.M. Watson for his help with the section on 'Dental implants'.

J.D.M.
B.M.E.

Preface to the first edition

There is now a considerable body of knowledge about the aetiology and pathogenesis of periodontal disease. Yet this knowledge is scarcely applied; chronic gingivitis and chronic inflammatory periodontal disease remain universal and tooth loss in the adult is still regarded by many people as an inevitable part of the ageing process. There are several reasons for this sorry state of affairs, including socioeconomic factors beyond the influence of the dental profession. One factor which is wholly dependent upon the profession is the standard of undergraduate teaching. Periodontics still occupies a minor position in the curriculum of many dental schools and is regarded by too many undergraduates and dentists as an esoteric subject peripheral to the main body of conservative dentistry.

This basic text has been written in an attempt to make our understanding of periodontal disease accessible to the undergraduate, to hygienists and to any interested reader. The main emphasis is on the plaque theory and on the prevention and early diagnosis of the disease. I have tried to avoid too great an emphasis on surgical techniques. Periodontics is not a surgical discipline; such techniques have to be resorted to only when prevention, early diagnosis and treatment techniques fail.

I am indebted to many of my colleagues, recognized in the text, for providing illustrative material, to Dr Barry Eley for his valuable comments, to Mr James Morgan of the Eastman Dental Hospital and Mr Peter Gordon for help with photography and to Mrs Jenny Halstead for her drawings without which this text would be incomplete.

J.D.M.

1

The periodontal tissues

The masticatory system consists of the mandible and maxilla, the muscles of mastication, the temporomandibular joints and associated ligaments, and the teeth plus the tooth-supporting or periodontal tissues.

It is essential to view this system as a functional unit in which all the parts are interdependent. Breakdown of the dentition may affect other components of the masticatory system; alterations in the functional activity of the muscles of mastication or temporomandibular joints can affect the dental tissues. Like all vital tissues, the tissues of the masticatory system are in a state of constant activity. Cells metabolize, reproduce, die and are replaced; non-cellular tissue components, e.g. collagen and ground substance, are synthesized, broken down and replaced. This activity is influenced by age, nutritional and hormonal status and by functional demand. It is also affected by disease.

The periodontium has four components: the gingivae, the alveolar bone, the periodontal ligament and the cementum. Knowledge of the periodontal tissue in health is essential to an understanding of its behaviour in disease.

The gingivae

Introduction

The gingiva is the part of the oral mucosa that surrounds the tooth and covers the alveolar ridge. It is part of the tooth-supporting apparatus, the periodontium, and by forming a connection with the tooth the gingiva protects the underlying tissues of the tooth attachment from the oral environment. The gingiva is tooth dependent; when there are teeth there are gingivae, and when teeth are extracted the gingivae disappear.

Like all vital tissues the gingiva can adapt itself to changes in its environment, and the mouth, which is the first part of the alimentary tract and the site of the initial preparation of food in digestion, may be regarded as a relatively hostile environment. The oral tissues are exposed to an enormous range of stimuli. The temperature and consistency of food and drink, its chemical composition, acidity and alkalinity vary considerably. The number of bacteria in the mouth is immense, and their variety is beyond exact definition. Add to this the insults and irritations of dental manipulations, and one can only be impressed by the sheer resilience of the oral mucosa and the efficiency of gingival defence mechanisms, which include:

1. The salivary flow and saliva contents, e.g. lysozyme, immunoglobulin (Ig) A
2. Cell turnover and surface desquamation
3. The activity of the immune mechanisms.

The junction between the tooth and the oral mucosa, the dentogingival junction, is unique and peculiarly vulnerable. It is the only attachment in the body between a soft tissue and a calcified tissue that is exposed to the external environment.

This junction is a highly dynamic tissue with its own battery of protective mechanisms.

Healthy gingiva is pink, firm, knife-edged and scalloped to conform to the contour of the teeth (*Figure 1.1*). Its colour may vary with the amount of melanin pigmentation in the epithelium, the degree of keratinization of the epithelium and the vascularity and fibrous nature of the underlying connective tissue. In Caucasian individuals, pigmentation is minimal; in patients of African or Asian origin, brown or blue-black areas of pigmentation may cover a great part of the gingiva; in Mediterranean races, occasional patches of pigmentation are found. It is important to distinguish physiological pigmentation from that which occurs in some diseases and with metal contamination.

The gingiva is divided into two zones: the marginal gingiva and attached gingiva (*Figure 1.2*).

Figure 1.1 Healthy gingivae in a girl of 19 years

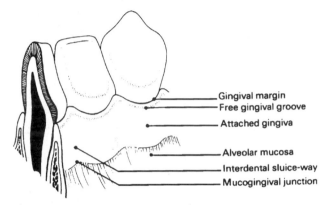

Figure 1.2 Diagram illustrating anatomical features of the gingiva

The gingival margin

The marginal gingiva forms a cuff 1–2 mm wide around the neck of the tooth and is the external wall of the gingival crevice, which is 0–2 mm deep. This cuff can be separated from the tooth by careful manipulation of a blunt probe. Between the teeth the margin forms a cone-shaped gingival papilla, the labial surface of which is frequently indented by a groove called a 'sluice-way'. The papilla fills the space in the interdental embrasure apical to the contact point, and its facial-lingual shape conforms to the curvature of the cemento-enamel junction to form the interdental col (*Figure 1.3*).

The surface of the gingival margin is smooth, in

Figure 1.3 The interdental gingiva in the shape of a 'col' reflects the contours of the tooth contact area

contrast to that of the attached gingiva, from which it is demarcated by an indentation called the 'free gingival' groove (see *Figure 1.2*).

Attached gingiva

The attached gingiva or 'functional mucosa' extends from the free gingival groove to the mucogingival junction, where it meets the alveolar mucosa (see *Figure 1.2*). The attached gingiva is a mucoperiosteum, which is tightly bound to the underlying alveolar bone. At the mucogingival junction the mucoperiosteum splits so that the alveolar mucosa is separated from the periosteum by a loose, highly vascular, connective tissue. Thus the alveolar mucosa is a relatively loose and mobile tissue, deep red in colour, in marked contrast to the pale pink attached gingiva (see *Figure 1.1*). The surface of the attached gingiva is stippled like orange peel. This stippling varies considerably. It is most prominent on facial surfaces, and often disappears in old age. There is some doubt about the cause of the stippling, but it appears to coincide with epithelial rete pegs.

The width of the attached gingiva can vary from about 0–9 mm. It is usually widest in the incisor region (3–5 mm) and narrowest over the mandibular canines and premolars. In the past it has been assumed that some attached gingiva is necessary to maintain the health of the gingival margin by separating the stable margin from the mobile alveolar mucosa, but this does not appear to be the case in the clean mouth. This variation in width has given rise to controversy about what form of anatomy is compatible with health, and techniques have been devised to widen areas of attached gingiva considered to be too narrow, irrespective of whether disease is present or not. Any width, even a zero width, is acceptable if the tissue is healthy.

Microscopic features of the gingiva

The gingival margin consists of a core of fibrous connective tissue covered by stratified squamous epithelium that, like all squamous epithelium, undergoes constant renewal by continuous cell reproduction in its deepest layers and shedding of the superficial layers. The two activities are held in balance so that the thickness of the epithelium remains constant. It has the characteristic layers of squamous epithelium:

1. The basal or formative cell layers of columnar or cuboidal cells
2. The prickle-cells or spinous layer (stratum spinosum) of polygonal cells
3. The granular layer (stratum granulosum), in which the cells are flatter and contain many particles of keratohyaline
4. The cornified layer (stratum corneum), in which the cells have become flat and shrunken, and keratinized or parakeratinized.

The mitotic rate of oral epithelium varies from place to place, with age, and also from one animal to another. Turnover times in the experimental animal are said to be 5–6 days for the palate, tongue and cheek, and 10–12 days for the gingiva.

Like all epithelial cells, gingival epithelium cells are connected to each other and to the underlying connective tissue corium by thickenings on the periphery of the cells called hemidesmosomes. The epithelium is joined to the underlying corium by a thin basal lamina made of a protein-polysaccharide complex which is permeable to fluid. Seen by electron microscopy it can be resolved into two layers: the lamina lucida and the lamina densa.

The epithelium of the outer or oral surface of the gingival margin is keratinized or parakeratinized, while the epithelium of the inner or crevicular surface is thinner and non-keratinized. Contrary to popular opinion, non-keratinized oral epithelium is not necessarily always more permeable than keratinized epithelium. Intact epithelium is an effective barrier against micro-organisms, which can breach damaged epithelium, but intact epithelium is permeable to many smaller substances, such as the molecules of skin antiseptics, topical anaesthetics and vasodilators (e.g. glyceryl trinitrate).

Pigmentation is produced by pigment-forming melanocytes. However, variation in pigmentation is not produced by variation in the number of these cells, but by genetically determined variation in their pigment-producing capacity. The ratio of melanocytes to the keratin-producing epithelial cells is relatively constant at 1 : 36 cells.

The gingival connective tissue is made up of a mesh of collagen fibre bundles running in a ground substance that contains blood vessels and nerves, plus fibroblasts, macrophages, mast cells, lymphocytes, plasma cells and other cells of the defence system, which are more numerous near the junctional epithelium, where immune activity is maintained. In common with other connective tissues, the gingival fibrous connective tissues are composed of specialized fibroblast cells and a collagenous fibrous network embedded in an extracellular matrix composed of proteoglycans and other matrix glycoproteins. The normal connective tissue function involves constant remodelling of the matrix components, and is dependent upon the interactions between the cells and the matrix molecules in their environment. This involves the production and attachment to their receptors of signal molecules such as growth and differentiation factors and cell adhesion molecules, and their interaction with components of the extracellular matrix. Various proteoglycans appear to play important role in tissue remodelling and the maintenance of structural integrity.

The ground substance

Connective tissue cells and fibres, together with vessels and nerves, are embedded in an amorphous, non-fibrous and non-cellular matrix made up of glycosaminoglycans (GAGs), proteoglycans and glycoproteins. All the components of the matrix are synthesized and secreted by fibroblasts. The most common GAG is hyaluronic acid (hyaluronan), large amounts of which are found in gingiva. Proteoglycans are composed of a central protein core, to which is attached a variable number of highly anionic GAG chains.

The structure of proteoglycans depends on the type of GAG chains attached to their protein core. The soft tissues, such as the gingival tissue and the periodontal ligament (see below), contain small dermatan sulphate proteoglycans and a larger molecular weight chondroitin sulphate proteoglycan, versican, which is capable of interacting with hyaluronan (Embery *et al.*, 1979, 1987; Purvis *et al.*, 1984; Pearson and Pringle, 1986; Larjava *et al.*, 1992). GAGs are long unbranched polysaccharides that can bind large amounts of water and, as a result of this, tissues containing large amounts of GAG resist compressive forces well. GAG also facilitates the transport of nutrients through the extracellular spaces. In addition, the matrix transports metabolic products, cells and chemical messengers known as cytokines, which moderate cellular function. Proteoglycans are also present on cell surfaces, for example syndecan and CD 44, where they function in the control of cell attachment, migration and proliferation and the binding of growth factors such as transforming growth factor beta (TGFβ) (Gallagher *et al.*, 1986).

One of the most important glycoproteins is fibronectin. This is a large protein that binds to cells, collagen and proteoglycans. It is important in promoting the adhesion of fibroblasts to the extracellular matrix, and also plays a role in the alignment of collagen fibres.

The gingival fibres (Figure 1.4)

The connective tissue of the gingiva is organized to keep the gingival margin tight around the neck of the tooth and to maintain the integrity of the dentogingival attachment. The arrangement of these fibres is complicated, but they have been described as being divided into several discernible groups of collagen fibre bundles:

1. *Dentogingival* or free gingival fibres, which are attached to cementum and fan out into the gingiva

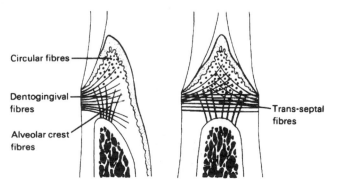

Figure 1.4 Gingival fibre groups: dentogingival, circular, alveolar crest and trans-septal fibres

and over the alveolar margin to merge with the periosteum of the attached gingiva

2. *Alveolar-gingival* or alveolar crest fibres, which arise from the alveolar crest and run coronally into the gingiva
3. *Circular* fibres, which encircle the tooth
4. *Trans-septal* fibres, which run from tooth to tooth coronally to the alveolar septum.

There is a great deal of interlinking between fibre groups, and special stains are needed to define the fibres.

Collagen is synthesized by fibroblasts and secreted in an inactive form, procollagen, which is then converted into tropocollagen. In the extracellular space, tropocollagen is polymerized into collagen fibrils, which are then aggregated into collagen bundles by the formation of cross-linkages. Different forms of collagen may be secreted, and each is based on variations in the composition of the basic tropocollagen molecule. The most common form found in the gingiva is Type I collagen, which forms the major fibre bundles and the loose collagenous fibres. Some Type III and V collagens are also present. Type VI collagen is present in the basement membranes of blood vessels and the overlying epithelium.

Gingival blood, lymph and nerve supply

The gingiva has a rich blood supply derived from three sources: supraperiosteal and periodontal ligament vessels, plus alveolar vessels, which emerge from the alveolar crest (*Figure 1.5*). These link in the gingiva to form capillary loops in the connective tissue papillae between the epithelial rete pegs. Lymphatic drainage starts in the connective tissue papillae and drains into regional lymph nodes: from the mandibular gingiva into the cervical, submandibular and submental nodes; from the maxillary gingiva into the deep cervical lymph nodes.

The nerve supply is derived from branches of the trigeminal nerve. A number of nerve endings have been identified in the gingival connective tissue as tactile corpuscles, and temperature and pain receptors.

The interdental gingiva

The gingiva between the teeth is concave and has been described as a 'col' that joins the facial and lingual papillae (see *Figure 1.3*). Where teeth make contact, the cols conform to the shape of the teeth apical to the contact area. Where neighbouring teeth do not make contact there is no col, and the interdental gingiva is flat or convex.

The epithelium of the col is very thin, non-keratinized, and made up of only a few cell layers. Its structure probably reflects its sheltered position. Turnover of interdental epithelial cells is the same as that of the rest of the gingiva.

The interdental region is of special importance, as it is the site of the most persistent bacterial stagnation and its structure makes it especially vulnerable. *It is the site of the initial lesion in gingivitis.*

The dentogingival junction

It is possible to define three zones of gingival epithelium (*Figure 1.6*). Oral epithelium extends from the mucogingival junction to the gingival margin, where crevicular (or sulcular) epithelium lines the gingival crevice (or sulcus). At the base of the crevice, the connection between the gingiva and the tooth is mediated by a special kind of epithelium called junctional epithelium.

In health, the junctional epithelium lies against enamel and extends to the cemento-enamel junction. If there is gingival recession, the junctional epithelium lies on cementum. Thus the base of the gingival crevice is the free surface of the junctional epithelium. It is said that in perfect health the depth of the crevice is zero, so there is

Figure 1.5 The rich gingival blood supply derives from: *(a)* periodontal ligament, *(b)* alveolar bone and *(c)* supraperiosteal vessels

Figure 1.6 The dentogingival junction. There are three zones of gingival epithelium: oral epithelium (O), crevicular (or sulcus) epithelium (C) and the junctional epithelium (J)

no crevicular epithelium and oral epithelium therefore merges directly into the junctional epithelium. This does not occur in humans.

At an ultrastructural level, a very thin basement lamina lies between the junctional epithelial cells and the connective tissue corium, and between the junctional epithelium and the tooth surface. The latter basement lamina and related hemidesmosomes form the 'epithelial attachment', which is a product of epithelial cells. If gingivectomy is carried out and the junctional epithelium is completely removed, a new gingival margin plus new junctional epithelium are formed on healing whether the gingiva is on enamel, dentine or cementum.

The junctional epithelium is very fragile, and does not form a barrier against probing. Its cells are larger than those of oral epithelium and are loosely connected together; indeed the cell-to-cell connection is more fragile than the attachment to the tooth surface. Unlike keratinized epithelial cells of the crevice, the cells of the junctional epithelium can attach via hemidesmosomes to tooth surface.

The junctional epithelium in adults is about 40 cells long from apex to crevicular surface, but it varies from 0.25 to 1.35 mm; in the young it is a narrow sleeve as thin as 3–4 cells, whereas in the adult it is 10–20 cells wide. Although it undergoes constant renewal, with cell division taking place throughout its structure, the junctional epithelium is relatively homogeneous and without any pattern of cell differentiation. Although the turnover time for human junctional epithelium is not known, in other primates it is said to be approximately 4–6 days – i.e. half that of oral epithelium, which is roughly 10–12 days. Desquamation of the junctional epithelium takes place through the small free area at the base of the gingival crevice. Listgarten (1972) has calculated that the rate of cellular exfoliation from a unit surface of junctional epithelium is 50–100 times as fast as that from a unit of oral gingival epithelium. A small number of leucocytes (neutrophils) are often found within the junctional epithelium.

In contrast to oral gingival epithelium and crevicular epithelium, the junctional epithelium is relatively permeable and allows a two-way movement of a variety of substances:

1. From corium into the crevice – gingival fluid exudate, polymorphonuclear leucocytes, various cells of the immune system plus immunoglobulins and complement. It is the exit point for most of the leucocytes found in saliva. In inflammation the movement of fluid and cells increases and, as the population of leucocytes increases, the junctional epithelium may degenerate and become even more permeable. Some research workers believe that in perfect health there is no passage of gingival fluid into the crevice.
2. From crevice into the corium – foreign materials such as carbon particles, trypan blue (mol.wt 960) and many other substances inserted into the gingival crevice are subsequently found in the gingival corium

and the bloodstream. *Micro-organisms cannot penetrate junctional epithelium*, but a large number of substances, some of them with high molecular weights, have been shown to pass through the intercellular spaces of the junctional epithelium. This is an extremely important finding, as it is believed that gingival inflammation is initiated by bacterial enzymes and metabolic products that diffuse from the crevice through the junctional epithelium into the gingival connective tissue.

Because of the permeability of junctional epithelium it is inevitable that the tissue defence mechanisms should be in a constant state of alertness, and this is manifested by an infiltration of inflammatory cells, lymphocytes and plasma cells in the underlying corium. This used to be interpreted as a sign of disease, but indicates the constant presence of the defence mechanisms in health.

Formation of the dentogingival attachment

There has been some controversy about the origin and structure of the attachment tissues but, using electron microscope findings and the results of autoradiographic studies of cellular activity, a consensus seems to have been achieved.

When enamel formation is complete, the reduced enamel epithelium is attached to enamel by a basal lamina and hemidesmosomes. As the tooth penetrates the oral mucosa the reduced enamel epithelium unites with the oral epithelium and, with continuing eruption, this epithelium condenses along the crown. Ameloblasts gradually atrophy and are replaced by squamous epithelium, i.e. the junctional epithelium, which forms a collar around the fully erupted tooth. As already described, junctional epithelium, like all squamous epithelium, is a constantly renewing structure with epithelial cells moving coronally to be shed at the free surface into the bottom of the crevice.

Gingival crevicular fluid

If a filter paper strip is inserted into the gingival crevice, it will absorb fluid already in the crevice and may also provoke an outward flow of fluid. This also happens in mastication, on toothbrushing and with any other stimulation of the gingivae; the flow is greatly increased when the gingivae are inflamed. Sex hormones, oestrogen and progesterone appear to increase the flow, perhaps by causing increased permeability of gingival blood vessels. Certain chemotactic factors found in plaque may also increase the flow. This fluid is an inflammatory exudate, and carries polymorphonuclear leucocytes and other antimicrobial substances. It forms part of the defence mechanism of the dentogingival junction. If a patient is on systemic tetracyclines, the drug finds its way via gingival blood vessels, connective tissue and junctional epithelium into the gingival crevice. In summary, the fluid performs the following functions:

1. It washes the crevice, carrying out shed epithelial cells, leucocytes, bacteria and other debris
2. The plasma proteins may influence the epithelial attachment to the tooth
3. It contains antimicrobial agents, e.g. lysozyme
4. It carries polymorphonuclear leucocytes and macrophages, which are capable of phagocytosing bacteria. It also transports immunoglobulins IgG, IgA, IgM and other factors of the immune system.

The amount of gingival crevicular fluid can be measured and used as an index of gingival inflammation. Its composition may also be determined by a variety of biochemical and immunocytochemical techniques, and may relate to the severity of the underlying periodontal pathology.

The periodontal ligament

A ligament is a bond, usually linking two bones together. The root of the tooth is connected to its socket in alveolar bone by a dense fibrous connective tissue, which can be regarded as a ligament. Above the alveolar crest it is continuous with the gingival connective tissue, and at the apical foramina with the pulp. Considerable research has been carried out into the structure, function and composition of the periodontal ligament for both functional and clinical reasons. It has the following functions:

*   It is the tissue of attachment between the tooth and alveolar bone; thus, it is responsible for resisting displacing forces and protects the dental tissues from the effects of excessive occlusal loads
*   It is responsible for maintaining the tooth in a functional position during tooth eruption and the changes in tooth position that follow tooth extraction, tooth attrition or excessive occlusal loading
*   Its cells form, maintain and repair alveolar bone and cementum
*   Its mechanoreceptors are involved in the neurological control of mastication
*   It has a rich blood supply, which anastomoses with that in the marrow spaces of the bone and the gingiva and facilitates these functions.

The periodontal ligament not only connects the tooth to the jaw bone but also supports the tooth in the socket and absorbs loads imposed on the tooth, thus protecting the tooth, especially at the root apex. The cells of the ligament maintain and repair alveolar bone and cementum. The ligament is a reservoir from which bone and cementum forming cells are derived; precursor cells are formed from stem cells in the bone marrow, and from there migrate into the periodontal ligament. The proprioceptor nerve endings in the ligament form part of the extremely refined neurological control of mastication, and the mechanoreceptors monitor changes in pressure within the ligament space. The anastomosis of the blood supply and tissue fluid between the bone marrow spaces is very important in the maintenance of an adequate supply during compression of the ligament during functional movements. All these points are more fully discussed below.

Structure and function

The thickness of the ligament varies from about 0.3–0.1 mm. It is widest at the mouth of the socket and at the apex, and narrowest at the level of the axis of rotation of the tooth, which is slightly apical to the middle of the root. In health there is a normal range of tooth mobility. Incisors are more mobile than posterior teeth; mobility is greatest on wakening and reduces through the day. As in other parts of the skeleton, functional stresses are essential to the maintenance of the periodontal ligament's tissues. When functional stresses are heavy the ligament becomes thicker, and when a tooth is functionless the ligament can become as thin as 0.06 mm. With ageing the ligament also becomes thinner.

The ligament consists of well-organized collagen fibre bundles, about 5 μm in diameter, in a ground substance matrix through which vessels and nerves course. The fibre bundles, which are inserted at one end into cementum and at the other into the socket wall as Sharpey's fibres, are usually described in identifiable groups according to their predominant orientation (*Figure 1.7*):

1. Alveolar crest fibres run from the cementum at the neck of the tooth to the alveolar crest
2. Horizontal fibres run from cementum to alveolar crest
3. Oblique fibres form the main component of the ligament and run from the bone in a slightly apical direction to be inserted in the cementum so that they appear to be suspending the tooth in its socket
4. Apical fibres radiate from the apex to the base of the socket. One can also include the inter-radicular

Figure 1.7 Periodontal ligament fibre bundles

fibres, which are found in the furcation of multi-rooted teeth and, like trans-septal fibres, run from root to root coronal to the alveolar crest.

A single fibre bundle is difficult to trace from tooth to bone. It has been claimed that an intermediate plexus is present in the midsection of the ligament during eruption, after which it disappears. However, this has more recently been questioned. It now appears that, in the fully erupted tooth, fibres cross the entire width of the periodontal space but branch en route and join neighbouring fibres to form a complex three-dimentional network. The principal fibres of the ligament do not run a straight course as they pass from bone to tooth, but appear to follow a wavy pathway. Apart from these major fibre bundles there are also less regularly orientated collagen fibre bundles.

Extracellular matrix components of the periodontium

Collagen

The periodontal ligament collagen is mostly Type I. This variety of collagen is the major protein component of most connective tissues, including skin, gingiva and bone. It contains two identical α_1 chains and a chemically different α_2 chain. It is low in hydrolysine and glycosylated hydroxylysine. The periodontal ligament is also relatively rich in Type III collagen (about 20%), which consists of three α_1 III chains. It is high in hydroxyproline, low in hydroxylysine and contains cysteine. Most major periodontal ligament fibres are composed of Type I collagen. Much of the collagen is gathered together to form bundles that are approximately 5 μm in diameter, and these are known as the principal fibres. The principal fibres appear to be more numerous, but smaller at their attachment to cementum than at the alveolar bone. Type III collagen is present in similar proportions to those found in embryonic tissues, and this probably reflects the high turnover rate within the ligament. Type III is more fibrillar and extensible than Type I, and may be important in maintaining the integrity of the ligament during the small vertical and horizontal movements that occur during chewing.

In addition to their structural role, collagens have also been shown to be involved either directly or indirectly in promoting cell attachment and differentiation, and as a chemotactic agent for both fibroblasts and macrophages (Hay, 1981).

Small amounts of other collagens are also present. Type IV is localized to basement membranes (Gage *et al.*, 1989) and type V is distributed in the matrix of the lamina propria, in close association with cells. Type VI collagen has a microfibrillar distribution (Romanos *et al.*, 1993). Types V and XII are co-distributed with type III collagen, which surrounds type I collagen in Sharpey's fibres (Bartold, 1995).

The main collagen in the organic matrix of bone and cementum collagen is type I, and this is virtually insoluble due to cross-links which provide the structural and mechanical stability for normal function (Bartold, 1995).

Oxytalan fibres

The human periodontal ligament also contains oxytalan fibres. The ultrastructural characteristics of these fibres suggest that they are immature elastic fibres. Their function remains unknown, but their fibres are thicker and more numerous in teeth that carry high loads, including abutment teeth for bridges and teeth being moved by orthodontic treatment. Thus, oxytalan fibres may have a role in tooth support. However, these fibres remain unchanged in the periodontal ligament of teeth with reduced masticatory loading. In humans, true elastic fibres are restricted to the walls of blood vessels.

Ground substance of the periodontal ligament

The ligament ground substance is an amorphous matrix of gycosaminoglycans (GAGs), proteoglycans and glycoproteins, and plays an extremely important role in the absorption of functional stresses. The GAGs are represented by several species, including chondroitin sulphate, dermatan sulphate, keratin sulphate and hyaluronan (Mariotti, 1993). The periodontal ligament ground substance composition is similar to that of gingival ground substance, and contains hyaluronic acid (hyaluronan), small dermatan sulphate proteoglycans and larger molecular weight chondroitin sulphate proteoglycans, versican, decorin, biglycan and syndecan, which are capable of interacting with hyaluronan (Embery *et al.*, 1979, 1987; Purvis *et al.*, 1984; Pearson and Pringle, 1986; Larjava *et al.*, 1992).

It is presumed that GAGs, proteoglycans and glycoproteins are secreted by fibroblasts. These molecules turn over at an even faster rate than collagen. They have many important functions, including ion and water binding and exchange, control of collagen fibrillogenesis and fibre orientation. Their water binding functions are thought to produce an hydraulic cushion in the periodontal ligament. This cushioning effect is probably more important in resisting the forces of mastication than traction on the ligament fibres. Proteoglycans also regulate cell adhesion and growth, and have capacity to bind and regulate growth factor activity (Bartold and Narayanan, 1998).

The glycoproteins include the high molecular weight, insoluble, fibre-forming glycoprotein fibronectin, which is present both intra- and extracellularly (Yamada and Olden, 1978). The structure consists of two identical disulphide-linked polypeptide chains and contains a sequence, aginine–glycine–aspartate (RGD), that binds to cells as well as other sites that bind to collagen, heparin and fibrin (Engel, 1991; Mariotti, 1993). This is thought to promote the attachment of cells to the substratum, and especially to collagen. Furthermore, cells preferentially adhere to fibronectin, which may be involved in cell migration and orientation (Berkowitz *et al.*, 1992). Fibronectin may have considerable biological significance within the ligament in view of its high rate of turnover. Immunochemical techniques have revealed that fibronectin is uniformly distributed throughout the periodontal ligament both during eruption and in fully erupted teeth (Tucker *et al.*, 1991; Steffensen *et al.*, 1992; Romanos *et al.*, 1993). However, fibronectin is expressed particularly strongly along attachment sites of the periodontal ligament collagen fibres to cementum but not to alveolar bone (Lukinmaa *et al.*, 1991; Matsuura *et al.*, 1995). It is also found in the endosseal spaces, periosteum and bone lining cells at their interface with alveolar bone (Steffensen *et al.*, 1992). In the cementum its expression is weaker than in the periodontal ligament (Zhang *et al.*, 1993). Fibronectin has been also localized in the basement membrane and lamina propria (Tucker *et al.*, 1991; Steffensen *et al.*, 1992) with a fibrillar and diffuse distribution (Romanos *et al.*, 1993).

Ultrastructural studies (Zhang *et al.*, 1993) have localized fibronectin over collagen fibres and at certain sites at the cell–collagen interface. As loss of fibronectin has been observed during the terminal maturation of many connective tissue matrices, its continued presence within the periodontal ligament may be indicative of either the ligament retaining immature characteristics or its high turnover.

In addition to its main function as an adhesive protein, fibronectin is involved in blood coagulation, wound healing and chemotaxis (Yamada and Olden, 1978; Mariotti, 1993).

Another glycoprotein, termed tenascin, has also been identified in the periodontal ligament, and this too is characteristic of immature connective tissue. It is a protein with six arms extending from a central core (Erikson and Inglesias, 1984). It was thought to play a prominent role in developmental processes, but it has been shown that transgenic mice in which the tenascin gene is not present nevertheless develop normally (Saga *et al.*, 1992). In contrast to other major extracellular matrix proteins, the expression of tenascin is only maintained during wound healing (Mackie *et al.*, 1987) and in a few adult tissues including bone marrow and the periodontal tissues. Unlike fibronectin, it is not uniformly localized throughout the periodontal ligament but is rather concentrated adjacent to the alveolar bone and the cementum (Lukinmaa *et al.*, 1991; Steffensen *et al.*, 1992; Becker *et al.*, 1993). It is found between less densely packed collagen fibrils of the periodontal ligament (Zhang *et al.*, 1993) and accumulated towards the alveolar bone and cementum (Lukinmaa *et al.*, 1991; Steffensen *et al.*, 1992), with only weak expression throughout the alveolar bone matrix. Cementum also shows weak expression of this protein, which may have been deposited prior to mineralization (Zhang *et al.*, 1993). It is also found in the basement membrane and lamina propria (Becker *et al.*, 1993).

Some elastic fibres are present in the gingival and periodontal connective tissue, and elastin, a very flexible and insoluble protein, is the major component of these (Hay, 1981; Mariotti, 1993; Bartold, 1995). Laminin is found exclusively in the basement membrane, where it is believed to mediate the attachment of epithelium cells to type IV collagen (Mariotti, 1993). In the periodontium, it has been located in the basal lamina of blood vessels and the oral, sulcus and junction epithelium (Steffensen *et al.*, 1992). Vitronectin is a protein that promotes the attachment and spreading of cells, and it has been found on the cells lining the alveolar bone and cementum (Steffensen *et al.*, 1992) and also associated with the connective tissue fibres of the the gingiva and periodontal ligament (Matsuura *et al.*, 1995).

Cells of the periodontal ligament

The periodontal ligament tissue is developmentally derived from the inner layer of the dental follicle shortly after root development starts (Ten Cate, 1994), but it is considered that cells migrating from the dental papilla to the dental follicle also have the potential to form periodontal ligament during odontogenesis (Palmer and Lubbock, 1995). Mature periodontal ligament is a highly vascular and cellular tissue.

Fibroblasts are the most abundant cell type in the periodontal ligament, and are aligned along and between the collagen fibres.

It is possible that the periodontal ligament fibroblasts are motile contractile cells and that they are capable of generating a force for tooth eruption (Berkovitz *et al.*, 1992). Much of the evidence for this comes from research on the behaviour and appearance of periodontal fibroblasts in cell culture. *In vitro* periodontal fibroblasts can organize a fibrous network and generate significant forces.

Under normal conditions, *in vivo* periodontal ligament fibroblasts are primarily involved in protein synthesis. They synthesize and secrete collagen, GAGs, proteoglycans and glycoproteins. Because of the high turnover of collagen and proteoglycan within the ligament, these cells are actively engaged in protein synthesis for long periods and appear plump with abundant cytoplasm.

In addition, there is evidence that fibroblasts are also responsible for collagen degradation within the ligament (Eley and Harrison, 1975). Periodontal ligament fibroblasts are also phagocytic and can take up damaged collagen fibrils. These fibrils can be seen within intracellular vacuoles in these cells at various levels of degradation (*Figures 1.8*, *1.9*). The time taken for intracellular degradation of collagen may be about 30 minutes.

While gingival fibroblasts maintain the synthesis and integrity of the gingival connective tissue, periodontal ligament fibroblasts have specialized functions that are concerned with the formation and maintenance of the periodontal ligament, including its repair or regeneration following damage (Berkovitz *et al.*, 1995). Although both gingival and periodontal ligament fibroblasts are similar in appearance when grown in culture, they have very important functional differences. Thus, in animal studies, it has been found that when tooth roots were covered with

Figure 1.8 An electron micrograph of a fibroblast containing multiple banded collagen fibrils within membrane-bound phagolysosomes

Figure 1.9 A higher power electron micrograph of a part of a fibroblast. It shows intracellular banded collagen fibrils within a membrane-bound vesicle (a phagolysosome)

periodontal ligament cells grown in culture and then re-implanted *in vivo*, they acted as progenitor cells and gave rise to the formation of new periodontal ligament tissue (Boyko *et al.*, 1981; Van Dijk *et al.*, 1991; Lang *et al.*, 1995, 1998). In marked contrast, gingival fibroblasts failed to produce new tissue (Boyko *et al.*, 1981). Also, the total protein and extracellular matrix protein production have been shown to be higher in periodontal ligament compared to gingival fibroblasts (Somerman *et al.*, 1988; Kuru *et al.*, 1998). Moreover, the response of these two cell types to attachment factors (Somerman *et al.*, 1989), extracellular matrix proteins (Giannopoulou and Cimasoni, 1996) and growth factors (Dennison *et al.*, 1994) have been found to be different.

In addition, some of the periodontal ligament cells have been shown to possess osteoblast-like characteristics, including the production of osteonectin (Somerman *et al.*, 1990; Nohutcu *et al.*, 1996), osteocalcin (Nojima *et al.*, 1990) and high levels of alkaline phosphatase (Kawase *et al.*, 1988). These studies indicate that phenotypically distinct and functional sub-populations of cells of both fibroblast and osteoblast/cementoblast lineage exist in the

periodontal ligament, and these cells probably include some stem and precursor cells important in repair and regeneration.

Osteoblasts, cementoblasts, osteoclasts and cementoclasts may also be found lining the endosteal and periosteal bone surfaces and the cementum surface. These cells are only conspicuous when active deposition of bone and cementum is taking place, at which time these cells also appear plump. Multinucleated cells (osteoclasts and cementoclasts) appear on bone and cementum surfaces when resorption is taking place, and indeed there appears to be no reason to differentiate between them since they both resorb mineralized tissue.

All of these cell types derive from stem and precursor cells in the ligament and/or alveolar bone marrow (see below). Osteoclasts and cementoclasts are derived from blood-borne precursors of marrow origin, which originate from mononuclear phagocyte cell precursors. Precursor and stem cells for all these connective cells are also present in the ligament (see below).

Groups of epithelial cells, the 'epithelial rests of Malassez', which are remnants of the Hertwig root sheath, are found close to the cementum. They may play a part in the formation of dental cysts. Histochemical and electron microscope studies reveal little activity in these cells. They may, however, proliferate to form cysts or tumours if appropriately stimulated (e.g. by chronic inflammation).

Defence cells may also be present in the periodontal ligament, including macrophages, mast cells and eosinophils, as in other connective tissues.

It is important to recognize that the collagen of the periodontal ligament undergoes constant remodelling, i.e. resorption of old fibres and formation of new ones, and the fibroblasts are involved in both processes. Autoradiographic studies demonstrate a high rate of collagen turnover, which is greatest at the alveolar crest and at the apex. The turnover of collagen in the periodontal ligament is said to be faster than in any other connective tissue. This probably reflects the constant functional demand placed on teeth.

Of major importance is the capacity of the periodontal ligament for repair and regeneration, which is reflected in the complex and heterogeneous sub-populations of cells of this tissue (Lekic and McCulloch, 1996). The cementoblasts, osteoblasts and osteoclasts, which maintain and remodel the cementum and alveolar bone on the borders of the periodontal ligament, are also considered part of this tissue (Berkovitz *et al.*, 1995). In addition, other mesenchymal cells (which may include stem and progenitor cells) are present and are key cells in the regenerative processes.

Stem and progenitor cells

The periodontal ligament and the marrow spaces of the alveolar bone contain stem and progenitor cells, which function as the precursor cells for the more specialized cells in the mesenchymal cell population that is continually renewing under physiological conditions due to cell death and terminal differentiation (Aukhil, 1991; Berkovitz *et al.*, 1995).

A number of recent studies have investigated the origin and location of the progenitor cell populations in the periodontal ligament. It has been suggested that, after the embryological development of the periodontal ligament from undifferentiated mesenchymal cells, some progenitor cells remain in the mature tissue (Hassell, 1993). It is thought that this progenitor population is located perivascularly, adjacent to blood vessels (McCulloch *et al.*, 1995; Lekic and McCulloch, 1996). In this regard, in a wound healing model, Gould *et al.* (1980) found that, following the partial removal of the periodontal ligament, the proportion of ^{3}H-thymidine-labelled perivascular cells in the adjacent periodontal ligament increased five-fold. The majority of such cells have been found to reside in the central part of the ligament (McCulloch and Melcher, 1983a), and it was suggested that they may give rise to periodontal ligament fibroblasts and also migrate towards the bone and cementum surfaces, where they may differentiate into osteoblasts or cementoblasts respectively (McCulloch and Melcher, 1983b; Lekic *et al.*, 1996).

The cells present in the vascular channels of the alveolar bone, which migrate towards the periodontal ligament, may be another source of progenitors (McCulloch *et al.*, 1987). This suggestion was supported by a study in which root slices were cultured *in vitro* with cells derived from the rat calvaria (Melcher *et al.*, 1987). It is also possible that separate precursor cells may be present for each distinct mature cell type (McCulloch, 1995).

These precursor cell populations undoubtedly play a major role in periodontal homeostasis and the regenerative healing process.

Blood supply

The rich blood supply to the periodontal ligament is mainly derived from the appropriate superior and inferior alveolar arteries, although arteries from the gingiva, such as the lingual and palatine arteries, may also be involved through anastomosis of the two supplies (*Figure 1.5*). The arteries supplying the ligament branch off from the artery supplying the pulp before it enters the apical foramina. The ligament also receives a secondary rich supply from the vessels supplying the alveolar bone, and there is massive anastomosis between vessels in the marrow spaces and the ligament via multiple foramina in the cribriform plate. This dual supply allows the ligament to survive following removal of the root apex during certain endodontic procedures.

Fenestrated capillaries are present in the periodontal ligament in contrast with other fibrous connective tissues, which usually have continuous capillaries. The presence of fenestrated capillaries in large numbers is therefore a specialized feature of the periodontal ligament. Fenestrated capillary beds differ from continuous capillary beds in that the diffusion and filtration capabilities are greatly increased. It is possible that the capillary fenestrations are related to the high metabolic requirements of the periodontal ligament and its high rate of turnover.

The dense anastomosis of deep and superficial vessels at the gingival margin leads to a crevicular plexus of capillary loops, which completely encircles each tooth within the connective tissue beneath the region of the gingival crevice. Each loop consists of one or two thin (8–10 μm in diameter) capillary ascending loops and one or two descending post-capillary venules. The crevicular capillary loops arise from a circular plexus, which is comprised of one to four intercommunicating vessels (6–30 μm in diameter) lying at the level of the junctional epithelium. They are separated from other more marginally situated loops just below the gingival surface.

The veins within the ligament do not usually accompany the arteries; instead, they pass through the cribriform plate to drain into intra-alveolar networks. Anastomoses with veins in the gingiva also occur, and a dense venous network is particularly prominent around the apex of the alveolus.

Nerve supply

The nerve supply to the periodontal ligament is of two types: sensory and autonomic. There are two types of sensory fibre, proprioceptive and pain, which supply the ligament's pressure and pain receptors. The pressure (proprioceptive) receptors are spindle-shaped structures, and this function is central to the control of the masticatory system in chewing, swallowing and talking. Pain fibres terminate as free nerve endings. The autonomic fibres are associated mainly with the supply of the periodontal blood vessels. Compared with other dense connective tissues, the periodontal ligament is well innervated.

Nerve bundles from the trigeminal nerve follow the blood vessels, and are derived from two sources. Some nerve bundles branch off the nerve supplying the pulp before it enters the apical foramen and supply the ligament directly. Other sensory fibres enter the middle and cervical portions of the ligament from the nerve supply to the alveolar bone, and enter the ligament as finer branches through the multiple foramina in the cribriform plate.

Periodontal nerve fibres are both myelinated and nonmyelinated. The myelinated fibres are 5–15 μm in diameter, and are all sensory fibres that respond to pressure. The non-myelinated fibres are about 0.5 μm in diameter, and are both sensory pain and autonomic fibres.

About 75% of the mechanoreceptors within the periodontal ligament have their cell bodies in the trigeminal ganglion, whilst the remaining 25% have cell bodies in the mesencephalic nucleus.

Most research has been carried out into the mechanoreceptors and the discharge of afferent impulses from single nerve fibres dissected free from the inferior alveolar nerve in animals (Berkovitz *et al.*, 1992). The discharge appears to vary according to the direction and amplitude of the displacing force. These fibres show directional sensitivity in that they respond maximally to a force applied to the tooth crown in one particular direction. Their conduction velocities place them within the A_β group of fibres. The response characteristics of these mechanoreceptors can vary from rapidly adapting through to slowly adapting, but it is not clear whether the rapidly, medium and slowly adapting mechanoreceptors are really different types of receptor. All of their sensory endings appear to be similar, and are encapsulated Ruffini-like terminals. Furthermore, the response characteristics appear to be dependent upon the position of the ending within the ligament relative to the position of loading.

The proprioceptor nerve endings in the ligament form part of the extremely refined neurological control of mastication. The mechanoreceptors in the periodontal ligament monitor changes in pressure within the ligament space and, as forces increase, greater numbers of mechanoreceptors are stimulated, resulting in increasing numbers of impulses passing via the sensory nerves to the trigeminal nuclei. This in turn results in inhibitory impulses passing to the motor nucleus, which reduces the number of motor impulses to the muscle fibres, reducing or stopping masticatory forces. A similar reflex arc passes from the muscle spindle receptors, which monitor muscle stretch. The loads in mastication, swallowing and speaking vary considerably in amount, frequency, duration and direction, and in normal function the structure of the ligament usually absorbs these variations effectively and transmits them to the supporting bone.

Little is known about pain fibres within the ligament, but it is presumed that they are fine non-myelinated nerves terminating in free nerve endings. There is a similar lack of information on the fine non-myelinated autonomic nerves. These fibres are $0.2-1$ μm in diameter, and are important in the control of the regional blood flow.

Tooth support mechanism

The proprioceptor nerve endings in the ligament form part of the extremely refined neurological control of mastication, and thus protect the ligament from damage (see above). In addition, blood supply, the ground substance and collagen bundles all take part in the absorption of functional stresses and their transmission to the bones.

There is some debate about the exact mechanism, but the system described by Parfitt (1967) appears to explain the observed behaviour of a tooth in function. He describes the vascular–ground substance complex as a shock-absorbing system and the fibre-bundle system as a suspensory system limiting tooth movement and transmitting strain to the supporting bone. Thus, when a force is applied to a tooth a series of events follow:

1. The initial displacement of the tooth is associated with intravascular and extravascular fluid movement through blood vessels and bone spaces

2. As the load increases, the collagen fibre bundles take the strain and become extended. They are not elastic and do not stretch
3. With further pressure, the alveolar process distorts
4. If the load is sufficiently powerful and prolonged, the tooth substance itself, i.e. the dentine, distorts.

This has been described as a visco-elastic system, in which the vascular, tissue fluid and ground substance components provide the viscous response while the fibrous tissue and bone provide elasticity. When an axial load is applied to a tooth there appears to be a biphasic response, with the elastic phase preceding the viscous phase. It is an extremely versatile and resilient system, which can cope with the variable loads imposed on the tissues by the mastication of a heterogeneous diet. However, it can break down if subject to abnormal loads or when involved in inflammation.

Axial forces are absorbed most readily. On loading, the wavy principal fibres assume their full length and the tooth is depressed in the socket. Lateral and rotational forces are absorbed less easily. On the tension side, fibres extend; on the pressure side, fibres are compressed. Further compression results in bone resorption and increased tension bone deposition.

All teeth are slightly mobile, and that mobility is influenced by:

1. The quantity and duration of the applied load
2. The length and shape of the root or roots, and therefore the position of the axis of rotation – inevitably, mobility of the lower incisor with a relatively short and conical root is easier to elicit than that of the multirooted upper first molar with its large root base
3. The status of the supporting tissues, i.e. thickness of collagen fibre bundles and proportion of mature collagen (the erupting tooth is more mobile than the fully erupted tooth), and the state of aggregation of the ground substance (in pregnancy, some increase in tooth mobility is caused by hormone-induced disaggregation).

Cementum

Cementum is the calcified connective tissue that covers the root dentine, and the periodontal fibre bundles are inserted into it. It can be regarded as a 'bone of attachment', and is the only specifically dental tissue of the periodontium. It is pale yellow and softer than dentine, and in some animals is present on the crowns of the teeth as an adaptation to a herbivorous diet. In humans its relationship to the enamel margin varies; it may abut or overlap enamel, but may also be separated from the enamel by a thin band of exposed dentine. The thickness of cementum varies considerably, and the coronal third may be only $16-60$ μm. When exposed by gingival recession or pocketing, this very thin layer of cervical cementum can be easily removed by the toothbrush or dental instrumentation so that the very sensitive dentine is exposed. In contrast, the apical third can be 200 μm or even thicker. Cementum is formed slowly throughout life, and is resistant to resorption. A layer of uncalcified matrix, the precementum, is laid down by the cementoblasts prior to calcification, and a layer of this uncalcified matrix is always present on its surface within the periodontium and may be responsible for its resistance to resorption. Cementum can triple its thickness throughout life, and is avascular and without enervation. It is more permeable than dentine, but this permeability decreases with age. Continual cemental formation is necessary to accommodate changes in fibre insertion within the periodontal ligament as a result of tooth movement and ligament turnover.

Like other calcified tissues, bone and dentine, it consists of collagen fibres embedded in a calcified organic matrix. It contains (by weight) 65% inorganic material, mainly hydroxyapatite, 23% organic material and 12% water. By volume, these proportions are 45%, 33% and 22% respectively.

There are two main types of cementum: cellular and acellular. The former contains cementocytes in lacunae which, like osteocytes in bone, communicate with each other through a network of canaliculi. Acellular cementum forms a thin surface layer, often confined to cervical portions of the root. It does not contain cementocytes within its substance, but as cementoblasts populate its surface the term 'acellular' may not be wholly appropriate. The degree of mineralization varies in different parts of the tissue, and some acellular zones may be as highly calcified as dentine. Cementoblasts are responsible for the synthesis and secretion of the components of organic matrix and also for its calcification, and are morphologically and functionally identical to osteoblasts. As cementum formation proceeds the cementoblasts become entrapped, and they are then referred to as cementocytes. It has been suggested that there may be two populations of cementoblasts, which can be distinguished by their phenotype and developmental origin (Ten Cate, 1997). Thus, while cells associated with acellular cementum may be derived from the dental follicle, cells from cellular cementum may originate from the progenitor cells migrating from the alveolar bone endosteal spaces (McCulloch *et al.*, 1987). It is probable that precursor and stems cells for cementoblasts are present in the periodontal ligament close to the cemental surface as well as the alveolar bone.

The principal inorganic component is hydroxyapatite, although other forms of calcium phosphate are present to a higher degree than in other calcified tissues. The organic content is primarily collagen, which is virtually all type I.

During calcification, hydroxyapatite crystals are firstly deposited on the surface of collagen fibrils parallel to their surface and then within the cementoid matrix. These crystals are similar to those seen in bone, and are thin and plate-like. They are, on average, 55 nm wide and 8 nm thick. The cementum surface is formed into conical projections about single fibrils or bundles.

The prime function of cementum is to give attachment to collagen fibres of the periodontal ligament. There are two arrangements of collagen fibrils in cementum. The principal fibrils are those of the periodontal ligament embedded as Sharpey's fibres in the calcified matrix and incorporated in the cementum as it is laid down. They are arranged at right angles to the cementum surface. The other fibrils form a dense and irregular meshwork within the matrix. In acellular cementum the Sharpey's fibres are closely packed and largely calcified; in cellular cementum they are more widely spaced and partly calcified.

Unlike in bone, there is no evidence of cementum remodelling (i.e. of internal resorption and deposition); however, there is continuous, slow apposition of surface cementum as cementoblast activity continues at a low level throughout life. Cementoid or precementum is the name given to the cementum matrix prior to calcification, and a layer of this is always present on its surface. Its resistance to resorption is a feature that allows orthodontic tooth movement. The precise reasons for its resistance to resorption are uncertain, but it may be related to differences between the physiochemical or biological properties of bone and cementum.

The greatest thickness of cementum is formed at the apex and in furcation areas. With attrition (i.e. wear of the occlusal surface of the tooth), compensatory deposition of apical cementum takes place which, together with bone deposition at the alveolar crest and at the socket fundus, maintains the vertical dimension of the face. At the tooth apex the cementum forms a constriction, so that the root canal exit is very narrow.

Excessive formation of cementum, hypercementosis, may follow pulp disease or occlusal stress. A generalized hypercementosis involving all teeth may be hereditary; it also occurs in Paget's disease. Occasionally cementicles, small spherical masses of cementum, may be found attached to the cementum surface or free in the periodontal ligament.

Cementum resorption can be a consequence of excessive occlusal stress, orthodontic movement, pressure from tumours or cysts or deficiencies of calcium or vitamins A and D. It is also found in metabolic diseases, but the pathogenesis is obscure. Repair of affected areas may occur if the cause is removed. Occasionally ankylosis of the cementum and socket bone takes place. Root fracture may be followed by the formation of a cementum callus, but this repair process does not demonstrate the highly organized remodelling capacity of bone.

Resorption is carried out by multinuclear cells resembling osteoclasts, termed cementoclasts or odontoclasts. These cells undoubtedly arise from myelo-monocytic cells in a similar way to osteoclasts. The resorptive lacunae resemble those seen in bone, and the cementoclasts are seen at the resorptive front. If the force is large, the resorption can also involve the underlying root dentine.

Areas of previous resorption can also be repaired by

the laying down of further cementum by cementoblasts, which probably develop from stem cells in the periodontal ligament. Repair cementum resembles cellular cementum.

Alveolar bone

The part of the maxilla and mandible that supports and protects the teeth is known as alveolar bone, and an arbitrary boundary at the level of the root apices separates alveolar bone from the body of the maxilla or mandible. Alveolar bone has its embryological origin from the initial condensation of ectomesenchyme around the early tooth germ (Ten Cate, 1997). The alveolar processes are tooth dependent, and are present as long as they house the teeth. It is comprised of the alveolar bone proper, in which the Sharpey's fibres are embedded, the compact bone, comprised of the oral and buccal cortical plates, and the cancellous bone located between them.

Apart from supporting the teeth, the bone of the maxilla and mandible also gives attachment to muscles, provides a framework for the bone marrow and acts as a reservoir for ions, in particular calcium. The alveolar bone is dependent on the presence of teeth for its development and maintenance, and thus after tooth extraction it atrophies and in anodontia it is absent.

Bone is a mineralized connective tissue and consists (by weight) of approximately 60% inorganic material, 25% organic material and 15% of water. By volume, these proportions are 36%, 36% and 28% respectively. The mineral fraction consists of hydroxyapatite, in the form of needle-like crystallites or thin plates about 8 nm thick and of variable length. About 90% of the organic material is in the form of type I collagen. In addition, there are small amounts of other proteins such as osteonectin, osteocalcin, osteopontin and proteoglycans. Two small molecular weight chondroitin sulphate proteoglycans have been identified in alveolar bone, namely decorin and biglycan, containing one and two chondroitin sulphate chains respectively (Waddington and Embery, 1991).

Osteoblasts synthesize and regulate the deposition of the bone organic matrix, including collagen type 1, proteoglycan, osteonectin, osteocalcin, bone sialoproteins and osteopontin (Gage *et al.*, 1989). They also express and release alkaline phosphatase, and this has been shown to be closely associated with new bone formation (Arnett, 1990). Osteoblasts also control the process of mineralization.

Anatomically, no distinct boundary exists between the body of the maxilla or mandible and their respective alveolar processes. However, as a result of functional adaption, two parts of the alveolar process can be distinguished. The first, the alveolar bone proper, consists of a thin lamella of bone that surrounds the root of the tooth. It gives attachment to the principal fibres of the periodontal ligament. The collagen fibres of the periodontal ligament are inserted into this bone to produce what is called 'bundle bone'. The periodontal ligament fibres embedded in bone are called Sharpey's fibres. This bone is also called the cribriform plate. As the name implies, the cribriform plate is perforated like a sieve so that a large number of vascular and neural connections can be made between the periodontal ligament and the trabecular spaces. The second part, the supporting bone, is the bone that surrounds the alveolar bone proper and gives support to the socket. This has facial and lingual plates of compact bone between which is cancellous trabeculation (spongy bone), and the cancellous bone is orientated around the tooth to form support for the alveolar bone proper.

The bone of the alveolar process is in no fundamental way different from bone in any other part of the body. In compact bone, the lamellae are arranged in two major patterns. At the periosteal or endosteal surfaces, they are arranged in concentric layers conforming to the bony surface contour. If the bone volume is sufficient, they may be also arranged as small concentric layers around a central vascular canal. This system is known as an haversian system, and may be comprised of up to 20 concentric layers. The central haversian canals are connected by transversely running Volkmann's canals. Spongy or cancellous bone consists of widely spaced concentric or transverse lamellae enclosing the marrow spaces.

The shape of the jaws and the morphology of the alveolar processes vary between individuals, and the size, shape and thickness of cortical plates and interdental septa vary in different parts of the same jaw. The margin of the alveolar crest usually runs parallel to the amelocemental junction at a remarkably constant distance of 1–2 mm, but this relationship may vary with the alignment of the tooth and the contour of the root surface. Where a tooth is displaced out of the arch, the overlying alveolar plate may be very thin or even perforated so that fenestrations (circumscribed defects) or dehiscence (splits) are formed. These defects occur more frequently in facial than in lingual bone and are more common over anterior than posterior teeth, although they are seen over the palatal root of the upper first molar if the roots are very divergent. They are very important clinically because, where they occur, the root of the tooth is covered only by mucoperiosteum, i.e. periosteum and the overlying gingiva, which may atrophy under irritation and thus expose the root. Where tooth roots approximate, interdental bone may be absent.

Five cell types can be identified in bone. Bone-forming cells, osteoblasts, are found on the surface of the bone. They become trapped in their own secretion and are subsequently incorporated in the matrix as osteocytes. Large multinucleated cells, osteoclasts, are responsible for resorbing bone. In addition, osteoprogenitor cells are present and appear as long, thin cells. These are a stem cell population to generate osteoblasts, and are situated close to the blood vessels of the marrow and periodontal ligament. When bone is not undergoing active deposition or resorption, its quiescent surface is lined by relatively undifferentiated cells known as bone lining cells, which may represent inactive osteoblasts. Active osteoblasts contain extensive rough endoplastic reticulum, numerous mitochondria and vesicles and an extensive Golgi apparatus. They manufacture and secrete type I collagen and proteoglycans, and bring about mineralization.

Like all bone, alveolar bone undergoes constant remodelling as a response to mechanical stress and the metabolic need for calcium and phosphorus ions. In health, the remodelling process maintains the total volume of bone and keeps its overall anatomy relatively stable. In the primate, the teeth drift mesially as interproximal tooth surface wear takes place, together with resorption on the mesial and deposition on the distal surfaces of the socket wall.

The resorbing surface of the bone shows resorption concavities, known as Howship's lacunae, in which lie osteoclasts. These vary in size, and may be up to 100 μm in diameter. The multinucleated osteoclast forms by the fusion of cells of the myelo-monocyte cell line. The part of the osteoclast that lies adjacent to the bone surface has a foamy, striated appearance, which is known as the brush border. Ultrastructurally, the brush border consists of many tightly packed microvilli coated with fine bristle-like structures. This zone may limit the diffusion of enzymes and ions to create an isolated microenvironment within which resorption can take place. These cells have less endoplastic reticulum than osteoblasts but a very prominent Golgi apparatus, and are also motile. They secrete cysteine- and metalloproteinases and hydrogen ions (see Chapter 5, *Figures 5.3 and 5.4*). Bone resorption takes place in two stages. Initially the mineral phase is removed, and later the organic matrix. The regulation of these events involves close co-operation between osteoblasts and osteoclasts (see Chapter 5).

Proteins mainly associated with bone and cementum

Osteonectin

Osteonectin is an acid phosphate containing glycoprotein rich in cysteine, which is mainly secreted by osteoblasts (Gage *et al.*, 1989). It is composed of a single polypeptide chain and has a strong affinity for calcium ions; (Sage and Borstein, 1991). It has been suggested that the phosphate groups may be crucial for initiating the mineralization process (Gage *et al.*, 1989). Osteonectin is one of the major non-collagenous proteins of bone, and has also been located in basal lamina (Bilezikian *et al.*, 1996). In addition, it has been found in the periodontal ligament, particularly strongly around the Sharpey's fibres, at the attachment sites between the ligament and alveolar bone and cementum (Matsuura *et al.*, 1995).

Osteocalcin

Osteocalcin, also called bone gla protein because it contains γ-carboxyglutamic acid (gla) residues, is a small protein that is mainly secreted by osteoblasts (Mariotti, 1993). It becomes incorporated in the mineralized matrix of bone soon after its secretion, and it has been suggested that it plays a crucial role in the mineralization process. It is probable that the gla sites on the protein act as calcium ion binding sites (Gage *et al.*, 1989). The expression of osteocalcin by the cells lining the tooth root surface has been shown during tooth root development in mice (D'Errico *et al.*, 1997).

Bone sialoprotein protein

Bone sialoprotein protein (BSP), also known as BSP II, is a phosphoglycoprotein containing up to 20% of sialic acid residues that also has an RGD sequence (Bilezikian *et al.*, 1996). It has a restricted pattern of expression and is primarily found in bone (Fujisawa *et al.*, 1995). BSP expression marks a late stage of osteoblast differentiation and an early stage of matrix mineralization (Lekic *et al.*, 1996). There is also weak expression in the periodontal ligament at attachment sites with alveolar bone and cementum (Matsuura *et al.*, 1995), and it is expressed by cells lining the root surface at early stages of cementogenesis during tooth development (MacNeil *et al.*, 1995, 1996). The cementoblasts appear to secrete this protein onto the root surface, which then becomes covered by cementum. Although the precise function of this protein is not yet known, it may serve as an attachment factor since it has an affinity for collagen fibres and enhances the attachment of osteoblasts and fibroblasts to plastic surfaces (Fujisawa *et al.*, 1995).

Osteopontin

Osteopontin is also termed BSP I due to its high sialic acid content, and is a glycophosphoprotein. It is found primarily in bone and in addition to an RGD cell attachment sequence it has an affinity for calcium ions (MacNeil *et al.*, 1995). Although its precise functions are unclear, it is expressed prior to mineralization and appears to be involved in the attachment and movement of osteoblasts and osteoclasts. It has also been suggested (MacNeil *et al.*, 1995) that it functions as an inhibitor of mineralization during periodontal ligament development. In this regard, it has been shown to be distributed in a non-specific fashion throughout the periodontal ligament of the developing mouse molar tooth germ between days 21 and 42 of development. However, in contrast, D'Errico *et al.* (1997) reported that osteopontin was not expressed in the periodontal ligament by day 41, but was expressed by the cells lining the tooth root surface. It has also been shown to be expressed in regenerating alveolar bone adjacent to a fenestration wound in rats, prior to the expression of BSP II (Lekic *et al.*, 1996).

Regulation of tissue turnover in the periodontium

The regulation of tissue turnover depends on the recruitment and stimulation of the appropriate cells at the requisite time, and often on the differentiation of appropriate stem and precursor cells in the functioning mature cells. Most of these functions are controlled by growth factors released by cells, and these are described below.

Growth factors in periodontal tissue turnover

Growth factors are proteins or polypeptides capable of initiating the proliferation of cells that are in a quiescent state (Hefti, 1993) by stimulating DNA synthesis and progression of the cell cycle (O'Neal *et al.*, 1994). They primarily have a paracrine or autocrine action, and exert their effects by binding to specific transmembrane receptors on target cells (Alexander and Damoulis, 1994) which generate a cascade of intracellular molecular signals (Sporn and Roberts, 1991). In this way they regulate the activation and proliferation of the signalled cells, and also a number of other factors including cell migration and cell synthesis, which are essential events in healing (Deuel *et al.*, 1991; Kiritsy *et al.*, 1993). It has also been suggested that the therapeutic topical application of growth factors could favourably affect periodontal regeneration (Terranover and Wikesjö, 1987).

Platelet-derived growth factor

Platelet-derived growth factor (PDGF) plays an important role not only in wound healing but also in normal tissue turnover (Sporn and Roberts, 1991). It is released primarily by platelets, but is also synthesized by macrophages, fibroblasts, osteoblasts, endothelial cells and myoblasts. It consists of a dimer of two glycoprotein subunits, A and B, and there are therefore three possible combinations: PDGF-AA, PDGF-BB and PDGF-AB. PDGF acts by binding to two distinct cell surface receptors, termed PDGF-receptor (PDGFR-α and PDGFR-β), on target cells.

A number of *in vitro* studies have demonstrated that PDGF can stimulate proliferation (Piche and Graves, 1989; Boyan *et al.*, 1994; Dennison *et al.*, 1994; Anderson *et al.*, 1998), DNA synthesis (Matsuda *et al.*, 1992; Oates *et al.*, 1993; Blom *et al.*, 1994) and collagen production (Matsuda *et al.*, 1992) by periodontal ligament cells. It is also chemotactic for these cells (Matsuda *et al.*, 1992; Boyan *et al.*, 1994; Nishimura and Terranova, 1996) and also for osteoblasts (Hughes *et al.*, 1992). PDGF-BB appears to be more effective than the other isoforms in promoting mitogenesis and chemotaxis of these cells *in vitro* (Boyan *et al.*, 1994), and it has also been shown to act synergistically with other growth factors both *in vitro* and *in vivo* (Lynch *et al.*, 1987; Matsuda *et al.*, 1992; Rutherford *et al.*, 1992; Hefti, 1993).

Transforming growth factors

Transforming growth factors (TGFs) are a family of structurally and functionally different proteins that have been isolated from normal and neoplastic tissues (Massagué *et al.*, 1987; Barnard *et al.*, 1990; Sporn and Roberts, 1991). The two best characterized are TGFα, primarily a growth stimulator, and TGFβ, primarily a growth inhibitor (Massagué *et al.*, 1987; Sporn and Roberts, 1991). TGFα stimulates epithelial and endothelial cells and acts through the receptor of another growth factor, epithelial growth factor (Hefti, 1993). TGFβ is encoded by five different genes yielding five isoforms, TGFβ1 to TGFβ5, which display different spatial and temporal patterns of expression during healing (Levine *et al.*, 1993; Frank *et al.*, 1996). TGFβ is present in high concentrations in platelets (Hefti, 1993), and is also produced by activated macrophages and neutrophils (Igarashi *et al.*, 1993). Three distinct receptors for these factors, type I, type II and type III, are present on almost all normal cells (Barnard *et al.*, 1990).

The biological effects of TGFβ are highly diverse. It has been shown to be chemotactic for macrophages (Barnard *et al.*, 1990) and gingival and periodontal ligament mesenchymal cells (Postlethwaite *et al.*, 1987; Nishimura and Terranova, 1996) to stimulate the proliferation of gingival and periodontal ligament mesenchymal cells (Postlethwaite *et al.*, 1987; Oates *et al.*,1993; Anderson *et al.*, 1998). It has also been shown selectively to stimulate the synthesis of extracellular matrix proteins such as collagen, fibronectin, tenascin and proteoglycans by these cells (Lynch *et al.*, 1989; Barnard *et al.*, 1990; Matsuda *et al.*, 1992; Irwin *et al.* 1994) and to inhibit the growth of epithelial, endothelial and certain mesenchymal cells (Lynch *et al.*, 1989; Barnard *et al.*, 1990; Matsuda *et al.*, 1992; Lu *et al.*, 1997). In addition, TGFβ1 alone or in combination with PDGF increases the proliferation of periodontal ligament mesenchymal cells more than those from gingival tissue (Dennison *et al.*, 1994).

Fibroblast growth factor

Fibroblast growth factors (FGFs) are a family of polypeptides that are potent mitogens and chemo-attractants for endothelial and mesenchymal cells (Caffesse and Quinones, 1993; Bilezikian *et al.*, 1996). The two most studied forms of this family are acid FGF (aFGF) and basic FGF (bFGF). Acid FGF stimulates endothelial cell proliferation. Basic FGF is widely distributed in nearly all tissues, including gingiva, periodontal ligament and bone (Hefti, 1993; Bilezikian *et al.*, 1996; Goa *et al.*, 1996; Murata *et al.*, 1997).

bFGF has been reported to stimulate periodontal ligament and endothelial cell migration (Terranova *et al.*, 1989). It has also been shown to increase DNA synthesis and enhance proliferation (Blom *et al.*, 1994; Takayama *et al.*, 1997) and inhibit the alkaline phosphatase production of periodontal ligament cells (Takayama *et al.*, 1997).

Epidermal growth factor

Epidermal growth factor (EGF) is a small polypeptide that stimulates the proliferation of epithelial, endothelial and mesenchymal cells (Caffesse and Quinones, 1993; Bilezikian *et al.*, 1996). It is present in most human extracellular fluids, including plasma, saliva, milk, amniotic fluid and urine (Sporn and Roberts, 1991). EGF is mitogenic for periodontal ligament cells (Matsuda *et al.*, 1992; Blom *et al.*, 1994), and was also found to stimulate the growth of gingival cells *in vitro* (Irwin *et al.*, 1994). In addition, it showed a slight chemotactic effect on periodontal ligament cells, but suppressed their collagen synthesis (Matsuda *et al.*, 1992).

Insulin-like growth factor

Insulin-like growth factors (IGFs) are a family of single chain proteins (Sporn and Roberts, 1991). IGF-I and IGF-II are anabolic peptides structurally and functionally related to insulin. They are synthesized in the liver, smooth muscle and placenta, and are transported via the plasma (Caffesse and Quinones, 1993). They are also present in bony tissues as a result of their synthesis by osteoblasts and the release of stored peptides from the bone matrix (Bilezikian *et al.*, 1996). Both gingival and periodontal mesenchymal cells show a dose-dependent migratory response to the presence of IGF-I and -II and IGF-I (Matsuda *et al.*, 1992; Nishimura and Terranova, 1996). They also increases DNA synthesis and protein production by periodontal ligament cells (Matsuda *et al.*, 1992; Blom *et al.*, 1994).

Bone morphogenic proteins

Bone morphogenic proteins (BMPs) are part of the large TGFβ superfamily (Wozney, 1995; Bilezikian *et al.*, 1996). Localization of members of the BMP family in the embryological development of the skeleton has provided strong evidence that they play an important role in mediating skeletal patterning as well as bone cell differentiation (Bilezikian *et al.*, 1996). Furthermore, the BMPs are considered to be responsible for the inductive abilities of demineralized bone allografts used in periodontal therapy (Urist, 1965; see also Chapter 17), and BMP-2 has been shown to stimulate osteocalcin and alkaline phosphatase expression by cultured periodontal ligament cells (Hughes, 1995). BMPs also have been shown to induce bone and cartilage formation when implanted subcutaneously (Wozney, 1995).

A description of the regulation of tissue turnover in the various periodontal tissues follows.

Epithelium

Stratified squamous epithelium continually renews itself by division of cells in the basal layer and shedding of keratinocytes from the surface. The turnover time for skin is 12–75 days, for oral epithelium 8–40 days and for junctional epithelium 4–11 days. Systemic hormones influence this process, with oestrogen stimulating cell division and corticosteroids inhibiting it. Local factors appear to play a more important role in its regulation. There is a negative feedback control system on keratinocytes by substances known as chalones. The precise nature of these is unknown, but their function could be due to one or more growth factors or cytokines. They act on cells in the basal layer and inhibit their division. Epithelial turnover is also affected by a number of growth factors, including epidermal growth factor (EGF), platelet-derived growth factor (PDGF) and transforming growth factors alpha (TGFα) and beta (TGFβ). EGF and TGFα are known to stimulate epithelial cell proliferation, whilst TGFβ appears to have an inhibitory effect.

The differentiation of epithelium is also profoundly affected by the underlying connective tissue lamina propria. The nature of the connective tissue or chemical messages from it determines the nature of the overlying epithelium – for instance, whether it is keratinized or not. Thus, in the free gingival graft it is the nature of the underlying connective tissue that determines the type of epithelium formed.

Periodontal ligament

The periodontal ligament is constantly breaking down and renewing its constituent tissues. In health, this process is carefully controlled and is in balance. The tooth responds to functional demands, and rates of turnover reflect increases or decreases in function.

Connective tissue turnover in the periodontium is five times higher than alveolar bone and fifteen times higher than the dermis of normal skin. Fibroblasts are responsible for both the synthesis and degradation of all components of the extracellular matrix. They secrete collagenolytic enzymes (collagenases), and these are part of a family of matrix metalloproteinases (MMPs) (*Table 1.1*) that require the presence of metallic cations such as magnesium and calcium for their activity (Birkedal-Hansen, 1993a, 1993b; Reynolds *et al.*, 1994; Reynolds, 1996). There are two distinct forms of collagenase, one originating from fibroblasts and other connective tissue cells of mesenchymal origin (MMP-1), and the other from polymorphs (MMP-8) (*Table 1.2*). Human tumours and bone cells also synthesize another collagenase (MMP-13 or collagenase 3). In addition, macrophages and monocytes synthesize and secrete in response to specific stimuli MMP-1 (Welgus *et al.*, 1990; Campbell *et al.*, 1991; Machein and Conca, 1997). The other proteinases in the group include the gelatinases, stromolysins, matrilysins, metalloelastases and membrane associated MMPs. Gelatinases A and B (MMP-2 and MMP-9), which degrade a specific locus on collagen IV, gelatins, collagens V, VII, X and XI, and elastin are also synthesized and secreted by connective tissue and inflammatory cells respectively. Macrophages produce and secrete mainly MMP-9, but

Table 1.1 The principal members of the family of metalloproteinases (MMPs), including the collagenases

MMP	Other name	Principal source	Main substrates
MMP-1	Collagenase 1	Fibroblasts and other CT cells of mesenchyme origin including macrophages	Helical region of collagen types I, II, III, VIII, X Gelatins (limited) Proteoglycan core protein (limited)
MMP-8	Collagenase 2	Inflammatory cells, e.g. PMNs	As above
MMP-13	Collagenase 3	Human tumours and bone cells	As above
MMP-2	Gelatinase A	Fibroblasts and other CT cells of mesenchyme origin	Gelatins Specific locus of collagen IV Collagens V, VII, X, XI Elastin
MMP-9	Gelatinase B	PMNs, macrophages and osteoclasts	As above
MMP-3	Stromolysin 1	Fibroblasts and other CT cells of mesenchyme origin	Proteoglycan core protein Non-helical regions of collagen IV Collagens X, XI Procollagens I, II, III Fibronectin Laminin Gelatins (limited) Elastin (limited)
MMP-10	Stromolysin 2	Inflammatory cells, e.g. PMNs	As above
MMP-11	Stromolysin 3	Fibroblasts and human breast tumour cells	As above
MMP-7	Matrilysin	Macrophages and fibroblasts	As for stromolysins
MMP-12	Metalloelastase	Macrophages	As for stromolysins Elastin
MMP-14	Membrane type	Cell membranes	Progelatinase A

Table 1.2 The mechanisms of expression, transcription, release and activation of metalloproteinases by various cell types

	Cell type						
	PMN	Macrophage	Fibroblast	Osteoblast	Osteoclast	Endothelial cell	Keratinocyte
Enzyme expressed	MMP 8,9	MMP-1,2,3,9,12	MMP-1,2,3,7,11	MMP-9	MMP-1,2,3,9	MMP-1,2,3,9	
Signals for transcription	Unknown	IL-1, TNFα, EGF, TGFα, PDGF	IL-1, TNFα, EGF, TGFα, PDGF	IL-1, TNFα, PGE2, Vitamin D₃	Signals from osteoblast	IL-1, TNFα, EGF, TGFα, PDGF	IL-1, TNFα, EGF, TGFα, PDGF
Release of enzyme	Granule release	Transcriptional activation	Transcriptional activation	Transcriptional activation	Transcriptional activation	Transcriptional activation	Transcriptional activation
Response time	Seconds	6–12 hours	6–12 hours	6–12 hours	6–12 hours	6–12 hours	6–12 hours
Duration of action	Minutes	Days	Days	Days	Days	Days	Days
Activation of pro-enzyme	Oxidative pathways in phagosome	Plasminogen activator, stromolysin and serine proteinases	Plasminogen activator, stromolysin and serine proteinases	Plasminogen activator, stromolysin and serine proteinases	Cysteine proteinases	Plasminogen activator, stromolysin and serine proteinases	Plasminogen activator, stromolysin and serine proteinases

Key: MMP matrix metalloproteinases
IL interleukin
TNF tumour necrosis factor
EGF epidermal growth factor
TGF transforming growth factor
PDGF platelet-derived growth factor

also some MMP-2 (Welgus *et al.*, 1990; Campbell *et al.*, 1991; Machein and Conca, 1997). Stromolysins 1 and 2 (MMP-3 and MMP-10) degrade proteoglycan protein core, the non-helical regions of collagen IV, X, XI, laminin, fibronectin and procollagens I, II and III. They are also found in fibroblasts and inflammatory cells respectively. Macrophages secrete only small amounts of MMP-3 when appropriately stimulated (Welgus *et al.*, 1990; Campbell *et al.*, 1991; Machein and Conca, 1997).

Another, possibly related, proteinase (MMP-11) with a similar substrate spectrum is secreted by human tumour cells. Matrilysin (MMP-7) is found in macrophages and has a similar action to the stromolysins. Another similar enzyme, with elastin as a primary substrate, is MMP-12, found in macrophages. Both of these proteinases are known as punctuated MMPs because they lack the C-terminal domain. The final proteinase in this group is a membrane-bound MMP (MMP-14), which seems to be involved in a pathway leading to the activation of gelatinase A.

During physiological turnover, the production and secretion of MMPs and other proteinases is carefully controlled by growth factors and cytokines (*Table 1.2*).

There are two main ways in which MMPs are generated by cells: transcriptional activation by growth factors, and triggered release from PMN lysosomal granules (Birkedal-Hansen *et al.*, 1993a; Ryan *et al.*, 1996). In mesenchymal cells and keratinocytes, certain growth factors (IL-1β, TNFα, PDGF, TGFα and EGF) appear to up-regulate collagenase expression, whilst other factors (interferon-gamma, TNFβ and glucocorticoids) down-regulate this process. The genetic regulation involves signal transduction mechanisms, leading to transactivation of the activator protein-1 element on the gene by transcription proto-oncogenes (Ryan *et al.*, 1996). Of relevance to bone resorption, parathyroid hormone and prostaglandin (PG) E$_2$ can also increase collagenase secretion in bone cells. In relation to other MMPs the process is probably very similar, and in this regard it has recently been shown that interleukin-1β can up-regulate MMP-3 (at both the mRNA and protein level) in periodontal ligament cells (Nakaya *et al.*, 1997), and may thus have this role for this proteinase.

Neutrophil MMP regulation is mediated primarily by granule release rather than transcriptional events, which results in a more immediate but less sustained response by this cell. MMPs are normally under tight regulation, not only at the level of gene expression but also extracellularly after secretion, and disruption of this regulation can lead to pathological breakdown of connective tissue.

The MMPs are characterized by a five domain molecular structure: the signal peptide, the propeptide, the catalytic site, the hinge region and the pexin-like domain (Ryan *et al.*, 1996). These enzymes are not stored in cells other than PMNs, but are secreted as inactive or latent pro-enzymes. In the activation process, the secreted pro-enzyme first loses its signal peptide. The function of the propeptide domain is to maintain enzyme latency until a signal is given for activation (Woessner, 1994). During activation, the propeptide domain is cleaved off in several steps.

In cells of mesenchymal origin, activation can be carried out by serine proteinases such as plasmin and elastase and other MMPs such as stromolysins, and only a small percentage of the enzyme may be activated to perform a designated physiological function. Neutrophil MMPs are activated within the phagosome by oxidative pathways (Sorsa *et al.*, 1994). PMN activation generates hydrogen peroxide, which in the presence of chlorine ions is converted by myeloperoxidase to hypochlorous acid. This reactive oxygen species then activates the pro-MMP.

The collagenases uniquely show specificity for the fibrillar collagens (Ryan *et al.*, 1996) whilst the gelatinases degrade denatured collagens and tissue constituents such as basement membrane type IV collagen (*Table 1.1*).

Inhibitors of MMPs play an important role in regulation, since an imbalance between the amount of activated enzyme and their inhibitors can lead to pathological breakdown of extracellular matrix. The natural inhibitors of MMPs are the tissue inhibitors of MMPs (TIMPs) and alpha-2-macroglobulin (α_2M) (Ryan *et al.*, 1996). TIMPs probably control MMP activities pericellularly, whereas α_2M functions as a regulator in body fluids. During inflammation, however, this large molecular weight protein leaves blood vessels and may be found in the exudate within the extracellular matrix. α_2M functions by entrapment of the susceptible proteinase, followed by cleavage of a peptide bond in the bait region – a venus flytrap-like mechanism (Birkedal-Hansen *et al.*, 1993). The TIMPs are widely distributed in tissue fluids, and are expressed by fibroblasts, keratinocytes, endothelial cells, monocytes and macrophages (Ryan *et al.*, 1996). They are capable of inactivating all the MMPs, binding strongly to their catalytic domains, and they may also prevent the activation of some latent MMPs. TIMP-1 is a glycoprotein, whereas TIMP-2 is its non-glycosylated counterpart. TIMP-3 has only just been isolated. TIMPs can be inactivated by reduction and alkylation, and by serine proteinase proteolysis. TIMP-1 is associated with MMP-1 and MMP-9, and TIMP-2 with MMP-2. TIMP-1 is up-regulated by retinoids, glucocorticoids, IL-1, EGF, TGFβ and TNFα, whereas TIMP-2 is down-regulated by TGFβ.

Other MMPs and cysteine and serine proteinases can also attack collagens, usually after primary cleavage by specific collagenases from fibroblasts and macrophages (MMP-1) or inflammatory cells (MMP-8). This type of collagen degradation takes place in the extracellular space, usually at times of major remodelling or during pathological states such as inflammation (see below). Elastase and cathepsin G (*Table 1.3*) are mainly produced by PMNs, but are also produced and secreted by monocytes and macrophages (Campbell *et al.*, 1989; Reilly *et al.*, 1989). Cathepsin B and L (*Table 1.3*) are synthesized and secreted mainly by monocytes and macrophages (Campbell *et al.*, 1989; Mørland, 1985; Reilly *et al.*, 1989; Reddy *et al.*, 1995). All of these proteinases are produced and secreted following the appropriate stimuli.

Active collagenase cleaves collagen at a specific site and separates small segments of fibrils from the fibre bundle. These small collagen segments may be further degraded in the extracellular environment by other MMPs or other proteinases, or they may be phagocytosed by fibroblasts or other phagocytic cells and degraded intracellularly by lysosomal enzymes (see below).

Under physiological conditions the normal turnover of soft connective tissue probably does not involve specific

Table 1.3 The cellular distribution of serine and cysteine proteinases in inflammatory cells

Proteinase	PMN	Macrophage
Serine		
Elastase	+++++	++
Cathepsin G	++	+
Cysteine		
Cathepsin B	+++	+++
Cathepsin L	+	+

collagenases (MMP-1 or MMP-8), since little or no collagenase can be detected in these tissues during health (Everts *et al.*, 1996). The normal turnover of soft connective tissue is likely to take place intracellularly within the lysosomal apparatus of fibroblasts after the phagocytosis of redundant collagen fibrils. This probably involves a multistep process as follows (See *Figures 1.8, 1.9, 1.10*):

1. The recognition of redundant collagen fibrils destined for degradation by membrane-bound receptors, probably integrens, on the surface of fibroblasts
2. Partial enclosure of the fibril by the fibroblast
3. Partial digestion of the fibril and its surrounding non-collagenous proteins by an MMP, probably gelatinase A (MMP-2)
4. Phagocytosis of the fibril and its segregation within a membrane-bound body (phagolysosome)
5. Fusion of a lysosome containing destructive enzymes with this vacuole to form a digestive lysosome
6. Final digestion of the enclosed collagen fibrils by cysteine proteinases such as cathepsins B and L.

The modulation of this process is carried out under the influence of growth factors and cytokines, including TGFα and IL-1α. In this regard, TGFα increases collagen fibril phagocytosis whilst IL-1α inhibits the process (Everts *et al.*, 1996).

The evidence for the precise mechanisms involved in these processes has built up over recent years, and is briefly described below.

First, membrane-bound intracellular collagen fibrils are frequently found in fibroblasts within two types of vacuole:

one where the space between the fibril is filled with electron-dense material, and the other with electron-lucent material (Beertsen *et al.*, 1978; Everts *et al.*, 1996). The number of these collagen-containing vacuoles in fibroblasts is greater in tissues with a high connective tissue turnover than those with a low one. In addition, these vacuoles have commonly been seen in fibroblasts in the human periodontal ligament (*Figure 1.8*) and gingival connective tissue (Eley and Harrison, 1975). Although these vacuoles are most common in fibroblasts, they have also been seen in epithelial cells, macrophages (*Figure 1.9*), osteoblasts, cementoblasts, chondrocytes, odontoblasts and smooth muscle cells, suggesting that this process goes on in many connective tissues (Everts *et al.*, 1996).

Secondly, these intracellular fibres cannot be newly synthesized collagen for the following reasons (Everts *et al.*, 1996):

- Procollagen is secreted into the extracellular space, and only then becomes aggregated into cross-banded fibrils
- Factors that block collagen synthesis have no influence on the number of intracellular collagen-containing vacuoles
- Factors that block phagocytosis completely inhibit the formation of intracellular collagen-containing vacuoles.

Thirdly, the recognition and internalization of collagen fibrils probably involves integrins on the surface of the fibroblasts. Fibrils destined for degradation are surrounded by a meshwork of non-collagenous proteins, including proteoglycans, glycoproteins and collagens V

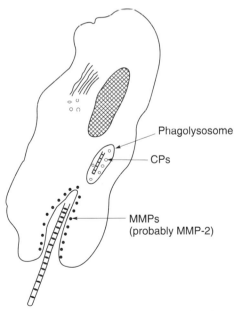

Key:

ⲭⲭⲭⲭⲭ	Banded collagen
⫽⫽	Endoplastic reticulum
CPs	Cysteine proteinases
MMPs	Matrix metalloproteinases

Phagolysosome

CPs

MMPs
(probably MMP-2)

Figure 1.10 A schematic presentation of the intracellular pathway of collagen degradation. Under physiological balanced conditions, this pathway is considered to be the major route of degradation. Collagen fibrils are engulfed by a fibroblast, and during this process the fibril is partially digested by a membrane-bound matrix metalloproteinase (MMP), probably gelatinase A (MMP-2). It is then taken up into a phagolysosome, where it is further degraded by cysteine proteinases (CPs) and VI. These may play a role in these processes because integrin recognizable sequences are present on several collagens and glycoproteins such as fibronectin (Everts *et al.*, 1996).

Fourthly, collagenase is not involved in processing these fibrils before they are internalized (Everts *et al.*, 1996) because:

• Factors that inhibit collagenase do not affect collagen fibril uptake by fibroblasts
• IL-1α, either alone or with EGF, stimulates the secretion of collagenase, whilst TGFβ inhibits its secretion
• TGFβ stimulates phagocytosis of collagen fibrils by fibroblasts, whilst IL-1α inhibits this process.

Therefore, there is an inverse relationship between collagenase secretion and phagocytosis of collagen fibrils by fibroblasts. However, selective inhibition of gelatinase A (MMP-2) does inhibit collagen fibril phagocytosis and prevent intracellular digestion. Thus, this enzyme may partially digest collagen fibrils prior to phagocytosis (Everts *et al.*, 1996).

Finally, the intracellular digestion of collagen fibrils involves cysteine proteinases such as cathepsins B and L (Everts *et al.*, 1996). This is because:

• Selective inhibition of cysteine proteinases increases the number of collagen-containing vacuoles in fibroblasts and prevents their digestion
• Selective inhibition of cysteine proteinases prevents the release of collagen degradation products into the culture medium

• Selective inhibition of individual cysteine proteinases has proved that cathepsin B is involved in this process (Van Noorden and Everts, 1991).

There are probably two pathways of collagen degradation:

1. The collagenase-independent intracellular route (*Figure 1.10*), of major importance in normal collagen turnover
2. The collagenase-mediated extracellular route (*Figure 1.11*), which is of importance in tissue remodelling involving large amounts of collagen breakdown and during inflammation. This involves the secretion of a number of MMPs by fibroblasts and other cells, including collagenases (MMP-1 and MMP-4), gelatinases A and B (MMP-2 and MMP-9) and stromolysins (MMP-3 and MMP-11).

The mechanisms controlling connective tissue turnover are only partly understood (see above). Some cytokines stimulate collagen, fibronectin and proteoglycan synthesis and secretion, and these include fibroblast growth factor (FGF), platelet-derived growth factor (PDGF) and transforming growth factors alpha (TGFα) and beta (TGFβ). Other cytokines such as interleukin-1 (IL-1) and interferon gamma (IFNγ), platelet-derived growth factor (PDGF) and transforming growth factor alpha (TGFα) can stimulate collagenase secretion (*Table 1.2*). However, the control mechanisms governing the secretion of these cytokines is not fully understood.

Key:

ⲭⲭⲭⲭⲭ	Banded collagen
⫻	Endoplastic reticulum
∘∘∘	Secretory vacuoles
MMPs	Matrix metalloproteinases

Figure 1.11 A schematic presentation of the extracellular pathway of collagen degradation. Digestion of relatively large amounts of collagen occurs primarily in the extracellular space, under the influence of a variety of enzymes secreted by the fibroblast. The most important of these are the metalloproteinases (MMPs), including gelatinase A (MMP-2), gelatinase B (MMP-9), collagenase (MMP-1) and stromolysin (MMP-3)

Bone

Bone turnover takes place continually throughout life, with bone deposition mediated by osteoblasts linked to bone resorption largely mediated by osteoclasts.

Osteoblasts are responsible for the synthesis of the bone matrix and its subsequent calcification. Initially uncalcified matrix or osteoid is formed, and this is mineralized as a result of deposition of crystals of hydroxyapatite.

Osteoclasts are only formed at bone surfaces undergoing resorption. However, bone resorption cannot take place unless both osteoclasts and osteoblasts are present (Dziak, 1993). Osteoblasts control the functions of osteoclasts through regulating hormones and local messengers (see Chapter 5). Stimulated osteoblasts secrete procollagenase which, when activated, can remove the non-mineralized collagenous surface of bone. Osteoclasts then spread over the bone surface and secrete acid beneath their ruffled borders, which dissolves the mineral phase (see *Figure 5.5*). They also secrete lysosomal cysteine proteinases such as cathepsins B and L, which are active at acid pHs and are probably responsible for removing the collagenous matrix.

This process is regulated by systemic hormones such as parathyroid hormone (PTH), vitamin D3 and calcitonin, and locally produced factors such as prostaglandin E_2 (PGE_2), leukotrienes and cytokines (such as IL-2, IL-3 and IL-6) and growth factors (such as $TNF\alpha$ and β, $TGF\beta$ and PDGF) (see *Figure 5.4*).

Radiographic appearance of the periodontal tissues

The radiographic image represents the product of the radiodensity of the various tissues that lie in the path of the X-ray beam, so that only the most radiodense tissues may be discernible. Thus, interdental bone registers while buccal and lingual plates of bone may be almost completely obscured by the image of the tooth (*Figure 1.12*).

There are a number of discernible anatomical features on the radiograph.

The socket walls and crest of the interdental septa register as linear radio-opacities, the white line of the lamina dura outlining the socket (*Figure 1.13*). The presence and clarity of these features reflect the contour of the alveolar crest and of the tooth socket, and variations in the thickness of these white lines, or their complete absence, do not necessarily mean that disease is present.

Because the facial–lingual width of the interdental septum between molars is substantial, the image of the crest is well-delineated. The interdental septa between premolars and incisors are much narrower, therefore they are more radiolucent and the images of the crests tend to be less well-defined (*Figure 1.14*).

The periodontal space between the calcified structures is extremely narrow, and shows as a thin dark line around

Figure 1.12 Radiographic appearance of healthy tooth-supporting tissue. The alveolar crest and sockets are delineated by a radio-opaque line. The images of buccal and lingual plates of bone are obscured by the image of the tooth

Figure 1.13 Radiograph of incisors shows that the image of the crest of alveolar septa is less well defined than between molars. (Courtesy Dr A Sidi)

the root. Where the proximal tooth surface is wide this line is likely to be clearer than where the interproximal dimension is narrow, and in some cases it may not be discernible at all. Increased functional stress produces a

Figure 1.14 Widened periodontal space at $\overline{1|1}$ indicating thickened ligament as a response to increased occlusal stress

thickened periodontal ligament, which is reflected on the radiographic film (*Figure 1.14*). A composite image of the cancellous bone trabeculation is projected on to the radiograph, and the image density reflects the density of the bone.

Cementum is discernible only when hypercementosis has taken place.

As the radiographic image can easily be distorted by variations in beam angle, exposure time and developing time, it is essential to use a completely standardized procedure. Lack of standardization makes comparison impossible and misdiagnosis possible.

Age changes in the periodontium

Because destructive periodontal disease tends to manifest itself most frequently in early middle age and is more advanced in the older individual, it has been regarded as part of the ageing process. This is not the case. Age changes do take place in the healthy periodontal tissues, but periodontal disease is not one of them. It is important to distinguish true age changes from the effects of trauma and disease that may accompany age.

The vasculature, gingiva, periodontal ligament, cementum and alveolar bone demonstrate age changes, and it is possible that the vascular changes (e.g. thickening of vessel walls, narrowing of the lumen and even arteriosclerosis) are central to changes in the tissues generally. Briefly, these consist of loss of cellularity and increasing

fibrosis. There may also be loss of ground substance and thickening of basement membranes.

In the periodontal ligament, fibre bundles are thicker and less distinct. Cementum, especially in the apical area, is thicker, largely as a compensation for attrition of occlusal tooth surfaces.

The alveolar bone becomes less vascular, and many haversian systems are closed. Some osteoporosis may be evident, but this is not usually as severe as in the long bones. Finally, wound healing may be slower in old age.

References

Alexander, M.B. and Damoulis, P.D. (1994) The role of cytokines in the pathogenesis of periodontal disease. *Current Opinions in Periodontology*, 39–53

Anderson, T.J., Lapp, C.A., Billman, M.A. and Schuster, G.S. (1998) Effects of transforming growth factor-β and platelet-derived growth factor on human gingival fibroblasts grown in serum-containing and serum-free medium. *Journal of Clinical Periodontology* **25**, 48–55

Arnett, T.R. (1990) Update on bone cell biology. *European Journal of Orthodontics* **12**, 81–90

Aukil, I. (1991) Biology of tooth-cell adhesion. *Dental Clinics of North America* **35**, 459–467

Barnard, J.A., Lyons, R.M. and Moses, H.L. (1990) The cell biology of transforming growth factor-β. *Biochimica Biophysica Acta* **1032**, 79–87

Bartold, P.M. (1995) Turnover in periodontal connective tissues: dynamic homeostasis of cells, collagen and ground substance. *Oral Diseases* **1**, 238–253

Bartold, P.M. and Narayanan, S. (1998) *Biology of the Periodontal Tissues*. Chicago: Quintessence Publishing Co. Ltd

Becker, J., Schuppan, D. and Muller, S. (1993) Immunohistochemical distribution of collagen types I, III, IV, VI, of undulin and tenascin in oral fibrous hyperplasia. *Journal of Oral Pathology and Medicine* **22**, 463–467

Beertsen, W., Brekelmans, M. and Everts, V. (1978) The site of collagen resorption in the periodontal ligament of the rat. *Anatomy Record* **192**, 305–318

Berkowitz, B.M.B., Holland, G.R. and Moxham, B.J. (1992) *A Colour Atlas and Textbook of Oral Anatomy, Histology and Embryology*, 2nd Edn. pp. 172–174, 182–183. London: Wolfe Publishing Ltd

Berkowitz, B.M.B., Moxham, B.J. and Newman, H.N. (1995) *Periodontal Ligament in Health and Disease*, 2nd Edn. Barcelona: Mosby-Wolfe

Bilezikian, J.P., Raisz, L.G. and Rodan, G.A. (1996) *Principles of Bone Biology*. San Diego: Academic Press

Birkedal-Hansen, H., Moore, W., Bodden, M. *et al.* (1993a) Matrix metalloproteinases: a review. *Critical Reviews of Oral Biology and Medicine* **4**, 197–250

Birkedal-Hansen, H. (1993b) Role of matrix metalloproteinases in human periodontal diseases. *Journal of Periodontology* **64**, 474–484

Blom, S., Holmstrup, P. and Dabelsteen, E. (1994) A comparison of the effect of epidermal growth factor, platelet-derived growth factor and fibroblast growth factor on rat periodontal ligament fibroblast-like cells' DNA synthesis and morphology. *Journal of Periodontology* **65**, 373–378

Boyan, L.A., Bhargava, G., Nishimura, F. *et al.* (1994) Mitogenic and chemotactic responses of human periodontal ligament cells to different isoforms of platelet-derived growth factor. *Journal of Dental Research* **73**, 1593–1600

Boyko, G.A., Melcher, A.H. and Brunette, D.M. (1981) Formation of new periodontal ligament by periodontal ligament cells implanted *in vivo* after culture *in vitro*. A preliminary study of transplanted roots in the dog. *Journal of Clinical Periodontology* **19**, 615–624

Caffesse, R.G. and Quinones, C.R. (1993) Polypeptide growth factors and attachment proteins in periodontal wound healing and regeneration. *Periodontology 2000* **1**, 69–79

Campbell, E.J., Silverman, E.K. and Campbell, M.A. (1989) Elastase and cathepsin G of human monocytes. Quantification of cellular content, release in response to stimuli, and heterogeneity in elastase-mediated proteolytic activity. *Journal of Immunology* **143**, 2961–2968

Campbell, E.J., Cury, J.D., Shapiro, S.D. *et al.* (1991) Neutral metalloproteinases produced by human mononuclear phagocytes. Cellular differentiation markedly alters cell phenotype for serine proteinases, metalloproteinases, and tissue inhibitor of metalloproteinases. *Journal of Immunology* **146**, 1286–1293

Dennison, D.K., Vallone, D.R., Pinero, G.J. *et al.* (1994) Differential effect of TGF-β1 and PDGF on proliferation of periodontal ligament cells and gingival fibroblasts. *Journal of Periodontology* **65**, 641–648

D'Errico, J.A., MacNeil, R.L., Takata, T. *et al.* (1997) Expression of bone associated markers by tooth root lining cells *in situ* and *in vitro*. *Bone* **20**, 117–126

Deuel, T.F., Kawahara, R.S., Mustoe, T.A. and Pierce, G.F. (1991) Growth factors and wound healing: platelet-derived growth factor as a model cytokine. *Annual Review of Medicine* **42**, 567–584

Dziak, R. (1993) Biochemical and molecular mediators of bone metabolism. *Journal of Periodontology* **64**, 407–415

Eley, B.M. and Harrison, J.D. (1975) Intracellular collagen fibrils in the periodontal ligament of man. *Journal of Periodontal Research* **10**, 168–170

Embery, G., Oliver, W.M. and Stanbury, J.B. (1979) The metabolism of proteoglycans and glycosaminoglycans in inflamed human gingiva. *Journal of Periodontal Research* **14**, 512–519

Embery, G., Picton, D. and Stanbury, J.B. (1987) Biochemical changes in the periodontal ligament ground substance associated with short-term intrusive loading in adult monkeys. *Archives of Oral Biology* **32**, 545–549

Engel, J. (1991) Common structural motifs in proteins in the extracellular matrix. *Current Opinions in Cell Biology* **3**, 779–785

Erikson, H.P. and Inglesias, J.L. (1984) A six-armed oligomer isolated from cell surface fibronectin preparations. *Nature* **311**, 267–269

Everts, V., Van der Zee, E., Creemers, L. and Beertsen, W. (1996) Phagocytosis and intracellular digestion of collagen, its role in turnover and remodelling. *Histochemical Journal* **28**, 229–245

Frank, S., Madlener, M. and Werner, S. (1996) Transforming growth factors β1, β2 and β3 and their receptors are differentially regulated during normal and impaired wound healing. *Journal of Biological Chemistry* **271**, 1018–1019

Fujisawa, R., Nodaska, Y. and Kuboki, Y. (1995) Further characterization of the interaction between bone sialoprotein (BSP) and collagen. *Calcifying Tissue International* **56**, 140–144

Gage, J.P., Francis, M.J.O and Triffitt, J.T. (1989) *Collagen and Dental Matrices*. London: Wright

Gallagher, J.T., Lyon, M. and Steward, W.P. (1986) Structure and function of heparin sulphate proteoglycans. *Biochemical Journal* **236**, 313–323

Giannopoulou, C. and Cimasoni, G (1996) Functional characteristics of periodontal and gingival fibroblasts. *Journal of Dental Research* **75**, 895–902

Goa, J., Jordan, T.W. and Cutress, T.W. (1996) Immunolocalization of basic fibroblast growth factor (bFGF) in human periodontal ligament (PDL) tissue. *Journal of Periodontal Research* **31**, 260–264

Gould, T.R.L., Melcher, A.H. and Brunette, D.M. (1980) Migration and division of progenitor cell populations in the periodontal ligament

after wounding. *Journal of Periodontal Research* **15**, 20–42

Hay, E.D. (1981) *Cell Biology of Extracellular Matrix*. New York: Plenum Press

Hassell, T.M. (1993) Tissues and cells of the periodontium. *Periodontology 2000* **3**, 9–38

Hefti, A.F. (1993) Aspects of cell biology of the normal periodontium. *Periodontology 2000* **3**, 64–75

Hughes, F.J. (1995) Cytokines and cell signaling in the periodontium. *Oral Diseases* **1**, 259–265

Hughes, F.J., Aubin, J.E. and Heersche, J.N.M. (1992) Differential chemotactic responses of different populations of fetal rat calvaria cells to platelet-derived growth factor and transforming growth factor β. *Bone Mineralisation* **19**, 63–74

Igarashi, A., Okochi, H., Bradham, D.M. and Grotendorst, G.R. (1993) Regulation of connective tissue growth factor gene expression in human skin fibroblasts and during wound repair. *Molecular Biology of the Cell* **4**, 637–645

Irwin, C.R., Schor, S.L. and Ferguson, M.W.J. (1994) Effects of cytokines on gingival fibroblasts *in vitro* are modulated by extracellular matrix. *Journal of Periodontal Research* **29**, 309–317

Kawase, T., Sato, S., Miake, K. and Saito, S. (1988) Alkaline phosphatase of human periodontal ligament fibroblast-like cells. *Advances in Dental Research* **2**, 234–239

Kiritsy, C.P., Lynch, A.B. and Lynch, S.E. (1993) Role of growth factors in cutaneous wound healing: a review. *Critical Reviews of Biological Medicine* **4**, 729–760

Kuru, L., Griffiths, G.S., Parkar, M.H. *et al.* (1998) Flow cytometry analysis of gingival and periodontal ligament cells. *Journal of Dental Research* **77**, 555–564

Lang, H., Schüler, N., Arnhold, S. *et al.* (1995) Formation of differentiated tissues *in vivo* by periodontal cell populations cultured *in vitro*. *Journal of Dental Research* **74**, 1219–1225

Lang, H., Schüler, N., and Nolden, R. (1998) Attachment formation following replantation of cultured cells into periodontal defects – a study in minipigs. *Journal of Dental Research* **77**, 393–405

Larjava, H., Häkkinen, L. and Rahemtulla, F. (1992) A biochemical analysis of human periodontal tissue proteoglycans. *Biochemical Journal* **284**, 267–274

Lekic, P. and McCulloch, C.A.G. (1996) Periodontal ligament cell populations: the central role of fibroblasts in creating a unique tissue. *Anatomical Record* **245**, 491–500

Lekic, P., Sodek, J. and McCulloch, C.A.G. (1996) Relationship of cellular proliferation to expression of osteopontin and bone sialoprotein in regenerating rat periodontium. *Cell and Tissue Research* **285**, 491–500

Levine, J.H., Moses, H.L., Gold, L.I. and Nanney, L.B. (1993) Spacial and temporal patterns of immunoreactive transforming growth factors β1, β2 and β3 during excisional wound repair. *American Journal of Pathology* **143**, 368–380

Listgarten, M.A. (1972) Normal development, structure, physiology and repair of the gingival epithelium. *Oral Science Review* **1**, 3–67

Lu, H., Mackenzie, I.C. and Levine, A.E. (1997) Transforming growth factor-β response and expression in junctional and oral gingival epithelial cells. *Journal of Periodontal Research* **32**, 682–691

Lukinmaa, P.L., Mackie, E.J. and Thesleff, I. (1991) Immunohistochemical localization of the matrix glycoproteins – tenascin and the ED-sequence-containing form of cellular fibronectin – in human permanent teeth and periodontal ligament. *Journal of Dental Research* **70**, 19–26

Lynch, S.E., Nixon, J.C., Colvin, R.B. and Antoniades, H.N. (1987) The role of platelet-derived growth factor in wound healing: synergistic effects with other growth factors. *Proceedings of the National Academy of Science USA* **84**, 7696–7700

Lynch, S.E., Colvin, R.B. and Antoniades, H.N. (1987) Growth factors in wound healing: single and synergistic effects on partial thickness porcine skin wounds. *Journal of Clinical Investigation* **84**, 640–646

Machein, N. and Conca, W. (1997) Expression of several matrix metalloproteinase genes in human monocytic cells. *Advances in Experimental Medicine and Biology* **421**, 247–251

Mackie, E.J., Thesleff, I. and Chiquet-Ehrismann, R. (1987) Tenascin is associated with chondrogenic and osteogenic differentiation *in vivo* and promotes chondrogenesis *in vitro*. *Journal of Cell Biology* **105**, 2569–2579

MacNeil, L.R., Berry, J., D'Errico, J. *et al.* (1995) Role of two mineral-associated adhesion molecules, osteopontin and bone sialoprotein, during cementogenesis. *Connective Tissue Research* **33**, 1–7

MacNeil, L.R., Berry, J., Strayhorn, C. and Somerman, M.J. (1996) Expression of bone sialoprotein mRNA by cells lining the mouse tooth root during cementogenesis. *Archives of Oral Biology* **41**, 827–835

Mariotti, A. (1993) The extracellular matrix of the periodontium; dynamic and interactive tissues. *Periodontology 2000* **3**, 39–63

Massagué, J. (1987) The TGF-β family of growth and differentiation factors. *Cell* **49**, 437–438

Matsuda, N., Lin, W.L., Kumar, H.M. *et al.* (1992) Mitogenic, chemotactic and synthetic responses of rat periodontal ligament fibroblastic cells to polypeptide growth factors *in vitro*. *Journal of Periodontology* **63**, 515–525

Matsuura, M., Herr, Y., Han, K.Y. *et al.* (1995) Immunochemical expression of extracellular matrix components of normal and healing periodontal tissues in the beagle dog. *Journal of Periodontology* **66**, 579–593

McCulloch, C.A.G. and Melcher, A.H. (1983a) Cell migration in the periodontal ligament of mice. *Journal of Periodontal Research* **18**, 339–352

McCulloch, C.A.G. and Melcher, A.H. (1983b) Cell density and cell generation in the periodontal ligament of mice. *American Journal of Anatomy* **167**, 43–58

McCulloch, C.A.G., Nemeth, E., Lowenberg, B. and Melcher, A.H. (1987) Paravascular cells in endosteal spaces of alveolar bone contribute to the periodontal cell ligament populations. *Anatomy Record* **219**, 233–242

McCulloch, C.A.G. (1995) Origins and functions of cells essential for periodontal repair: the role of fibroblasts in tissue homeostasis. *Oral Diseases* **1**, 271–278

Melcher, A.H., McCulloch, C.A.G., Cheong, T. *et al.* (1987) Cells from bone synthesize cementum-like and bone-like tissue *in vitro* and may migrate into the periodontal ligament *in vivo*. *Journal of Periodontal Research* **22**, 246–247

Mørland, B. (1985) Cathepsin B activity in human blood monocytes during differentiation *in vitro*. *Scandinavian Journal of Immunology* **22**, 9–16

Murata, M., Hara, K. and Saku, T. (1997) Dynamic distribution of basic fibroblast growth factor during epulis formation: an immunohistochemical study in an enhanced healing process in the gingiva. *Journal of Oral Pathology and Medicine* **26**, 224–232

Nakaya, H., Oates, T.W., Hoany, H.M. *et al.* (1997) Effects of interleukin-1β on matrix metalloproteinase-3 levels in human periodontal ligament cells. *Journal of Periodontology* **68**, 517–533

Nishimura, F. and Terranova, V.P. (1996) Comparative study of the chemotactic responses of periodontal ligament cells and gingival fibroblasts to polypeptide growth factors. *Journal of Dental Research* **75**, 986–992

Nohutcu, R.M., McCauley, L.K., Shigeyama, Y. and Somerman, M.J. (1996) Expression of mineral-associated proteins by periodontal ligament cells: *in vitro* vs *in vivo*. *Journal of Periodontal Research* **31**, 369–372

Nojima, N., Kobayashi, M., Shionome, M. *et al.* (1990) Fibroblast cells derived from bovine periodontal ligaments have the phenotypes of osteoblasts. *Journal of Periodontal Research* **25**, 179–185

Oates, T.W., Rouse, C.A. and Cochran, D.L. (1993) Mitogenic effects of growth factors on human periodontal ligament cells *in vitro*. *Journal of Periodontology* **64**, 142–148

O'Neal, R., Wang, H.I., MacNeil, R.I and Somerman, M.J. (1994) Cells and materials involved in guided tissue regeneration. *Current Opinions in Periodontology* 141–156

Palmer, R.M. and Lubbock, M.J. (1995) The soft tissues of the gingiva and periodontal ligament: are they unique? *Oral Diseases* **1**, 230–237

Parfitt, G.J. (1967) The physical analysis of the tooth-supporting structures. In *The Mechanisms of Tooth Support* (D.J. Anderson *et al.*, eds), pp. 154–160. Bristol: Wright

Pearson, C.H. and Pringle, G.A. (1986) Chemical and immunochemical characteristics of proteoglycans in bovine gingiva and dental pulp. *Archives of Oral Biology* **31**, 541–548

Piche, J.E. and Graves, D.T. (1989) Study of growth factor requirements of human bone-derived cells: a comparison with human fibroblasts. *Bone* **10**, 131–138

Postlethwaite, A.E., Keski-Oja, J., Moses, H.L. and Kang, A.H. (1987) Stimulation of the chemotactic migration of human periodontal fibroblasts by transforming growth factor β. *Journal of Experimental Medicine* **165**, 251–256

Purvis, J.A., Embery, G. and Oliver, W.M. (1984) Molecular size distribution of proteoglycans in human inflamed gingival tissue. *Archives of Oral Biology* **29**, 573–579

Reddy, V.Y., Zhang, Q.-Y. and Weiss, S.J. (1995) Pericellular mobilization of tissue-destructive cysteine proteinases, cathepsins B, L, and S, by human monocyte-derived macrophages. *Proceedings of the National Academy of Science USA* **92**, 3849–3853

Reilly, J.J., Mason, R.W., Chen, P. *et al.* (1989) Synthesis and processing of cathepsin L, an elastase, by human alveolar macrophages. *Biochemical Journal* **257**, 493–498

Reynolds, J.J. (1996) Collagenases and tissue inhibitors of metalloproteinases; a functional balance in tissue degradation. *Oral Diseases* **2**, 70–76

Reynolds, J.J., Hembry, R.M. and Meikle, M.C. (1994) Connective tissue degradation in health and periodontal disease and the role of matrix metalloproteinases and their natural inhibitors. *Advances in Dental Research* **8**, 312–319

Romanos, G.E., Strub, J.R. and Bernimoulin, J.P. (1993) Immunochemical distribution of extracellular proteins as a diagnostic parameter in healthy and diseased gingival tissue. *Journal of Periodontology* **64**, 110–119

Rutherford, R.B., Trailsmith, M.D., Ryan, M.E. and Charette, M.F. (1992) Synergistic effects of dexamethazone on platelet-derived growth factor mitogenesis *in vitro*. *Archives of Oral Biology* **37**, 139–145

Ryan, M.E., Ramamurthy, S and Golub, L.M. (1996) Matrix metalloproteinases and their inhibition in periodontal treatment. *Current Opinion in Periodontology* **3**, 85–96

Saga, Y., Yagi, T., Ikawa, Y. *et al.* (1992) Mice develop normally without tenascin. *Genes Development* **6**, 1821–1831

Sage, E.H. and Borstein, P. (1991) Extracellular proteins that modulate cell-matrix interactions. SPARC, tenascin, and thrombospondin. *Journal of Biological Chemistry* **266**, 14831–14834

Somerman, M.J., Archer, S.Y., Imm, G.R. and Foster, R.A. (1988) A comparative study of periodontal ligament cells and gingival fibroblasts *in vitro*. *Journal of Dental Research* **67**, 66–70

Somerman, M.J., Foster, R.A., Imm, G.R. *et al.* (1989) Periodontal ligament cells and gingival fibroblasts respond differently to attachment factors *in vitro*. *Journal of Periodontology* **60**, 73–77

Somerman, M.J., Young, M.F., Foster, R.A. *et al.* (1990) Characteristics of human periodontal ligament cells *in vitro*. *Archives of Oral Biology* **35**, 241–247

Sorsa, T., Ding, Y., Sato, T. *et al.* (1994) Effects of tetracyclines on neutrophil, gingival and salivary collagenases: a functional and Western blot assessment with special reference to their cellular sources in periodontal disease. *Annals of the New York Academy of Science* **732**, 112–131

Sporn, M.B. and Roberts, A.B. (1991) Polypeptide growth factors and their receptors. New York: Springer-Verlag

Steffensen, B., Duong, A.H., Milam, S.B. *et al.* (1992) Immunohistochemical localization of cell adhesion proteins and integrins in the periodontium. *Journal of Periodontology* **63**, 584–592

Takayama, S., Murakami, S., Miki, Y. *et al.* (1997) Effects of basic fibroblast growth factor on human periodontal ligament cells. *Journal of Periodontal Research* **32**, 667–675

Ten Cate, A.R. (1994) *Oral Histology. Development, Structure and Function*, 4th Edn. St. Louis: Mosby.

Ten Cate, A.R. (1997) The development of the periodontium – a largely ectomesenchymally derived unit. *Periodontology 2000* **13**, 9–19

Terranover, V.P. and Wikesjö, U.M.E. (1987) Extracellular matrices and polypeptide growth factors as mediators of functions of cells of the periodontium. A review. *Journal of Periodontology* **58**, 371–380

Terranover, V.P., Odziemiec, C., Tweden, K.S. and Spadone, D.P. (1989) Repopulation of dentin surfaces by periodontal ligament cells and endothelial cells. Effects of basic fibroblast growth factor. *Journal of Periodontology* **60**, 293–301

Tucker, J.E., Lemon, R., Mackie, E.J. and Tucker, R.P. (1991) Immunohistochemical localization of tenascin and fibronectin in the dentine and gingiva of *Canis familiaris*. *Archives of Oral Biology* **36**, 165–170

Urist, M.R. (1965) Bone formation by autoinduction. *Science* **150**, 833–899

Van Dijk, L.J., Schakenraad, J.M., Van der Voort, H.M. *et al.* (1991) Cell-seeding of periodontal ligament fibroblasts. A novel technique to create new attachment. A pilot study. *Journal of Clinical Periodontology* **18**, 196–199

Van Noorden, C.J.F. and Everts, V. (1991) The selective inhibition of cysteine proteinases by Z-Phe-AlaCH$_2$F suppresses digestion of collagen by fibroblasts and osteoclasts. *Biochemical and Biophysiological Research Communications* **178**, 178–184

Waddington, R.J. and Embery, G. (1991) Structural characterization of human alveolar bone proteoglycans. *Archives of Oral Biology* **36**, 859–866

Welgus, H.G., Campbell, E.J., Cury, J.D. *et al.* (1990) Neutral metalloproteinases produced by human mononuclear phagocytes. Enzyme profile, regulation, and expression during cellular development. *Journal of Clinical Investigation* **86**, 1496–1502

Woessner, J. Jnr (1994) The family of matrix metalloproteinases. *Annals of the New York Academy of Science* **732**, 11–21

Wozney, J.M. (1995) The potential role of bone morphogenic proteins in periodontal reconstruction. *Journal of Periodontology* **66**, 506–510

Yamada, K.M. and Olden, K. (1978) Fibronectins – adhesive glycoproteins of cell surface and blood. *Nature* **275**, 179–184

Zhang, X., Schuppan, D., Becker, J. *et al.* (1993) Distribution of undulin, tenascin, and fibronectin in the human periodontal ligament and cementum: comparative immuno-electron microscopy with ultra-thin cryosections. *Journal of Histochemistry and Cytochemistry* **41**, 245–251

Further reading

Berkowitz, B.M.B., Moxham, B.J. and Newman, H.N. (1995) *Periodontal Ligament in Health and Disease*, 2nd Edn. Barcelona: Mosby-Wolfe.

Berkowitz, B.M.B., Holland, G.R. and Moxham, B.J. (1992) *A Colour Atlas and Textbook of Oral Anatomy, Histology and Embryology*, 2nd Edn. London: Wolfe Publishing Ltd

Williams, D.M., Hughes, F.J., Odell, E.W. and Farthing, P.M. (1992) The normal periodontium. In *Pathology of Periodontal Disease*, pp. 17–31. Oxford: Oxford Medical Press

2

The oral environment in health and disease

The oral mucosa is bathed in saliva and is exposed to the passage of food, the oral flora and stimulus or injury from toothbrushes and oral hygiene aids, as well as the other objects that people put in their mouths – such as cigarettes, pipes, hair-grips and so on. Considering these different factors, the variations in temperature and pH values, the range of textures and the diversity of oral habits, the oral mucosa demonstrates remarkable adaptability and resistance.

The tooth surface, which is also exposed to these factors, may become covered wholly or in part by a number of deposits: pellicle, plaque, food debris, calculus, materia alba and stains.

Saliva

Saliva plays a vital role in maintaining the integrity of the oral tissues, in food digestion and in speech. As every clinician knows, there is considerable variation in the rate of secretion from the several salivary glands. This is influenced by neurotransmission mechanisms in response to olfactory, gustatory and masticatory stimuli, and even the thought of food can increase secretion. The average unstimulated or resting flow rate is about 0.3–0.4 ml/min, but in some people can reach about 2 ml/min. The stimulated flow rate can vary between 0.2–6.0 ml/min.

Composition

Saliva is 99.5% water plus 0.5% organic and inorganic substances. The organic fraction contains both large and small molecules; the former are mainly protein in the form of glycoproteins together with some gammaglobulins, serum albumin and enzymes, and the latter include glucose, urea and creatinine. The inorganic fraction consists of calcium, phosphorus, sodium, potassium and magnesium as well as dissolved carbon dioxide, oxygen and nitrogen. The main salivary enzyme is amylase, but in disease many enzymes produced by bacteria are found, along with leucocytes. Most of the organic fraction is produced by the salivary gland cells, and the remainder is transported into the saliva from the blood. Among the compounds transported from the blood are the electrolytes, albumin, immunoglobulins G, A and M, and vitamins, drugs and hormones. Indeed, there is a good correlation between plasma and salivary levels of hormones and medications.

Function

Saliva has a number of functions:

1. In the digestive process it helps to form the food bolus and provides amylase for the digestion of starch.
2. The flow of viscous fluid helps to remove bacterial and food debris.
3. Bicarbonates and phosphates buffer food and bacterial acids.
4. Salivary mucin and other constituents protect the oral mucosa and tooth surfaces in a variety of ways:
   (a) Salivary glycoproteins cover and lubricate the mucosa. This protective action becomes more obvious when it is removed, as in xerostomia (dry mouth) caused by pathology of the salivary glands. The oral mucosa becomes dry and red, bleeds readily and is prone to infection.
   (b) The antibacterial enzyme lysozyme splits bacterial cell walls and acts as a scavenger.
   (c) Antibacterial gammaglobulin (antibody), mostly immunoglobulin A (IgA), appears to have two forms of protective action:
      (i) It prevents the attachment of bacteria and viruses to the tooth surface and oral mucosa.
      (ii) It reacts with food antigens to neutralize their effect.

(d) Saliva contains a large number of leucocytes, which migrate through the junctional epithelium, and the number of salivary leucocytes increases when there is gingival inflammation.

(e) The enzyme sialoperoxidase has antibacterial activity, especially against lactobacilli and streptococci.

(f) The mineral components, in particular calcium and phosphorus ions, act to maintain tooth integrity by modulating ion diffusion and preventing the loss of mineral ions from the tooth tissue. The interchange of minerals between tooth structure and saliva goes on constantly, and decalcification of enamel may be remineralized.

5. The water and mucin (glycoprotein) form the lubricant essential for speech, smoothing the movements and contacts of the lips, and of the tongue against the teeth and palate, that enable us to form consonants.

Oral bacteria

At birth the mouth is sterile, but within a few hours micro-organisms appear, mainly *Streptococcus salivarius*. By the time the deciduous teeth erupt, a complex flora is present. Bacteria are present in saliva, on the tongue and cheeks, on tooth surfaces, especially in fissures, and in the gingival crevice. The number of bacteria in saliva can be measured in thousands of millions per millilitre, but the largest population of bacteria is found on the dorsum of the tongue. Even the healthy gingival crevice contains more bacteria than saliva, and in periodontal disease the crevicular population multiplies.

The various parts of the mouth – the tongue, cheeks, tooth fissures, saliva and gingival crevices – can be regarded as consisting of different ecosystems in which varieties of bacteria are found in balance with one another and with the tissues. The dominant organisms are streptococci. The number and variety vary from person to person, from one part of the mouth to another, even on different surfaces of the same tooth, and before and after eating or toothbrushing. Age, diet, composition of saliva and its rate of flow, as well as systemic factors, influence the oral flora (see Chapters 3, 4 and 5).

Tooth deposits

Acquired salivary pellicle

Within seconds of tooth cleaning a thin layer of salivary protein, largely glycoprotein, is deposited on to the tooth surface (as well as on to restorations and dentures). This layer, called pellicle, is thin (0.5 μm), smooth, colourless and translucent. It adheres firmly to the tooth surface and can be removed only by positive friction. There appears to be an electrostatic affinity between hydroxyapatite and glycoprotein. Initially it is bacteria free.

The function of salivary pellicle is protective. Salivary glycoproteins and salivary calcium phosphate are adsorbed on to the enamel surface and help to reduce tooth wear. Pellicle also restricts the diffusion of acid products of sugar breakdown. It can bind various inorganic ions, e.g. calcium, phosphate and fluoride, and contains antibacterial factors, including IgG, IgA, IgM, complement and lysozyme.

Dental plaque

Very soon, indeed within minutes of being deposited, the pellicle is populated by bacteria. Bacteria may deposit directly on to enamel, but usually they attach to pellicle and the bacterial aggregates may be coated in salivary glycoprotein. In primitive peoples on a 'natural' diet of hard and fibrous food, occlusal surfaces and contact areas are subject to considerable wear so that bacterial deposition is minimal. On a soft 'civilized' diet, tooth wear is slight or absent and bacterial deposition is encouraged. Accumulations are greatest in sites sheltered from functional friction and tongue movement. The interdental region below the contact area is the site of greatest plaque thickness.

Plaque formation

Within the first few hours, species of *Streptococcus* and (a little later) *Actinomyces* attach to the pellicle. During the first few days this bacterial population grows along and spreads out from the tooth surface so that, under electron microscopy, palisades of organisms rather like skyscrapers can be seen, one layer on top of another radiating from the surface. Plaque grows by internal multiplication and surface deposition. Different varieties of bacteria attach to these columns and multiply so that after 3–4 weeks a complex microflora is established, which represents a balanced equilibrium of organisms or a microbial ecosystem on the tooth surface (*Figure 2.1*).

Supragingival plaque formation is pioneered by bacteria with an ability to form extracellular polysaccharides, which allow them to adhere to the tooth and each other. The first colonizing bacteria are *Streptococcus mitior*, *S. sanguis*, *Actinomyces viscosus* and *A. naeslundii*. If these bacteria grow unchecked for a few days, gingival inflammation will develop. During this process the environmental conditions will gradually change, causing a selective overgrowth. This results in a shift in the bacterial composition and, after 2–3 weeks of uninhibited growth, a complex flora develops, including Gram negative anaerobes, motile bacteria and spirochaetes. Moore *et al.* (1982) have isolated 166 bacterial species from supragingival plaque.

At a clinical level, dental plaque is a soft, non-calcified layer of bacteria that accumulates on and adheres to teeth and other objects in the mouth, e.g. restorations, dentures and calculus. In thin layers it is scarcely visible and can be revealed only by the use of a disclosing agent

Figure 2.1 Scanning electron micrograph of organisms in mature plaque (×1400). (Courtesy Dr H N Newman and the publishers of the *British Dental Journal*)

(a)

(b)

Figure 2.2 *(a)* Plaque deposits seen prior to the use of a disclosing agent; *(b)* as revealed by disclosing agent

(*Figure 2.2*). In thick layers it can be seen as a yellowish or grey deposit that cannot be removed with mouthwash or by irrigation, but can be brushed off. It is unusual to find it on the masticatory surface of the tooth unless that tooth is out of function, when gross deposits may form.

Composition of mature plaque

Approximately 70% of plaque is microbial, and the rest represents extracellular products of plaque bacteria, cell remnants and glycoprotein derivatives. Protein, carbohydrate and lipids are found. The most common carbohydrate is bacteria-produced dextran; there is also some levan and galactose. The principal inorganic components are calcium, phosphorus, traces of magnesium, potassium and sodium. The inorganic salt content is highest on the lingual surface of the lower incisors. Calcium ions may actually aid adhesion between bacteria, and between bacteria and the pellicle.

Plaque deposition and food intake

Plaque will form in patients and animals fed by stomach tube, although in diminished amounts. There is some debate as to whether the frequency of meals or the amount of food eaten influences the amount of plaque deposited. However, plaque bacteria do use nutrients that can diffuse easily into the plaque, e.g. soluble sugars, sucrose, fructose, glucose, maltose and lactose. Starches may also serve as a bacterial substrate.

Dextran is the most important extracellular bacterial product because of its relative insolubility and adhesive properties. It can be produced from sucrose in the diet, and influences plaque deposition and metabolism. Plaque forms more rapidly during sleep than following meals because the mechanical action of eating plus the stimulated salivary flow deters plaque deposition. Eating hard, coarse and fibrous food deters plaque formation, and this fact is used in the experimental production of plaque. Gingivitis can be produced in a dog by feeding it a soft diet for as short a time as 4 days.

Although some debate still lingers about the benefits of finishing meals with apples, celery and carrots, these are preferable to the usual very sweet dessert offerings. Certainly vigorous mastication, which produces natural tooth wear on both occlusal and interproximal surfaces, minimizes plaque deposition.

Materia alba (Figure 2.3)

This is a yellowish or whitish, soft, loose deposit found in neglected mouths. It consists of a mass of micro-organisms, desquamated epithelial cells, food debris and leucocytes plus salivary deposits. Its structure is amorphous and, unlike plaque, it can be removed easily and washed away with a water spray.

Figure 2.3 Soft deposits of material alba in a very dirty mouth. Deposits of plaque and subgingival calculus are also present

Figure 2.4 Supragingival calculus lingual to lower incisors

Dental calculus (tartar)

Calculus, the 'stony crust' that forms on teeth, has long been associated with periodontal disease. Along with other pathological calcifications, e.g. kidney stones and gallstones, dental calculus is described in ancient medical writings. Calculus is a calcified mass that forms on and adheres to the surface of teeth and other solid objects in the mouth, e.g. restorations and dentures, that are not exposed to friction. *Calculus is calcified plaque.* Stages in its formation can be studied by collection on plastic veneers attached to teeth or dentures.

Calculus is rarely found on deciduous teeth and is not common on the permanent teeth of young children. However, by the age of 9 years it is found frequently, and it is present in virtually all adult mouths.

Deposits are classified according to their relationship to the gingival margin, i.e. they are either supragingival or subgingival.

Supragingival calculus (*Figure 2.4*)

By definition, this is found coronal to the gingival margin. It is deposited first on tooth surfaces opposite salivary ducts, on the lingual surfaces of lower incisors and the buccal surfaces of upper molars, but it may be deposited on any tooth or denture not adequately cleaned – for example, the occlusal surface of an unopposed tooth. It is light yellow unless stained by other factors (such as tobacco, wine or betel nut), fairly hard, brittle and easily detached from the tooth by a suitable instrument.

Subgingival calculus

This is attached to root surfaces and its distribution is not related to the salivary glands but to the presence of gingival inflammation and pocketing, a fact reflected by its old name of 'seruminal calculus'. It is dark green or black, much harder than supragingival calculus and more tightly adherent to the tooth surface. It may be found on roots close to the apical limit of a deep pocket, in severe cases as far down as the apex of the tooth. It can be difficult to detect on clinical examination. Sometimes its presence can be seen as a darkening of the thin overlying layer of gingiva, and its presence can be revealed directly by detaching the gingiva with a carefully directed blast of warm air. Cautious probing along the root surface with a fine probe will reveal deposits; if thick enough these may be seen on radiographs.

Composition of calculus

The composition of calculus varies slightly with the age of the deposit, its position in the mouth and even the geographical location of the individual.

It consists of 80% inorganic matter, some water and an organic matrix of protein and carbohydrate, which includes desquamated epithelial cells, Gram positive filamentous bacteria, cocci and leucocytes. The proportion of filamentous forms in calculus is greater than in the rest of the mouth. The inorganic fraction consists mainly of calcium phosphate as hydroxyapatite, brushite, whitlockite and octacalcium phosphate. There are also small amounts of calcium carbonate, magnesium phosphate and fluoride. The fluoride content of calculus is many times higher than in plaque.

The surface of calculus is covered by bacterial plaque, but the centre of thick deposits may be sterile.

The obvious differences in appearance and distribution of supragingival and subgingival calculus suggest that their composition and mode of deposition may be different.

The composition of subgingival calculus is very similar to that of supragingival calculus except that its Ca/P ratio is higher and its sodium content greater. Salivary proteins are not found in subgingival calculus, indicating a non-salivary source for this deposit.

The deposition of calculus

Calculus is mineralized bacterial plaque, but not all plaque mineralizes. Supragingival calculus is rarely seen on the facial surface of the lower molars, but is common on the facial surfaces of the upper molars, which are opposite the mouth of the parotid ducts. Perhaps 90% of all supragingival calculus on a dentition is on the lower incisors, which are bathed in saliva directly from the submandibular and sublingual salivary glands. Precipitation of mineral salts into plaque may be seen only hours after plaque deposition, but is more usual 2–14 days after plaque is formed. Minerals in supragingival calculus derive from saliva, those in subgingival calculus from gingival fluid exudate. In early plaque, concentrations of calcium and phosphorus ions are high; indeed, the concentration of calcium in plaque is about 20 times that in saliva, but no apatite crystals are present. Furthermore, there is no evidence that hydroxyapatite crystals form spontaneously in saliva. A trigger appears to be necessary, and it is generally believed that some element in plaque acts as a seeding or nucleation site where crystallization can start. Electron microscope studies suggest that apatite crystals are formed either in or on filamentous microorganisms, but as calculus can be formed in germ-free animals it is likely that other factors can act as a seed. Once calcification is started, it can continue by crystal growth.

Various theories have been put forward for the mechanism of initial mineralization:

1. Saliva can be regarded as an unstable, supersaturated solution of calcium phosphate. As CO_2 tension is relatively low in the mouth, CO_2 can be lost from saliva, with deposition of insoluble calcium phosphate.
2. During sleep salivary flow is reduced and ammonia is formed from salivary urea, producing a rise in pH, which favours precipitation of calcium phosphate.
3. Protein may hold calcium in high concentrations, but when saliva contacts the teeth the protein comes out of solution, leading to precipitation of calcium and phosphate ions.

Whichever of these mechanisms operates, the calcified deposit fixes the plaque in position against the tooth and gingiva. Calculus is attached to pellicle, to irregularities in the tooth surface, or via filamentous organisms that penetrate the surface of cementum.

Tooth stains

Many substances form stains that are tenaciously fixed to the tooth surface and require professional cleaning for removal. Tobacco, wine, metal salts, chlorhexidine mouthwash, etc., all produce characteristic stains. A green stain is found on children's teeth that may be the pigmentation of salivary pellicle by chromogenic bacteria.

Stains are unsightly, but there is no evidence that they cause gingival irritation or act as a focus for plaque deposition.

The subgingival flora

Subgingival bacterial colonization only occurs if supragingival plaque and gingivitis are present. It does not occur as a simple apical downgrowth of plaque but rather by the slow apical movement of pioneer bacteria, which may be attracted by nutrient and oxygen tension gradients (Newman, 1977). This initial pioneering growth is followed by progressive colonization by other indigenous bacteria and multiplication of those species that are particularly well adapted to the subgingival conditions, such as Gram negative rods and spirochaetes. This is partly due to the environment, but also to symbiotic relationships between different bacterial species and selective inhibition of some species by others. Anaerobic *Actinomyces* species are associated with the root surface, forming discrete colonies or continuous layers. Other bacteria remain unattached and free within the protected environment of the pocket, which provides them with many of the trace substances that they require. The subgingival flora is a very complex community of many different species.

Methods of investigating subgingival flora

The composition of dental plaque and the identification of individual bacterial species can be partially or fully determined in a number of ways. These methods include dark ground or phase contrast microscopy (Listgarten, 1986), culture techniques, immunological techniques including immunofluorescence (Zambon *et al.*, 1985; Zambon *et al.*, 1986) or enzyme linked immunosorbent assay (ELISA) (Ebersole *et al.*, 1984), DNA probes (French *et al.*, 1986) and other molecular biological techniques, and enzyme-based assays (Loesche, 1986). These are more fully described in Chapter 13. Precise speciation of bacteria in culture can be carried out with a variety of laboratory-based methods, including selective sub-cultures, biochemical tests, SDS PAGE, gene probes, ribotyping, DNA fingerprinting and cell wall long chain fatty acid analysis (Genco *et al.*, 1986; Greenstein, 1988).

However, it must be realized that, whatever techniques are used to determine the bacteria present in the subgingival flora, the picture will always be incomplete and can sometimes be very misleading. It will also depend on the methods used for collection. The flora contains either facultative or strict anaerobic bacteria, and many bacteria will only be preserved if strict anaerobic conditions are adhered to during both collection and culture. Furthermore, it is estimated that less than 50% of the bacteria in the subgingival flora are culturable even with special selective culture conditions. The best examples of this are the spirochaetes, which may account for 40–60% of the total flora. In addition, a considerable number of both Gram positive and Gram negative bacterial species can only be cultured with difficulty using very selective techniques. Also, some Gram positive bacteria may appear as Gram negative when grown in poor cultural conditions.

The latest molecular techniques, which detect bacteria on the basis of their genetic composition, have yielded very different compositions compared to cultural techniques using the same sample. Thus, knowledge of the composition of the subgingival flora is still incomplete, and it may appear different as these new techniques yield information.

Finally, DNA and RNA probes and monoclonal antibodies are available for some subgingival bacteria and can detect these species when they are present. They are very specific and can only detect the species to which they are directed, and will thus only detect bacteria already suspected to be present.

Nomenclature of anaerobic rods in the subgingival flora

The nomenclature of oral black-pigmented Gram negative anaerobic rods has recently changed as a result of extensive investigations of these bacteria. The principal changes have been reviewed by Van Steenbergen *et al.* (1991), and are shown in *Table 2.1*.

For the moment *Bacteroides forsythus* retains its present name, but *Wolinella recta* has been renamed *Campylobacter recta*. Subdivision of some current species will probably occur soon as our knowledge increases, and the next likely division will probably affect *Fusobacterium nucleatum*.

Several new species with very fastidious growth requirements, making them difficult to cultivate routinely, are beginning to be reported from subgingival plaque samples (Tanner, 1991). These include Gram positive bacteria such as *Eubacterium* species, including *E. timidum*, *E. brachy* and *E. nodatum* (Holdeman *et al.*, 1980), *Streptococcus oralis* and *S. gordonii* (Kilian *et al.*, 1989) and *Actinomyces georgiae* and *A. genencseriae* (Johnson *et al.*, 1990). Fastidious Gram negative bacteria reported include *Fusobacterium alocis* and *F. sulci* (Cato *et al.*, 1985), *Mitsuokella dentalis*, a motile *Selenomonas* (Moore *et al.*, 1987), *Treponema socranskii* sub-species

(Smibert *et al.*, 1984) and *B. forsythus* (Tanner *et al.*, 1986).

Subgingival flora in health and disease

Dark ground and phase contrast microscopy studies have shown that in periodontal health there is a very scant subgingival flora consisting of non-motile rods and cocci (Listgarten and Hellden, 1987; Listgarten, 1992). In gingivitis there is a marked decrease in the proportion of cocci, and a parallel increase in motile rods and spirochaetes. In chronic adult periodontitis, the number of motile rods and spirochaetes show further increases. There is also evidence that the numbers of spirochaetes and motile rods are greater in pockets with recurrent periodontitis than in those that remain inactive (Listgarten, 1984; Listgarten *et al.*, 1984).

Cultural studies have identified about 300 bacterial species in the periodontal pocket, some of which occur infrequently and in low numbers (Slots and Listgarten, 1988). The healthy gingival sulcus contains a scant microflora dominated by Gram positive facultative species of *Streptococcus* and *Actinomyces*, and a similar flora is found in successfully treated periodontal pockets. In chronic gingivitis, Gram negative anaerobic bacteria make up about 45% of the culturable flora (Slots, 1979). The predominating bacteria are *Actinomyces* species, *Streptococcus* species, *Fusobacterium nucleatum*, *Prevotella intermedia* and various non-pigmenting *Bacteroides* species. In advancing adult periodontitis, the proportions of these bacteria continue to increase until Gram negative bacteria form about 75% and anaerobic and facultative bacteria about 90% of the cultural flora. Common Gram negative bacteria in chronic adult periodontitis include *P. gingivalis*, *P. intermedia*, *F. nucleatum*, *Capnocytophaga* species, *Campylobacter* (formerly *Wolinella*) *recta*, *Eikenella corrodens* and *Actinobacillus actinomycetemcomitans*, seen in cultural studies (Slots, 1979; Slots and Genco, 1984), and spirochaetes, seen by dark ground microscopy.

The description of the precise bacterial species present in the subgingival flora associated with health, gingivitis and progressive periodontitis has been refined as the speciation of the flora has developed in recent years.

Table 2.1 The nomenclature of black pigmented anaerobes

Former name	New name
Black-pigmented *Bacteroides*	Black-pigmented anaerobic rods
Bacteroides gingivalis	*Porphyromonas gingivalis*
Bacteroides endodontalis	*Porphyromonas endodontalis*
Bacteroides corporis	*Porphyromonas corporis*
Bacteroides melaninogenicus	*Porphyromonas melaninogenicus*
Bacteroides denticola	*Porphyromonas denticola*
Bacteroides loescheii	*Porphyromonas loescheii*

Table 2.2 Bacterial species associated with health

Gram positive rods	
Actinomyces israelli	*Rothia dentocariosa*
Actinomyces naeslundii	*Actinomyces gerencseriae*
Actinomyces odontolyticus	
Gram positive cocci	
Streptococcus mitis	*Streptococcus sanguis*
Streptococcus oralis	*Streptococcus gordonii*
Peptostreptococcus micros	
Gram negative rods	
Selenomonas sputigena	*Prevotella intermedia*
Capnocytophaga gingivalis	*Fusobacterium nucleatum* subsp. *vincentii*

Table 2.3 Bacterial species associated with gingivitis

Similar proportions in health, gingivitis and periodontitis	Elevated in gingivitis	Elevated in gingivitis and periodontitis
Actinomyces gerencseriae	Actinomyces naeslundii III	Prevotella intermedia
Actinomyces naeslundii	Campylobacter concisus	Eubacterium timidum
Bacteroides gracilis	Streptococcus anginosis	Fusobacterium nucleatum
Capnocytophaga ochracea	Streptococcus sanguis	Campylobacter recta
Haemophilus aphrophilus		
Proprionibacter acnes		
Gamella (Streptococcus) morbillorula		
Veillonella parvula		

These bacterial species have recently been reviewed and described by Tanner (1991), and are listed in *Tables 2.2, 2.3* and *2.4*. Various combinations of the bacteria shown in *Table 2.4* have been reported as increasing at sites with progressive periodontitis in many studies on patients in different parts of the world. In this regard, a recent study of 148 Chinese adult patients aged 30–59 years with chronic periodontitis found an increase in a number of these species, notably *P. gingivalis, T. denticola, B. forsythus* and *C. recta*, at sites with progressive periodontitis (Papapanou *et al.*, 1997).

The composition of the pocket flora may vary from one individual to another, and from one tooth site to another. The predominance of certain bacteria in the pocket does not necessarily indicate that these bacteria are exclusive pathogens, since all the different bacterial species that exist in the pocket flora in various proportions and frequencies originate from the normal oral flora (Theilade, 1986).

Table 2.4 Bacterial species associated with progressive periodontitis

Gram positive rods	Gram positive cocci
Eubacterium brachy	Peptostreptococccus micros
Eubacterium nodatum	Peptostreptococccus anaerobius
Eubacterium timidum	Peptostreptococccus acnes
Proprionibacter acnes	
Lactobacillus minutus	

Gram negative rods	Gran negative spiochaetes
Porphyromonas gingivalis	Borrelia vincentii
Prevptella intermedia	Treponema denticola
Prevotella denticola	Trepanema macrodentium
Prevotella oralis	Treponema oralis
Bacteroides forsythus	Treponema socaranskii
Actinobacillus actino-mycetemcomitans	
Eikenella corrodens	
Campylobacter recta	
Fusobacterium nucleatum subsp. nucleatum	
Fusobacterium alocis	
Selenomonas sputigena	
Selenomonas flueggei	

References

Cato, E.P., Moore, L.V.H. and Moore, W.E.C. (1985) *Fusobacterium alocis* sp. nov. and *Fusobacterium sulci* sp. nov. from the human gingival sulcus. *International Journal of Systematic Bacteriology* 35, 475–477

Ebersole, J.L., Frey, D.E., Taubman, M.A. *et al.* (1984) Serological identification of oral *Bacteroides* sp. by enzyme-linked immunosorbent assay. *Journal of Clinical Microbiology* 19, 639–644

French, C.K., Savitt, E.D., Simon, S.L. *et al.* (1986) DNA probe detection of periodontal pathogens. *Oral Microbiology and Immunology* 1, 58–62

Genco, R.J., Zambon, J.J. and Christersson, L.A. (1986) Use and interpretation of microbiological assays in periodontal disease. *Oral Microbiology and Immunology* 1, 73–79

Greenstein, G. (1988) Microbiological assessments to enhance periodontal disease diagnosis. *Journal of Periodontology* 59, 508–515

Holdeman, V., Cato, E.P., Burnmeister, J.A. and Moore, W.E.C. (1980) Description of *Eubacterium timidum* sp. nov., *Eubacterium brachy* sp. nov. and *Eubacterium nodatum* sp. nov. isolated from human periodontitis. *International Journal of Systematic Bacteriology* 30, 163–169

Johnson, J.L., Moore, L.V.H., Kaneko, B. and Moore, W.E.C. (1990) *Actinomyces georgiae* sp. nov., *Actinomyces genencseriae* sp. nov., designation of two genospecies of *Actinomyces naeslundii*, and inclusion of *A. naeslundii* serotypes II and III and *Actinomyces viscosus* serotype II in *A. naeslundii* genospecies II. *International Journal of Systematic Bacteriology* 40, 273–286

Kilian, M., Mikkelson, L. and Henrichsen, J. (1989) Taxonomic study of viridans streptococci: description of *Streptococccus gordonii* sp. nov. and embedded description of *Streptococcus sanguis* (White and Niven, 1946), *Streptococcus oralis* (Bridge and Neath, 1982) and *Streptococcus mitis* (Andrews and Horder, 1996). *International Journal of Systematic Bacteriology* 39, 471–484

Listgarten, M.A. (1984) Subgingival microbiological differences between periodontally healthy sites and diseased sites prior to and after treatment. International Journal of Periodontics and Restorative Dentistry 4, 27

Listgarten, M.A. (1986) Direct microscopy of periodontal pathogens. *Oral Microbiology and Immunology* 1, 31–36

Listgarten, M.A. (1992) Microbial testing in the diagnosis of periodontal disease. *Journal of Periodontology* 63, 332–337

Listgarten, M.A. and Hellden, L. (1987) Relative distribution of bacteria at clinically healthy and periodontally diseased sites in humans. *Journal of Clinical Periodontology* 5, 115–132

Listgarten, M.A., Levin, S., Schifter, C.C. *et al.* (1984) Comparative differential dark-field microscopy of subgingival bacteria from tooth surfaces with recent evidence of recurring periodontitis and from non-affected sites. *Journal of Periodontology* **55**, 398–401

Loesche, W.J. (1986) The identification of bacteria associated with periodontal disease and dental caries by enzymatic methods. *Oral Microbiology and Immunology* **1**, 65–70

Moore, W.E.C., Holdeman, L.V., Smibert, R.M. *et al.* (1982) Bacteriology of experimental gingivitis in young adult humans. *Infection and Immunity* **38**, 651–667

Moore, L.V.H., Johnson, J.L. and Moore, W.E.C. (1987) *Selenomonas noxia* sp. nov., *Selenomonas flueggei* sp. nov., *Selenomonas infelix* sp. nov., *Selenomonas dianae* sp. nov. and *Selenomonas artemidis* sp. nov. from human gingival crevice. *International Journal of Systematic Bacteriology* **36**, 271–280

Newman, H.N. (1977) Ultrastructure of the apical border of dental plaque. In *The Borderland between Caries and Periodontal Disease* (T. Lehner, ed.), pp. 79–103. London: Academic Press

Papapanou, P.N., Baelam, V., Luan, W.-M *et al.* (1997) Subgingival microbiota in adult Chinese: prevalence and relation to periodontal disease progression. *Journal of Periodontology* **68**, 651–666

Slots, J. (1979) Subgingival microflora and periodontal disease. *Journal of Clinical Periodontology* **6**, 351–352

Slots, J. and Genco, R.J. (1984) Black-pigmented *Bacteroides* species, *Capnocytophaga* species and *Actinobacillus actinomycetemcomitans* in human periodontal disease: virulence factors, colonization, survival and tissue destruction. *Journal of Dental Research* **63**, 412–421

Slots, J. and Listgarten, M.A. (1988) *Bacteroides gingivalis, Bacteroides intermedius* and *Actinobacillus actinomycetemcomitans* in human periodontal diseases. Journal of Clinical Periodontology **15**, 85–93

Smibert, R.M., Johnson, J.L. and Ranney, R.R. (1984) *Treponema socranskii* subsp. *socranskii* subsp. nov., *Treponema socranskii* subsp. *buccule* subsp. nov. and *Treponema socranskii* subsp. *paerdis* subsp. nov. isolated from human periodontitis. *International Journal of Systematic Bacteriology* **34**, 457–462

Tanner, A.C.R. (1991) Microbial succession in the development of periodontal disease. In *Periodontal Disease: Pathogens and Host Immune Responses* (S. Hamada, S.C. Holt and J.R. McGhee, eds), pp. 13–25. Tokyo: Quintessence Publishing Co. Ltd

Tanner, A.C.R., Listgarten, M.A., Ebersole, J.L. and Strzempko, M.N. (1986) *Bacteroides forsythus* sp. nov., a slow-growing fusiform *Bacteroides* sp. from the human oral cavity. *International Journal of Systematic Bacteriology* **36**, 213–221

Theilade, E. (1986) The non-specific theory in microbial etiology of inflammatory periodontal diseases. *Journal of Clinical Periodontology* **13**, 905–911

Van Steenbergen, T.J.M., van Winkelhoff, A.J. and de Graaff, J. (1991) Black-pigmented oral anaerobic rods: Classification and role in periodontal disease. In *Periodontal Disease: Pathogens and Host Immune Responses* (S. Hamada, S.C. Holt and J.R. McGhee, eds), pp. 41–52. Tokyo: Quintessence Publishing Co. Ltd

Zambon, J.J., Reynolds, H.S., Chen, P. and Genco, R.J. (1985) Rapid identification of periodontal pathogens in subgingival dental plaque. Comparison of indirect immunofluorescence microscopy with bacterial culture for detection of *Bacteroides gingivalis*. *Journal of Periodontology* **56** (special issue), 32–40

Zambon, J.J., Bochacki, V. and Genco, R.J. (1986) Immunological assays for putative periodontal pathogens. *Oral Microbiology and Immunology* **1**, 39–44

3

Host–parasite interaction

The description of periodontal anatomy in Chapter 1 provides little idea of the continuous activity of living tissue. Health is not a static condition; it is a dynamic state in which the living and functioning organism or tissue remains in balance with a constantly changing environment. These changes in the environment provoke corresponding alterations in tissue activity so that normal function can continue. This constant process of readjustment to maintain normal tissue activity, normal function and ultimately the continuity of life is known as homeostasis. If an environmental change is so great that homeostasis cannot be maintained, the activity of the tissues becomes abnormal, normal function cannot be continued and the change in tissue activity is perceived as disease.

Bacteria constitute an important part of our environment; indeed, life without bacteria would be impossible. Usually all external surfaces in nature, including those of living tissues, are covered by bacteria. The skin and the gut are no exception, and the oral mucosa as part of the gut is covered by many species of bacteria – the oral flora. Bacteria attach themselves to surfaces by a number of means: by the microscopic roughness of the surface, by hairlike extensions on the surface of the bacteria, and by natural glues made of proteins and polysaccharides, as in the glycoprotein of the salivary pellicle described in Chapter 2.

Where different life forms exist together there is competition for existence; therefore, mechanisms have evolved that help one form to protect itself from another. As the tissues of the body have evolved together with their micro-organisms over millions of years, one would expect that these defence mechanisms would have been perfected and that a state of harmony or balance between the host and its bacteria would have been achieved. If such a balance had not been established, at least one of the species involved would have died out, as explained by Darwin's theory of natural selection. In fact we live quite happily in a state of partnership (symbiosis) with most of the bacteria on our bodies, and only under certain circumstances do we suffer from their presence. For example, both dental caries and periodontal disease are caused by bacteria that are normally resident in our mouths. In primitive man and in so-called 'primitive' communities today the prevalence of dental disease is very low, and bacterial plaque occurs in much smaller quantities and only rarely apical to the tooth-contact area. By contrast, in 'civilized' man bacterial plaque may be found on almost all tooth surfaces, and dental disease is rampant. The change in texture of our diet and its large component of refined and easily fermentable carbohydrate have altered the oral environment in such a way that bacterial stagnation takes place around the teeth and gum margin, with resultant imbalance in the bacteria–tissue relationship and the production of substances with the capacity to damage the tissues. This is amply demonstrated in animals, which do not normally suffer from dental diseases but do develop periodontal disease and caries when fed on a soft, sticky diet rich in carbohydrate.

Defence mechanisms

A number of mechanisms operate to protect the body from attack by foreign bodies and toxins, including infection by bacteria (*Figure 3.1*). These mechanisms can be classed as:

1. Non-specific mechanisms
2. Mechanisms specific to invading foreign proteins called antigens, which stimulate the immune system.

Non-specific protection mechanisms

There are five non-specific protection mechanisms.

1. Bacterial balance

The mouth as a whole and various zones in the mouth, including what has been called the 'crevicular domain',

Microorganisms
Saliva (lysozyme)
Antibody (IgA)
Shedding epithelial layer

Reproducing epithelial layer

Lymphokines

Key

M	Macrophage		Polymorphonuclear leucocyte
	Microorganism		Red blood cell
	Antigen		Plasma cell
	Antibody		Lymphocyte
C	Complement	P	Prostaglandin

Figure 3.1 Diagram to show the multiplicity of factors that take place in the tissue defence system

can be viewed as ecosystems in which a balance exists between the different species of micro-organisms and between the flora and the tissues. Upset in this balance is most commonly seen after prolonged use of antibiotics, which suppress some types of bacteria and allow others to flourish to the detriment of the tissues – for example, the fungal infection *Candida* (thrush) may occur after the use of some antibiotics.

2. Surface integrity

The surface integrity of skin and mucous membrane barriers, including the gingiva, is maintained by the continuing renewal of the epithelium from its base and desquamation of the surface layers. These two activities balance so that the thickness of the epithelium remains constant. The efficiency of the surface barrier is enhanced by keratinization and parakeratinization. The junctional epithelium, although semi-permeable, has a very high rate of cell turnover.

3. Surface fluid and enzymes

All vital surfaces are washed by fluids, which are the products of surface glands and contain substances capable of attacking foreign material, e.g. gastric acid in the stomach, lysozyme in tears and sebum from skin hair follicles. Saliva bathes the oral mucosa and contains antibacterial substances. The gingival fluid exudate flows

through the junctional epithelium into the gingival crevice, and this fluid contains phagocytic leucocytes and their enzymes.

4. Phagocytosis

Certain cells in the bloodstream and in the tissues are capable of engulfing and digesting foreign material. The two most important phagocytic cells are the polymorphonuclear leucocyte and the macrophage (Greek: big eater) (M in *Figure 3.1*).

Polymorphonuclear leucocytes (PMNs, neutrophils)

PMNs are the most common of the white blood cells. Produced in the bone marrow, they are the most important blood cells for protecting the body against acute invasion by bacteria. Because they possess an amoeba-like ability to change shape and move rapidly they can pass through the walls of capillaries and move through the tissues, including gingival connective tissue and junctional epithelium. The direction in which they move is determined by chemical substances, mainly derived from bacteria or the complement cascade. These attract PMNs to the site of damage, where foreign particles are engulfed and digested. While their role is primarily defensive, PMNs can also produce proteolytic enzymes, which can destroy the surrounding tissue.

Macrophages (monocytes)

The macrophage is an indiscriminate scavenger of foreign material. It starts life as a monocyte, which moves into the tissues and matures to become the extremely efficient phagocyte, the macrophage, which is capable of digesting large foreign particles. If a bacterial disease lasts more than a few days, the number of monocytes in the tissues increases until there may be as many monocytes as PMNs. Unlike PMNs, monocytes are capable of several divisions within the tissues, which progressively increases the number of macrophages.

While PMNs are the main line of defence in acute infection, the monocytes are more important in long-term chronic infection. The macrophages also take up antigens from the circulating fluid for processing and presentation to the lymphocytes.

Phagocytosis is aided by a battery of nine related proteins, known as 'complement'. The complement cascade is initiated by the combination of immunoglobulin and the C1 component. The final product of the cascade is an esterase, which damages cell membranes and leads to bacteriolysis. Two intermediary products, C3a and C5a, are produced, which attach to receptor sites on mast cells and inflammatory cells. They release histamine and other substances from mast cells and prostaglandins from inflammatory cells, and these released substances increase vascular permeability. They are also chemotactic to PMNs. C3a also aids phagocytosis by attaching the antigen to the phagocyte via the C3 receptor on the surface of PMNs and macrophages (monocytes).

In addition, after detecting infection macrophages can secrete interleukin (IL)-6 (see *Table 3.1*), which can stimulate hepatocytes in the liver to secrete a mannose-binding protein that can bind to some bacterial capsules resistant to complement binding (Janaway, 1993). After binding it can activate the complement cascade.

There are diseases in which leucocyte-forming tissues become deficient and the number of PMNs may fall to almost zero (leucopenia).

Phagocytic cells in the gingival crevice

Both PMNs and macrophages migrate from the gingival tissues through the junctional epithelium into the gingival crevice/periodontal pocket. The rate of this cellular migration increases with increasing inflammation within the tissues. It is known, however, that the phagocytic capacity of PMNs and probably macrophages is much less within the crevice than in the tissues. The presence on the surface of the phagocytic cells of immunoglobulin type II and III receptors (Fcγ R II and III) is essential for phagocytosis to occur. In this regard it has been shown that there appears to be a down-regulation of Fcγ R III in

PMNs harvested from gingival crevicular fluid (GCF) (Sugita *et al.*, 1993). More recent studies have compared the presence and synthesis of these receptors in both GCF and peripheral blood (Miyazaki *et al.*, 1997). They found that the synthesis and expression of both Fcγ R II and III were lower in GCF PMNs than in peripheral blood PMNs. In addition, the down-regulation of these receptors in GCF PMNs significantly correlated with their reduced phagocytic capacity. Thus, it appears that GCF PMNs are characterized by reduced surface expression and synthesis of Fcγ receptors, and this appears to be responsible for their lack of phagocytic capacity.

5. The inflammatory reaction

The inflammatory reaction is stimulated by tissue injury and infection, and leads to changes in the local microcirculation. This produces hyperaemia, increased vascular permeability and the formation of a fluid and cellular exudate. In this way serum proteins and phagocytic cells accumulate around the irritant.

Innate immunity cannot protect against all infections, as microbes evolve rapidly, enabling them to devise means of evading these defence mechanisms. To counter these changes, vertebrates have developed a unique

Table 3.1 Lymphokines and cytokines

Cytokines	Cell source(s)	Main cell target(s)	Main actions
IFNγ	T cells	Lymphocytes	Immunoregulation
	NK cells	Macrophages	B cell differentiation
		Tissue cells	Some antiviral action
IL-1α	Macrophages	Thymocytes	Immunoregulation
IL-1β	Dendritic cells	Neutrophils	Inflammation
	Some B cells	T and B cells	Fever
	Fibroblasts		Protein synthesis
	Epithelial cells		
	Endothelium		
	Astrocytes		
IL-2	T cells	T cells, B cells	Proliferation
	NK cells	Macrophages	Activation
IL-3	T cells	Stem and progenitor cells	Pan-specific colony-stimulating factor
IL-4	T cells	B cells	Division and differentiation
		T cells	
IL-5	T cells	B cells	Differentiation
		Eosinophils	
IL-6	T cells	T cells, B cells	Differentiation
	Macrophages	Thymocytes	Acute phase protein synthesis
	Fibroblasts	Hepatocytes	
	Some B cells		
IL-8 (family)	Macrophages	Granulocytes	Chemotaxis
	Skin cells	T cells	
IL-10	T cells	Macrophages	Inhibits antigen presentation,
		T cells	production of INFγ and macrophage production of IL-1, IL-6 and TNFα
TNFα	Macrophages	Fibroblasts	Inflammation
TNFβ (lymphotoxin)	Lymphocytes	Endothelium	catabolism, fibrosis, production of other cytokines (IL-1, IL-6, GM-CSF) and adhesion molecules

system of adaptive immunity which enables the body to recognize, remember and respond to any bacteria, virus or cancer cell, even if it has never faced it before.

Specific protective mechanisms

The adaptive immune system

The unique surveillance and attack system developed to the full by mammals has three main characteristics:

1. It can distinguish between itself and the enemy, i.e. between 'self' and 'non-self', so that it does not attack itself. This recognition system can go wrong and in certain diseases, known as auto-immune diseases, the defence system attacks parts of its own body.
2. The defences contain elements specific against any given antigen. This is possible because each antigen contains specific amino acid sequences, or 'flags', which the immune system uses to recognize 'non-self'. Antigens are proteins, and because of their novelty the body does not resist their invasion on the first attack of bacteria or viruses containing them However, within a few days or weeks the immune system will have developed specific 'answers' to each antigen. Certain non-protein substances, known as haptens, can become antigenic by associating with proteins.
3. The system has a memory. The first contact with the antigen produces a primary response in which the uneducated or virgin lymphocytes (the main cell in the immune system) proliferate and mature, and the antigen is memorized so that further contact provokes a ready secondary response.

Overview

The adaptive immune system is brought about by the actions of an array of cells, which take up, process, present and react to foreign proteins known as antigens (Nossal, 1993). Antigen-presenting cells such as macrophages roam the body, ingesting the antigen they find and fragmenting it into antigenic peptides. Within the cell these species of peptide are joined to the major histocompatibility complex (MHC) molecules and displayed on the surface of the cell. Thymus-dependent (T) lymphocytes have antigenic surface receptors, which recognize the specific antigenic peptide–MHC combinations. The T-lymphocytes are activated by that process, and divide to produce memory and effector cells. The effector cells secrete chemical signals (lymphokines), which mobilize other components of the immune system. One set of cells that responds to these signals are B-lymphocytes, which also have specific receptor molecules on their surface but, unlike T-lymphocytes, can recognize parts of the whole antigen free in solution. When activated they differentiate into plasma cells that secrete specific antibodies, which are soluble forms of their receptors. By binding to anti-

gen, the antibodies can neutralize them or precipitate their destruction by activating the complement cascade or enabling phagocytic cells to destroy them. Some B-lymphocytes also persist as memory cells.

Development of immune cells

It is known that the cells concerned with immunity all develop from stem cells in the bone marrow (Weissman and Cooper, 1993). One group of these cells, T-lymphocytes, is dependent on the thymus gland for its development, and if this gland is removed in a foetal animal, T-cell immunity does not develop. In birds, another group of cells is similarly dependent on a sac in the hind gut known as the bursa of Fabricius, and these are known as bursal dependent or B-lymphocytes. In mammals, B-lymphocyte development takes place in the bone marrow.

Cells destined to become T-lymphocytes migrate early in foetal life to the thymus, where they divide and differentiate. They give rise to successive bands of cells, which migrate to the lining epithelia of body orifices and later to the lymphoid organs. The first cells going to the epithelia develop T-cell receptors (TCR) with gamma-delta chains, whereas the later ones going to the lymphoid organs develop TCRs with alpha-beta chains and will develop into helper (T4) and killer (T8) lymphocytes.

B-lymphocytes develop under the influence of the stromal cells, which produce factors needed for their growth and development. They develop interleukin (IL)-7 receptors, which are stimulated by IL-7 from the stromal cells. They then progressively develop and express specific antibody receptors. They form the heavy chain first, then add the light chain and ultimately express the complete specific immunoglobulin (Ig) receptor. They produce additional Ig alpha and beta chains, which associate with the Ig molecule to produce the complete receptor. If the developing B-lymphocytes react with large amounts of self-antigens, they are signalled to undergo programmed death (apoptosis). The clones that survive this process migrate to the lymphoid organs.

The T-lymphocyte pathway is more complex, and they pass through a number of challenges in their development. As they develop, they make and express either CD4 or CD8 receptors. CD4 cells react with Class II MHC and become T4 helper cells, and CD8 cells react with Class I MHC and become T8 killer cells. Following this, the cells make and express the specific TCR. They are first tested to see whether they detect antigens presented by other cells, an essential feature of T cells. Cells that react with self-MHC survive, and those that do not undergo apoptosis. They also die if they react with large amounts of self-antigen. The surviving T-lymphocytes migrate to the lymphoid organs, and these are the cells that can recognize both foreign peptides and self-MHC.

Development of the specific receptors

There is tremendous diversity of both the TCR and Ig receptors on T and B cells respectively (Janaway, 1993;

Marrak and Kappler, 1993). This is determined during their development in a unique way. Both the antibody and TCR genes are inherited as gene fragments known as mini genes, which are functional only after they join together to form complete genes. This process only occurs in individual lymphocytes as they develop. The order in which they join and the joining process itself produce immense diversity. Immunoglobulins consist of heavy and light chains joined together to form a Y shape. Each cell produces one type of heavy and one type of light chain to produce together the unique Ig receptor. Each chain consists of combinations of the products of mini genes, which are shuffled to produce a myriad of different combinations. Diversity springs from the size of the mini gene families, which are divided into variable (V), of which there are more than 100, diversity (D), of which there are 12, and joining (J), of which there are 4 sets. There are also constant (C) mini genes, which only vary slightly to affect the function of the antibody and not its specificity. During development, the shuffling of these mini genes into different VDJC combinations produces 4800 different heavy chains and 400 VDJ combinations in the light chains, making 1 920 000 antibody genes. In addition, special enzymes insert a few extra DNA coding units at VD or DJ junctions, which further increases diversity.

The alpha-beta or gamma-delta chains of the TCR of T-lymphocytes are constructed in a similar way, producing comparable levels of diversity.

Lymphoid tissues

Nearly all the T-lymphocytes in the lymphoid organs and over 90% of those in the blood have alpha-beta TCRs, whereas virtually all such cells associated with epithelia have gamma-delta TCRs (Lydyard and Grossi, 1993). In the lymphoid organs, T and B cells that have matured but are not associated with immune responses reside in separate domains. After stimulation by antigen, the cells that will participate in antibody production form new structures known as germinal centres. Three types of cells, T4 helper lymphocytes, B-lymphocytes and dendritic cells, which are types of antigen-presenting cell, predominate in the interface between B and T cell domains.

Lymphocyte circulation

Lymphocytes constantly circulate around the body to provide each lymphoid organ with a rapid sampling of all the lymphocytes that may possess receptors for foreign antigens already attracting the body's attention (Weissman and Cooper, 1993). They pass into the lymphoid organs through a specialized blood vessel known as a high endothelial venule (HEV). Only lymphocytes expressing homing receptors that match the receptors on the HEV can pass through. There are two types of receptors, one that matches lymph nodes and one that matches lymphoid organs of the gastro-intestinal tract. When T and B cells become activated they stop producing these homing markers and produce another integrin, VCAM-1, which matches receptors on blood vessels so that they can pass through inflamed vessels into infected tissues.

The immune response and function (*Figure 3.2*)

Antigens are first taken up by antigen presenting cells (Janaway, 1993; Marrak and Kappler, 1993; Paul, 1993). These include macrophages throughout the body, follicular dendritic cells in lymphoid organs, and dendritic and Langerhans cells present throughout the mucosal surfaces. All these cells carry the CD4 surface marker. Antigens, usually in the form of infecting organisms, are phagocytosed by these cells and broken down within phagolysosomes into their constituent peptides. A Class II MHC molecule made in the endoplasmic reticulum (ER) is transported to the vesicle. A covering protein chain keeps the molecule inactive until it reaches the antigenic peptide within its processing vesicle. In this vesicle the chain falls away, enabling the MHC molecule to bind to any antigenic peptides there. The complex then moves to the cell surface where it is presented so that it can be detected by T and B cells with the appropriate specific antigen receptor.

Antigenic peptides held in the groove of the Class II MHC molecule are recognized by T4 helper lymphocytes carrying CD4 marker and the appropriate TCR. The binding of the antigen to the receptor interacts with the biochemical message system in the T4 cell, which will tell the cell to divide, grow, differentiate and produce its products. The lymphocyte must also receive a second message at the same time for these events to occur, and if this is not received the cell will be programmed to die rather than develop. A molecule known as B7 serves this purpose, and is presented at the same time by the antigen-presenting cell and reacts with a CD28 receptor on the T-helper cell. B7 is only produced by infected cells, and thus protects against stimulation by auto-antigens.

During this process, IL-1 is also produced by the macrophage (*Table 3.1*) and reacts with its receptor on the T4 cell (Rook, 1993). This activates the appropriate genes in the T4 cell to produce IL-2 and IL-2 receptor. Stimulation by IL-2 and other cytokines causes cell division and results in the production of a clone of memory T4 cells and effector T4 cells. The effector T4 helper lymphocytes produce helper lymphokines, which stimulate T4, T8 and B-lymphocytes reacting to the same antigen.

T4 immunity controlling intracellular parasites (*Figure 3.2*)

Effector T4-lymphocytes produce lymphokines, which activate macrophages containing the antigens to destroy the material within their vesicles (Paul, 1993). This response occurs with intracellular bacterial or protozoan infections, such as tuberculosis, leprosy, Leishmania, etc. The T4 cells consist of two subsets of cells; one (TH1)

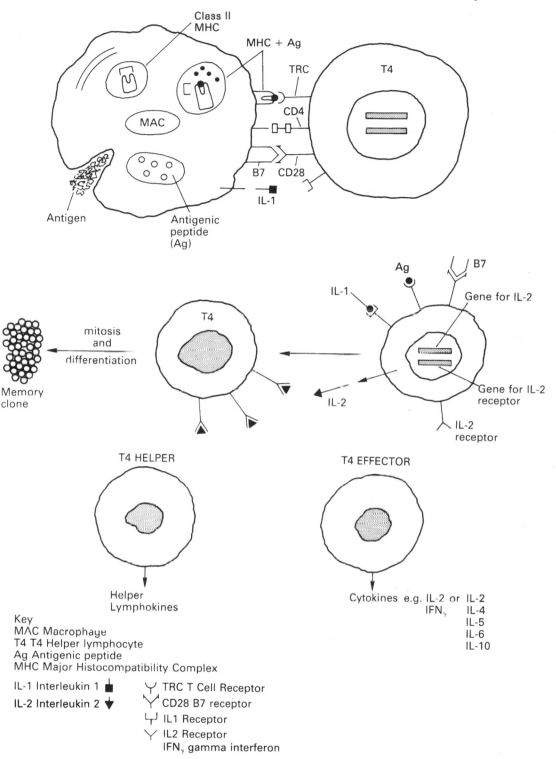

Figure 3.2 Diagram to show primary stages in the immune reaction

secretes predominantly IL-2 and gamma interferon (IFNγ) and the other (TH2) IL-2, IL-4, IL-5, IL-6 and IL-10 (*Table 3.1*). The type of T4 response may affect the outcome. IFNγ induces macrophages to produce tumour necrosis factors (TNF) and chemicals such as nitric oxide and toxic forms of oxygen, which lead to microbial destruction in the phagosome. The other response activates B-lymphocytes.

Humoral immunity (*Figure 3.3*)

The antibody receptor on the surface of a B-lymphocyte can recognize a foreign antigen in the bloodstream and bind to it (Paul, 1993). The antigen is taken into the cell and placed with a vesicle inside the cell. Class II MHC

molecules made in the ER are delivered to the vesicle as previously described. It is then presented on the cell surface, where it is detected by the appropriate clone of T4 helper lymphocytes. The TCR and CD4 bind to the antigen and MHC respectively. B cells also need a second signal from the T-helper cell. This comes from the

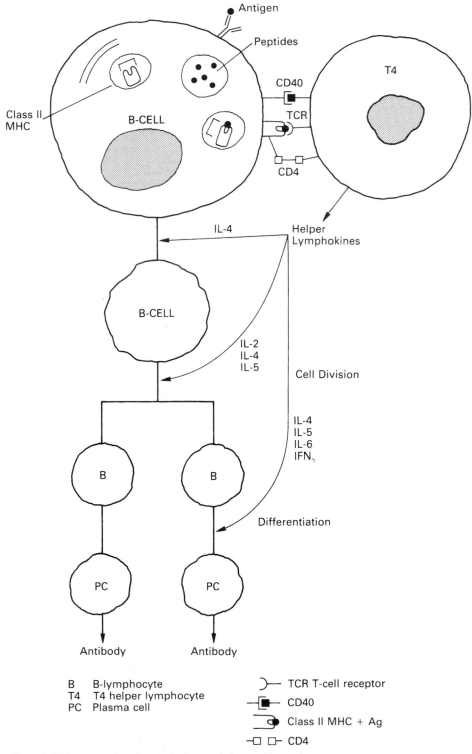

Figure 3.3 Diagram to show the principal events in humoral immunity

production and presentation of CD40 by the helper cell, which binds to the CD40 receptor on the B cell. The T4 cell produces helper lymphokines, which then switch on the signal system, resulting in division, differentiation to plasma cells and antibody production. These helper lymphokines include IL-2, IL-4, IL-5, IL-6 and IFNγ (*Table 3.1*) (Feldmann, 1993).

When differentiation of B-lymphocytes begins, they cease to display their antibody receptor molecule and prepare for antibody production. The antibodies produced by the cell are the same as those that are presented by the cell as antigen receptors. Different kinds of antibody are made, each with the same specificity, by a different variation of the antibody molecule during development. This is done by altering the so-called constant part of the heavy chain, again by gene rearrangement, which creates different receptor areas on this part of the molecule and enables the antibodies to go to different parts of the body. After binding to antigens on the microbe, these different antibody types can activate complement, promote phagocytosis (opsonization) or activate mast cells.

All antibody molecules have the same basic structure, with two specific antigen-combining sites and a single receptor-binding site. There are five types of antibody molecule, each made by a separate group of plasma cells: IgG, IgM, IgA, IgE and IgD. IgG and IgM are found mainly in blood and inflammatory exudates. IgG is the most abundant, and is a single Ig molecule with a receptor area for the C3 and Ig gamma receptors on macrophages and polymorphs. IgM is a polymer of five Ig molecules with the same receptors as IgG. IgA is a dimer and has a secretory piece added between the two molecules by cells in secretory glands, which allows it to pass through glandular epithelium into the secretion, where it binds to the surface of mucous membranes. IgE binds to receptors on mast cells and basophils, and causes a release of mediators.

The main function of these antibody types is as follows:

IgG • Antitoxin
  • Opsonin
  • Complement activation
  • Neutralizes virus in blood
IgM • Opsonin
  • Bacterial agglutination
IgA • Prevents viral attachment
  • Neutralizes virus on mucous membrane
  • Prevents bacterial adherence on mucous membrane
  • Antitoxin
IgE • Degranulates mast cells
  • Promotes inflammation
  • Stimulates the production of some factors that may be lethal to parasites
  • Attaches to macrophages and may bind parasites
IgD • Possible role in B cell function.

In terms of humoral immune function in periodontal disease, it has been shown that the serum level of anti-*Porphyromonas gingivalis* titre significantly correlated with the detection and number of *P. gingivalis* at periodontitis sites in patients with both adult periodontitis and early onset periodontitis (Kajima *et al.*, 1997). There were higher levels of *P. gingivalis* at early onset periodontitis sites compared to adult periodontitis sites, but no differences in the serum IgG titres.

T8 immunity controlling viral infection (*Figure 3.4*)

Class I MHC molecules are manufactured by practically all body cells in their ER, and they bind to peptides that originate from proteins in the cytosolic compartment of the cell (Paul, 1993). Viruses infect this area of the cell, and some of the viral proteins are broken down to peptides. They are pumped by a transport system into the ER. There the Class I MHC molecules are synthesized as long chains of amino acids, which shape themselves around the antigenic peptide to form the complete molecule. This signals to be transported to the surface in a vesicle to be displayed on the surface of the cell. Here it can be detected by a killer T8-lymphocyte, which expresses the CD8 protein. Again, two stimuli are needed to activate the cell; one from the Class I MHC and antigen and the other from B7, which is synthesized and expressed by the body cell when it presents a foreign peptide. This links to the CD28 receptor on the T8 cell.

When activated, the killer T8-lymphocyte acts directly and indirectly to kill the infected cells. They secrete perforin and other proteins that disrupt the cellular membrane, and may also release molecules that promote programmed cell death or apoptosis. They also release IFNγ and TNF (*Table 3.1*), which limit viral multiplication inside a cell and also attract macrophages and other phagocytes, which can destroy the cell.

Hypersensitivity

Although the activity of the immune system has the primary function of defending the body, once set in motion its activity can become excessive and lead to gross tissue damage. This excessive activity is called hypersensitivity (Lichenstein, 1993).

There are four main types of hypersensitivity. Types I, II and III are called immediate reactions, and depend on antibody–antigen reactions. Type I is related to the production of IgE antibodies, which attach to receptors on mast cells and basophils, resulting in the release of the contents of their granules and membranes, which mediate the allergic responses. The granular mediators are histamine and platelet activating factor, and the lipid mediators are leukotrienes and prostaglandin D. These dilate and increase the permeability of blood vessels, stimulate mucus production and constrict bronchial smooth muscle. Conditions caused by these reactions include hay fever, asthma, urticaria and anaphylaxis.

Type II reactions involve the production of IgG antibody, which activates complement on cell surfaces harbouring the antigen and causes cell damage.

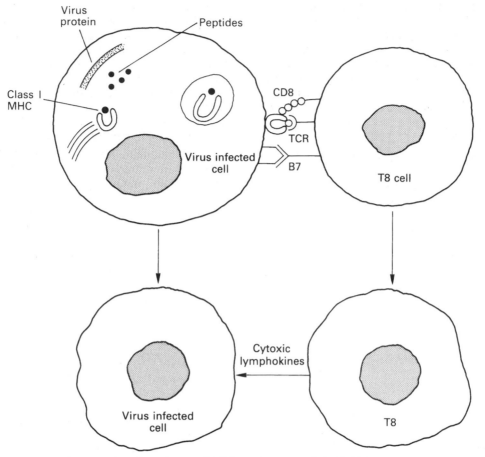

Figure 3.4 Diagram to show the main stages in T8 immunity to control viral infections

Type III (Arthus) reactions involve IgG antibody–antigen complexes reacting within blood vessel walls. The resulting activation of complement damages the vessel wall.

Type IV hypersensitivity is termed delayed, and is essentially the cell-mediated immune reaction described in the last section.

Periodontal pathology

The periodontal tissues are subject to two types of environmental factors:

1. A mechanical system in which the varying stresses of mastication demand constant modulation of the periodontal ligament, alveolar bone and cementum
2. Those oral factors described in Chapter 2; in particular, the bacterial ecosystem of the gingival crevice.

In health, the periodontal tissues metabolize and function normally in harmony with these two milieux and, because of the adaptability of vital tissues, a balance can be maintained within broad environmental limits.

The periodontal tissues may undergo a variety of pathological changes; inflammatory, degenerative and neo-plastic. They may also be involved in auto-immune diseases. Inflammation is by far the most common form of periodontal pathology. This may be restricted to the gingivae (gingivitis), or involve the deeper periodontal tissues (periodontitis). Inflammation may be acute or chronic. By definition, acute inflammation comes on suddenly, is painful and of short duration. Chronic inflammation comes on slowly, is rarely painful and is of long duration. Acute gingivitis is usually caused by specific infection or injury. Acute periodontitis may follow a blow to a tooth, or develop as a complication of chronic periodontitis. Chronic gingivitis and chronic periodontitis are successive stages in chronic inflammatory periodontal disease, and although gingival inflammation is the essential precursor to chronic periodontitis, this progression is not inevitable.

Epidemiological studies indicate that this progression seems to take place in a much smaller proportion of individuals than was previously believed. Unfortunately, we cannot yet predict in which individual the progression from gingivitis to periodontitis will take place, and much current research is directed to trying to define the person who is 'at risk'. A great deal of epidemiological and clinical research in the past decade has highlighted considerable variation in clinical features and rates of disease progression, and although all periodontitis involves loss of connective tissue attachment to the root surface in the presence of gingival inflammation (Papapanou, 1994), it is now common practice to speak of periodontal diseases in the plural. This is not only because of the considerable variation in most features of the disease, even in the otherwise healthy individual, but also because this variation in the periodontal lesion does not appear to bear a clear and simple relationship to the causal agent, i.e. to the quantity of related bacterial plaque or the types of bacteria in the plaque.

These variables include:

1. The distribution, extent and severity of gingival inflammation.
2. The presence or absence of gingival ulceration.
3. The quantity of plaque and its bacterial constituents.
4. The extent and distribution of areas of loss of periodontal attachment, i.e. periodontitis.
5. The rapidity of loss of attachment and alveolar bone.
6. The form of the bone lesion.
7. The humoral and cellular component of the lesion described above.

This variation is further confused in the presence of systemic factors – genetic, hormonal, nutritional, haematological and pharmaceutical – as described in Chapter 6.

On classifications

Many forms of classification have been devised in attempting to provide the clinician with some rationale for making a differential diagnosis and arriving at a reasonable prediction of how the tissues will respond to treatment. Some classifications have used variation in clinical presentation as parameters; others, in trying to provide some understanding of the causes of disease, have included both aetiological factors and clinical features. The results have been confusion rather than clarification.

A classification should be a systematic arrangement of groups (plants, animals, diseases, etc.) that possess common attributes. This arrangement should provide insight into the relationship between groups, and between members of the same group. This requires some form of homogeneity within the group, and clear delineation between different groups. A very simple example of this process is to put dogs and cats in different animal groups because dogs of all kinds can interbreed but cannot mate with cats of any kind.

In the host–parasite interaction that results in periodontal pathology, many factors enter the equation to produce a variety of tissue changes and, therefore, clinical features. On one side lie the rich oral flora plus any 'secondary' factors described in subsequent chapters; on the other side of the equation are a multiplicity of host or systemic factors. Also, there are wide quantitative variations rather than a simple present or absent situation in the different parameters connected with periodontal diseases. Thus, clear correlation between the severity of periodontal tissue destruction and, for example, specific bacterial species, or deficiencies in neutrophil activity, or even oral hygiene status, become difficult to define. Establishing a simple cause and effect relationship is impossible, and drawing the lines that a classification demands becomes a matter of approximation and, therefore, of probable confusion. Given our present knowledge this would not help to bring rationality to bear on our clinical problems.

References

Feldmann, M. (1993) Cell co-operation in the antibody response. In *Immunology*, 3rd Edn (I. Roitt, J. Brostoff and D. Male, eds), pp. 7.1–7.16. St. Louis: Mosby

Janaway, C.A. (1993) How the immune system recognizes invaders. *Scientific American* (Sept.) pp. 41–47

Kajima, T., Yano, K. and Ishikawa, I. (1997) Relationship between serum antibody levels and subgingival colonization of *Porphyromonas gingivalis* in patients with various types of periodontitis. *Journal of Periodontology* **68**, 618–625

Lichenstein, L.M. (1993) Allergy and the immune system. *Scientific American* (Sept.) pp. 85–91

Lydyard, P. and Grossi, C. (1993) Cells involved in the immune response. In *Immunology*, 3rd Edn (I. Roitt, J. Brostoff and D. Male, eds), pp. 2.1–2.20. St. Louis: Mosby

Marrak, P. and Kappler, J.W. (1993) How the immune system recognizes the body. *Scientific American* (Sept.) pp. 49–55

Miyazaki, A., Kobayashi, T., Suzuki, T. *et al.* (1997) Loss of Fc$_\gamma$ receptors and impaired phagocytosis of polymorphonuclear leucocytes in gingival crevicular fluid. *Journal of Periodontal Research* **32**, 439–446

Nossal, G.V.A. (1993) Life, death and the immune system. *Scientific American* (Sept.) pp. 21–30

Papapanou, P.N. (1994) Epidemiology and natural history of periodontal disease. In *Proceedings of the 1st European Workshop on Periodontology* (N.P. Lang and T. Karring, eds), pp. 23–41. London: Quintessence Publishing Co. Ltd

Paul, W. (1993) Infectious disease and the immune system. *Scientific American* (Sept.) pp. 57–63

Rook, R. (1993) Cell-mediated immune reactions. In *Immunology*, 3rd Edn (I. Roitt, J. Brostoff and D. Male, eds), pp. 2.1–2.20. St. Louis: Mosby

Sugita, N., Suzuki, T., Yoshi, H. *et al.* (1993) Differential expression of CR3, Fc$_\varepsilon$RII and Fc$_\gamma$RIII on polymorphonuclear leukocytes. *Journal of Periodontal Research* **28**, 363–372

Weissman, I.L. and Cooper, M.D. (1993) How the immune system develops. *Scientific American* (Sept.) pp. 33–39

4

The aetiology of periodontal disease

Primary factors

The primary cause of periodontal disease is bacterial irritation. However, small amounts of plaque are compatible with gingival and periodontal health (Lang *et al.*, 1973), and some patients can resist larger amounts of plaque for long periods without developing destructive periodontitis although they exhibit gingivitis.

A number of other factors, local and systemic, predispose towards plaque accumulation or alter the gingival response to plaque. These may be regarded as secondary aetiological factors.

The plaque theory

A relationship between oral hygiene and gingival disease is described in ancient writings. Today, a great deal of evidence has been amassed to support this idea.

The evidence stems from clinical observation, epidemiological studies, clinical and microbiological research and, most recently, immunological investigations. This evidence can be summarized as follows:

1. The number of bacteria in the inflamed gingival crevice or periodontal pocket is greater than in a healthy crevice.
2. In the presence of gingival inflammation or periodontal pocketing, the number of organisms in the mouth increases.
3. Injection of human oral bacteria into guinea pigs produces abscess formation, i.e. these bacteria can be pathogenic.
4. Epidemiological studies of many population groups in different parts of the world demonstrate a direct correlation between the amount of bacterial deposit as measured by oral hygiene indices (see Chapter 9) and the severity of gingival inflammation.
5. Epidemiological data show a direct correlation between oral hygiene status and the degree of perio-

dontal destruction as indicated by radiographic evidence of alveolar bone loss.

6. The experimental production of gingival inflammation by the withdrawal of all forms of oral hygiene. Löe *et al.* (1965) showed that, when 12 students stopped cleaning their teeth, thus allowing plaque to accumulate around the gingival margin, gingival inflammation always appeared. When tooth cleaning was resumed and the plaque removed, the inflammation disappeared (*Figure 4.1*).
7. The above experiment repeated in Beagle dogs produced the same result. Indeed, feeding experimental animals on a soft, sticky diet is sufficient to produce periodontal disease.
8. Epidemiological studies demonstrated that oral hygiene control reduced the incidence of gingivitis.
9. Gingival inflammation produced by the withdrawal of oral hygiene measures can be prevented by the use of non-specific antiseptic mouthwashes, e.g. chlorhexidine gluconate, in both humans and experimental animals (see Chapter 15).

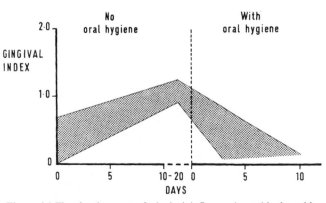

Figure 4.1 The development of gingival inflammation with the withdrawal of oral hygiene measures, followed by resolution of inflammation as plaque control is resumed. (Courtesy Dr H Löe)

10. Topical or systemic antibiotics will reduce gingival inflammation (see Chapter 15).
11. Mechanical irritants, such as rough or overhanging filling margins, do not produce persistent gingival inflammation unless the fillings are covered by bacterial plaque.
12. In germ-free animals, mechanical abuse of the gingivae by placing silk ligatures between the teeth does not appear to produce gingival inflammation or alveolar bone loss. When bacteria are introduced, both gingival inflammation and bone loss result.
13. Cultures of bacteria from human periodontal pockets can produce enzymes that can degrade gingival and periodontal connective tissue (see Chapter 5).
14. In periodontal disease, there is a raised antibody titre to plaque bacteria. These antibodies can be detected in blood and crevicular fluid.
15. Lymphocytes and immunoglobulin-producing plasma cells are present in gingival connective tissue and gingival fluid, and increase in amount where there is evidence of gingival inflammation.
16. *In vitro* lymphocytes are activated by plaque deposits, and there is a direct correlation between the severity of periodontal disease and lymphocyte transformation.
17. When healthy young adults abstained from oral hygiene measures for 28 days, the resultant accumulation of bacterial plaque and associated gingival inflammation were correlated with an increase in lymphocyte transformation and release of migration inhibition factor. These cellular responses returned to base-line values 28 days after plaque was removed (Lehner *et al.*, 1974).

Although each piece of evidence taken by itself might be questioned, the aggregate provides powerful support for the plaque theory. A further conclusion from the evidence is that it takes a certain minimum amount of time for plaque products to produce inflammation. Lang *et al.* (1973) showed that if teeth are cleaned at intervals of 48 hours, no gingivitis results; however, if cleaning is delayed for 72 hours, gingival inflammation is produced.

Specific and non-specific bacterial theories of the aetiology of periodontal disease

Recently it has become popular to speak of different periodontal diseases with possible different causes. However, only three inflammatory periodontal diseases – adult chronic periodontitis (Chapter 8), juvenile periodontitis (Chapter 20) and acute ulcerative gingivitis (Chapter 21) – can be recognized as distinctive. Chronic periodontal disease includes conditions ranging from gingivitis to advanced periodontitis, with varying rates of progression and a diversity of clinical forms. The condition may or may not progress, and when it does it may go through periods of progression, inactivity and regression (Goodson *et al.*, 1982). The controversy between the specific and non-specific theories of the microbial aetiology of inflammatory periodontal disease has continued for nearly 100 years, and is discussed below.

Specific theory

According to the pure specific theory, a single specific pathogen is the cause of inflammatory periodontal disease – as in the case of the well-known exogenous bacterial infections of man, such as pneumococcal pneumonia, typhoid, tuberculosis and syphilis. If this were the case, treatment would be directed towards the elimination of the specific pathogen from the mouth with the appropriate narrow-spectrum antibiotic. Following this, plaque control would no longer be necessary, since plaque without the specific pathogen would be non-pathogenic (Theilade, 1986). However, no one single pathogen has been found and many suspected periodontal pathogens have been suggested, including *Actinomycetes*, spirochaetes and a number of Gram negative anaerobic rods (Socransky *et al.*, 1982). Much recent work has centred around three bacterial species – *Porphyromonas gingivalis, Prevotella intermedia* and *Actinobacillus actinomycetemcomitans* – (Slots, 1986) and spirochaetes (Listgarten and Levin, 1981; Loesche, 1988). However, none of these bacteria are foreign invaders, since they are all members of the normal oral flora. Although they often make up a larger proportion of the subgingival flora in diseased sites with recent evidence of progression, they are also present in smaller numbers in non-progressive pockets and in the absence of disease (Chapter 2). Several of these organisms fulfil some of the criteria set up by Socransky (1979) to indicate pathogenicity, including quantitative association with disease, altered immune response, animal pathogenicity and the possession of virulence factors. However, none have yet been shown to fulfil Socransky's other criteria, that disease should be cured by eliminating the suspected species without otherwise changing plaque. Such specific treatment is not effective, and even the strongest supporters of the specific theory (Goodson *et al.*, 1979) advocate non-specific plaque control with subgingival scaling supplemented by the most broad-spectrum antibiotic, tetracycline (Chapter 15). It should also be noted that over 50% of the subgingival flora cannot be cultivated, and modern genetic methods of detecting bacteria have yielded different compositions from cultural techniques (Chapter 2). Thus the bacteria detected from any given site at any given time depend on the methods used for collection and detection.

Studies of the bacteria associated with active stages of chronic periodontitis are hampered by the fact that the disease is a dynamic condition, and may have short periods of active disease progression and long periods of inactivity (Goodson *et al.*, 1982). The chances of taking a bacterial sample from the right place at the right time, coinciding with active disease, are therefore very small, and probably have never been achieved.

Non-specific theory

According to pure non-specific theory, the indigenous oral bacteria colonize the gingival crevice to form plaque in the absence of effective oral hygiene (Theilade, 1986). Inflammatory periodontal disease develops when bacterial proliferation exceeds the threshold of host resistance, and is caused by the effects of the total plaque flora. All plaque bacteria are thought to have some virulence factors, causing gingival inflammation and periodontal destruction. It is implied that plaque will cause disease regardless of its composition. Total plaque control is therefore considered necessary in the prevention and treatment of inflammatory periodontal diseases. This traditional measure, combined where necessary with subgingival scaling and root planing, has proved effective. However, the pure non-specific theory does not consider that variations in the composition of the subgingival flora may have implications for its pathogenic potential. Moreover, it does not explain why some patients or tooth sites have lifelong contained gingivitis, whereas others experience slowly or rapidly progressive periodontitis. This may, however, be due to differences in the general or local host resistance rather than changes in the bacterial flora.

It seems likely, therefore, that a modern theory of the microbial aetiology of periodontal diseases should be a compromise between the extreme versions of the specific and non-specific theories.

Unified theory of the bacterial aetiology of chronic periodontitis

The modern version of the specific theory (Socransky, 1979) has abandoned the idea of a single periodontal pathogen, and states that periodontal disease can be initiated by any of a number of different pathogens. It states that 6–12 bacterial species may be responsible for the majority of cases of destructive periodontitis, and additional species may be responsible for a small number of other cases. On the other hand, the supporters of the non-specific theory agree that some indigenous bacteria are more commonly associated with disease than others and possess important virulence factors. The modern versions of two theories therefore appear to have much in common, and a unified theory is possible (Theilade, 1986).

All bacterial plaque may contribute to the pathogenic potential of the subgingival flora to a greater or lesser degree by its ability to colonize and evade host defences and provoke inflammation and tissue damage. Any composition of plaque in sufficient quantity in the gingival crevice causes gingivitis, but only in some cases does it lead to destructive periodontitis.

Different combinations of bacteria may be present in individual lesions, and together produce the necessary virulence factors. As over 300 species of bacteria make up the oral flora, it is not surprising that different indigenous bacteria predominate in different stages of disease and in different persons and different sites within the same mouth. The increased virulence of the subgingival flora seems to be due to the emergence of a plaque ecology unfavourable to the host but favourable to the growth of bacteria with pathogenic potential (Theilade, 1986).

Over the last 25 years, a selected number of bacteria from the subgingival flora have been shown to relate positively to periodontal disease progression (Socransky, 1970; Van Palenstein Heldermann, 1981; Genco *et al.*, 1988; Loesche, 1988; Socransky and Haffajee, 1990; Zambon, 1990). These studies showed positive correlations between their presence and numbers and signs of disease such as inflammation, increased probing depth and loss of attachment. There is also accumulated evidence that the microflora of the periodontal pocket at possible active sites, i.e. those that have shown significant attachment and bone loss within short time intervals, is characterized by the presence of *Porphyromonas gingivalis*, *Prevotella intermedia*, *Bacteroides forsythus*, *Peptostreptococcus micros*, *Campylobacter recta*, *Fusobacterium nucleatum* and *Actinobacillus actinomycetemcomitans* (Tanner *et al.*, 1984; Dzink *et al.*, 1985, 1988; Slots *et al.*, 1986, 1996; Moore *et al.*, 1991). Furthermore, other retrospective studies (Slots *et al.*, 1986; Bragd et al., 1987; Wennström *et al.*, 1987; Slots and Listgarten, 1988) have suggested that microbiological assays for critical levels of the target bacteria *A. actinomycetemcomitans*, *P. gingivalis* and *P. intermedia* at subgingival sites might be of diagnostic value. However, it should be noted that in these studies the samples were taken after breakdown had occurred and, although they showed an association between the number of these bacteria and previous attachment loss at the site, they were not shown to be predictive of future attachment loss.

Other retrospective studies using the BANA test have shown that higher numbers of *Treponema denticola*, *Porphyromonas gingivalis* and *Bacteroides forsythus* correlate with apparent periodontal progression (Schmidt *et al.*, 1988). However, the retrospective nature of the correlation in these studies cannot be related to prospective disease activity.

In a prospective study of a population on maintenance following treatment for periodontitis, the percentage of spirochaetes and motile rods at baseline were shown to be predictive of future disease progression occurring during the 1-year study (Listgarten and Levin, 1981). In a further 3-year prospective study (Listgarten *et al.*, 1986), similar findings were found for patients receiving irregular widely spaced maintenance visits, but not for a control group receiving regular 3-monthly maintenance. Similar lack of reliability was found in attempting to predict future episodes of periodontal breakdown using *Porphyromonas gingivalis*, *Prevotella intermedia* and *Actinobacillus actinomycetemcomitans* as indicators in a 3-year prospective study of patients on regular maintenance following treatment of periodontitis (Listgarten *et al.*, 1991).

Similar findings have been reported in different parts of the world, and a recent retrospective study of 148 Chinese adult patients aged 30–59 years with chronic periodontitis found an increase in certain species, notably *P. gingivalis*, *T. denticola*, *B. forsythus and C. recta*, at sites with progressive periodontitis (Papapanou *et al.*, 1997). This type of study, however, does not show that any of these bacteria are predictive of periodontal progression.

It should also be realized that the correlations in all these studies do not distinguish between bacteria that may be pathogenic and non-pathogens that have proliferated because of disease-associated tissue change such as deepened pockets, increased serum factors from exudate and blood or bacterial shifts, which may have promoted their growth (Listgarten, 1992). Unfortunately it is not possible to determine in any particular patient which of the many bacteria colonizing their pockets are pathogenic or contributing to disease at any one point in time. Furthermore, the pathogenicity of bacterial species may differ at different stages of periodontal disease, and a sequence of different bacteria may succeed one another as the conditions for their optimum growth alter.

Having outlined the theories of bacterial involvement, it needs to be emphasized that disease is produced by the interaction of oral bacteria with the tissue defences, i.e. host factors (Chapter 6).

Secondary factors

Secondary factors may be local or systemic. A number of local factors, in the gingival environment, predispose towards the accumulation of plaque deposits and prevent their removal. These are called plaque-retention factors. The systemic or host factors modify the response of the gingivae to local irritation.

Local factors

These include:

1. Faulty restorations
2. Carious cavities
3. Food impaction
4. Badly designed partial dentures
5. Orthodontic appliances
6. Malalignment of teeth
7. Lack of lip-seal, or mouth breathing
8. Developmental grooves on cervical enamel or root surface
9. Tobacco smoking – this may have both local and systemic effects.

Faulty restorations

Faulty restorations are probably the most common factor favouring plaque retention. Overhanging filling margins are extremely frequent, and result from careless use of matrix bands and the failure to polish margins (*Figure*

4.2). At one time it was assumed that rough filling margins in proximity to the gingival margin actually irritated the tissue, but there is no evidence for this. If there is no plaque accumulation on the restoration margin, inflammation does not occur.

Badly contoured restorations, particularly overcontoured and bulbous crowns and fillings, may impede effective toothbrushing.

Carious cavities

Carious cavities, particularly those close to the gingival margin, encourage plaque stagnation.

Food impaction

Food impaction is the forceful wedging of food against the gingiva between teeth. Where teeth have drifted apart food wedging can take place, especially in the presence of

(a)

(b)

Figure 4.2 *(a)* Overhanging restoration margins. *(b)* Gingival inflammation in relation to edge of crown on 1|

an opposing 'plunger cusp'. It is questionable whether actual physical trauma occurs, but food impaction sites are usually sites of plaque stagnation.

Badly designed partial dentures

Dentures are foreign bodies, which can cause tissue irritation in a number of ways. Ill-fitting or inadequately polished dentures will tend to act as foci for plaque collection. Tissue-borne dentures frequently sink into the mucosa and compress the gingival margins, causing inflammation and tissue destruction. These effects are compounded when the dentures are inadequately cleaned and worn during sleep. A further consequence of the badly designed partial denture is excessive occlusal stress on abutment teeth, and this, together with plaque-induced gingival inflammation, is an extremely common cause of tooth loss.

Orthodontic appliances

Orthodontic appliances are worn both at night and by day, and unless the patient is instructed in cleaning the appliance, plaque accumulation is inevitable. As most orthodontic patients are young, a severe inflammation with gingival swelling can occur.

Tooth malalignment

Tooth malalignment predisposes to plaque retention and makes plaque removal difficult (*Figure 4.3*). Unless the patient's oral hygiene technique is very thorough, tooth malalignment is frequently accompanied by gingival inflammation and may provide a case for orthodontic treatment. However, it is important to be certain that orthodontic movement is justified. If a patient's oral hygiene is poor, it may be just as bad if the teeth are straight. On the other hand, if a patient's oral hygiene

overcomes the difficulties caused by malalignment, no orthodontic treatment is required, at least on periodontal grounds. Orthodontic treatment is indicated where the patient's home care is effective in all areas except where there is malalignment. It is then likely that creating a good alignment will also be followed by gingival health.

Other discrepancies in tooth and jaw relationship may also produce gingival inflammation. In a very deep overbite, upper incisors may impinge on lower labial gingiva or lower incisors on upper palatal gingiva, causing inflammation and tissue destruction in the presence of plaque.

Failure to replace a missing tooth may result in plaque and calculus accumulations on the non-functional opposing teeth.

Lack of lip-seal

There is some uncertainty about the influence of lip posture on gingival health, but a commonly occurring clinical phenomenon is a hyperplastic gingivitis in anterior segments, usually the upper incisor regions, where there is lack of lip-seal. Indeed, in many cases the area of hyperplasia is clearly delineated by the lip line (*Figure 4.4*). Although lack of lip-seal is frequently associated with mouth breathing, inadequate lip-seal may be present even when the patient breathes through the nose. With the lips apart, the gingivae in the front of the mouth are not bathed in saliva. This seems to have two effects: (i) the normal cleansing action of saliva is diminished so that plaque accumulation is encouraged; (ii) dehydration of the tissues may impair their resistance.

Developmental grooves

Grooves on the root surface or the cervical crown lead to plaque accumulation and are impossible to clean. This may result in local areas of gingivitis and pocketing, most

Figure 4.3 Gingival inflammation and pocketing in relation to maligned lower incisors

Figure 4.4 Hyperplastic gingivitis in relation to plaque deposits and lack of lip-seal

commonly seen palatal to the upper incisors. The canine fossa on the mesial surface of the upper first premolar may also act in this way.

Tobacco smoking

The most obvious effect of tobacco smoking is tooth staining, but a large number of studies have shown that tobacco smoking has an influence on the prevalence and severity of periodontal diseases, including gingivitis, periodontitis and acute ulcerative gingivitis. The effect of smoking on plaque and calculus deposition, gingival inflammation and bleeding, pocket depth and bone loss, as well as the bacteriology of plaque and features of the tissue response, have been investigated. Pindborg (1947) found that smokers had more calculus than non-smokers, and this was confirmed by many other studies such as those by Ainamo (1971) and Sheiham (1971), who also found that plaque deposits were greater in smokers. These early studies showed that the standard of oral hygiene in smokers was significantly poorer than in non-smokers, and Macgregor (1984, 1985) found that smokers spend less time brushing their teeth than non-smokers.

Young smokers appear to have the same degree of, or slightly more, gingival inflammation than non-smokers, but in older age groups signs of inflammation are less in smokers. Bergström and Floderus-Myrhed (1983) and other workers have found less gingival bleeding in smokers than non-smokers, a finding that Palmer (1987) suggests could be due to vasoconstriction of gingival vessels, but may also be attributable to the heavier keratinization of the gingivae in smokers. The gingivae of smokers contain an increased number of keratinized cells (Calonius, 1962). Pocket depth is greater in smokers (Feldman *et al.*, 1983; Stoltenberg *et al.*, 1993), as is alveolar bone loss (Arno *et al.*, 1959; Bergström *et al.*, 1991). A study of 70-year-old Swedes demonstrated that toothlessness was higher in smokers and former smokers than in non-smokers (Österberg and Mellström, 1986). Furthermore, refractory periodontitis (i.e. where there has been persistent failure of periodontal treatment) is found more commonly in smokers than in non-smokers (MacFarlane *et al.*, 1992).

The relationship between smoking and poor oral hygiene and its consequences is well established, but where smokers and non-smokers with comparable levels of oral hygiene are studied it is found that smoking *per se* has a marginal but significant harmful effect on the periodontal tissues. Ismail *et al.* (1983) looked at data from epidemiological studies of 3000 individuals in the USA, adjusting the data for age, sex, race, socio-economic status, oral hygiene and frequency of toothbrushing, and found that smokers had a higher Periodontal Index score in all age groups. They suggest that, although the strongest correlation is with poor oral hygiene, smoking has a weaker but independent direct relation to periodontal disease. Bergström *et al.* (1991) examined alveolar bone loss in 210 subjects aged 24–60 years – smokers, former smokers and non-smokers – and found a correlation between bone loss and smoking that was not plaque related.

Several investigations have been made into the nature of this direct effect, possible changes in plaque and pocket flora, and various components of the tissue reaction. Bacteriological studies (Bastiaan and Waite, 1978; Bardell, 1981) have produced rather unclear results about differences in the make-up of plaque flora or in the rate of plaque formation in smokers and non-smokers. However, several changes in the tissue response have been noted.

Smoking appears to produce vasoconstriction of the gingival vasculature and, as Palmer (1987) points out, a 'reduction in the vascular component of the inflammatory response may reduce the availability of serum-derived protective factors such as antibodies and a decrease in the passage of leucocytes into the periodontal tissues'. McLaughlin *et al.* (1993) found that smoking produces a marked but transient initial increase in gingival fluid flow rate, which they felt might reflect changes in the blood flow known to be produced by nicotine. Armitage and Turner (1970) showed that nicotine from cigarettes and cigars could pass through the oral mucosa and also, in a study of the toxicity of nicotine from cigarettes, they showed a 50% or more inhibition of function of oral neutrophils (Armitage *et al.* 1975). In an earlier study, Eichel and Shahrick (1969) reported that tobacco smoke produced 50–100% inhibition of oral leucocytes due to loss of motility, which they ascribed to such substances as acrolein and cyanide in tobacco smoke.

Oral keratinocytes are the first cells to come into contact with tobacco products from smoking. A recent study by Johnson and Organ (1997) investigated the effects of nicotine on human gingival keratinocytes (obtained from healthy gingival tissue) in culture in respect of their release of inflammatory mediators. They found that exposure to nicotine did not alter the production of prostaglandin E_2; it did, however, produce an increase in the level of interleukin (IL)-1α both in the supernatant and lysed cells. This may have significance, since IL-1α is known to play a central role in the regulation of inflammation.

In the study of refractory periodontitis by MacFarlane *et al.* (1992), abnormal PMN phagocytosis was found. Both the motility and chemotactic ability of PMNs can be impaired by even small amounts of tobacco smoke (Bridges *et al.*, 1977). Peacock *et al.* (1993) have shown that, in tissue cultures of human gingival fibroblasts, continuous nicotine exposure enhances attachment of the fibroblasts, and at low concentrations of nicotine cell replication is stimulated.

The role of smoking in the aetiology of acute necrotizing ulcerative gingivitis (ANUG) has been much discussed. When this form of periodontal disease was very common, many studies found a relationship between the prevalence and severity of ANUG (or AUG, Vincent's disease, trench mouth, etc.; see Chapter 22) and smoking. Stammers (1944) examined 1017 cases of ANUG and found that almost all of them were smokers and, in looking at 3880 naval recruits aged 17–21 years, Ludwick and Massler (1952) found 20 cases of ANUG, 19 of them smokers, a finding more recently confirmed in an Edinburgh study in which Kowolik and Nisbet (1983) found that 98 out of 100 individuals with ANUG were smokers. No mechanism has so far been defined to explain this relationship, but there is little doubt that smoking has multiple deleterious effects on the tissues, vascularity and the immune system. In a study of the effects of cigarette smoking on healing following periodontal surgery, Preber and Bergström (1990) suggested that smoking may impair the outcome of surgical treatment.

A large amount of research indicates that tobacco use is directly related to the prevalence and incidence of a whole variety of medical problems including lung and possibly other cancers, pulmonary, cardiovascular and gastrointestinal disease, and low birth weight (Bartecchi *et al.*, 1994). Over the last 50 years, evidence has accumulated that smoking is also related to the prevalence and severity of periodontal diseases (Haber *et al.*, 1993; Ryder, 1996) and subsequent tooth loss (Mohlin *et al.*, 1979; Alvesalo *et al.*, 1982; Österberg and Mellström, 1986; Ryder, 1986; Ahlquist *et al.*, 1989; Ragnarsson *et al.*, 1992; Holm, 1994). Furthermore, recent studies have shown that smoking may be one of the most significant risk factors in the development and progression of periodontal disease (Beck *et al.*, 1990; Horning *et al.*, 1992; Locker and Leake, 1993; Grossi *et al.*, 1994, 1995).

In Europe and the USA more than a quarter of the adult population smoke, and in many other countries the proportions are even higher (Council on Scientific Affairs, 1990; Centers for Disease Control and Prevention, 1993; Bartecchi *et al.*, 1994; MacKenzie *et al.*, 1994). Thus, the association between cigarette smoking and periodontal disease represents a significant problem. Although the percentage of male adults who smoke appears to be gradually declining in developed countries, the percentage of females is increasing (Bartecchi *et al.*, 1994; MacKenzie *et al.*, 1994). Furthermore, the use of tobacco products by young people appears to be increasing again (Centers for Disease Control, 1989).

The relationship between tobacco products and periodontal diseases can be considered in six areas:

1. The effect on the prevalence and severity of periodontal diseases
2. The possible association with refractory periodontitis
3. The role of smokeless tobacco products on the periodontal tissues
4. The possible mechanisms of its effects on the periodontal tissues
5. The effects on the response to periodontal treatment
6. Smoking cessation in periodontal disease prevention.

Those sections dealing with its response to treatment will also be covered in Chapters 14, 16, 17 and 18.

The effect on the prevalence and severity of periodontal diseases

Acute necrotizing ulcerative gingivitis (ANUG) (see also Chapter 22)

A clear association between smoking and ANUG was demonstrated over 50 years ago (Stammers, 1944; Pindborg, 1947, 1949). Stammers (1944) examined 1017 cases of ANUG, and found that nearly all of them were smokers. More recently, in a study in Edinburgh, Kowolik and Nisbet (1983) found that 98 out of 100 individuals with ANUG were smokers. This evidence has been reviewed by Macgregor (1992). More recently, a similar association has been found between smoking and the ANUG-like lesions of HIV infected individuals (Swango *et al.*, 1991).

Chronic gingivitis and periodontitis

Earlier cross-sectional studies of the relationship between smoking and the severity of periodontal disease were contradictory and inconclusive (Ludwick and Massler, 1952; Arno *et al.*, 1958; Schei *et al.*, 1959; Solomon *et al.*, 1968; Sheiham, 1971; Preber and Kant, 1973; Preber *et al.*, 1980; Bergström, 1981; Bergström and Floderus-Myrhed, 1983; Macgregor *et al.*, 1985; Preber and Bergström, 1986a). Some investigators reported less gingival inflammation and, particularly, less gingival bleeding in smokers compared to non-smokers (Ludwick and Massler, 1952; Bergström and Floderus-Myrhed, 1983; Preber and Bergström, 1985; Bergström, 1990) whilst other studies (Arno *et al.*, 1958; Preber and Kant, 1973; Preber *et al.*, 1980) showed more gingival inflammation in smokers. There were also reports of an increase (Sheiham, 1971; Preber and Kant, 1973; Preber *et al.*, 1980; Bergström, 1981; Bergström and Floderus-Myrhed, 1983) or no difference (Macgregor *et al.*, 1985; Preber and Bergström, 1986a; Bergström, 1990) in the amounts of plaque in smokers compared to non-smokers. Gingival crevicular fluid (GCF) flow was reported to increase immediately following smoking (McLaughlin *et al.*, 1993). However, it was found to be diminished in chronic smokers (Bergström and Preber, 1986).

A clear correlation between probing depths and alveolar bone loss was reported by most earlier researchers (Arno *et al.*, 1959; Shei *et al.*, 1959; Solomon *et al.*, 1968; Summers and Oberman, 1968; Ismail *et al.*, 1983; Bergström and Floderus-Myrhed, 1983), but some others (Sheiham, 1971; Preber and Kant, 1973) reported no clear relationship. Some workers (Shei *et al.*, 1959; Sheiham, 1971; Preber *et al.*, 1980; Ismail *et al.*, 1983) have suggested that the differences in attachment loss between smokers and non-smokers may be due to poor oral hygiene in smokers.

However, over the last 10–12 years cross-sectional studies on much larger groups of subjects have demonstrated a much clearer relationship between smoking and periodontal disease (Ryder, 1996). In a number of these studies, the plaque accumulation levels were either balanced between the groups of smokers and non-smokers (Bergström and Elíasson, 1987a, 1987b; Bergström,

1989; Linden and Mullally, 1994) or plaque levels were minimal in both groups (Grossi *et al.*, 1994, 1995). In both of these situations the smoking group was found to have deeper periodontal pockets and greater probing attachment loss (Bergström and Elíasson, 1987a; Bergström, 1989; Linden and Mullally, 1994; Grossi *et al.*, 1994; Martinez-Canut *et al.*, 1995) and/or alveolar bone loss (Bergström and Elíasson, 1987a; Grossi *et al.*, 1995) than the non-smoking group. Similar findings have also been reported from other large cross-sectional studies (Feldman *et al.*, 1983; Anerud *et al.*, 1991) and several longitudinal studies (Bolin *et al.*, 1986; Grossi *et al.*, 1994, 1995; Bergström and Preber, 1994). The number of cigarettes smoked per day and the number of years an individual has smoked impacts on the severity of periodontitis suffered (Martinez-Canut *et al.*, 1995). The term 'pack years' is currently used to quantify this effect.

From all these more recent studies a general pattern has emerged, with smokers suffering the following effects more than non-smokers:

- Greater alveolar bone loss
- Increased numbers of deep pockets
- Increased calculus formation
- Less clinically apparent gingival inflammation
- Less gingival bleeding.

This pattern of effects from smoking was also shown in recent studies in which general disease categories were assigned and the risk of developing the disease was calculated using odds ratios (Ismail *et al.*, 1983; Haber and Kent, 1992; Jette *et al.*, 1993; Grossi *et al.*, 1994, 1995). In one of these studies (Haber and Kent, 1992), current and former smokers were found to be more prevalent in a population of patients with moderate to advanced periodontitis from American periodontal practices when compared to the referring general practice or the general population.

A relationship has also been found between the prevalence of moderate to advanced periodontitis and the number of cigarettes smoked per day (Brandzaeg and Jamison, 1964; Ismail *et al.*, 1983; Haber and Kent, 1992; Haber *et al.*, 1993; Grossi *et al.*, 1994, 1995) and the number of years that the patients had smoked (Haber and Kent, 1992; Jette *et al.*, 1993; Grossi *et al.*, 1994, 1995).

The possible association with refractory periodontitis

Tobacco smoking may play a significant role in the development of refractory periodontitis (Adams, 1992; MacFarlane *et al.*, 1992), and this is shown by the fact that an unusually high percentage of refractory periodontitis patients have been found to be smokers (MacFarlane *et al.*, 1992).

The role of smokeless tobacco products on the periodontal tissues

The use of tobacco products such as snuff and chewing tobacco are popular in many countries in Asia, and may often be combined with other products such as betel nut. The relationship between these products and oral leukoplakia and carcinoma is well known and documented (Ernster *et al.*, 1990; Creath *et al.*, 1991; Wray and McGuirt, 1993), and these lesions are commonly found in areas of the mouth where the tobacco product is placed. Their use has also been related to cardiovascular mortality (Bolinger *et al.*, 1994).

Although individual cases of ANUG, chronic periodontitis and gingival recession have been reported in smokeless tobacco users (Christen *et al.*, 1979; Hoge and Kirkham, 1983; Offenbacher and Weathers, 1985), a clear relationship to chronic periodontitis has not been demonstrated. In one study of large numbers of smokeless tobacco users (Robertson *et al.*, 1990) there was a significant increase in localized gingival recession and attachment loss, and this was found in buccal areas, adjacent to where the product was placed.

Some investigators have proposed that local exposure to high concentrations of tobacco products may play a role in local attachment loss and this could be due to their effects on local defence mechanisms (Robertson *et al.*, 1990; Ernster *et al.*, 1990; Payne *et al.*, 1994). In addition, the high concentrations of nicotine from these products could alter the local gingival blood flow (Johnson *et al.*, 1991). Finally, it has been shown that smokeless tobacco extracts affect the secretion of monocyte inflammatory mediators (Payne *et al.*, 1994).

The possible mechanisms of its effects on the periodontal tissues

Microbiology

One possible hypothesis for these effects is that smoking acts on plaque growth and maturation, leading either to more plaque or to the presence of different or more virulent bacteria. In this regard, the earlier studies (Pindborg, 1947, 1949; Ainamo, 1971; Sheiham, 1971) found that plaque deposits were greater in smokers than non-smokers and that their standard of oral hygiene was significantly poorer. In addition, Macgregor (1984, 1985) found that smokers spend less time brushing their teeth than non-smokers. However, later studies (Bastiaan and Waite, 1978; Feldman *et al.*, 1983; Bergström and Elíasson, 1987a; Bergström, 1989; Bergström *et al.*, 1991) have shown little difference in the levels of plaque accumulation in smokers compared to non-smokers. This may reflect better standards of oral hygiene in the population as a whole in more recent times. Furthermore, in respect of the possible role of smoking alone, cross-sectional studies where plaque levels were controlled to a minimum in both the smoking and non-smoking groups studied showed that alveolar bone loss was greater in the smoking group (Bergström and Elíasson, 1987a; Bergström, 1989; Bergström *et al.*, 1991). Similar results were found in the retrospective study of Ismail *et al.* (1983) described earlier. They looked at data from epidemiological studies of 3000 individuals in the USA, adjusting the data for age, sex and socio-economic status and oral hygiene and frequency of toothbrushing. They found that smokers had a higher Periodontal Index score in all age groups, and found evidence for a direct correlation between smoking and this score. Thus, the amount of plaque present does not seem to be responsible for the differences.

On the other hand, several studies have shown that greater quantities of supra- and subgingival calculus does appear to form in smokers compared to non-smokers (Pindborg, 1947, 1949; Ainamo, 1971; Feldman *et al.*, 1987; Linden and Mullally, 1994). Subgingival calculus might act as a tissue irritant as a result of substances absorbed into its surface, or might create a local environment that promotes the growth of pathogenic bacteria. In this regard, it has been shown that the periodontal pockets of smokers are more anaerobic than those of non-smokers (Kenny *et al.*, 1975). This profound anaerobic environment could promote the growth of periodontopathic Gram negative anaerobic species. However, neither earlier (Kenny *et al.*, 1975; Bardell, 1981) nor later studies (Preber *et al.*, 1992; Stoltenberg *et al.*, 1993) have supported this view. Cultural and microscopic studies (Kenny *et al.*, 1975) showed no differences in the bacterial composition of subgingival plaque between smokers and non-smokers. Furthermore, more recent studies (Preber *et al.*, 1992; Stoltenberg *et al.*, 1993) showed no significant differences in the recovery of *Porphyromonas gingivalis*, *Prevotella intermedia*, *Bacteroides forsythus* and *Actinobacillus actinomycetemcomitans* from deep pockets in the two groups. Therefore, to date there is no evidence to support the view that smoking adversely effects the periodontal tissues by altering the composition of plaque.

Effects on the local and general host response

A number of investigators have examined the role of smoking in altering the host response by:

1. Impairing the response of the host against infection (Seymour, 1991)
2. Changing the response so that it was more destructive to the tissues (Lamster, 1992).

In the first regard, smokers have been found to have decreased levels of salivary IgA antibodies (Bennet and Read, 1982) and serum IgG antibodies to *P. intermedia* and *Fusobacterium nucleatum* (Haber, 1994). In addition, smokers appear to have depressed numbers of T-helper lymphocytes, which are key components of the immune system (Ginns *et al.*, 1982; Costabel *et al.*, 1986). Fully functional phagocytes are also a key component of the defence system against infections, and it has been shown that smoking can have deleterious effects on various neutrophil functions (Eichel and Shahrik, 1969; Armitage *et al.*, 1975; Bridges *et al.*, 1977; Kenny *et al.*, 1977; Codd *et al.*, 1987; Nowak *et al.*, 1990; Kalra *et al.*, 1991; Lannan *et al.*, 1992; Selby *et al.*, 1992; Ryder, 1994; Totti *et al.*, 1994). In this regard, it has been shown that tobacco smoke can impair the motility and chemotaxis of oral (Eichel and Shahrik, 1969; Kenny *et al.*, 1977) and peripheral (Bridges *et al.*, 1977; Lannan *et al.*, 1992;

Selby *et al.*, 1992) neutrophil polymorphonuclear leucocytes (PMNs). Impaired phagocytosis has also been shown in PMNs from patients with refractory periodontitis (MacFarlane *et al.*, 1992). In addition, smoking has been shown to either stimulate (Kalra *et al.*, 1991) or impair the oxidative burst of PMNs. Similar effects have been observed with higher concentrations of individual tobacco components such as nicotine, acrolein and cyanide (Eichel and Shahrik, 1969).

It has also been shown that the GCF levels of the pro-inflammatory cytokine TNFα were significantly higher in both untreated and treated smoking chronic periodontitis patients in comparison with corresponding non-smoking patients (Boström *et al.*, 1998a, 1998b). This suggests that smoking is associated with the local production of greater quantities of this cytokine, which could in turn lead to more severe destructive inflammation in the periodontal tissues.

The most researched tobacco component is undoubtedly nicotine. Armitage and Turner (1970) showed that nicotine from cigarettes and cigars could pass through the oral mucosa. At low concentrations nicotine appears to stimulate PMN chemotaxis (Totti *et al.*, 1994), but at higher concentrations it impairs motility, chemotaxis and phagocytosis of PMNs (Armitage *et al.*, 1975; Ryder, 1994). However, nicotine is only one of over 2000 potentially toxic substances in tobacco smoke (International Agency for Research on Cancer, 1986), and many of these could have harmful effects on the periodontal tissues.

It has been shown that low doses of nicotine can be stored in and released by periodontal fibroblasts (Hanes *et al.*, 1991) but it is not clear as to whether fibroblasts exposed to nicotine have impaired (Raulin *et al.*, 1989) or enhanced (Peacock *et al.*, 1993) function. In addition, nicotine has been shown to suppress the proliferation of cultured osteoblasts, but stimulate their production of alkaline phosphatase (Fang *et al.*, 1991). However, all these changes have been demonstrated *in vitro* and therefore their effects on the cells of the normal periodontium can only be surmised.

It has been known for some time that both tobacco smoke and tobacco components may reduce gingival blood flow and gingival bleeding (Bergström and Floderus-Myrhed, 1983). This could either be due to vasoconstriction of gingival vessels or to the heavier keratinization of the gingiva in smokers and, in this last regard, the gingiva of smokers has been shown to contain an increased number of keratinized cells (Calonius, 1962). It has also been suggested (Palmer, 1987) that a reduction in the vascular component of the inflammatory response may reduce the availability of serum-derived protective factors such as antibodies and could also impede the passage of leucocytes into the periodontal tissues.

Earlier studies of the effects of nicotine on gingival blood flow using a heat diffusion technique showed a decrease in flow (Clarke *et al.*, 1981). However, more recent studies in the effects of cigarette smoking on gingival blood flow using laser Doppler probes has yielded contradictory results (Baab and Oberg, 1987).

Inconclusive results have also been obtained in studies of possible thermal damage by cigarette smoke (Bastiaan, 1979).

A relationship between cigarette smoking and bone mineral content, particularly osteoporosis, has also been found (Daniell, 1983; Hollenbach *et al.*, 1993); however, the possible effects of this on the alveolar bone is unclear.

Thus, tobacco smoke may induce or exacerbate periodontal disease by direct local damage, altering the host response or altering the normal repair mechanisms of the periodontal tissues.

The effects on the response to periodontal treatment

It is known that smoking has a very significant adverse effect on the response to all forms of periodontal treatment (Preber and Bergström, 1986b, 1990; Miller, 1987; Goultshin *et al.*, 1990; Jones and Triplett, 1992; Ah *et al.*, 1994; Newman *et al.*, 1994), and this will be fully described in Chapters 14, 16, 22.

Smoking cessation in periodontal disease prevention

Informing patients about the dangers of smoking and encouraging them to stop smoking is an important function in preventing periodontal disease initiation and progression (Telivuo *et al.*, 1992; Bolin *et al.*, 1993), and this will be described in Chapter 10.

Host factors affecting susceptibility to periodontal disease

Genetic factors

Genetic susceptibility to chronic periodontitis may greatly increase its rate of progression, such that destructive disease occurs in the early adult years. Some of these cases may be termed rapidly progressive periodontitis (see Chapter 20). Conversely, patients genetically resistant to periodontitis show little or no signs of attachment loss throughout their lives (*Figure 4.5*), and may keep well-supported teeth into old age with little or no periodontal treatment. In this regard, epidemiological studies have shown that the amount of periodontal attachment loss is greater in some patients than others, even when differences of oral hygiene are taken into account (Löe *et al.*, 1978). In addition, other epidemiological studies from a number of different countries have indicated that approximately 10% of subjects experience severe periodontal destruction with rapid progression and tooth loss, whilst about 10% appear to be resistant to destructive periodontitis despite the continued presence of plaque and gingivitis (Löe *et al.*, 1978; Page and Schroeder, 1986; Papapanou *et al.*, 1989). The remaining 80% of subjects appear to be susceptible to slowly progressive periodontitis, which rarely results in tooth loss if they receive adequate periodontal treatment. Their rate of disease

Figure 4.5 An 85-year-old woman with minimal attachment loss. She has only attended a dentist on four occasions during her life and has lost one tooth, a lower first molar, due to caries when she was 30 years of age. She has relatively poor oral hygiene and has gingivitis and supragingival calculus deposits. However, the only attachment loss found was slight buccal gingival recession on a few teeth. All the probing depths were minimal, and there was no radiographic evidence of alveolar bone loss. Her younger sister, aged 81 years, had all her teeth and a similar periodontal condition.

progression depends much more on their individual oral hygiene status. Thus it is important to identify each patient's individual susceptibility to periodontitis, since this will determine the type and frequency of treatment that they will require.

Twin studies have shown that a significant variance in the susceptibility to chronic periodontitis may be attributable to genetic factors (Michalowicz *et al.*, 1991; Michalowicz, 1994), but attempts to identify specific genetic markers have proved difficult (Hart and Kornman, 1997).

One type of genetic marker tested recently has been those coding for proteins of the pro-inflammatory cytokines such as interleukin (IL)-1 and tumour necrosis factor alpha (TNFα), which are key regulators of host responses to microbial infection (Kornman *et al.*, 1997). IL-1 is also a major modulator of extracellular matrix degradation and bone resorption (see Chapter 5). It has been shown that the specific genotype of the polymorphic IL-1 gene cluster was associated with the severity of chronic periodontitis in a group of non-smokers, and statistically significantly distinguished individuals with severe periodontitis from those with mild disease. Functionally, the specific periodontitis-associated IL-1 genotype comprised a variant of the IL-1B gene that is associated with high levels of IL-1 production. The specific association found in this study was with the presence of allele 2 of the IL-1A with allele 2 of the IL-1B gene, and this composite genotype has been found to occur in 29.1% of Northern European subjects. No association was found either for single alleles of this gene or for alleles of the TNF genes (Kornman *et al.*, 1997).

In this study (Kornman *et al.*, 1997) the smokers were put into a separate group to the non-smokers because of the known association between tobacco smoking and the severity of periodontitis (see above). They found that in smokers severe periodontitis was not associated with the genotype. However, 86% of the severe periodontitis patients were accounted for by either smoking or the IL-1 genotype.

In addition, in this regard, another research group (Gore *et al.*, 1998) have determined the distribution of IL-1α and -β genotypes in patients with adult chronic periodontitis and their matched healthy controls. The subjects were 32 Caucasian adult periodontitis patients matched for sex and age with 32 control Caucasian subjects with no clinical signs of periodontal disease. They found that the frequency of IL-1β genotypes including allele 2 of the IL-$1\beta^{+3953}$ restriction length bi-allelic polymorphism was significantly increased in patients with advanced adult periodontitis compared to those with early and moderate disease. Furthermore, the presence of allele 2 of this type was associated with increased production of IL-1β by activated peripheral blood polymorphonuclear leucocytes from patients with advanced disease, although this increase did not reach statistical significance. The findings also showed a significant linkage disequilibrium between allele 2 of the IL-$1\beta^{+3953}$ polymorphism and allele 2 of the bi-allelic IL-$1\alpha^{-889}$ polymorphism in both periodontitis patients and healthy controls. These findings support further the possible role of IL-1α and -β gene polymorphisms in the susceptibility to adult chronic periodontitis.

It is likely that, in the future, other genes coding for alternative key factors that play a role in the pathogenesis of periodontal disease will be investigated for their possible association with the susceptibility to chronic periodontitis.

Psychological stress factors

Psychological stress can play a role in many conditions, and probably mediates its effects both biochemically and behaviourally; the first by affecting the immune system, and the second through altered compliance and health behaviour (Andersen *et al.*, 1994). It could affect the course of periodontal disease in both these ways.

It has already been shown that negative life events may play a role in acute or chronic oral symptoms (Marcenes *et al.*, 1993), and it has been suggested that such factors could also play a role in the patient's susceptibility to periodontal disease progression, although this has been questioned (Wilton *et al.*, 1988; Sculley *et al.*, 1991). It has, however, been suggested that the apparent lack of relationship could have been due to small sample size, unsuitable selection criteria and the recording of one rather than several life events (Marcenes and Sheiham, 1992). In this regard, a recent case control study has investigated the possible role of several life events on chronic periodontitis (Croucher *et al.*, 1997). One hundred dental patients, matched for age and sex, were used in the study, and they reported 43 life events on a positive–negative impact scale. These were then compared with the periodontal status, along with oral health beha-

viour, tobacco use and socio-demographics. The study showed that the severity of chronic periodontitis significantly correlated with the negative impact of life events, the number of negative life events, high level of dental plaque, tobacco smoking and being unemployed. Conversely, positive life events were associated with better periodontal health. The negative life event variables remained statistically significant after adjusting for oral health behaviour and socio-demographic variables, but not tobacco smoking.

It has been postulated by Locker (1989) that factors in the social environment that lead to stress, which then impacts on psychological process and behaviour, may lead to an increase in disease susceptibility. It is also possible that negative life events are important determinants of smoking, which is itself a major risk factor for periodontitis (see above). The study of Croucher *et al.* (1997) would suggest that psychological factors and oral health risk behaviours cluster together as important determinants of susceptibility to periodontitis.

The role of psychological stress producing a poor response to treatment of chronic periodontitis has also been investigated (Axtelius *et al.*, 1988). Two groups of patients, one responding well to periodontal treatment (respondent group) and one failing to respond (non-respondent group), were compared. Somatic and psychological data were obtained by interviews and psychological tests, and these variables were then statistically compared in the two groups. The results showed that the non-respondent group patients demonstrated a passive, dependent personality and indications of more psychological strain, whereas those in the respondent group displayed a more rigid personality and had experienced less stressful events in the past.

All other host factors are described in Chapter 6.

References

Adams, D.F. (1992) Diagnosis and treatment of refractory periodontitis. *Current Opinions in Dentistry* **2**, 33–38

Ah, M.K.B., Johnson, G.K., Kaldahl, W.B. *et al.* (1994) The effect of smoking on the response to periodontal therapy. *Journal of Clinical Periodontology* **21**, 91–97

Ahlquist, M., Bengtsson, C., Hollender, L. *et al.* (1989) Smoking habits and tooth loss in Swedish women. *Community Dentistry and Oral Epidemiology* **17**, 144–147

Ainamo, J. (1971) The seeming effect of tobacco consumption on the occurrence of periodontal disease and caries. *Suomen Hammaslaakariseeuran Toimituksia* **67**, 87–94

Alvesalo, I., Reisin, S, Hay, J. and Bailit, H. (1982) Effects of fluoride and regular dental care on personal dental expenditures of young adults in Finland. *Community Dentistry and Oral Epidemiology* **10**, 15–22

Andersen, B.L., Kiecolt-Glaser, J.K and Glaser, R. (1994) A biobehavioural model of cancer stress and disease course. *American Psychologist* **49**, 389–404

Anerud, A., Löe, H. and Boysen, H. (1991) The natural history and clinical course of calculus formation in man. *Journal of Clinical*

Periodontology **18**, 160–170

Armitage, A.K., Dollery, C.T., George, C.F. *et al.* (1975) Absorption and metabolism of nicotine from cigarettes. *British Medical Journal* **4**, 313–316

Armitage, A.K. and Turner, D.M. (1970) Absorption of nicotine in cigarette and cigar smoke through oral mucosa. *Nature* **226**, 1231–1232

Arno, A., Waerhaug, J., Lovdal, A. and Schei, O. (1958) Incidence of gingivitis as related to sex, occupation, tobacco consumption, tooth-brushing and age. *Oral Surgery, Oral Medicine, Oral Pathology* **11**, 587–595

Arno, A., Schei, O., Lovdal, A. and Waerhaug, J. (1959) Alveolar bone loss as a function of tobacco consumption. *Acta Odontologica Scandinavica* **17**, 3–10

Axtelius, B., Soderfeldt, B., Nilsson, A. *et al.* (1988) Therapy-resistant periodontitis. Psychological characteristics. *Journal of Clinical Periodontology* **25**, 482–491

Baab, D.A. and Oberg, P.A. (1987) The effect of cigarette smoking on the gingival blood flow in humans. *Journal of Clinical Periodontology* **14**, 418–424

Bardell, D. (1981) Viability of six species of normal oropharyngeal bacteria to cigarette smoke *in vitro*. *Microbios* **32**, 7–13

Bartecchi, C.E., MacKenzie, T.D. and Schrier, R.W. (1994) The human costs of tobacco use. *New England Journal of Medicine* **331**, 907–912

Bastiaan, R.J. (1979) The effects of tobacco smoking on the periodontal tissues. *Journal of the Western Society of Periodontology, Periodontal Abstracts* **27**, 120–125

Bastiaan, R.J. and Waite, I.M. (1978) Effects of tobacco smoking on plaque development and gingivitis. *Journal of Periodontology* **49**, 480–482

Beck, J.D., Koch, G.C., Rozier, R.G and Cohen, M.E. (1990) Prevalence and risk indicators for periodontal attachment loss in a population of older community-dwelling blacks and whites. *Journal of Periodontology* **61**, 521–528

Bennett, K.R. and Read, P.C. (1982) Salivary immunoglobulin A levels in normal subjects, tobacco smokers, and patients with minor aphthous ulceration. *Oral Surgery, Oral Medicine, Oral Pathology* **53**, 461–465

Bergström, J. (1981) Short-term investigation on the influence of cigarette smoking upon plaque accumulation. *Scandinavian Journal of Dental Research* **89**, 235–238

Bergström, J. (1989) Cigarette smoking as a risk factor in chronic periodontitis. *Community Dentistry and Oral Epidemiology* **17**, 245–247

Bergström, J. (1990) Oral hygiene compliance and gingivitis expression in cigarette smokers. *Scandinavian Journal of Dental Research* **98**, 497–503

Bergström, J. and Elíasson, S. (1987a) Noxious effect of cigarette smoking and periodontal health. *Journal of Periodontal Research* **22**, 513–517

Bergström, J. and Elíasson, S. (1987b) Cigarette smoking and alveolar bone height in subjects with a high standard of oral hygiene. *Journal of Clinical Periodontology* **14**, 466–469

Bergström, J. and Elíasson, S. (1989) Cigarette smoking as a risk factor in chronic periodontal disease. *Community Dentistry and Oral Epidemiology* **17**, 245–247

Bergström, J. and Floderus-Myrhed, B. (1983) Co-twin study of the relationship between smoking and some periodontal disease factors. *Community Dentistry and Oral Epidemiology* **11**, 113–116

Bergström, J. and Preber, H. (1986) Influence of cigarette smoking on the development of experimental gingivitis. *Journal of Periodontal Research* **21**, 668–676

Bergström, J. and Preber, H. (1994) Tobacco use as a risk factor. *Journal of Periodontology* **65**, 545–550

Bergström, J., Elíasson, S. and Preber, H. (1991) Cigarette smoking and periodontal bone loss. *Journal of Periodontology* **62**, 242–246

Bolin, A., Lavsted, S., Frithiof, L. and Hendrikson, C.O. (1986) Proximal alveolar bone loss in a longitudinal radiographic investigation. IV. Smoking and some other factors influencing the progress of individuals with at least 20 remaining teeth. *Acta Odontologica Scandinavica* **44**, 263–269

Bolin, A., Eklund, G., Frithiof, L. and Lavsted, S. (1993) The effects of changed smoking habits on marginal alveolar bone loss. *Swedish Dental Journal* **17**, 211–216

Bolinger, G., Alfredsson, L., Englund, A. and de Faire, U. (1994) Smokeless tobacco use and increased cardiovascular mortality amongst Swedish construction workers. *American Journal of Public Health* **84**, 399–404

Boström, L., Linder, L.E. and Bergström, J. (1998a) Influence of smoking on the outcome of periodontal surgery. A 5-year follow-up. *Journal of Clinical Periodontology* **25**, 194–201

Boström, L., Linder, L.E. and Bergström, J. (1998b) Clinical expression of TNF-α in smoking-associated periodontal disease. *Journal of Clinical Periodontology* **25**, 767–773

Bragd, L., Dahlén, G., Wikström, M. and Slots, J. (1987) The capability of *Actinobacillus actinomycetemcomitans*, *Bacteroides gingivalis* and *Bacteroides intermedius* to indicate progressive periodontitis. *Journal of Clinical Periodontology* **14**, 95–99

Brandtzaeg, P. and Jamison, H.C. (1964) A study of periodontal health and oral hygiene in Norwegian army recruits. *Journal of Periodontology* **35**, 302–307

Bridges, R.D., Kraal, J.H., Huang, L.J.T. and Chancellor, M.B. (1977) The effects of tobacco smoke on chemotaxis and glucose metabolism of polymorphonuclear leucocytes. *Infection and Immunology* **15**, 115–123

Calonius, P.E.B. (1962) A cytological study on the variation of keratinization in the normal oral mucosa of young males. *Journal of the Western Society of Periodontology* **10**, 69–74

Centers for Disease Control (1989) Tobacco use among high school students–United States *Morbidity and Mortality Weekly Report* **40**, 617–619

Centers for Disease Control and Prevention (1993) *Morbidity and Mortality Weekly Report* **42**, 230–232

Christen, A.G., Armstrong,W.R. and McDaniel, R.K. (1979) Intra-oral leukoplakia, abrasion, periodontal breakdown and tooth loss in a snuff dipper. *Journal of the American Dental Association* **98**, 584–586

Clarke, N.G., Shephard, B.C. and Hirsch, R.S. (1981) The effects of intra-arterial epinephrine and nicotine on gingival circulation. *Oral Surgery, Oral Medicine, Oral Pathology* **52**, 577–582

Codd, E.E., Swim, A.T. and Bridges, R.B. (1987) Tobacco smokers' neutrophils are desensitized to chemotactic peptide-stimulated oxygen uptake. *Journal of Laboratory and Clinical Medicine* **110**, 648–652

Council on Scientific Affairs (1990) The world-wide smoking epidemic. Tobacco trade, use and control. *Journal of the American Medical Association* **263**, 3312–3318

Costabel, U., Bross, K.J., Reuter, C. *et al.* (1986) Alterations in immunoregulatory T-cell subsets in cigarette smokers. A phenotypic analysis of broncho-alveolar and blood lymphocytes. *Chest* **90**, 39–44

Creath, C.J., Cutter, G., Bradley, D.H. and Wright, J.T. (1991) Oral leukoplakia and adolescent smokeless tobacco use. *Oral Surgery, Oral Medicine, Oral Pathology* **72**, 35–41

Croucher, R., Marcenes, W.S., Torres, M.C.M.B. *et al.* (1997) The relationship between life-events and periodontitis. A case–control study. *Journal of Clinical Periodontology* **54**, 481–487

Daniell, H.W. (1983) Post-menopausal tooth loss. Contribution to edentulism by osteoporosis and cigarette smoking. *Archives of Internal Medicine* **143**, 1678–1682

Dzink, J.L., Tanner, A.R.C., Haffajee, A.D. and Socransky, S.S. (1985)

Gram negative species associated with active destructive periodontal lesions. *Journal of Clinical Periodontology* **12**, 648–659

Dzink, J.L., Haffajee, A.D. and Socransky, S.S. (1988) The predominant cultivable microbiota of active and inactive lesions of destructive periodontal diseases. *Journal of Clinical Periodontology* **15**, 316–323

Eichel, G. and Shahrick, H.A. (1969) Tobacco smoke toxicity: loss of human oral leucocyte function and fluid cell metabolism. *Science* **166**, 1424–1428

Ernster, V., Grady, D.G., Green, J.C. *et al.* (1990) Smokeless tobacco use and health effects amongst baseball players. *Journal of the American Medical Association* **264**, 218–224

Fang, M.A., Frost, P.J., Iida-Klein, A. and Hahn, T.J. (1991) Effects of nicotine on cellular function in UMR 106-01 osteoclast-like cells. *Bone* **12**, 283–286

Feldman, R.S., Bravacos, J.S. and Rose, C.L. (1983) Association between smoking different tobacco products and periodontal disease indexes. *Journal of Periodontology* **54**, 481–487

Feldman, R.S., Alman, J.E. and Chauncey, H.H. (1987) Periodontal disease indexes and tobacco smoking in healthy aging men. *Gerodontics* **3**, 43–46

Genco, R.J., Zambon, J.J. and Christersson, L.A. (1988) The role of specific bacteria in periodontal disease: The origin of periodontal infections. *Advances in Dental Research* **2**, 245–259

Ginns, L.C., Goldenheim, P.D. and Miller, L.G. (1982) T-lymphocyte subsets in smoking and lung cancer. Analysis of monoclonal antibodies and flow cytometry. *American Review of Respiratory Disease* **126**, 265–269

Goodson, J.M., Haffajee, A.D. and Socransky, S.S. (1979) Periodontal therapy by local delivery of tetracycline. *Journal of Clinical Periodontology* **6**, 83–92

Goodson, J.M., Tanner, A.C.R., Haffajee, A.D. *et al.* (1982) Patterns of progression and regression of advanced destructive periodontal disease. *Journal of Clinical Periodontology* **9**, 472–481

Gore, E.A., Sanders, J.J., Pandey, J.P. *et al.* G.M.P. (1988) Interleukin-$1\beta^{+3953}$ allele 2: association with disease status in adult periodontitis. *Journal of Clinical Periodontology* **25**, 781–795

Goultschin, J., Sgan Cohen, H.D., Donchin, M. *et al.* (1990) Association of smoking with periodontal treatment needs. *Journal of Periodontology* **61**, 364–367

Grossi, S.G., Zambon, J.J., Ho, A.W. *et al.* (1994) Assessment of risk for periodontal disease. I. Risk indicators for attachment loss. *Journal of Periodontology* **65**, 260–267

Grossi, S.G., Genco, R.J., Machtei, E.E. *et al.* (1995) Assessment of risk for periodontal disease. I. Risk indicators for alveolar bone loss. *Journal of Periodontology* **66**, 23–29

Haber, J. (1994) Cigarette smoking: a major risk factor for periodontitis. *Compendium of Continuous Education in Dentistry* **15**, 1002–1014

Haber, J. and Kent, R.L. (1992) Cigarette smoking in periodontal practice. *Journal of Periodontology* **63**, 100–106

Haber, J., Wattles, J., Crowley, M. *et al.* (1993) Evidence for cigarette smoking as a major risk factor for periodontitis. *Journal of Periodontology* **64**, 16–23

Hanes, P.J., Schuster, G.S. and Lubas, S. (1991) Binding, uptake, and release of nicotine by human gingival fibroblasts. *Journal of Periodontology* **62**, 147–152

Hart, T.C. and Kornman, K.S. (1997) Genetic factors in the pathogenesis of periodontitis. *Periodontology 2000*, **14**, 202–215

Hoge, H.W. and Kirkham, D.B. (1983) Clinical management and soft tissue reconstruction of periodontal damage resulting from habitual use of snuff. *Journal of American Dental Association* **107**, 744–745

Hollenbach, K.A., Barrett-Connor, E., Edelstein, S.L. and Holbrook, T. (1993) Cigarette smoking and bone mineral density in older men and women. *American Journal of Public Health* **83**, 1265–1270

Holm, G. (1994) Smoking as an additional risk for tooth loss. *Journal of Periodontology* **65**, 996–1001

Horning, G.M., Hatch, C.L. and Cohen, M.E. (1992) Risk indicators for periodontitis in a military treatment population. *Journal of Periodontology* **63**, 297–302

International Agency for Research on Cancer (1986) Chemistry and analysis of tobacco smoke. In: *IARC Monographs on the Evaluation of the Carcinogenic Risk of Chemicals to Humans. Tobacco Smoking*, pp. 86–89. Lyon: IARC

Ismail, A.I., Burt, B.A. and Eklund, S.A. (1983) Epidemiologic patterns of smoking and periodontal disease in the United States. *Journal of the American Dental Association* **106**, 617–621

Jette, A.M., Feldman, H.A. and Tennstedt, S.L. (1993) Tobacco use: a modified risk factor for dental disease among the elderly. *American Journal of Public Health* **83**, 1271–1276

Johnson, C.K. and Organ, C.C. (1997) Prostaglandin E_2 and interleukin-1 concentrations in nicotine-exposed oral keratinocyte cultures. *Journal of Periodontal Research* **32**, 447–454

Johnson, C.K., Todd, G.L., Johnson, W.T. *et al.* (1991) Effects of topical and systemic nicotine on gingival blood flow in dogs. *Journal of Dental Research* **70**, 906–909

Jones, J.K. and Triplett, R.G. (1992) The relationship of cigarette smoking to intra-oral wound healing: a review of evidence and implications for patient care. *Journal of Maxillofacial Surgery* **50**, 237–239

Kalra, J., Chandhary, A.K. and Prasad, K. (1991) Increased production of oxygen free radicals in cigarette smokers. *International Journal of Experimental Pathology* **72**, 1–7

Kenny, E.B., Saxe, S.R. and Bowles, R.D. (1975) The effect of cigarette smoking on anaerobosis in the oral cavity. *Journal of Periodontology* **46**, 82–85

Kenny, E.B., Kraal, J.H., Saxe, S.R. and Jones, J. (1977) The effects of cigarette smoke on human polymorphonuclear leukocytes. *Journal of Periodontal Research* **12**, 227–234

Kornman, K.S., Crane, A., Wang, H.-Y. *et al.* (1997) The interleukin-1 genotype as a severity factor in adult periodontal disease. *Journal of Clinical Periodontology* **24**, 72–77

Kowolik, M.J. and Nisbet, T. (1983) Smoking and acute ulcerative gingivitis. *British Dental Journal* **154**, 241–242

Lamster, I.B. (1992) The host response in gingival crevicular fluid: potential applications in periodontitis clinical trials. *Journal of Periodontology* **63**, 1117–1123

Lang, N.P., Cumming, B.R. and Löe, H. (1973) Toothbrushing frequency as it relates to plaque development and gingival health. *Journal of Periodontology* **44**, 396–405

Lannan, S., McLean, A., Drost, E. *et al.* (1992) Changes in neutrophil morphology and morphometry following exposure to cigarette smoke. *International Journal of Experimental Pathology* **73**, 183–191

Lehner, T., Wilton, J.M.A., Challacombe, S. *et al.* (1974) Sequential cell mediated immune responses in experimental gingivitis in man. *Clinical and Experimental Immunology* **16**, 481–492

Linden, G.J. and Mullally, B.H. (1994) Cigarette smoking and periodontal destruction in young adults. *Journal of Periodontology* **65**, 718–723

Listgarten, M.A. (1992) Microbial testing in the diagnosis of periodontal disease. *Journal of Periodontology* **63**, 332–337

Listgarten, M.A. and Levin, S. (1981) Positive correlation between proportions of subgingival spirochaetes and motile bacteria and susceptibility of human subjects to periodontal deterioration. *Journal of Clinical Periodontology* **8**, 122–138

Listgarten, M.A., Schifter, C.C., Sulivan, P. *et al.* (1986) Failure of a microbial assay to reliably predict disease recurrence in a treated periodontitis population receiving regularly scheduled prophylaxes. *Journal of Clinical Periodontology* **13**, 768–773

Listgarten, M.A., Slots, J., Nowotny, A.H. *et al.* (1991) Incidence of periodontitis recurrence in treated patients with and without cultivable *Actinobacillus actinomycetemcomitans*, *Porphyromonas gingivalis* and *Prevotella intermedia*: a prospective study. *Journal of Periodontology* **62**, 377–386

Locker, D. (1989) Stress in dental practice. In *An Introduction to Behavioural Science*, pp. 21–38. Tavistock: Routledge

Locker, D. and Leake, J.L (1993) Risk indicators and risk markers for periodontal disease experience in a population of older adults living independently in Ontario. *Journal of Dental Research* **72**, 9–17

Löe, H., Theilade, E. and Jensen, S.B. (1965) Experimental gingivitis in man. *Journal of Periodontology* **36**, 177–187

Löe, H., Anerud, A., Boysen, H. and Smith, M. (1978) The natural history of periodontal disease in Man. *Journal of Periodontology* **49**, 607–620

Loesche, W.J. (1988) The role of spirochaetes in periodontal disease. *Advances in Dental Research* **2**, 275–283

Ludwick, W. and Massler, M. (1952) Relation of dental caries experience and gingivitis to cigarette smoking in males 17 to 21 years old (at the Great Lakes Naval Training Center). *Journal of Dental Research* **31**, 319–322

MacFarlane, G.D., Herzberg, M.C., Wolff, L.F. and Hardie, N.A. (1992) Refractory periodontitis associated with abnormal polymorphonuclear leucocyte phagocytosis and cigarette smoking. *Journal of Periodontology* **63**, 908–913

Macgregor, I.D.M. (1984) Toothbrushing efficiency in smokers and non-smokers. *Journal of Clinical Periodontology* **11**, 313–320

Macgregor, I.D.M. (1985) Survey of toothbrushing habits in smokers and non-smokers. *Clinical Preventive Dentistry* **7**, 27–30

Macgregor, I.D.M., Edgar, W.M. and Greenwood, A.R. (1985) Effects of cigarette smoking on the rate of plaque formation. *Journal of Clinical Periodontology* **12**, 259–263

Macgregor, I.D.M. (1992) Smoking and periodontal disease. In *Drugs, Diseases and the Periodontium* (R.A. Seymour and P.A. Heasman, eds), pp. 118–119. Oxford: Oxford University Press

MacKenzie, T.D., Bartecchi, C.E. and Schrier, R.W. (1994) The human costs of tobacco use. *New England Journal of Medicine* **331**, 975–980

Marcenes, W.S. and Sheiham, A. (1992) The relationship between work stress and oral health status. *Social Science and Medicine* **35**, 1511–1520

Marcenes, W.S., Croucher, R., Sheiham, A. and Marmot, M. (1993) The association between self reported oral symptoms and life-events. *Psychology and Health* **8**, 123–134

Martinez-Canut, P., Lorca, P. and Magan, R. (1995) Smoking and periodontal disease severity. *Journal of Clinical Periodontology* **22**, 743–749

McLaughlin, W.S., Lovat, F.M., Macgregor, I.D.M. and Kelly, P.J. (1993) The immediate effects of smoking on gingival fluid flow. *Journal of Clinical Periodontology* **20**, 448–451

Michalowicz, B.S. (1994) Genetic and heritable risk factors in periodontal disease. *Journal of Periodontology* **65**(5th Suppl.), 479–488

Michalowicz, B.S., Aeppli, D., Virag, J.G. *et al.* (1991) Periodontal findings in adult twins. *Journal of Periodontology* **62**, 293–299

Miller, P.D. Jnr (1987) Root coverage with free gingival graft. Factors associated with incomplete coverage. *Journal of Periodontology* **58**, 674–681

Mohlin, B., Ingervall, B., Hedegård, B. and Thilander, B. (1979) Tooth loss, prosthetics and dental treatment habits in a group of Swedish men. *Community Dentistry and Oral Epidemiology* **7**, 101–106

Moore, W.E.C., Moore, L.H. and Ranney, R.R. (1991) The microflora of periodontal sites showing active destruction progression. *Journal of Clinical Periodontology* **18**, 729–739

Newman, M.G., Kornman, K.S. and Holzman, S. (1994) Association of clinical risk factors with treatment outcomes. *Journal of Periodontology* **65**, 489–497

Nowak, D., Ruta, U. and Piasecka, G. (1990) Nicotine increases human polymorphonuclear leukocytes' chemotactic response – possible additional mechanism of lung injury in cigarette smokers. *Experimental Pathology* **39**, 37–43

Offenbacher, S. and Weathers, D.R. (1985) Effects of smokeless tobacco on the periodontal and caries status of adolescent males. *Journal of Oral Pathology* **14**, 169–181

Österberg, T. and Mellström, D. (1986) Tobacco smoking: a major risk factor for loss of teeth in three 70-year-old cohorts. *Community Dentistry and Oral Epidemiology* **14**, 367–370

Page, R.C. and Schroeder, H.E. (1986) *Periodontitis in Man and Other Animals*. Basel: Karger

Palmer, R.M. (1987) Tobacco Smoking and Oral Health. Health Education Authority. Occasional Paper No. 6

Papapanou, P.N., Wennström, J.J. and Gröndahl, K. (1989) A 10-year retrospective study of periodontal disease progression. *Journal of Clinical Periodontology* **16**, 403–411

Papapanou, P.N., Baelam, V., Luan, W.-M. *et al.* (1997) Sub-gingival microbiota in adult Chinese: prevalence and relation to periodontal disease progression. *Journal of Periodontology* **68**, 651–666

Payne, J.B., Johnson, G.K., Reinhardt, R.A. *et al.* (1994) Smokeless tobacco effects on monocyte secretion of PGE$_2$ and IL-1β. *Journal of Periodontology* **65**, 937–941

Peacock, M.E., Sutherland, D.E., Schuster, G.S. *et al.* (1993) The effect of nicotine on reproduction and attachment of human gingival fibroblasts *in vitro*. *Journal of Periodontology* **64**, 658–665

Pindborg, J.J. (1947) Tobacco and gingivitis. I. Statistical examination of the significance of tobacco in the development of acute ulceromembranous gingivitis and in the formation of calculus. *Journal of Dental Research* **26**, 261–264

Pindborg, J.J. (1949) Tobacco and gingivitis. II. Correlation between consumption of tobacco, acute ulceromembranous gingivitis and calculus. *Journal of Dental Research* **28**, 460–463

Preber, H. and Bergström, J. (1985) Occurrence of gingival bleeding in smoker and non-smoker patients. *Acta Odontologica Scandinavica* **43**, 315–320

Preber, H. and Bergström, J. (1986a) Cigarette smoking in patients referred for periodontal treatment. *Scandinavian Journal of Dental Research* **94**, 102–108

Preber, H. and Bergström, J. (1986b) The effect of non-surgical treatment on periodontal pockets in smokers and non-smokers. *Journal of Clinical Periodontology* **13**, 319–323

Preber, H. and Bergström, J. (1990) Effect of cigarette smoking on periodontal healing following surgical therapy. *Journal of Clinical Periodontology* **17**, 324–328

Preber, H. and Kant, T. (1973) Effect of tobacco smoking on the periodontal tissue of 15-year-old children. *Journal of Periodontal Research* **8**, 278–283

Preber, H., Kant, T. and Bergström, J. (1980) Cigarette smoking, oral hygiene and periodontal health in Swedish army conscripts. *Journal of Clinical Periodontology* **7**, 106–113

Preber, H., Bergström, J. and Linder, L.E. (1992) Occurrence of periopathogens in smoker and non-smoker patients. *Journal of Clinical Periodontology* **19**, 667–671

Ragnarsson, E., Elíasson, S.T. and Ólafsson, S.H. (1992) Tobacco smoking: a factor in tooth loss in Reykjavíc, Iceland. *Scandinavian Journal of Dental Research* **100**, 322–326

Raulin, L.A., McPherson, J.C., McQuade, M.J. and Hanson, B.S. (1989) The effect of nicotine on the attachment of human fibroblasts to glass and human root surfaces *in vitro*. *Journal of Periodontology* **59**, 318–325

Robertson, P.B., Walsh, M., Greene, J. *et al.* (1990) Periodontal effects associated with the use of smokeless tobacco. *Journal of Periodontology* **61**, 438–443

Ryder, M.I. (1994) Nicotine effects on neutrophil F-actin formation and calcium release: implications for tobacco use and respiratory disease. *Experimental Lung Research* **20**, 283–296

Ryder, M.I. (1996) Position paper. Tobacco use and the periodontal patient. *Journal of Periodontology* **67**, 51–56

Schei, O., Waerhaug, J., Lovdal, A. *et al.* (1959) Alveolar bone loss as a function of tobacco consumption. *Acta Odontologica Scandinavica* **17**, 3–10

Schmidt, E.F., Bretz, W.A., Hutchinson, R.A. and Loesche, W.J. (1988) Correlation of the hydrolysis of benzoyl-arginine-naphthylamide (BANA) by plaque with clinical parameters and subgingival levels spirochaetes in periodontal patients. *Journal of Dental Research* **67**, 1505–1509

Sculley, C., Porter, R. and Mutlu, S. (1991) Changing subject bases risk factors in for destructive disease. In *Risk Markers for Periodontal Diseases, Vol. 3. Periodontal Diseases* (N. Johnson, ed.), pp. 139–179. Cambridge: Cambridge University Press

Selby, C., Drost, E., Brown, D. *et al.* (1992) Inhibition of neutrophil adherence and movement by acute cigarette smoke exposure. *Experimental Lung Research* **18**, 813–827

Seymour, G.L. (1991) Importance of host response in the periodontium. *Journal of Clinical Periodontology* **18**, 421–426

Sheiham, A. (1971) Periodontal disease and oral cleanliness in tobacco smokers. *Journal of Periodontology* **42**, 259–263

Slots, J. (1986) Bacterial specificity in adult periodontitis. A summary of recent work. *Journal of Clinical Periodontology* **13**, 912–917

Slots, J. and Listgarten, M.A. (1988) *Bacteroides gingivalis, Bacteroides intermedius* and *Actinobacillus actinomycetemcomitans* in human periodontal disease. *Journal of Clinical Periodontology* **15**, 85–93

Slots, J., Emrich, L.J. and Genco, R. (1985) Relationship between some subgingival bacteria and periodontal pocket depth and gain or loss of attachment after treatment of adult periodontitis. *Journal of Clinical Periodontology* **12**, 540–552

Slots, J., Bragd, L., Wikström, M. and Dahlén, G. (1986) The occurrence of *Actinobacillus actinomycetemcomitans, Bacteroides gingivalis* and *Bacteroides intermedius* in destructive periodontal disease in adults. *Journal of Clinical Periodontology* **13**, 570–577

Socransky, S.S. (1970) Relationship of bacteria to the aetiology of periodontal disease. *Journal of Dental Research* **49**, 203–222

Socransky, S.S. (1979) Criteria for infectious agents in dental caries and periodontal disease. *Journal of Clinical Periodontology* **6**, 16–21

Socransky, S.S., Tanner, A.C.R., Haffajee, A.D. *et al.* (1982) Present status of studies on the microbial etiology of periodontal diseases. In *Host–Parasite Interactions in Periodontal Diseases* (R.J. Genco and S.E. Mergenhagen, eds), pp. 1–12. Washington DC: American Society for Microbiology

Socransky, S.S. and Haffajee, A.D. (1990) Microbial risk factors for destructive periodontal diseases. In *Risk Assessment in Dentistry* (J.D. Bader, ed.), pp. 79–90. Chapel Hill: University of North Carolina Dental Ecology

Solomon, H.A., Prior, R.L. and Bross, I.D. (1986) Cigarette smoking and periodontal disease. *Journal of the American Dental Association* **77**, 1081–1084

Stammers, A. (1944) Vincent's infection: observations and conclusions regarding the aetiology and treatment of 1017 civilian cases. *British Dental Journal* **76**, 147–155

Stoltenberg, J.L., Osborn, J.B., Philstrom, B.L. *et al.* (1993) Association between cigarette smoking, bacterial pathogens and periodontal status. *Journal of Periodontology* **64**, 1225–1230

Summers, C.J. and Oberman, A. (1968) Association of oral disease with 12 selected variables: II. Edentulism. *Journal of Dental Research* **47**, 594–598

Swango, P.A., Kleinman, D.V. and Konzelman, J.L. (1991) HIV and periodontal health. A study of military personnel with HIV. *Journal of the American Dental Association* **122**, 49–54

Tanner, A.R.C., Socransky, S.S. and Goodson, J.M. (1984) Microbiota of periodontal pockets losing alveolar crestal bone. *Journal of Periodontal Research* **19**, 279–291

Telivuo, M., Murtomaa, H. and Lahtinen, A. (1992) Observations and concepts of the oral health consequences of tobacco use of Finnish periodontists and dentists. *Journal of Clinical Periodontology* **19**, 15–18

Theilade, E. (1986) The non-specific theory in microbial etiology of inflammatory periodontal diseases. *Journal of Clinical Periodontology* **13**, 905–911

Totti, N., McCuster, K.T., Campbell, E.J. *et al.* (1994) Nicotine is chemotactic for neutrophils and enhances neutrophil responsiveness to chemotactic peptides. *Science* **227**, 169–171

Van Palenstein Helderman, W.H. (1981) Microbial etiology of periodontal disease. *Journal of Clinical Periodontology* **8**, 261–280

Wennström, J.L., Dahlén, G., Swensson, J. and Nyman, S. (1987) *Actinobacillus actinomycetemcomitans, Bacteroides gingivalis* and *Bacteroides intermedius*: predictors of attachment loss? *Oral Microbiology and Immunology* **2**, 158–163

Wilton, J., Griffiths, G., Curtis, M. *et al.* (1988) Detection of high risk groups and individuals for periodontal disease. Systemic predisposition and markers of general health. *Journal of Clinical Periodontology* **15**, 339–346

Wray, A. and McGuirt, E. (1993) Smokeless tobacco usage associated with oral carcinoma. Incidence, treatment and outcome. *Archives of Otolaryngology and Head and Neck Surgery* **119**, 929–933

Zambon, J.J. (1990) Microbial risk factors in human periodontal disease. In *Risk Assessment in Dentistry* (J.D. Bader, ed.), pp. 91–93. Chapel Hill: University of North Carolina

5

Mechanisms of disease production

Bacteria are the primary cause of periodontal disease, but are rarely found in the tissues in chronic periodontitis except during abscess formation. Only in acute necrotizing ulcerative gingivitis are spirochaetes seen to invade the tissues on a regular basis, and they only penetrate superficially. Intact crevicular epithelium is not permeable to bacteria, but it is permeable to bacterial antigens, metabolites and enzymes. It is assumed that inflammation and tissue destruction are brought about by these products.

Plaque bacteria produce a number of factors, which may operate on the tissues directly or indirectly by stimulating the immune and inflammatory reactions.

Direct effects of bacteria

In order to cause damage, bacteria must:

- Colonize the gingival crevice by evading host defences
- Damage the crevicular epithelial barrier
- Produce substances that can either directly or indirectly cause tissue damage.

These will be discussed separately below.

Evasion of host defences

A number of the putative periodontal pathogens possess potent mechanisms of evading or damaging host defences, including the following.

Direct damage to polymorphonuclear leucocytes (PMNs) and macrophages

The leucotoxin (see Chapter 20) produced by some strains of *Actinobacillus actinomycetemcomitans* can damage PMNs and macrophages (Tsai *et al.*, 1979).

Reduced PMN chemotaxis

A number of bacterial species, including *Porphyromonas gingivalis*, *Actinobacillus actinomycetemcomitans* and *Capnocytophaga* species, can reduce PMN chemotaxis and decrease phagocytosis and intracellular killing (Slots and Genco, 1984).

Degradation of immunoglobulins

A number of Gram negative black-pigmented anaerobes and *Capnocytophaga* species produce proteases, which can degrade IgG and IgA (Slots and Genco, 1984; Kilian, 1981; Jansen *et al.* 1995).

Modulation of cytokine function

Cytokines are the major controlling factors of the inflammatory and immune systems (see Chapter 3). There is now growing evidence that infectious agents are able to modify cytokine networks to their advantage (Henderson *et al.*, 1996a, 1996b; Takahashi and Earnshaw, 1996). There is also now evidence that some of the putative periodontal pathogens may have this ability. In this regard, the R1 proteinase (see below) of *Porphyromonas gingivalis* can both cleave and activate certain pro- and anti-inflammatory cytokines, and activate others (Aduse-Opoku *et al.*, 1995, 1996; Rangarajan *et al.*, 1997). The balance between these two opposing functions may influence the inflammatory status of the local cytokine network in the periodontal tissues.

Degradation of fibrin

Some Gram negative black-pigmented anaerobes possess fibrinolytic activity (Slots and Genco, 1984), which will reduce the trapping of bacteria by fibrin for surface phagocytosis.

Altered lymphocyte function

A number of Gram negative bacteria and spirochaetes in the subgingival flora can alter lymphocyte function and produce immunosuppression (Schenker, 1987). It has been suggested that these mechanisms could produce a temporary delay in the local immune response, which might lead to enhanced colonization, possible invasion and tissue injury, and account for the episodic nature of periodontal disease progression.

Damage to crevicular epithelium

Many bacteria in the subgingival flora seem capable of directly or indirectly damaging crevicular epithelium. Factors directly toxic to epithelium are produced by *P. gingivalis*, *Prevotella intermedia*, *A. actinomycetemcomitans*, *Treponema denticola* and *Capnocytophaga* species (Slots and Genco, 1984). This would increase the permeability of the crevicular epithelium to bacterial products and, possibly, to the bacteria themselves.

Production of volatile sulphur compounds

Volatile sulphur compounds comprise hydrogen sulphide, H_2S, methyl mercaptan, CH_3SH, dimethyl sulphide, $(CH_3)_2S$, and dimethyl disulphide, $(CH_3)_2S_2$. They are all thiols containing a characteristic -SH group, which is formed when the oxygen atom in the hydroxl group (-OH) is replaced by sulphur. Oral thiols are all toxic byproducts of Gram negative anaerobic bacterial metabolism of sulphur-containing amino acids (cystine, cysteine and methionine) that are present in saliva, gingival crevicular fluid, the gingival and periodontal pockets and the tongue surface. This bacterial metabolism is of a putrefactive nature, and leads to oxygen depletion (Tonzetich and Carpenter, 1971; Tonzetich and Catherall, 1976; Tonzetich, 1977; Nara, 1977; Persson *et al.*, 1989; Kleinberg and Westbay, 1992).

Porphyromonas gingivalis, *Prevotella intermedia*, *Prevotella melaninogenicai*, *Bacteroides forsythus*, *Treponema denticola* and *Fusobacterium nucleatum* have all been shown to be capable of producing volatile sulphur compounds through their metabolic pathways (Sawyer *et al.*, 1962; Tonzetich and McBride, 1981; Pianotti *et al.*, 1986; Claesson *et al.*, 1990; Persson *et al.*, 1989, 1990; Kleinberg and Westbay, 1992). They are all strictly anaerobic Gram negative bacteria.

It has been shown that volatile sulphur compounds, and especially CH_3SH, increase the permeability of the oral mucosa and crevicular epithelium (Ng and Tonzetich, 1984). Furthermore, proteoglycans and glycoproteins in the extracellular matrix are held in an aggregated state via disulphide bonds, and volatile sulphur compounds can induce their disaggregation by breaking these bonds (Ng and Tonzetich, 1984).

Volatile sulphur compounds also impair oxygen utilization by host cells, react with cellular proteins, interfere with collagen maturation, increase collagen solubility, decrease DNA synthesis and proline transport, and reduce the total protein content and collagen synthesis of fibroblasts (Horowitz and Folke, 1972; Tonzetich and Lo, 1978; Johnson and Tonzetich, 1979, 1982; Johnson *et al.*, 1992a).

In addition, volatile sulphur compounds, especially CH_3SH, incite the secretion of collagenase and prostaglandins from human fibroblasts, stimulate mononuclear cells to produce interleukin-1, augment the activity of cathepsin B, and convert mature collagen to a product more susceptible to enzymic degradation (Johnson *et al*, 1992b; Ratkay *et al.*, 1995). Volatile sulphur compounds, especially CH_3SH, also reduce intracellular pH, inhibit cell growth periodontal ligament cell migration (L'Allemain *et al.*, 1984; Simchowitz and Cragoe, 1986; Lancero *et al.*, 1996). Volatile sulphur compounds thus have the capacity to contribute to periodontal pathology.

Finally, volatile sulphur compounds are also related to the production of oral malodour or halitosis. Although it had been previously assumed that indole and amines were the main malodorous components in mouth air (Fosdick *et al.*, 1953), it is now established that volatile sulphur compounds are the malodorous substances primarily responsible for unpleasant oral breath (Tonzetich and Kesterbaum, 1969; Tonzetich, 1971, 1978; Miyaki *et al.*, 1995; Scully *et al.*, 1997). However, it has also been postulated that another possible component of oral malodour may be cadaverine, a malodorous diamine produced from fish and meat by BANA-hydrolysing Gram negative anaerobic bacteria (Goldberg *et al.*, 1994). Finally, the possible contribution of volatile fatty acids (butyrate, propionate, valerate) and putrescine (another diamine) to oral malodour remains unclear (Scully *et al.*, 1997).

Degradation of periodontal tissues by bacterial enzymes

The subgingival Gram negative bacteria use proteins for their nutrition and therefore possess proteolytic enzymes to break down proteins to peptides and amino acids, which they can absorb. A number of these proteases can degrade proteins essential to the host. In this respect, a number of the putative pathogens in the subgingival flora produce enzymes that can degrade components of the periodontal tissues and proteins essential to the defence system, and these are described below.

Proteolytic enzymes from putative periodontal pathogens

A number of the putative periodontal pathogens have been shown to produce proteases that are capable of degrading periodontal tissues. The main structural proteins of gingival connective tissue and periodontal ligament are collagen and proteoglycans. An early and persistent feature of periodontal disease is breakdown of connective tissue composed of these proteins (Page and Schroeder, 1976), which can be attacked by proteases of bacterial or host origin. The bacteria associated with periodontal disease produce a variety of proteolytic enzymes, which may participate in tissue breakdown. These include: collagenases, mainly from *Porphyromonas gingivalis* but also from *Actinobacillus actinomycetemcomitans* and spirochaetes (Robertson *et al.*, 1982); an elastase-like enzyme from spirochaetes (Uitto *et al.*, 1986) and *Capnocytophaga* species (Gazi *et al.*, 1987, 1996); trypsin-like enzymes from *P. gingivalis*, *Bacteroides forsythus*, *Treponema denticola* and other spirochaetes (Suido *et al.*, 1986; Gazi *et al.*, 1997); chymotrypsin-like enzymes from *T. denticola* and *Capnocytophaga* species (Uitto *et al.*, 1988a, 1988b, 1989a; Gazi *et al.*, 1997); aminopeptidases from *Capnocytophaga* species (Suido *et al.*, 1986; Gazi *et al.*, 1997) and *Treponema denticola* (Mäkinen *et al.*, 1986; Gazi *et al.*, 1997) and dipeptidyl peptidases from *P. gingivalis*, *P. intermedia* and *Capnocytophaga* species (Cox *et al.*, 1993; Gazi *et al.* 1995, 1997) (*Table 5.1*).

The amount of enzyme produced by each bacterial species varies considerably. A recent study has investigated the bacterial proteases from cell sonicates of putative periodontal pathogens using selective peptide substrates with appropriate inhibitors and activators (Cox *et al.*, 1993; Gazi *et al.*, 1994, 1996, 1997). Strong trypsin-like activity was found in *P. gingivalis*, moderate activity from *T. denticola* and *C. gingivalis*, and weak activity from *C. ochracea*, *C. sputigena* and *Prevotella intermedia*. The activity from *P. gingivalis* and *P. intermedia* had the characteristics of a cysteine proteinase, and in the case of *P. gingivalis* there appeared to be two separate cysteine proteinases, one cleaving arginine substrates and one lysine substrates (Gazi *et al.*, 1994, 1996, 1997) (see below). Weak chymotrypsin-like activity was found in *C. gingivalis*, *C. ochracea* and *T. denticola* (Gazi *et al.*, 1996, 1997). Weak elastase-like activity was only found in *C. sputigena*, and very weak activity in *C. gingivalis* and *C. ochracea* (Gazi *et al.*, 1996). Moderate DPP-like activity was found in *P. gingivalis*, *P. intermedia*

and *C. gingivalis*, and weak activity in *C. ochracea*, *C. sputigena and T. denticola* (Cox *et al.*, 1993; Gazi *et al.*, 1995, 1997) (*Table 5.1*).

These proteases can degrade all the elements of periodontal connective tissue, including Type I collagen, basement membrane Type IV collagen, elastin, proteoglycans and fibronectin. They can also degrade components of the host defence systems such as immunoglobulin and complement (see previous section and below), inactivate key components of the plasma proteinase cascade systems involved in the inflammatory response and blood clotting, and degrade the serum proteinase inhibitors α1-antiproteinase and α2-macroglobulin. Furthermore, some bacteria have fibrinolytic activity and some can also degrade haemoglobin (see below).

Other hydrolytic enzymes from putative periodontal pathogens

These bacteria also produce enzymes capable of degrading the non-proteinaceous elements of the periodontal connective tissue. Hyaluronidase and chondroitinase activities are produced by *C. ochracea*, *F. nucleatum*, *P. gingivalis* and *T. denticola* (Steffan and Hengtes, 1981; Tipler and Embery, 1985; Fiehn, 1986; Seddon and Shah, 1989). These could hydrolyse the glycosaminoglycan components of proteoglycans in the extracellular matrix. Neuraminidase (sialidase) activity, which is found in *B. forsythus*, *P. melaninogenicus* and *P. gingivalis* (Moncla *et al.*, 1990), might attack sialoproteins in the epithelium, thereby increasing its permeability to bacterial products. Damage to the surface of epithelial and other cells could result from the action of phospholipases from *Porphyromonas*, *Prevotella* and *Bacteroides* species (Bulkacz *et al.*, 1979, 1985). Finally, strong acid and alkaline phosphatase activities are present in *Porphyromonas*, *Prevotella*, *Bacteroides* and *Capnocytophaga* species (Slots, 1981; Laughton *et al.*, 1982a). These could contribute to alveolar bone breakdown, but probably only if bacterial invasion advances to this site.

Table 5.1 Bacterial protease

Bacteria	AminoP	DPP	Elastase	Trypsin	ChymoT	Collagenase
P. gingivalis	−	++	−	++++	−	++++
P. intermedia	−	++	−	±	−	±
A. actino	−	−	−	−	−	+
C. gingivalis	++	++	±	++	+	±
C. ochracea	++	+	+	+	±	−
C. sputigena	++	+	+	+	±	−
T. denticola	+	±	−	++	++	+
F. nucleatum	−	−	−	−	−	−
C. recta	+	−	−	−	−	−
E. corrodens	−	−	−	−	−	−

A. actino	− *Actinobacillus actinomycetemcomitans*	++++	Strong activity
AminoP	− Aminopeptidase	++	Moderate activity
DPP	− Dipeptidyl peptidase	+	Weak activity
ChymoT	− Chymotrypsin-like protease	±	Very weak activity
Trypsin	− Trypsin-like protease	−	No activity
Elastase	− Elastase-like protease		

The proteolytic and hydrolytic enzymes from individual putative periodontal pathogens are described in more detail below.

Porphyromonas gingivalis

Proteolytic enzymes

P. gingivalis produces by far the greatest proteolytic activity of any periodontal bacteria (Courant and Bader, 1966). It produces a variety of proteases, which differ in size, pH optima, sensitivity to inhibitors, ability to hydrolyse specific substrates and location within or on the surface of the bacterial cell (Lawson and Meyer, 1992). When separated by gel electrophoresis, a total of eight distinct bands of proteolytic activity are seen, each with different properties (Grenier *et al.*, 1989a). All these proteases are produced in large quantities by this bacteria and are recognized as important factors because of their potential to favour bacterial growth and cause damage to host tissues (Loesche *et al.*, 1985). A number of important proteins are hydrolysed by proteases from this bacteria. These include collagen (Toda *et al.*, 1984; Birkedal-Hansen *et al.*, 1988), basement membrane collagen IV (Uitto *et al.*, 1988a, 1988b), fibronectin (Uitto *et al.*, 1989b; Lantz *et al.*, 1991a), immunoglobulins A1, A2 and G (Kilian, 1981; Mortensen and Kilian, 1984; Sato *et al.*, 1987; Grenier *et al.*, 1989b), complement factors (Sundqvist *et al.*, 1985; Schenkein, 1988), iron-binding proteins (Carlsson *et al.*, 1984a), plasma proteinase inhibitors, α_1-proteinase inhibitor and α_2-macroglobulin (Carlsson *et al.*, 1984b), some key factors in the plasma proteinase cascade systems (Nilsson *et al.*, 1985) and salivary lysozyme (Endo *et al.*, 1989).

These proteinases are produced in cell associated and secretory forms (Grenier and McBride, 1987). They could play an important role in periodontal pathology as they have the potential to degrade connective tissues and basement membrane, and to interfere with host defences by degrading immunoglobulins and complement and degrading or activating inflammatory proteins (Sojar *et al.*, 1993).

Nakamura *et al.* (1991) separated the proteases in supernatants from *P. gingivalis* cultures into four separate activities, which they called proteases A, B and C and a Gly-Pro dipeptidyl peptidase. Proteases B and C were thiol-dependent cysteine proteinases and had trypsin-like activity. Protease A was neither a cysteine proteinase nor had trypsin-like activity. Protease C was the most abundant and had a large molecular size, and they felt that it could have represented a mixture of two or three enzymes. All the collagenolytic activity was present in this fraction. However, they stated that it could well result from a separate enzyme or enzymes from the trypsin-like proteinase.

Trypsin-like proteinases

In surveys of the proteolytic activity of oral bacteria, *P. gingivalis* was found to have a particular ability to cleave peptide substrates with arginine terminal groups such as benzoyl-arginine-2-naphthylamide (BANA) or benzoyl-arginine-p-nitroanilide (BAPNA), and this activity was termed trypsin-like (Slots, 1981; Laughton *et al.*, 1982b). In cultures of *P. gingivalis*, the relative amount of trypsin-like activity in bacterial cells and medium depends on the stage of growth and growth rate. During high growth rates the enzyme is mainly associated with the cells, but as the culture ages or at low growth rates the proportion of activity in the medium increases (Suido *et al.*, 1987; Tsutsui *et al.*, 1987; Fujimura and Nakamura, 1989; Minhas and Greenman, 1989). Most of the activity is associated with bacterial membranes (Yoshimura *et al.*, 1984; Tsutsui *et al.*, 1987; Fujimura and Nakamura, 1989), and the enzymes are located at the inner membrane and cell surface (Lantz *et al.*, 1993). Activity has also been found in extracellular outer membrane vesicles (Grenier and Mayrand, 1987; Smalley and Birss, 1987), with the relative amount varying in similar way to that in the supernatant (Minhas and Greenman, 1989).

The purified enzyme is inhibited by thiol-blocking agents and enhanced by sulphydryl compounds (Yoshimura *et al.*, 1984; Fujimura and Nakamura, 1987; Otsuka *et al.*, 1987; Smalley and Birss, 1987; Sorsa *et al.*, 1987; Suido *et al.*, 1987; Sundqvist *et al.*, 1987; Tsutsui *et al.*, 1987; Shah *et al.*, 1991; Lantz *et al.*, 1993). It is similar in its actions to other cysteine proteinases like papain and, by analogy, it has been proposed that it is either known as gingivain or gingipain (see below).

There have also been some conflicting reports on other properties of the trypsin-like activities. Some workers have found them sensitive to the serine protease inhibitors (Sorsa *et al.*, 1987; Suido *et al.*, 1987; Sundqvist *et al.*, 1987; Tsutsui *et al.*, 1987) whilst others have not (Fujimura and Nakamura, 1987; Otsuka *et al.*, 1987; Lantz *et al.*, 1993). Also, some have found a requirement for metal ions (Yoshimura *et al.*, 1984; Fujimura and Nakamura, 1987; Sorsa *et al.*, 1987; Sundqvist *et al.*, 1987; Tsutsui *et al.*, 1987), but others have found the opposite (Otsuka *et al.*, 1987; Suido *et al.*, 1987). In addition, the figures for pH optimum range from 6.0–8.5 (Yoshimura *et al.*, 1984; Fujimura and Nakamura, 1987; Otsuka *et al.*, 1987; Suido *et al.*, 1987; Sundqvist *et al.*, 1987; Tsutsui *et al.*, 1987), whilst estimates for molecular weight range from 18–300 kDa (Fujimura and Nakamura, 1987; Otsuka *et al.*, 1987; Smalley and Birss, 1987; Sorsa *et al.*, 1987; Tsutsui *et al.*, 1987; Lantz *et al.*, 1993).

The most likely explanation for these variations is that there is more than one trypsin-like enzyme. In this regard, one study obtained four distinct factions of trypsin-like activity, all of which appeared to be cysteine proteinases (Fujimura and Nakamura, 1989). Another separated two cysteine proteinases, both of which cleaved arginine bonds and one of which also cleaved lysine bonds, and a third serine proteinase (Hinode *et al.*, 1991). Similar findings (Nakamura *et al.*, 1991) have been reported by other workers. In addition, many reports on trypsin-like proteinases include descriptions of collagenase activity, which is almost certainly due to separate proteinases (see below).

Shah *et al.* (1991) separated the trypsin-like activity from *P. gingivalis* outer membrane vesicles and culture supernatant. They showed that it was a thiol-dependent cysteine proteinase, which cleaved synthetic arginine substrates. They proposed the name gingivain for this enzyme. A similar and probably identical proteinase was isolated from the culture supernatant by Chen *et al.* (1992), and they gave it the name of gingipain. They showed that it had a narrow spectrum of activity against peptide bonds containing arginine, was resistant to inhibition by serine proteinase inhibitors, and was activated by glycine-containing dipeptidides. They also found that it had a molecular weight of 50 kDa and a pH optimum of 6.0. This enzyme may either be referred to as arggingipain or as gingipain-R.

Pike *et al.* (1994) separated the trypsin-like activity in *P. gingivalis* culture supernatants and found that there were two separate cysteine proteinase activities, one with arginine and one with lysine specificity. The argininespecific proteinase was a high molecular weight form of gingipain and proved to be 50 kDa gingipain complexed with 44 kDa binding proteins, which were shown to be haemagglutinins. The lysine-specific activity had a molecular weight of 60 kDa and a pH optimum of 8.0–8.5, and was also complexed with haemagglutinin binding proteins. They called this enzyme lys-gingipain, but it is also referred to as gingipain-K. They thought that these proteinase/haemagglutinin complexes might be involved in the uptake of haemin, which is a vital metabolite for *P. gingivalis*, by haemagglutination and subsequent haemolysis of erythrocytes.

Scott *et al.* (1993) also isolated and identified this lysine specific activity, and called the enzyme lys gingivain. They showed that it was capable of cleaving high molecular weight kininogens to generate bradykinin, and could degrade fibrinogen. In addition, this protease has been shown to be capable of activating fibroblast and neutrophil interstitial collagenases (Sorsa *et al.*, 1992; De Carlo *et al.*, 1997). Thus, *P. gingivalis* produces two cysteine proteinases with trypsin-like activity. One of these is arginine specific and is called either gingivain or gingipain, and the other is lysine specific and is called lys-gingivain or lys-gingipain.

A significant proportion of the arginine-specific proteinase activity from the human *P. gingivalis* strain, W52, has been shown to be associated with an adhesin component (Curtis *et al.*, 1993; Aduse-Opoku *et al.*, 1995), and the arginine-specific gene *prpR1*, which encodes for the polyprotein of this enzyme, Arg I (PrpRI), has been cloned and sequenced (Aduse-Opoku *et al.*, 1995). The enzyme product of this gene has been found in both heterodimeric ($\alpha\beta$) and monomeric (α) forms in which only the α component is proteolytically active, and together these forms comprise the majority of the arginine-specific activity from *P. gingivalis*. The structure of the arginine-specific proteinase has recently been determined, and is schematically represented in *Figure 5.1* (Curtis *et al.*, 1993; Aduse-Opoku *et al.*, 1995, 1996; Rangarajan *et al.*, 1997).

P. gingivalis produces three isoforms of the protein (PrpR1) from the *prpR1* gene, which have been termed the R1, R1A and R1B proteins. The full length translation product of the full *prp R1* gene is a large precursor protein consisting of 1706 amino acid residues, which contains four domains: i) a propeptide, ii) a catalytic (α) domain, iii) an adhesin (β) domain and iv) a long C-terminal (γ) domain (*Figure 5.1*). This precursor protein is either processed to a heterodimeric protease (R1) containing the α and β chains in non-covalent association, or to two monomeric forms, R1A and R1B. The second monomeric form (R1B) has extensive lipid modification, represented in *Figure 5.1* as lipopolysaccharide (LPS).

Preliminary studies have shown that the Arg1 proteinase is capable of cleaving and inactivating certain pro- and anti-inflammatory cytokines (Fletcher *et al.*, 1997, 1998). In addition, a 16 KDa protein from the outer

Figure 5.1 A schematic representation of the prpR1 protein produced by the *PrpR1* gene of *Porphyromonas gingivalis*. The protein consists of 1706 amino acid residues and is organized into four major domains: Pro, α, β and γ. The propeptide is preceded by a typical *E. coli* signal sequence. The presence of arginine residues at the junctions of these domains suggests autolytic processing of the polyprotein indicated by the vertical arrows to give either dimeric Arg 1 (α β) or monomeric Arg 1A (α). The LPS annotation to Arg 1B denotes the extensive lipid modification to this form

surface membrane of this bacterium has been found to have cytokine-inducing function with regard to IL-6 (Sharp *et al.*, 1998). This protein shares the sequence of part of the β chain of the R1 proteins and thus appears to be a cleaved fragment from this chain. Therefore, the RI proteinase appears to have a dual action in both activating and inactivating certain cytokines.

Thus, as well as being essential for the nutrition of *P. gingivalis*, these trypsin-like proteinases could be involved in periodontal tissue degradation. They degrade protein substrates such as albumin (Fujimura and Nakamura, 1987; Otsuka *et al.*, 1987; Tsutsui *et al.*, 1987; Hinode *et al.*, 1992), as well as fibronectin and other cell surface glycoproteins (Smalley *et al.*, 1988a; Uitto *et al.*, 1989b; Lantz *et al.*, 1991b), immunoglobulin A (Sato *et al.*, 1987) and lysozyme (Endo *et al.*, 1989). In addition, they are capable of modulating cytokine function (Fletcher *et al.*, 1997, 1998; Sharp *et al.*, 1998).

The reports of the collagenolytic activity of these proteinases (Sorsa *et al.*, 1987; Tsutsui *et al.*, 1987; Smalley *et al.*, 1988a) probably reflect contamination of the enzyme preparation with the true collagenases (Fujimura and Nakamura, 1987) (see below). However, there is some evidence that the breakdown of Type I collagen by *P. gingivalis* may involve the concerted action of both a collagenase and trypsin-like enzyme (McDermid *et al.*, 1988).

Possible pathophysiological roles for gingipains in periodontitis

Both the membrane-bound and secreted forms of *P. gingivalis* arg-gingipain have been found potently to enhance vascular permeability. They induce this effect by the production of plasma kallikrein through activation of prokallikrein, which then leads to the release of vasoactive bradykinin (Travis *et al.*, 1997). It has been found that it can only induce these changes in human plasma when working in concert with lys-gingipain. In this way these enzymes increase gingival crevicular fluid production and thus provide a continuous supply of nutrients for the bacterium, enhancing its growth and virulence.

Arg-gingipain has also been found to be a very efficient enzyme for the production of the potent chemotactic factor C5a by directly cleaving the C5 component of complement (Travis *et al.*, 1997). At the same time this enzyme also degrades C3, and in this way eliminates the creation of C3-derived opsonins. This renders *P. gingivalis* more resistant to phagocytosis by neutrophils. These combined effects result in a massive accumulation of neutrophils in the tissues, which then produce an array of proteinases that can degrade connective tissue. The resulting production of peptides in turn allows these bacteria to thrive.

Fibrinogen is a major target for lys-gingipain and it thus increases the local clotting time, leading to gingival bleeding. The bleeding of periodontal sites is of primary importance for the growth of *P. gingivalis*, since it ensures the rich source of haem and iron that it requires for survival.

Gingipains act as adhesins and have a strong binding affinity for fibrinogen, fibronectin and laminin. This interaction inhibits haemagglutination (Travis *et al.*, 1997). All the bound proteins are then easily degraded by the functional proteinase domain. Arg-gingipain is more active on fibronectin and laminin, and lys-gingipain is more active on fibrinogen. Thus both of these enzymes may progressively attach to, degrade and detach from their target proteins. Since these complexes are present on the surfaces of both the vesicles and membranes of *P. gingivalis*, they may play an important role in the attachment of this bacterium to host cells.

Collagenolytic proteinases

Collagenolytic activity has frequently been reported in *P. gingivalis* (Robertson *et al.*, 1982; Toda *et al.*, 1984; Birkedal-Hansen *et al.*, 1988). The activity is usually described as cell bound, and has also been found in extracellular outer membrane vesicles (Grenier and Mayrand, 1987). Unlike mammalian collagenase, it degrades collagen into multiple fragments (Robertson *et al.*, 1982; Toda *et al.*, 1984; Sundqvist *et al.*, 1987; Birkedal-Hansen *et al.*, 1988), but the initial attack is in the triple helical region, indicating that it is a true collagenase (Birkedal-Hansen *et al.*, 1988). Further breakdown probably involves other proteases. The activity is activated by sulphydryl compounds and inhibited by thiol-blocking agents and metal-chelating agents (Robertson *et al.*, 1982; Toda *et al.*, 1984; Sundqvist *et al.*, 1987; Birkedal-Hansen *et al.*, 1988). Thus, it appears to be a cysteine proteinase with a requirement for metal ions, and it probably has a binding specificity for arginine residues (Toda *et al.*, 1984; Birkedal-Hansen *et al.*, 1988). Type IV collagen is also degraded by *P. gingivalis*, but its activity is not affected by thiol-blocking agents, indicating that another enzyme is involved (Uitto *et al.*, 1988a, 1988b).

The separate collagenolytic enzymes from *P. gingivalis* have been investigated by several workers, and separate proteinase activities have been only recently isolated.

Lawson and Meyer (1992) purified the collagenolytic activities from *P. gingivalis* using electrophoretic techniques. They showed that the enzymes were present in the bacterial cell wall and were released into the culture medium. The purified enzyme was capable of cleaving basement membrane collagen Type IV and synthetic substrates for bacterial collagenases. The activity had the characteristics of a cysteine proteinase and appeared to exist as an active precursor protein of 94 kDa molecular weight, which undergoes proteolytic cleavage to 75, 56 and 19 kDa forms. It appeared to function also as an adhesin, permitting the bacteria to attach to collagenous tissue.

Sojar *et al.* (1993) purified the proteases from *P. gingivalis* that were capable of cleaving the bacterial collagenase substrate called the pZ-peptide. They showed that the purified enzyme activity was present in the bacterial cell wall and was also released into the culture medium. The purified enzyme was capable of hydrolysing salt-solubilized Type I collagen, kininogen and transferrin in the presence of both calcium and dithiothreitol (a reducing agent required by cysteine proteinases), and could also function as a gelatinase. However, it failed to degrade acid-soluble Type I or Type IV collagens and fibrinogen, and also did not cleave either terminal arginine or lysine or glycyl-prolyl synthetic peptide substrates. It thus appeared to be a collagenolytic cysteine proteinase with no trypsin-like or dipeptidyl peptidase activities, which had a calcium and salt requirement for its activity. The native enzyme had a molecular weight of 120 kDa, and its range of activity suggested that it had specificity for the Pro−X−Gly sequence found on several proteins including collagen.

Kato *et al.* (1992) isolated a gene (*prt C*) from *P. gingivalis* that coded for a protein with collagenolytic activity. They cloned the gene into *Escherichia coli* and harvested the resultant protein, which was purified by gel filtration and ion exchange chromatography. The purified enzyme had a molecular weight of 35 kDa, and the active enzyme behaved as a dimer. It degraded soluble and reconstituted fibrillar Type I collagen, heat denatured Type I collagen, but did not degrade gelatin or synthetic substrates for bacterial collagenases. Its activity was not dependent on reducing agents, and was enhanced by calcium ions and inhibited by chelating agents. It was therefore not a cysteine proteinase, and had some properties of a metalloproteinase.

The three collagenolytic proteinases described above all differ from one another in important respects, so it appears that at least three distinct collagenolytic proteinases are produced by *P. gingivalis*. These enzymes are also distinct from the two trypsin-like cysteine proteinases, the dipeptidyl peptidase and probably other proteinases degrading other proteins such as fibrinogen.

Other proteases

Another protease coding gene (*tpr*) has been isolated from *Porphyromonas gingivalis* and cloned into *Escherichia coli*. The resultant enzyme had a molecular weight of 64 kDa, and was active against general protein substrates but not collagen (Bourgeau *et al.*, 1992). In addition, two proteinases of 120 and 150 kDa that degraded fibrinogen (Lantz *et al.*, 1991a) and fibronectin (Lantz *et al.*, 1991a, 1991b) and a 70 kDa collagenase-like neutral protease (Sorsa *et al.*, 1987) have been isolated from *P. gingivalis*. The 150 kDa fraction has been shown to be a cysteine proteinase with trypsin-like activity, and to bind to both fibrinogen and fibronectin prior to degrading them (Lantz *et al.*, 1991b). It has also been shown to be located on the outer cell membrane and to mediate attachment of the bacteria to these proteins (Lantz *et al.*, 1993). Since it cleaves fibrinogen in an identical way to plasmin, it may also activate procollagenase and degrade fibrin and glycoproteins in the extracellular matrix and basement membrane.

Finally, *P. gingivalis* produces dipeptidyl peptidase

activity against glycyl-prolyl and alanyl-prolyl dipeptides (Suido *et al.*, 1986; Nakamura *et al.*, 1991; Cox *et al.*, 1993; Gazi *et al.*, 1995). Glycyl-prolyl arylamidase activities have also been studied by several groups (Abiko *et al.*, 1985; Grenier and McBride, 1987; Suido *et al.*, 1987; Barua *et al.*, 1989; Kay *et al.*, 1989). These are serine proteases with a pH optima of 7.5−8.5. These activities are found in bacterial cells in association with the outer membrane, and are also present in extracellular outer membrane vesicles (Grenier and McBride, 1987; Kay *et al.*, 1989).

All of the collagenolytic trypsin-like dipeptidyl peptidases and other proteases described above (*Table 5.1*) would appear to be located in the cell wall, concentrated in outer membrane vesicles and released into the surrounding environment in extracellular vesicles. Thus, they could enter the periodontal tissues and play a role in periodontal pathology. In summary, these proteases could:

- Degrade basement membrane and extracellular matrix proteins, including collagen, proteoglycans and glycoproteins such as fibronectin. This would both destroy periodontal connective tissue and facilitate bacterial invasion of the host tissues.
- Interfere with tissue repair by inhibiting clot formation or lysing the fibrin matrix in periodontal lesions.
- Activate latent host tissue collagenases, which would enhance host tissue enzyme-mediated tissue destruction.
- Inactivate proteins important in host defence.

Other hydrolytic enzymes

P. gingivalis also produces hyaluronidase and chondroitinase activities (Steffen and Hengtes, 1981; Tipler and Embery, 1985; Fiehn, 1986; Seddon and Shah, 1989) which could hydrolyse the glycosaminoglycan components of proteoglycans. These activities could be present in the outer membrane vesicles (Smalley *et al.*, 1988b). It also produces neuraminidase activity (Moncla *et al.*, 1990) which might attack sialoproteins in the epithelium. Finally, it produces strong acid and alkaline phosphatase activities (Slots, 1981; Laughton *et al.*, 1982b).

Prevotella intermedia and nigrescens

Proteolytic enzymes

P. intermedia and *nigrescens* are capable of degrading a number of tissue proteins, including collagen, fibronectin, fibrin and immunoglobulins (Kilian, 1981; Wikström and Lindhe, 1986; Larjava *et al.*, 1987; Smalley *et al.*, 1988a; Uitto *et al.*, 1989b; Jansen *et al.*, 1995), and proteolytic activity has also been demonstrated against gelatin (Uitto *et al.*, 1989b; Seddon and Shah, 1989). However, this proteolytic activity only showed weak trypsin-like activity (Gazi *et al.*, 1994, 1996, 1997), and this has been shown to be a cysteine protease (Gazi *et al.*, 1997). It has no aminopeptidase, chymotrypsin- or elastase-like activity

(Slots, 1981; Laughton *et al.*, 1982a; Suido *et al.*, 1988a, 1988b; Seddon and Shah, 1989), but has been shown to have moderate dipeptidyl peptidase activity (Suido *et al.*, 1986; Cox *et al.*, 1993; Gazi *et al.*, 1995, 1997).

Other hydrolytic enzymes

This bacteria also produces strong acid and alkaline phosphatases (Slots, 1981; Laughton *et al.*, 1982a).

Treponema species

Proteolytic enzymes

Treponema denticola shows significant proteolytic activity against a range of host components such as collagens Types I and IV, fibronectin, keratin and fibrin (Wikström and Lindhe, 1986; Larjarva *et al.*, 1987; Mikx and De Jong, 1987; Smalley *et al.*, 1988a; Uitto *et al.*, 1988a, 1988b; Lantz *et al.*, 1991b). These proteases have also been shown to be capable of activating fibroblast and neutrophil interstitial collagenases (Sorsa *et al.*, 1992). This species also hydrolyses a number of synthetic peptide substrates including those from aminopeptidase, trypsin-, chymotrypsin- and bacterial collagenase-like activities (Laughton *et al.*, 1982a; Mäkinen et al., 1986; Uitto *et al.*, 1988a, 1988b) (*Table 5.1*). In contrast, *T. vincentii* has negligible trypsin- and chymotrypsin-like activities (Laughton *et al.*, 1982a; Mäkinen *et al.*, 1986; Uitto *et al.*, 1988b), though it does possess collagenase-like and aminopeptidase activities (Mäkinen *et al.*, 1986). These proteases are also found in the outer sheath and extracellular vesicles from this bacteria (Rosen *et al.*, 1995).

The capacity of *T. denticola* to degrade proteins appears mostly to be associated with its chymotrypsin-like activity. The partially purified activity has a molecular weight of 95 kDa, a pH optimum of 7.5 and the characteristics of a cysteine proteinase (Uitto *et al.*, 1988a, 1988b). The enzyme has a broad range of proteolytic activity, and extensively breaks down transferrin, fibrinogen and gelatin. It also produces a limited cleavage of α_1-antiproteinase inhibitor and immunoglobulins. It has also been found to attack the basement membrane components collagen type IV, fibronectin and laminin, and this ability, together with location on the outside of the cell envelope, indicates a possible role in destruction and invasion of the epithelium by *T. denticola* (Grenier *et al.*, 1990).

The gene coding for the *T. denticola* chymotrypsin-like activity has been inserted into *E. coli* and the protein product (the cloned enzyme) showed similar properties to the bacteria itself (Que and Kuramitsu, 1990).

The trypsin-like proteinases of *T. denticola* are active against BANA and BAPNA substrates, and there is evidence that two different enzymes cleave each of these substrates and, furthermore, the activity may vary in different strains of this bacterium. The activity against BAPNA has a molecular weight in the range of 40–69 kDa and a pH optimum of about 8.5 (Ohta *et al.*, 1986). It had the characteristics of a serine proteinase, but was not able to degrade protein substrates such as haemoglobin or gelatin.

Both *T. denticola* and *T. vincentii* are able to cleave synthetic substrates for bacterial collagenase activity (Mäkinen *et al.*, 1988). Cell extracts from *T. vincentii* yielded two fractions active against this substrate, with molecular weights of 23 and 75 kDa and pH optima of 7.0–8.0 and 6.5–7.5 respectively (Mäkinen *et al.*, 1988). Both activities have the characteristics of metalloproteinases, and the 75 kDa fraction hydrolysed gelatin at a low rate. The gene coding for the *T. denticola* collagenase-like activity has been inserted into *E. coli* and the cloned enzyme purified and characterized (Que and Kuramitsu, 1990). This has a molecular weight of 36 kDa and a pH optimum of 7.5. Like the *T. vincentii* collagenase enzyme, it has the characteristics of a metalloproteinase. However, it is unable to hydrolyse collagens Type I and IV or gelatin.

T. denticola produces both an iminopeptidase and aminopeptidase. The iminopeptidase has a molecular weight of 100 kDa, a pH optimum of 7.5 and the characteristics of a cysteine protease (Mäkinen *et al.*, 1986, 1987). As collagen is rich in proline, it is possible that the enzyme acts on degradation products to provide nutrition for the organism. Some *T. denticola* strains also produce an aminopeptidase cleaving terminal aspartic acid residues (Mäkinen *et al.*, 1986). *T. vincentii* gave the highest aminopeptidase activity, cleaving terminal arginine residues, and this has a molecular weight of about 200 kDa and a pH optimum of 7.0–8.0 (Mäkinen *et al.*, 1988). Finally, *T. denticola* has also been shown to produce dipeptidylpeptidase activity (Gazi *et al.*, 1997).

Other hydrolytic enzymes

Hyaluronidase and chondroitinase activities are produced by *T. denticola* (Steffen and Hengtes, 1981; Tipler and Embery, 1985; Fiehn, 1986; Seddon and Shah, 1989), and these could hydrolyse the glycosaminoglycan components of proteoglycans.

Capnocytophaga species

Proteolytic enzymes

Capnocytophaga species show low to moderate activity against host proteins, and may degrade collagen Types I and IV and immunoglobulins (Kilian, 1981; Seddon and Shah, 1989). In a recent study, both smooth and rough surfaced strains were found to possess weak to moderate activity against Type I collagen, gelatin, collagen polypeptides and synthetic bacterial collagenase substrates (Söderling *et al.*, 1991). The main fraction of the separated sample that contained these activities had a molecular weight of 54 kDa. The cleavage of IgA1 by *C. gingivalis*, *C. ochracea* and *C. sputigena* protease was inhibited by metal chelators, suggesting that metalloproteinases were involved.

Weak trypsin-like activity has been shown in *C. gingivalis*, *C. ochracea* and *C. sputigena* by a number of studies (Slots, 1981; Laughton *et al.*, 1982a; Nakamura and Slots, 1982; Suido *et al.*, 1986; Seddon and Shah, 1989; Söderling et al., 1991; Gazi *et al.*, 1994, 1996, 1997). However, more recently this activity has been shown to consist of two separate proteases, one specific for arginine and the other for lysine substrates (Gazi *et al.*, 1997). Weak chymotrypsin-like activity has also been detected in various *Capnocytophaga* species (Gazi *et al.*, 1996, 1997). In addition, weak elastase activity has been found in *C. sputigena*, and very weak activity in *C. gingivalis* and *C. ochracea* (Gazi *et al.*, 1996, 1997).

A number of studies have found that all *Capnocytophaga* strains and species possess high aminopeptidase (Slots, 1981; Suido *et al.*, 1986; Söderling *et al.*, 1991) and dipeptidylpeptidase (Gazi *et al.*, 1997) activity.

Other hydrolytic enzymes

Hyaluronidase and chondroitinase activities are produced by *C. ochracea* (Steffen and Hengtes, 1981; Tipler and Embery, 1985; Fiehn, 1986; Seddon and Shah, 1989), which could hydrolyse the glycosaminoglycan components of proteoglycans. Strong acid and alkaline phosphatase activities are also present in *Capnocytophaga* species (Slots, 1981; Laughton *et al.*, 1982b).

Actinobacillus actinomycetemcomitans

Proteolytic enzymes

Some studies have shown that *A. actinomycetemcomitans* is able to degrade native Type I collagen (Robertson *et al.*, 1982; Rozanis and Slots, 1982; Rozanis *et al.*, 1983) and a synthetic substrate for bacterial collagenases (Rozanis *et al.*, 1983). The activity is found both in the bacterial cell and the culture medium (Robertson *et al.*, 1982, Rozanis and Slots, 1982), and it produces multiple scissions in the collagen molecule (Robertson *et al.*, 1982). The activity has the characteristics of a metalloproteinase (Robertson *et al.*, 1982; Rozanis and Slots, 1982; Rozanis *et al.*, 1983). Weak gelatinase activity has also been reported. However, surveys with a variety of other substrates have shown that this bacteria produces no trypsin-, chymotrypsin-, elastase-, dipeptidylpeptidase- or aminopeptidase-like activity (Slots, 1981; Laughton *et al.*, 1982a; Suido *et al.*, 1986; Seddon and Shah, 1989). However, a unified alanine/lysine activity has been detected (Gazi *et al.*, 1997).

Fusobacterium nucleatum

Proteolytic enzymes

F. nucleatum appears to have little ability to degrade proteins or synthetic substrates for trypsin-, chymotrypsin-, elastase-, dipeptidylpeptidase-, or aminopeptidase-like activity (Suido *et al.*, 1986).

Other hydrolytic enzymes

Hyaluronidase and chondroitinase activities are produced by *F. nucleatum* (Steffen and Hengtes, 1981; Tipler and Embery, 1985; Fiehn, 1986; Seddon and Shah, 1989).

Campylobacter recta

Proteolytic enzymes

C. recta produces aminopeptidases, but so far no proteinases have been detected (Umemoto *et al.*, 1991).

Eikenella corrodens

Proteolytic enzymes

E. corrodens produces proteases connected with its nutritional use of protein, but these have not yet been characterized.

Bacterial metabolites and toxic factors

There are many bacterial metabolites and toxic products that can damage the tissues or stimulate inflammation. They include ammonia, toxic amines, indole, organic acids, hydrogen sulphide, methylmercaptan and dimethyl disulphide (Slots and Genco, 1984).

Gram negative bacterial cell walls contain lipopolysaccharides (LPS, endotoxins) which are released when they die. Distinct LPSs are produced by individual species, but they share common properties, including activating complement by the alternative pathway and stimulating bone resorption in tissue culture. Lipoteichoic acid and peptidoglycans present in Gram positive bacterial cell walls also stimulate bone resorption (Meikle *et al.*, 1986). Extracts from Gram negative bacteria isolated from periodontal pockets can cause polyclonal B-cell activation, which could contribute to periodontal pathology by inducing B-lymphocytes to produce antibodies with determinants unrelated to the activating agent. They can also induce the release of lymphokines that mediate inflammation and bone resorption.

Bacterial antigens

Each bacterial species contains many antigens that can stimulate the immune system and lead to a variety of immune and hypersensitivity reactions, which may contribute to both host protection and tissue damage. It has been established that patients with chronic inflammatory diseases have raised serum antibodies to a variety of periodontopathic bacteria (Taubman *et al.*, 1992). One such bacteria, *Actinobacillus actinomycetemcomitans*, has been found to have 13 major antigen bands, which are recognized by sera from patients with juvenile periodontitis and rapidly progressing periodontitis (Watanabe *et al.*, 1989). Patients with juvenile periodontitis also produce serum antibodies against its leucotoxin (see Chapter 20).

It is known that many important antigen sites are located on or close to the bacterial outer cell membrane, and it has been shown that components of the surface associated material (SAM) (see below) can provoke an immune response. It has been established that one of the main components of SAM from many bacteria is the chaperonins (Coates, 1996), and these, in particular chaperonin 60, are important immunodominant antigens in bacterial infections. In this regard it has been found that a proportion of localized juvenile periodontitis patients have serum antibodies to *A. actinomycetemcomitans* SAM, which can inhibit the osteolytic activity of this material (Meghji *et al.*, 1993). It is probable that the immunodeterminant antigen in these cases is chaperonin 60. It is also known that about half of the patients with localized juvenile periodontitis also produce serum antibodies that neutralize the cell cycle inhibitory activity of gapstatin (White *et al.*, 1995).

Sites of periodontal infections

The sites of periodontal infection are shown in *Figure 5.2* and listed below:

1. Supragingival plaque
2. Subgingival flora which are:
    (a) Attached to the root surface
    (b) Free within the pocket
    (c) Within radicular cementum or dentine
    (d) Attached to the lining of the pocket
    (e) Within the soft tissue wall of the pocket.

In all stages of periodontitis, bacteria are present on the root surface, on the surface of the soft tissue wall of the pocket and free within the pocket. From these sites

bacterial products may enter the tissues through the pocket epithelium, which is often ulcerated.

Bacterial penetration of the radicular cementum and dentine

Actinomyces species may penetrate small distances into cementum, and bacterial products such as LPS may contaminate it. However, the penetration of these products into cementum appears superficial (Moore *et al.*, 1986).

Many Gram negative bacteria have the ability to attach to Gram positive bacteria and epithelial cells (Slots and Genco, 1984). This ability is an important factor in their colonization of the subgingival environment, and also allows them to colonize the surface cells of the pocket epithelium.

Bacterial invasion of the cementum and radicular dentine was thought by early investigators to be an important factor in the pathogenesis of periodontal disease, and Miller (1890) described bacteria invading the the radicular dentine of periodontally diseased teeth. More recently, observations using light microscopy, scanning electron microscopy and bacterial culture have suggested that some bacteria invade cementum and radicular dentine, and that the dentinal tubules may act as reservoirs of putative periodontal pathogens (Adriaens *et al.*, 1984, Adriaens *et al.*, 1987, 1988a, 1988b).

Another recent study (Giuliana *et al*, 1997) attempted to determine the bacterial species which invade the root dentine. Samples of the middle layer of the radicular dentine of 26 periodontally diseased teeth and 14 healthy teeth were taken, and these were further divided into outer, middle and inner parts. All of these samples were cultured anaerobically, and the bacterial concentrations at these sites were expressed as colony forming units (CFU) per mg of tissue. Bacteria were detected in 14 (54%) of the periodontally diseased teeth and in none of the healthy teeth. The concentrations of bacteria ranged from 831–11971 CFU/mg, and the bacteria detected included many of the putative periodontal pathogens such as *Porphyromonas gingivalis*, *Prevotella intermedia*, *Bacteroides forsythus*, *Fusobacterium nucleatum*, *Peptostreptococcus micros* and *Streptococcus intermedius*.

All these findings suggest that radicular dentine could act as a bacterial reservoir from which periodontal pathogens can recolonize treated periodontal pockets, and could thus contribute to the recurrence of disease.

Bacterial invasion

It can be shown from evidence of transient bacteraemias that can follow gingival trauma that, from time to time, bacteria penetrate into the soft tissues of the pocket. However, infection of the soft tissue appears to be rare because of the ability of the immune and inflammatory systems to destroy bacteria in the tissues.

Bacterial invasion of the tissues in periodontitis has mainly been described in cases of advanced chronic periodontitis (Takeuchi *et al.*, 1974; Frank, 1980; Saglie *et al.*,

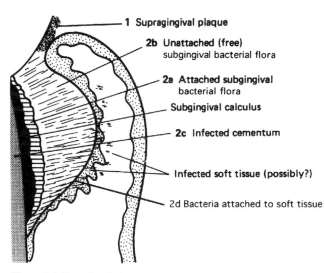

Figure 5.2 Sites of periodontal infection

1982a, 1982b, 1985; Manor *et al.*, 1984) and juvenile periodontitis (Gillett and Johnson, 1982, Carranza *et al.*, 1983; Christersson *et al.*, 1987). Some studies have indicated that putative periodontal pathogens may penetrate epithelium, epithelial cells and connective tissue (Saglie *et al.*, 1986, 1988a, 1988b; Wolinsky *et al.*, 1987, Papapanou *et al.*, 1994; Sandros *et al.*, 1994). On the other hand, another study of advanced chronic and juvenile periodontitis (Liakoni *et al.*, 1987) has concluded that the few bacteria found in the tissues were more likely to result from passive entry in tissue processing than from active invasion.

It has been suggested that bacterial invasion could be a factor in the production of an acute episode of progression in chronic periodontitis (Pertuiset *et al.*, 1987; Saglie *et al.*, 1987, 1988c). In this regard, it has been suggested that the mechanism involved might be the production of local necrosis or microabscesses (Allenspach-Petrzilka and Guggenheim, 1983).

Saglie *et al.* (1987) attempted to test this hypothesis by monitoring 20 patients with advanced chronic periodontitis for episodic progression. When active sites were detected by significant attachment loss, periodontal surgery was performed. Biopsies of the active sites and control inactive sites in the same patient with similar pocket depths were obtained. These tissues were examined by a number of electron microscopical and immunocytochemical techniques. They found statistically significant higher numbers of bacteria in the gingival connective tissue in active as opposed to control sites. *Porphyromonas gingivalis* and *Actinobacillus actinomycetemcomitans* were found most frequently at active sites.

Several recent studies have specifically identified bacterial species in the periodontal tissues of patients with advanced chronic periodontitis or juvenile periodontitis using immunofluorescent techniques or DNA probes (Chapter 13). These are listed in *Table 5.2*.

In these studies, care was taken to avoid translocation of bacteria during the surgery and tissue processing. Saglie *et al.* (1987) claimed that translocation was ruled out in their work because control biopsies did not contain bacteria, a pattern of invasion of the gingival connective tissue was seen in the intercellular spaces, bacteria were seen in the same plane as the tissue elements and bacteria were also seen within phagocytic cells.

Animal studies using normal and immunosuppressed rats (Savani *et al.*, 1985) showed that bacterial invasion of the gingiva only occurred when virulent bacteria overcame normal host defences or when the host defences were compromised by immunosuppression.

Saglie *et al.* (1988b) have also studied the cellular infiltration associated with bacterial invasion of the gingival connective tissue. On the basis of their findings they postulated that inactive periods were associated with T-helper lymphocytes, NK-cells and macrophages and active periods with B-lymphocytes, T-cytotoxic/suppressor lymphocytes, Langerhans cells, pan-lymphocytes and polymorphs. In addition, it has also been shown that bacteria in gingival connective tissue were always associated with specific antibodies, and often also complement (Pekovic and Fillery, 1984). This indicates that a strong immune reaction is mounted against bacteria invading the gingiva. In most situations, the local defence mechanisms will rapidly kill invading bacteria and prevent any multiplication. It would seem that bacteria only rarely multiply in the gingival tissues, and usually in advanced periodontitis. Multiplication of bacteria within the tissues may lead to the formation of a lateral periodontal abscess.

Indirect tissue damage

Immunity

The role of the immune system in tissue degradation

Bacterial antigens penetrate the crevicular epithelium to enter the tissue and stimulate immunity. Both arms of the immune system have the potential for host protection and

Table 5.2 Specific identification of bacteria in gingival tissue

Author	Year	Method	Bacteria	Disease
Courant and Bader	1966	Immunofluorescence	*Bacteroides melaninogenicus*	Chronic periodontitis
Takeuchi *et al.*	1974	Immunofluorescence	*Bacteroides melaninogenicus* *Corynebacterium*	Chronic periodontitis
Saglie *et al.*	1882a	Immunoperoxidase	*Actinobacillus actinomycetemcomitans* *Capnocytophaga sputigena*	Juvenile periodontitis Chronic periodontitis
Pekovic and Fillery	1984	Immunofluorescence	*Actinomyces viscosus* *A. naeslundii* *Porphyromonas gingivalis* *Prevotella intermedia*	Chronic periodontitis
Saglie *et al.*	1988b	Immunoperoxidase	*Porphyromonas gingivalis* *Actinobacillus actinomycetemcomitans* *Capnocytophaga* *Fusobacterium nucleatum* *Bacterionema matruchotii*	Chronic and juvenile periodontitis
Saglie *et al.*	1988a	DNA probes	*Mycoplasma pneumoniae*	Chronic and juvenile periodontitis
Christersson *et al.*	1987	Immunofluorescence	*Actinobacillus actinomycetemcomitans*	Juvenile periodontitis
Wolinsky *et al.*	1987	Immunoperoxidase	*Treponema vincentii*	Chronic periodontitis

tissue damage. Activation of humoral immunity leads to an accumulation of plasma cells and the production of immunoglobulins, which will activate the complement cascade and lead to inflammation and generation of prostaglandins. The accumulated inflammatory cells can release tissue destructive enzymes (see below).

Stimulation of cellular immunity leads to the production of lymphokines from activated T-lymphocytes, which modulate macrophage activity. Activated macrophages (Chapter 3) release a number of cytokines and these can affect other cells, leading to tissue damage. The cytokines released include interleukin-1 (IL-1), tumour necrosis factor (TNF) and gamma interferon (IFNγ) (*Table 5.3*). IL-1 can induce the release of collagenase from a variety of connective tissue cells, including fibroblasts. Osteoclast activation factor (see below) has now been shown to be identical to IL-1 (Dewhirst *et al.*, 1985). Activated T8-lymphocytes (Chapter 3) also release cytotoxic lymphokines known as perforins, which disrupt cell membranes, and connective tissue cells close to activated T-8 cells could be damaged. Some clinical findings support the idea that immune responses take part in the pathogenesis of periodontal disease:

1. Patients receiving immunosuppressive drugs or who have immunodeficiency diseases have less gingival inflammation than might be expected from their oral hygiene status.
2. When drugs that enhance the immune response are given, the severity of gingivitis increases.
3. Patients with a deficiency of white cells (agranulocytosis) have much more severe periodontal disease.
4. Patients with immunosuppression are prone to develop to acute ulcerative gingivitis. This can occur as a complication of HIV infections, and these patients are also prone to develop an aggressive form of periodontitis (Winkler *et al.*, 1988).

Table 5.3 Host and bacterial factors involved in bone resorption

Bacterial
Capsular and surface associated material
Lipopolysaccharides
Lipoteichoic acids
Peptidoglycan
Muramyl dipeptide
Lipoprotein
Host
Inflammatory mediators
Prostaglandins, e.g. PGE_2
Leukotrienes
12-HETEs
Heparin
Thrombin
Bradykinin
Cytokines
Interleukin-1
Interleukin-6
Tumour necrosis factors
Transforming growth factor β
Platelet derived growth factor

Inflammation

Inflammation leads to the accumulation of PMNs, macrophages and mast cells, which are very important in protecting against infection. They do, however, contain destructive enzymes within lysosomes, normally used to degrade phagocytosed material, which are capable of damaging tissue if released. Such enzymes may be released by inflammatory cells during function, or when they degenerate and die.

In addition, inflammatory cells (in particular PMNs) also produce reactive oxygen species (ROS) via the metabolic pathway of the respiratory burst, which occurs in the process of phagocytosis. These include the superoxide anion (O_2^-) and hydrogen peroxide (H_2O_2), which further react together in the presence of transitional metal ions to produce the hydroxyl radical (-OH). The production of these highly reactive oxygen species provides inflammatory cells with a host protective role, killing invading pathogens. However, evidence suggests that ROS can cause connective tissue destruction (Freeman and Crapo, 1982), resulting in the loss of structural integrity and function of the periodontal tissues, when these substances leak into the tissues. The generation of ROS during periodontal disease could be associated with degradation of the connective tissue of the gingiva and periodontium. In this connection, ROS released by PMNs has been shown to damage proteoglycans (Moseley *et al.*, 1995). Cells and tissues in the vicinity of inflammatory cells will be damaged by these processes, and this type of damage around these cells is known as bystander damage.

As ROS can also be produced by osteoclasts and osteoblasts, they may play a role in bone resorption during disease. Bone cells are probably involved in the pathological destruction of the mineralized matrix as a consequence of their altered metabolic activity during active disease, following stimulation by factors from bacteria and mediators such as prostaglandins and IL-1 from gingival fibroblasts and circulating monocytes (Hausmann, 1974; Reynolds *et al.*, 1994). Osteoclasts, stimulated with parathyroid hormone and IL-1, have been shown to produce superoxide anions (Garrett *et al.*, 1990). Moreover, bone resorption by osteoclasts was inhibited by superoxide dismutase, an enzyme that scavenges superoxide (see below).

In order to understand the possible roles of these enzymes and ROS it is necessary briefly to consider collagen and proteoglycan degradation.

Collagen degradation

Collagen degradation is a multistage process (*Figure 5.3*). Each collagen molecule consists of two distinct regions. The larger (96% by weight) part is the triple helical region, which is resistant to attack by most proteinases except collagenase. The smaller terminal regions consist of peptides, known as the terminal peptides, which contain the sites of intra- and intermolecular cross-links. These areas can be attacked by a number of proteinases.

Figure 5.3 A diagram of collagen degradation showing the proteolytic enzymes and inhibitors involved

Collagen fibrils, with intermolecular cross-links, are resistant to the action of collagenases, and under physiological conditions a number of enzymes may act in concert (Harris and Cartwright, 1977). Mammalian collagenases are metalloproteinases, which act at neutral pH in the presence of metal ions to cleave the triple helix into two fragments. They cannot cleave the molecule further, but expose it to the action of other proteinases in the tissues or within cells. Collagenases now known as matrix metalloproteinases (MMPs) 1 and 8 are present in many cells and tissues as latent enzymes, either as pro-enzymes or enzyme inhibitor complexes (Meikle *et al.*, 1986; Birkedal-Hansen, 1993; Birkedal-Hansen *et al.*, 1993; Reynolds *et al.*, 1994; Reynolds, 1996), and need to be activated by other proteinases. Under physiological conditions the tissues are at neutral pH, and neutral proteinases are most likely involved.

The evidence for the possible role of MMPs, and particulary inflammatory cell derived MMPs, MMP-8 and -9, is quite strong (Birkedal-Hansen, 1993; Birkedal-Hansen *et al.*, 1993; Vernillo *et al.*, 1994; Ryan *et al.*, 1996). This includes the production of elevated levels by diseased gingival tissue in culture, the detection of active rather than latent collagenase in GCF, and extracts of adjacent gingival tissue in patients with chronic periodontitis (Fullmer and Gibson, 1966; Golub *et al.*, 1985; Lee *et al.*, 1995) and the presence of MMP messenger RNA in the cells of the periodontal lesion as well as periodontal ligament and gingival fibroblasts, keratinocytes, endothelial cells osteoblasts and osteoclasts. Inflammatory cells, particularly PMNs, are thought to play a major role in the MMP-mediated destructive lesion (Golub *et al.*, 1995, 1998; Lee *et al.*, 1995). Additional evidence for this pathogenic pathway is the presence of elevated MMP protein in periodontal lesions, shown by immunocytochemical studies (Birkedal-Hansen, 1993; Ryan *et al.*, 1996). Moreover, the ability of MMP inhibitors such as doxycycline to retard periodontal breakdown (see Chapter 17) further supports the possible pathogenic role of these proteinases.

Other proteinases, such as the serine proteinase elastase, could also play a role in these processes (Eley and Cox, 1996a). Furthermore, in inflammatory states the tissues surrounding inflammatory cells may be acidified and could also provide suitable conditions for the action of acid proteinases such as cathepsin B (Burleigh, 1977; Eley and Cox, 1996b).

Proteoglycan degradation

When connective tissue is degraded in disease, the catabolism of collagen is often preceded by that of proteoglycans. Proteoglycans are composed of a central protein core to which is attached a variable number of highly anionic glycosaminoglycan (GAG) chains (Bartold, 1987). The structure of proteoglycans (*Figure 5.4*) depends on the type of GAG chains attached to its protein core (see Chapter 1). Several interactions occur between individual proteoglycans and cell surfaces, basal lamina and collagen. The most common GAG in the gingiva and periodontal ligament is hyaluronic acid (hyaluronan), and large amounts of this are found in gingiva. The main proteoglycans in these tissues are small dermatan sulphate proteoglycans and a larger molecular weight chondroitin sulphate proteoglycan, versican, which is capable of interacting with hyaluronan (Embery *et al.*, 1979, 1987; Purvis *et al.*, 1984; Pearson and Pringle, 1986; Larjava *et al.*, 1992). In bone and cementum the principal proteoglycans are two small molecular weight chondroitin sulphate (CS) proteoglycans, named decorin and biglycan, which contain one and two CS chains respectively (Waddington and Embery, 1991).

In proteoglycan degradation (*Figure 5.4*), protein cleavage occurs first to release GAGs from the protein core. A number of metallo-, serine and cysteine proteinases can do this. The metalloproteinases with this function (Birkedal-Hansen, 1993; Reynolds *et al.*, 1994; Reynolds, 1996) are known as stromolysins (MMP-3, -10, -11). The released GAG usually remains intact, but may be further degraded. The role of the hydrolytic enzymes, such as

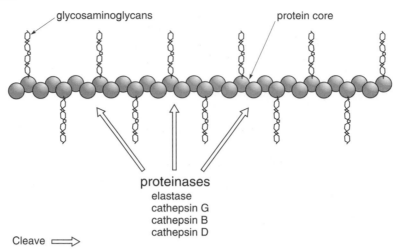

glycosaminoglycans   protein core

proteinases
elastase
cathepsin G
cathepsin B
cathepsin D

Cleave ⟹

Figure 5.4 A diagram of proteoglycan degradation showing the proteolytic enzymes involved

hyaluronidase, chondroitinases, aryl sulphatase and glucuronidases, in degrading proteoglycans is confusing, since none of them are proteolytic. They could be involved in the subsequent degradation of the released GAGs, but observations of GAGs isolated from inflamed gingiva indicate that they remain intact despite the abundance of hydrolytic enzymes in the tissues.

Reactive oxygen species (ROS) have also been shown to damage proteoglycans (Moseley *et al.*, 1995). Both ROS generated by chemical means and from stimulation of isolated polymorphonuclear leucocytes *in vitro* have been shown to produce chain depolymerization, modification of hexuronic acid and hexuronic residues and limited desulphation. These effects were more evident following exposure to -OH radicles, and non-sulphated GAGs were more susceptible than sulphated GAGs to this damage.

Proteolytic enzymes with inflammatory cells (*Figure 5.5*)

The proteolytic enzymes present within inflammatory cells will now be considered. PMNs, macrophages and mast cells will be discussed separately.

Neutrophil polymorphonuclear leucocytes (Figure 5.5a)

PMNs contain and release acid and neutral proteinases (Baggiolini *et al.*, 1980). Four distinct types of cytoplasmic body – azurophilic, specific, C-particles and secretory vacuoles – are formed during polymorph maturation.

The azurophil granules contain neutral serine proteinases, the most important of which are elastase and cathepsin G and small amounts of acid proteinases. The specific granules contain collagenase (MMP-8) and other metalloproteinases, known as gelatinases and stromolysins. The latter enzymes can degrade collagen further once it has been cleaved by collagenase, and also basement membrane collagens and proteoglycans. Of these,

PMNs contain gelatinase B (MMP-9) and some stromolysins (MMP-3 and possibly also MMP-10 and -11) (Birkedal-Hansen, 1993; Reynolds *et al.*, 1994; Reynolds, 1996). The C-granules contain the acid hydrolases cathepsins B and D. Plasminogen activator is stored in secretory vacuoles. While the granule-bound proteinases are only released during phagocytosis, plasminogen activator is secreted. Proteinases can leak from the cells into the tissues during the process of phagocytosis, and are also released when cells degenerate.

Elastase can only occasionally be detected in PMNs in inflamed human gingiva using histochemical peptide substrates that only detect active enzyme (Kennett *et al.*, 1995). In contrast, elastase can be immunocytochemically detected in all gingival PMNs using a monoclonal antibody that can detect both active and inactive enzyme. This suggests that the vast majority of gingival PMNs contain inactive elastase. Using immunocytochemistry, PMNs containing elastase are found throughout the periodontal lesion and in the junctional epithelium migrating into the crevice. Numerous PMNs containing elastase can also be found in the crevice (Kennett *et al.*, 1997a). Occasional PMNs containing active elastase were only seen in a few individuals with severe periodontitis (Kennett *et al.*, 1995), and were found in the junctional epithelium and at the active front of the lesion and could have been associated with disease activity.

PMNs also produce reactive oxygen species (ROS) via the metabolic pathway of the respiratory burst, which occurs in the process of phagocytosis (Freeman and Crapo, 1982). These can leak out of these cells during phagocytosis or when these cells die and degenerate, and can be one cause of bystander damage (see above).

Macrophages (Figure 5.5b)

Macrophages synthesize a variety of proteinases (Baggiolini *et al.*, 1980). The levels are usually low compared

Figure 5.5 Release of proteolytic enzymes and vasoactive substances from inflammatory cells: *(a)* neutrophil polymorphonuclear leucocyte; *(b)* macrophage; *(c)* mast cell; *(d)* fibroblast

with those in PMNs, but the amounts produced become sizeable with time. Acid and neutral proteinases are confined to different intracellular compartments. Acid proteinases (cathepsins B and D) are found in lysosymes, and neutral proteinases in secretory vacuoles. The major neutral proteinase of activated inflammatory macrophages is plasminogen activator. The other neutral proteinases are present in small amounts, and include the metalloproteinase macrophage elastase (MMP-12) and other metalloproteinases collagenase (MMP-1) and gelatinase (MMP-9). The acid lysosomal proteinases are released during phagocytosis and, although small quantities may leak out during this process, they are generally confined to the cell. The neutral proteinases are all secreted. Enzyme secretion, in particular of plasminogen activator, is a characteristic property of activated macrophages.

Cathepsin B can be detected in both macrophages and fibroblasts in human gingiva, either histochemically using peptide substrates detecting only active enzyme, or immunocytochemically using an antibody that detects both active and inactive enzyme (Kennett *et al.*, 1994). This suggests that lysosomal cathepsin B in gingival cells is in an active form. Ultrastructural studies have also shown this proteinase localized within lysosomes and associated with the surface membrane of macrophages (Kennett *et al.*, 1997b). In addition, cathepsin B was seen on the surface of collagen fibrils in the adjacent connective tissue to these cells, and this suggests that it could play a role in connective tissue degradation around these infiltrating cells. In this connection, macrophages containing the enzyme were seen in areas of inflammatory cellular infiltration and also within the junctional epithelium migrating into the crevice. Furthermore, cells containing these enzymes are present in the crevice (Kennett *et al.*, 1997a).

Macrophages also produce reactive oxygen species (ROS) in the process of phagocytosis (Freeman and Crapo, 1982), which may leach from the cells to cause bystander damage. Less ROS is released from these cells than PMNs. Macrophages live for much longer than PMNs, and therefore the release of ROS from dying and degenerating macrophages is much less.

Mast cells (Figure 5.5c)

Mast cells are important in inflammation because they release histamine and other vasoactive compounds. They also contain heparin and a number of proteinases, which are associated with heparin as active tetramers. In the absence of heparin, the enzymes dissociate into inactive monomers. The principal proteolytic enzymes are tryptase and a chymotrypsin-like enzyme.

Tryptase can be histochemically detected in mast cells in the healthy and inflamed human gingiva using synthetic peptide substrates (Kennett *et al.*, 1993). Mast cells are mainly present in the lamina propria, but were also found in the junctional epithelium migrating into the crevice. Greater numbers of these cells are found in inflamed as compared to healthy gingiva. Mast cells

containing tryptase are also found in the gingival crevice (Kennett *et al.*, 1997a).

Fibroblasts (Figure 5.5d)

Fibroblasts are found throughout the connective tissues and are the main cells secreting and degrading collagen under physiological conditions (Everts *et al.*, 1996). Small amounts of collagen are phagocytosed and degraded intracellularly, primarily by cysteine proteinases (see Chapter 1). Larger amounts of collagen may be degraded by these cells extracellularly as a result of their secretion of metalloproteinases. They contain two forms of lysosomes, one containing cathepsin B, cathepsin L and dipeptidylpeptidase (DPP) II, and the other, collagenase (MMP-1), other MMPs (MMP-2, MMP-3, -10, -11), α_1 antiproteinase inhibitor, α_2 macroglobulin and TIMP (*Figure 5.3d*). All of these enzymes and inhibitors may be secreted by these cells when suitably stimulated.

Control of proteolytic enzymes

Macrophages, fibroblasts and the extracellular environment contain the proteinase inhibitors alpha-1-proteinase inhibitor (α_1PI) and alpha-2-macroglobulin (α_2M), which are responsible for inactivating proteinases in the tissues (Kennett *et al.*, 1995). Active enzyme in the tissues can only cause damage if there is an enzyme/inhibitor imbalance. This could take place in the close environment of these cells, where bystander damage could occur. It might also be a local feature of episodic periodontal disease activity.

The synthesis and secretion of proteinases in both health and disease is controlled by the activation of the appropriate gene(s) by the cellular messenger system, which itself is under the control of the activation of cell surface receptors by the appropriate growth factor or cytokine. In this regard, it has recently been shown that interleukin (IL)-1β can upregulate MMP-3 (at both the mRNA and protein level) in periodontal ligament cells (Nakaya *et al.*, 1997), and may control the release of this proteinase in both health and disease. In addition, IL-1β and tumour necrosis factor (TNF) have also been shown to stimulate the release of cathepsin B (Hussain *et al.*, 1997), and TNF α dipeptidylpeptidase IV (Kennett *et al.*, 1997c), from cultured gingival fibroblasts.

Connective tissue degradation by inflammatory cell proteinases

Proteoglycans can be degraded at neutral pH by elastase and cathepsin G (serine proteinases, SP), and at acid pH by cathepsin B (cysteine proteinase, CP) and cathepsin D (carboxylproteinase).

Collagenase (matrix metalloproteinase, MMP) can be activated at neutral pH by tryptase and plasmin (SP), and at acid pH by cathepsin B (CP). The terminal peptide regions of collagen can be cleaved at neutral pH by elastase, and at acid pH by cathepsin B.

The triple helix of collagen is specifically cleaved by specific collagenases (MMP-1, -8) and further degraded at neutral pH by gelatinases (MMP-3, -9) and elastase (SP), and at acid pH by cathepsin B (CP).

Proteoglycans, basement membrane collagens (type IV, X and XI), laminin and fibronectin can be degraded at neutral pH by stromolysins (MMP-3, -10, -11) and elastase (SP), and at acid pH by cathepsins B and L (CP).

Tryptase (SP) can also cleave complement to generate C3a and thus increase vascular permeability; mast cell chymase (SP) can attack basal lamina, increasing epithelial permeability.

The degradation products of proteoglycans (GAGs) have been found in crevicular fluid (Embery *et al.*, 1982); collagenase, elastase, cathepsins B, D and G, tryptase, chymotrypsin and aminopeptidases have been found in gingival tissue and/or crevicular fluid (Meikle *et al.*, 1986; Cox and Eley, 1987, 1989a, 1989b, 1989c). The activity of a number of crevicular fluid proteases have been positively correlated with the severity of chronic periodontitis, and also significantly decrease following basic periodontal treatment and periodontal surgery (Cox and Eley, 1992; Eley and Cox, 1992a, 1992b, 1992c). To date, elastase, cathepsin B and dipeptidylpeptidases II and IV have been shown to be predictors of disease activity in longitudinal studies (Eley and Cox, 1995, 1996a, 1996b) (see also Chapter 13).

Bone resorption

The host and bacterial factors involved in bone resorption are summarized in *Table 5.3*. Understanding of how these work requires a knowledge of the physiology of bone resorption, which is briefly described in this section.

Bone resorption is probably the most critical factor in periodontal attachment loss leading to eventual tooth loss. Substances produced by the subgingival bacterial flora and the tissues during inflammation and immune reactions may affect bone turnover, either by causing the differentiation and stimulation of osteoclasts or by inhibiting bone formation by osteoblasts.

Host and bacterial factors involved in bone resorption

The factors thought to be involved in bone resorption have been studied with tissue culture systems using embryonic bone labelled with radioactive calcium, and bone loss can be detected and measured by the release of this marker. The substances that can induce resorption in periodontal disease come from two sources:

1. Subgingival bacteria
2. Periodontal tissues.

Bacterial factors

Substances from bacteria include lipopolysaccharides (LPS) from Gram negative bacteria (Hausmann *et al.*, 1970; Hausmann, 1974), lipoteichoic acid from *Actinomyces viscosus* (Hausmann, 1974; Hausmann *et al.*, 1975), peptidoglycan (Lensgraf *et al.*, 1979), muramyl dipeptide (MDP) (Dewhirst, 1982), bacterial lipoprotein (Millar *et al.*, 1986), and capsular or surface associated material (SAM) from Gram negative bacteria (Wilson *et al.*, 1985), which can stimulate bone resorption *in vitro* using the murine calvaria model. The potency to cause resorption *in vitro* varies with each source; LPS is 10 times more potent than lipoteichoic acid, and capsular material is 1000 times more potent than the corresponding LPS (Hopps and Sisney-Durrant, 1991). Peptidoglycan, MDP and bacterial lipoprotein are all less potent than the three materials above.

There are also different effects due to the different bacterial sources of these materials. In this regard, LPS from *P. gingivalis* is more active than that from *A. actinomycetemcomitans*, *C. ochracea* or *F. nucleatum*. Some bacterial LPS, such as that from *E. corrodens*, also release cytokines such as IL-1 and/or IL-6 from osteoblasts and fibroblasts, but most do not (Reddi *et al.*, 1995a; Wilson, 1995). However, LPS is known to activate the complement cascade by the alternative pathway, which in turn generates prostaglandins.

It has been shown during the last decade that proteins associated with the outer surfaces of some, but not all, periodontopathogens are potent inducers of cell and tissue pathology *in vitro* (Wilson *et al.*, 1985, 1993; Meghji *et al.*, 1992; Wilson and Henderson, 1995). Capsular material or surface-associated material (SAM) can stimulate the production of prostaglandin E$_2$ (PGE$_2$) and collagenase from bone cells (Harvey *et al.*, 1987).

The SAMs from *P. gingivalis* and *Eikenella corrodens* appear to achieve this by first releasing IL-1, which then stimulates the release of PGE$_2$ and collagenase (Henderson and Blake, 1992). Inhibition of bone DNA and collagen production by osteoblasts in murine calvaria is produced by low titres of SAM from *P. gingivalis* and *E. corrodens*, and this may be due to this mechanism because it is blocked by indomethacin, an inhibitor of prostaglandins (Meghji *et al.*, 1992).

The SAM from *A. actinomycetemcomitans* is most potent in stimulating bone resorption *in vitro*. However, it appears to produce this effect by mimicking the action of IL-1. The main cytokine released from connective tissue and bone cells by SAMs is IL-6, and it seems that this release may either be stimulated by IL-1 or stimulated directly. This is of particular relevance because IL-6 has been shown to stimulate the formation of osteoclasts (Löwick *et al.*, 1989).

The constituents of the SAM from *A. actinomycetemcomitans* have been recently characterized (Wilson and Henderson, 1995). This SAM is made up of a number of proteins and peptides with potent biological actions that are relevant to the pathology of both chronic periodontitis and juvenile periodontitis (Wilson and Henderson, 1995). These include: first, a protein with potent osteolytic activity that has close homology to the molecular chaperone from *Escherichia coli*, known either as chaperonin 60 or GroEL (Meghji *et al.*, 1994; Kirby *et al.*, 1995); secondly, a protein with anti-mitotic activity, which has been termed gapstatin (White *et al.*, 1995); and thirdly, a potent cytokine-inducing peptide, which acts by stimulating IL-6 gene transcription (Nair *et al.*, 1996). This cytokine is pro-inflammatory and plays a role in the differentiation and maturation of T- and B-lymphocytes (see Chapter 3 and *Table 3.1*). These proteins are active in the picogram to nanogram per ml concentration range, and it is presumed that their actions are important in the pathogenesis of chronic periodontitis and juvenile periodontitis by stimulating alveolar bone resorption (Wilson *et al.*, 1985, 1993; Kirby *et al.*, 1995; Reddi *et al.*, 1995b), inhibiting bone and periodontal ligament regeneration and repair (Kamin *et al.*, 1986; Wilson *et al.*, 1988; Meghji *et al.*, 1992) and promoting B-lymphocyte and plasma cell proliferation (Reddi *et al.*, 1995c, 1996a, 1996b; Henderson *et al.*, 1996; Wilson *et al.*, 1996).

Host factors

The main host-derived bone-resorbing factors appear to be the eicosanoids and cytokines, which are generated in the gingiva and periodontium during the inflammatory and immune reactions.

Eicosanoids

Prostaglandins, hydroxyeicosatetraenoic acids (HETEs) and leukotrienes are inflammatory mediators derived from cell membrane phospholipids by the action of cyclooxygenase or lipoxygenases on arachadonic acid. These compounds are secreted by cells involved in inflammatory and immune reactions, such as macrophages, PMNs and endothelial cells. These are also released by some cells during normal function, such as fibroblasts and osteoblasts. Many of these compounds have been implicated in the pathogenesis of periodontal diseases (Seymour and Heasman, 1988).

The prostaglandins (PG) were the first mediators of local bone resorption to be discovered, and may be one of the most important factors in periodontal bone loss. PGE_1, PGE_2 and prostacyclin (PGI_2) all stimulate bone resorption in tissue culture systems, but PGE_2 is the most potent and stimulates increasing resorption in concentrations ranging from 1 nM–10 μM (Dietrich *et al.*, 1975). The levels of PGE_2 found in inflamed gingival tissue (Ohm *et al.*, 1984) and GCF from inflamed sites (Offenbacher *et al.*, 1984) fall well within the levels stimulating bone resorption *in vitro*. The GCF levels of PGE_2 also correlate with the periodontal disease status, and have been claimed to predict periodontal attachment loss (Offenbacher *et al.*, 1986).

The role of prostaglandins in alveolar bone loss is supported by numerous experiments in which the effects of non-steroidal anti-inflammatory drugs (NSAIDs) on periodontal bone loss have been studied. Drugs such as indomethacin and flurbiprofen, which inhibit the synthesis of prostaglandins, markedly reduce bone loss in experimental periodontitis in animals induced by ligaments (Nyman *et al.*, 1979; Weakes-Dybvig *et al.*, 1982; Williams *et al.*, 1988) or diet (Lasfargues and Saffir, 1983).

In addition, lipo-oxygenase products of arachidonic acid also stimulate bone resorption in tissue culture experiments (Meghji *et al.*, 1988). Leukotrienes and 12-HETE are potent stimulators of bone resorption at picomolar or nanomolar concentrations. Relatively high levels of leukotrienes and HETEs are present in inflamed gingival tissue (Sighagen *et al.*, 1982; El Attar and Lin, 1982) and diseased periodontal pocket tissue (El Attar *et al.*, 1986). These experiments also showed that gingival tissue in culture metabolized arachidonic acid, mainly through the lipo-oxygenase pathway, and if this also occurs *in vivo* then these would be important bone resorbing factors.

Other products of inflammation

Heparin from mast cell can enhance bone resorption in tissue culture systems induced by LPS and lipoteichoic acid, but cannot induce bone resorption on its own. Thrombin, an inflammatory mediator and end product of the blood coagulation cascade, is a potent bone resorbing agent (Dziak, 1993). Another inflammatory agent, bradykinin, evokes similar effects, and in both cases these effects are independent of prostaglandin production.

Cytokines

Several cytokines produced during inflammation stimulate bone resorption *in vitro*, and these represent a potentially important major group of host-derived bone resorbing factors that may play a role in alveolar bone loss in periodontal disease. The cytokines that have been shown to stimulate bone resorption *in vitro* include interleukin (IL)-1α and -β (Gowen and Munday, 1986), tumour necrosis factor (TNF) α and β (Bertolini *et al.*, 1986), transforming growth factor (TGF) (Tashjian *et al.*, 1985) and platelet derived growth factor (PDGF) (Tashjian *et al.*, 1982). In addition, IL-6 produced by fibroblasts, endothelial cells and osteoblasts may stimulate the formation of osteoclasts from precursor cells (Löwick *et al.*, 1989). Out of all these cytokines, IL-1 and TNF are the most potent stimulators of bone resorption and are the only ones so far to be implicated in periodontal pathology (Hopps and Sisney-Durrant, 1991). IL-1 has widespread effects on non-immune cells, and these are shown in *Table 5.4*.

IL-1 is 100 times more potent than TNF, and can produce resorption in picomolar concentrations. Osteoclast activation factor (OAF) has now been shown to be identical with IL-1β (Dewhirst *et al.*, 1985). IL-1β has been found in significant amounts in inflamed gingiva, but has not been detected in healthy gingiva (Hönig *et al.*,

Table 5.4 Action of IL-1 on non-immune cells

Tissue/cell type	Prostaglandin synthesis	Proliferation	Protein synthesis	Other effects
Brain	+	−		Fever
Synovial cells	+	−	Collagenase	Proteolytic enzyme release
Bone/osteoblasts	−	−	Collagenase	−
Cartilage/chondrocytes	+	−	Plasminogen activator	−
Muscle cells	+	−	−	Proteolytic enzyme release
Fibroblasts	+	+	Collagenase	−
Endothelium	+	+	Pro-coagulant activity	Boosts macrophage and PMN adhesion
Epithelium	−	−	Type IV collagen	−
Liver/hepatocytes	−	−	Acute phase proteins	−

1989). Both IL-1α and -β have been found in GCF from diseased sites in nanomolar concentrations that are sufficient to cause bone loss *in vitro* (Masada *et al.*, 1990). TNFα has also been detected in GCF but in low levels which are below those necessary for bone resorption *in vitro* (Rossomando *et al.*, 1990).

The mechanism of bone resorption

The account below is based upon a wealth of experimental evidence reviewed in articles by Vaes (1988), Dziak (1993) and Meghji (1992).

Bone is continually remodelled by the combined activities of osteoblasts and osteoclasts, and in pathological situations like chronic periodontitis there may be a preponderance of bone resorption over formation due to a variety of factors discussed in the previous section. The bone loss in periodontal disease occurs at local sites, but it is regulated by both systemic and local factors.

Osteoclasts are the main effector cells in the resorptive process, but it has been shown in tissue culture experiments that bone resorption cannot occur without the presence of both osteoblasts and osteoclasts. All systemic and local bone resorbing factors exert their influence by stimulating the osteoblast (*Figure 5.3*). Osteoblasts are involved in the regulation of osteoclast function at several levels. Osteoblasts have receptors for systemic factors such as parathormone (PTH) and 1,25(OH)$_2$(vitamin D$_3$), which affect general remodelling, and locally produced factors such as prostaglandins, leukotrienes and cytokines, which affect local changes, and all exert their influence by stimulating the osteoblast in a specific way (Meikle *et al.*, 1986). In distinction, the systemic hormone, calcitonin, which favours bone deposition directly inhibits osteoclasts and causes their disaggregation into mononuclear cells. Osteoclasts have numerous receptors for calcitonin (*Figure 5.6*).

As explained in the previous section, several of the locally produced factors are increased by the inflammatory and immune reactions of chronic periodontitis, and some are produced by subgingival bacteria. Osteoblasts stimulated by these factors (*Figure 5.6*) mediate their response through a series of intracellular secondary messenger systems. One pathway involves cyclic AMP, and a second involves membrane phospholipids, dicycloglycerol, protein kinase C and cystolic calcium. Both of these mechanisms are stimulated by PGE$_2$ and prostocyclin (PGI$_2$), and thrombin and bradykinin. The leukotrienes and cytokines (IL-1, TNFs) do not appear to affect these intracellular mechanisms, and must involve others at present unknown. In response to this stimulus, osteoblasts secrete factors that both prepare the bone surface for osteoclastic resorption and stimulate the development of functional osteoclasts.

Osteoclast production involves the formation of precursor cells from stem cells in the bone marrow and the migration of these to the bone surface, where they remain as pre-osteoclasts until they receive the appropriate stimulus (*Figure 5.6*). Osteoblasts stimulate osteoclast formation by the secretion of cytokines and cell-to-cell contact. Osteoblasts secrete growth factors, in particular granulocyte/macrophage colony stimulating factor (GM-CSF) and macrophage colony stimulating factor (M-CSF), and IL-6. IL-6 secretion is stimulated by IL-1 attachment to its osteoblast receptor. In combination with GM-CSF, and by the attachment of IL-1, M-CSF and IL-3, it can stimulate the development of precursor cells in the marrow. IL-6 also stimulates the differentiation and maturation of these cells into osteoclasts. It cannot, however, stimulate the mature osteoclast.

Stimulated osteoblasts secrete prostaglandins and a protein made of two components (activation factor), which is responsible for activating the mature osteoclast (*Figure 5.6*). Prostaglandins also modulate osteoclast function. The pre-osteoclasts divide and fuse into multinucleated osteoclasts, and spread over the bone surface prior to resorption. Stimulated osteoblasts also secrete pro-collagenase and plasminogen activator. Plasminogen activator generates plasmin from plasminogen, and this activates pro-collagenase. This is then responsible for removing the non-mineralized collagenous surface layer, which covers most bone surfaces in preparation for osteoclastic resorption.

Osteoclastic resorption involves first, a solubilization of the mineral phase and secondly, a dissolution of the organic matrix, and these processes take place extracellularly (*Figure 5.7*). The resorption area is defined beneath

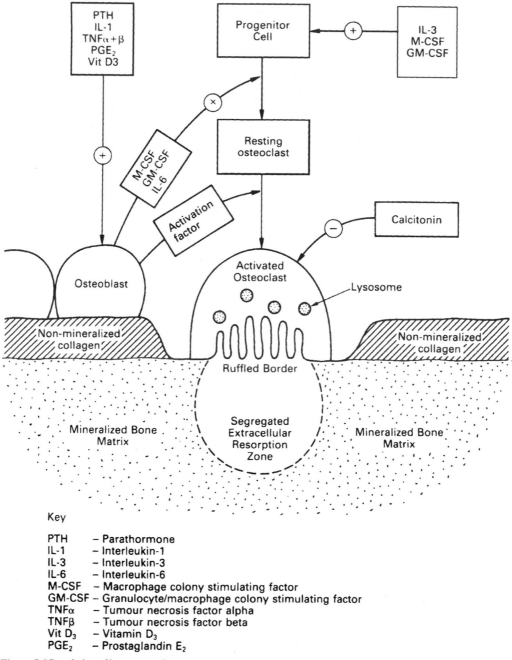

Figure 5.6 Regulation of bone resorption

the ruffled border of the osteoclast. This is a highly specialized region of cytoplasmic infolding of the plasma membrane, below which is outlined a sealing or clear zone. This contains podosomes, which are specialized protrusions of the ventral membrane of the osteoclast, which adhere directly to the bone surface being broken down.

The mineral is dissolved by acid secretion, which is brought about by an electrogenic hydrogen ion transporting system. This is an ATPase-driven proton pump (*Fig-*

ure 5.7). Intracellular pH regulation is achieved by carbonic anhydrase, which is abundant in the osteoclast cytoplasm. Bicarbonate, generated by carbonic anhydrase, appears to be secreted from the basal outer membrane via HCO_3/Cl^- exchange. The hydrogen ions are released into the functionally extracellular lysosomal compartment, and here they solubilize the mineral.

Osteoclasts also produce reactive oxygen species (ROS), which may play a role in the pathological demineralization of bone during disease (Garrett *et al.*, 1990).

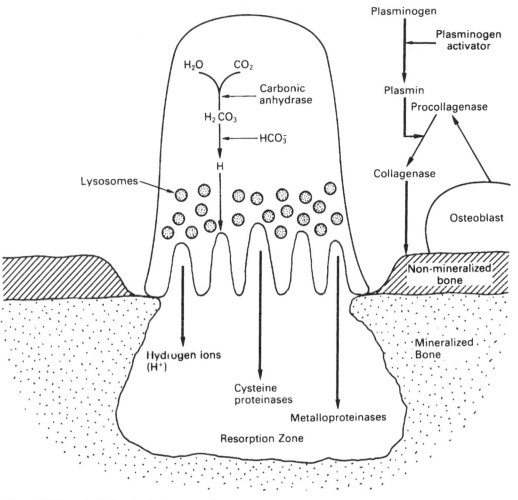

Figure 5.7 Osteoclastic function in bone resorption

Osteoclasts involved in the pathological destruction of the mineralized matrix may have altered metabolic activity during active disease, following stimulation by factors from bacteria and inflammatory mediators such as prostaglandins and IL-1 released by gingival fibroblasts and circulating monocytes (Hausmann, 1974; Reynolds *et al.*, 1994). In this regard, osteoclasts stimulated with parathyroid hormone and IL-1 have been shown to produce superoxide anions (Garrett *et al.*, 1990). In addition, bone resorption by osteoclasts has been shown to be inhibited by superoxide dismutase, an enzyme that scavenges superoxide.

Hydrogen ions and/or ROS create a suitable pH for the lysosomal cysteine proteinase enzyme activity that is involved in the first stage of the degradation of the demineralized bone matrix. This involves the secretion of acid cysteine proteinases, including cathepsins B, L and N, which have been shown to be capable of degrading collagen and proteoglycans under these conditions (*Figure 5.7*). However, recently it has been shown that the degradation of the demineralized organic matrix of bone by osteoclasts involves the production, secretion and function of both cysteine- and metalloproteinases (Everts *et al.*, 1992; Everts *et al.*, 1994). Using a bone tissue culture system they showed that, when selective inhibitors of either cysteine proteinases or metalloproteinases were separately added to the system, bone demineralization occurred, but there was no degradation of the remaining organic bone matrix. Therefore, degradation of the organic matrix involves both cysteine proteinases and metalloproteinases (*Figure 5.7*). It seems likely that the cysteine proteinases are responsible for the first stage of degradation, when the environment within the bone-resorbing compartment below the ruffled border of the osteoclast is acid. They probably degrade the proteoglycans of the bone matrix and attack the non-helical terminal portions of the collagen molecules. In addition, they may also function to activate the metalloproteinase pro-enzymes. As the pH in this environment increases, the metalloproteinase may become functional and then attack the helical portion of the collagen molecules.

References

Abiko, Y., Hayakawa, M., Murai, S. and Takiguchi, H. (1985) Glycylprolyl dipeptidyl aminopeptidase from *Bacteroides gingivalis*. *Journal of Dental Research* **64**, 106–111

Adriaens, P.A., Claeys, G.W. and De Boever, J.A. (1984) Colonization of human dentin by a mixed flora of oral bacteria *in vitro*. *Caries Research* **18** Abstr. 21, 160

Adriaens, P.A., Loesche, W.J. and De Boever, J.A. (1987) Bacteriology of the flora present in the roots of periodontally diseased teeth. *Journal of Dental Research* **66** Abstr. 1855, 338

Adriaens, P.A., De Boever, J.A. and Loesche, W.J. (1988a) Bacterial invasion in root cementum and radicular dentin of periodontally diseased teeth in humans. *Journal of Periodontology* **59**, 222–230

Adriaens, P.A., Edwards, C.A., De Boever, J.A. and Loesche, W.J. (1988b) Ultrastructural observations on bacterial invasion in cementum and radicular dentin of periodontally diseased human teeth. *Journal of Periodontology* **59**, 493–503

Aduse-Opoku, J., Muir, J., Slaney, J.M. *et al.* (1995) Characterization, genetic analysis and expression studies of a protease antigen (PrpR1) of *Porphyromonas gingivalis* W50. *Infection and Immunity* **63**, 4744–4754

Aduse-Opoku, J., Slaney, J.M., Rangarajan, M., Booth, V., Cridland, J., Shepherd, P. and Curtis, M.A. (1996) Characterization of an adherence and antigen determinant of the Arg 1 protease *Porphyromonas gingivalis* which is present on multiple gene products. *Infection and Immunity* **64**, 2532–2539

Allenspach-Petrzilka, G.E. and Guggenheim, B. (1983) Bacterial invasion of the periodontium; an important factor in the pathogenesis of periodontitis? *Journal of Clinical Periodontology* **10**, 609–617

Baggiolini, M., Schnyder, J., Bretz, U. *et al.* (1980) Cellular mechanisms of proteinase release from inflammatory cells and degradation of extracellular proteins. In *Protein Degradation in Health and Disease* (D. Evered and J. Whelan, eds), pp. 105–121. Ciba Foundation Symposium 75

Bartold, P.M. (1987) Proteoglycans in the periodontium. Structure, role and function. *Journal of Periodontal Research* **22**, 431–444

Barua, P.K., Neiders, M.E., Topolnyeky, A. *et al.* (1989) Purification of an 8000 Mr glycylprolyl peptidase from *Bacteroides gingivalis*. *Infection and Immunity* **57**, 2522–2528

Bertolini, D.R., Nedwin, G.E., Bringman, T.S. *et al.* (1986) Stimulation of bone resorption *in vitro* by human tumour necrosis factors. *Nature* **319**, 516–519

Birkedal-Hansen, H. (1993) Role of matrix metalloproteinases in human periodontal diseases. *Journal of Periodontology* **64**, 474–484

Birkedal-Hansen, H., Moore, W., Bodden, M. *et al.* (1993) Matrix metalloproteinases: a review. *Critical Reviews of Oral Biology and Medicine* **4**, 197–250

Birkedal-Hansen, H., Taylor, R.E., Zambon, J.J. *et al.* (1988) Characterization of collagenolytic activity from strains of *Bacteroides gingivalis*. *Journal of Periodontal Research* **23**, 258–264

Bourgeau, G., Laponte, H., Péloquin, P. and Maryland, D. (1992) Cloning, expression and sequencing of a protease gene (tpr) from *Porphyromonas gingivalis* W83 in *Escherichia coli*. *Infection and Immunity* **60**, 3186–3192

Bulkacz, J., Newman, M.G., Socransky, S.S. *et al.* (1979) Phospholipase A activity of micro-organisms from dental plaque. *Microbiology Letters* **10**, 79–88

Bulkacz, J., Schuster, G.S., Singh, B. and Scott, D.F. (1985) Phospholipase A activity of extracellular products from *Bacteroides melaninogenicus* on epithelial tissue cultures. *Journal of Periodontal Research* **20**, 146–153

Burleigh, M.C. (1977) Degradation of collagen by non-specific proteinases. In *Proteinases in Mammalian Cells and Tissues* (A.J. Barrett, ed.), pp. 185–209. Amsterdam: Elsevier/North-Holland Biomedical Press

Carlsson, J., Hofling, J.F. and Sundqvist, G.K. (1984) Degradation of albumin, haemopexin, heptoglobin and transferrin by black-pigmented *Bacteroides* species. *Journal of Medical Microbiology* **18**, 39–46

Carlsson, J., Hermann, B.F., Hofling, J.F. and Sundqvist, G.K. (1984) Degradation of the human proteinase inhibitors alpha-1-antitrypsin and alpha-2-macroglobulin by *Bacteroides gingivalis*. *Infection and Immunity* **43**, 644–648

Carranza, F.A., Saglie, F.R., Newman, M.G. and Valentin, P.L. (1983) Scanning and transmission electron microscopic study of tissue-invading microorganisms in localised juvenile periodontitis. *Journal of Periodontology* **54**, 598–617

Chen, Z., Potempa, J., Polanowski, A. *et al.* (1992) Purification and characterization of a 50-kDa cysteine proteinase (gingipain) from *Porphyromonas gingivalis*. *Journal of Biological Chemistry* **267**, 18896–18901

Christersson, L.A., Wikesjö, U.M.A., Albini, B. *et al.* (1987) Tissue localization of *Actinobacillus actinomycetemcomitans* in human periodontitis. 1. Light, immunofluorescent and electron microscopic studies. *Journal of Periodontology* **58**, 529–539

Claesson, R., Edlund, M.B., Persson, S. and Carlsson, J. (1990) Production of volatile sulphur compounds by various *Fusobacterium* species. *Oral Microbiology and Immunology* **5**, 137–142

Coates, A.R.M. (1996) In *The Chaperonins* (R.J. Ellis, ed.), pp. 267–296. London: Academic Press

Courant, P. and Bader, H. (1966) *Bacteroides melaninogenicus* and its products in the gingiva of man. *Periodontics* **4**, 131–136

Cox, S.W. and Eley, B.M. (1987) Preliminary studies on cysteine and serine proteinase activities in inflamed human gingiva using different 7-amino-4-trifluoromethyl coumarin substrates and protease inhibitors. *Archives of Oral Biology* **32**, 599–605

Cox, S.W. and Eley, B.M. (1989a) Identification of a tryptase-like enzyme in extracts of inflamed human gingiva by effector and gel filtration studies. *Archives of Oral Biology* **34**, 219–221

Cox, S.W. and Eley, B.M. (1989b) Tryptase-like activity in crevicular fluid from gingivitis and periodontitis patients. *Journal of Periodontal Research* **24**, 41–44

Cox, S.W. and Eley, B.M. (1989c) The detection of cathepsin B and L-, elastase-, tryptase-, trypsin-, and dipeptidyl peptidase IV-like activities in crevicular fluid from gingivitis and periodontitis patients with peptidyl derivatives of 7-amino-4-trifluoromethyl coumarin. *Journal of Periodontal Research* **24**, 353–361

Cox, S.W. and Eley, B.M. (1992) Cathepsin B/L-, elastase-, tryptase-, trypsin- and dipeptidylpeptidase IV-like activities in gingival crevicular fluid: a comparison of levels before and after basic periodontal treatment. *Journal of Clinical Periodontology* **19**, 333–339

Cox, S.W., Gazi, M.I., Clark, D.T. and Eley, B.M. (1993) Host tissue and *Porphyromonas gingivalis* dipeptidyl peptidase activities in gingival crevicular fluid. *Journal of Dental Research* **72**, 705

Curtis, M.A., Ramakrishnan, M and Slaney, J.M. (1993) Characterization of the trypsin-like enzymes of *P. gingivalis* W83 using a radio-labelled active-site-directed inhibitor. *Journal of General Microbiology* **139**, 949–955

De Carlo, A.A. Jnr, Windsor, L.J., Boden, M.K. *et al.* (1997) Activation and novel processing of matrix metalloproteinases by a thiol-proteinase from the oral anaerobe *Porphyromonas gingivalis*. *Journal of Dental Research* **76**, 1260–1270

Dewhirst, F.E. (1982) N-acetyl muramyl dipeptide stimulation of bone resorption in tissue culture. *Infection and Immunity* **35**, 133–137

Dewhirst, F.E., Stashenko, P.P., Mole, J.E. and Tsurumachi, T. (1985) Purification and partial sequence of osteoclast-activation factor: identity with interleukin-1-beta. *Journal of Immunology* **135**, 2562–2568

Dietrich, F.E., Goodson, J.M. and Raisz, L.G. (1975) Stimulation of bone resorption by various prostaglandins in organ culture. *Prostaglandins* **10**, 231–240

Dziak, R. (1993) Biochemical and molecular mediators of bone metabolism. *Journal of Periodontology* **64**, 407–415

El Attar, T.M.A. and Lin, H.S. (1982) Relative conversion of arachidonic acid through lipo-oxygenase and cyclo-oxygenase pathways by homogenates of diseased periodontal tissues. *Journal of Oral Pathology* **12**, 7–10

El Attar, T.M.A., Lin, H.S., Killoy, W.J. *et al.* (1986) Hydroxy fatty acid and prostaglandin formation in diseased periodontal pocket tissue. *Journal of Periodontal Research* **21**, 169–176

Eley, B.M. and Cox, S.W. (1992a) Cathepsin B/L-, elastase-, tryptase-, trypsin- and dipeptidylpeptidase IV-like activities in gingival crevicular fluid: correlation with clinical parameters in untreated chronic periodontitis patients. *Journal of Periodontal Research* **27**, 62–69

Eley, B.M. and Cox, S.W. (1992b) Correlation of gingival crevicular fluid proteases with clinical and radiological measurements of periodontal attachment loss. *Journal of Dentistry* **20**, 90–99

Eley, B.M. and Cox, S.W. (1992c) Cathepsin B/L-, elastase-, tryptase-, trypsin- and dipeptidylpeptidase IV-like activities in gingival crevicular fluid: a comparison before and after periodontal surgery. *Journal of Periodontology* **63**, 412–417

Eley, B.M. and Cox, S.W. (1995) Correlation between gingival crevicular fluid dipeptidyl peptidase II and IV and periodontal attachment loss. *Oral Diseases* **1**, 201–213

Eley, B.M. and Cox, S.W. (1996a) A 2-year longitudinal study of elastase in gingival crevicular fluid and periodontal attachment loss. *Journal of Clinical Periodontology* **23**, 681–692

Eley, B.M. and Cox, S.W. (1996b) The relationship between gingival crevicular fluid cathepsin B and periodontal attachment loss in chronic periodontitis patients. A 2-year longitudinal study. *Journal of Periodontal Research* **31**, 381–392

Embery, G., Oliver, W.M. and Stanbury, J.B. (1979) The metabolism of proteoglycans and glycosaminoglycans in inflamed human gingiva. *Journal of Periodontal Research* **14**, 512–519

Embery, G., Olivier, W.M., Stanbury, J.B. and Purvis, J.A. (1982) The electrophoretic detection of acid glycosaminoglycans in human gingival sulcular fluid. *Archives of Oral Biology* **27**, 177–179

Embery, G., Picton, D. and Stanbury, J.B. (1987) Biochemical changes in the periodontal ligament ground substance associated with short-term intrusive loading in adult monkeys. *Archives of Oral Biology* **32**, 545–549

Endo, J., Otsuka, M., Ohara, E. *et al.* (1989) Cleavage action of a trypsin-like protease from *Bacteroides gingivalis* 381 on reduced egg-white lysozyme. *Archives of Oral Biology* **34**, 911–916

Everts, V., Delaissé, J.M., Korper, W. *et al.* (1992) Degradation of collagen in the bone-resorbing compartment of the osteoclast involves both cysteine-proteinase and matrix metalloproteinases. *Journal of Cell Physiology* **150**, 221–231

Everts, V., Creemers, L. and Beertsen, W. (1994) The use of selective inhibitors in the study of collagen breakdown. *Proceedings of Royal Microscopical Society* **29** Abstr. 7c, 216

Everts, V., Van der Zee, E., Creemers, L. and Beertsen, W. (1996) Phagocytosis and intracellular digestion of collagen, its role in turnover and remodelling. *Histochemical Journal* **28**, 229–245

Fiehn, N.-E. (1986) Enzyme activities from eight small-sized oral spirochaetes. *Scandinavian Journal of Dental Research* **94**, 132–140

Fletcher, J., Reddi, K., Poole, S. *et al.* (1997) Interactions between periodontopathic bacteria and cytokines. *Journal of Periodontal Research* **32**, 200–205

Fletcher, J., Nair, S., Poole, S. *et al.* (1998) Cytokine degradation by biofilms of *Porphyromonas gingivalis* **36**, 216–219

Fosdick, L.S., Blackwell, R.Q. and Carter, W.J. (1953) Chemical studies on periodontal disease. *Journal of Dental Research* **32**, 646–651

Frank, R.M. (1980) Bacterial penetration in the apical pocket wall of advanced human periodontitis. *Journal of Periodontal Research* **15**, 563–573

Freeman, B.A. and Crapo, J.C. (1982) Biology of disease. Free radicals and tissue injury. *Laboratory Investigations* **47**, 421–426

Fujimura, S. and Nakamura, T. (1987) Isolation and characterization of a protease from *Bacteroides gingivalis*. *Infection and Immunity* **55**, 716–720

Fujimura, S. and Nakamura, T. (1989) Multiple forms of proteases of *Bacteroides gingivalis* and their cellular location. *Oral Microbiology and Immunology* **4**, 227–229

Fullmer, H. and Gibson, W. (1966) Collagenolytic activity of gingivae of man. *Nature* **209**, 728–729

Garrett, I.R., Boyce, B.F., Oreffo, R.O.C. *et al.* (1990) Oxygen-derived free radicals stimulate osteoclastic bone resorption in rodent bone *in vitro* and *in vivo*. *Journal of Clinical Investigation* **85**, 632–639

Gazi, M.I., Cox, S.W., Clark, D.T. and Eley, B.M. (1994) Cathepsin B, tryptase and *Porphyromonas gingivalis* trypsin-like activities in gingival crevicular fluid. *Journal of Dental Research* **73**, 799

Gazi, M.I., Cox, S.W., Clark, D.T. and Eley, B.M. (1995) Comparison of host tissue and bacterial dipeptidylpeptidases in human gingival crevicular fluid by analytical isoelectric focusing. *Archives of Oral Biology* **40**, 731–736

Gazi, M.I., Cox, S.W., Clark, D.T. and Eley, B.M. (1996) A comparison of cysteine and serine proteinases in human gingival crevicular fluid with host tissue, saliva and bacterial enzymes by analytical isoelectric focusing. *Archives of Oral Biology* **41**, 393–400

Gazi, M.I., Cox, S.W., Clark, D.T. and Eley, B.M. (1997) Characterization of protease activities in *Capnocytophaga* spp., *Porphyromonas gingivalis*, *Prevotella* spp., *Treponema denticola* and *Actinobacillus actinomycetemcomitans*. *Oral Microbiology and Immunology* **12**, 240–248

Gillett, R. and Johnson, N.W. (1982) Bacterial invasion of the periodontium in a case of juvenile periodontitis. *Journal of Clinical Periodontology* **9**, 93–100

Giuliana, G., Ammatuna, P., Pizzo, G. *et al.* (1997) Occurrence of invading bacteria in radicular dentin of periodontally diseased teeth: microbiological findings. *Journal of Clinical Periodontology* **24**, 478–485

Goldberg, S., Kozlovsky, A. and Gordon, D. (1994) Caderverine as a putative component of oral malodour. *Journal of Dental Research* **73**, 1168–1172

Golub, L., Wolff, M., Lee, H. *et al.* (1985) Further evidence that tetracyclines inhibit collagenase activity in human crevicular fluid and other mammalian sources. *Journal of Periodontal Research* **20**, 12–23

Golub, L., Sorsa, T., Lee, H.M. *et al.* (1995) Doxycycline inhibits neutrophil (PMN) -type matrix metalloproteinases in human adult periodontitis gingiva. *Journal of Clinical Periodontology* **21**, 1–9

Golub, L., Lee, H.M., Ryan, M.E. *et al* (1998) Tetracyclines inhibit connective tissue breakdown by multiple non-antimicrobial mechanisms. *Advances in Dental Research* **12**, 12–26

Gowen, M. and Mundy, G.R. (1986) Actions of recombinant interleukin 1, interleukin 2 and interferon γ on bone resorption *in vitro*. *Journal of Immunology* **136**, 2478–2482

Grenier, D. and Mayrand, D. (1987) Functional characterization of extracellular vesicles produced by *Bacteroides gingivalis*. *Infection and Immunity* **55**, 111–117

Grenier, D. and McBride, B. (1987) Isolation of membrane-associated *Bacteroides gingivalis* glycylprolyl protease. *Infection and Immunity* **55**, 3131–3136

Grenier, D., Chao, D. and McBride, B.C. (1989a) Characterization of sodium dodecyl sulfate-stable *Bacteroides gingivalis* proteases by polyacrylamide gel electrophoresis. *Infection and Immunity* **57**, 95–99

Grenier, D., Mayrand, D. and McBride, B.C. (1989b) Further studies on the degradation of immunoglobulins and black-pigmented *Bacteroides*. *Oral Microbiology and Immunology* **4**, 12–18

Grenier, D., Uitto, V.-J. and McBride, B.C. (1990) Cellular location of a *Treponema denticola* chymotrypsin-like protease and the importance of the protease in migration through basement membrane. *Infection and Immunity* **58**, 347–351

Harris, E.D. and Cartwright, E.C. (1977) Mammalial collagenases. In *Proteinases in Mammalian Cells and Tissues* (A.J. Barrett, ed.), pp. 247–283. Amsterdam: Elsevier/North-Holland Biomedical Press

Harvey, W., Kamin, S., Meghji, S. and Wilson, M. (1987) Interleukin 1-like activity in capsular material from *Haemophilus actinomycetemcomitans*. *Immunology* **60**, 415–418

Hausmann, E. (1974) Potential pathways for bone resorption in human periodontal disease. *Journal of Periodontology* **45**, 338–343

Hausmann, E., Raisz, L.G. and Miller, W.A. (1970) Endotoxin: stimulation of bone resorption in tissue culture. *Science* **168**, 862–864

Hausmann, E., Ludereitz, E.O., Knox, K. and Weinfeld, N. (1975) Structural requirements for bone resorption by endotoxin and lipoteichoic acid. *Journal of Dental Research* **54**, 94–99

Henderson, B. and Blake, S. (1992) Therapeutic potential of cytokine manipulation. *Trends in Pharmacological Science* **13**, 145–152

Henderson, D., Poole, S and Wilson, M. (1996a) Bacterial modulins: a novel class of virulence factors which cause host tissue pathology by inducing cytokine synthesis. *Microbiological Reviews* **60**, 316–341

Henderson, D., Poole, S and Wilson, M. (1996b) Microbial/host interactions in health and disease: who controls the cytokine network? *Immunopharmacology* **35**, 1–21

Hinode, D., Hayashi, H. and Nakamura, R. (1991) Purification and characterization of three types of proteases from culture supernatants of *Porphyromonas gingivalis*. *Infection and Immunity* **59**, 3060–3068

Hinode, D., Nagata, A., Ichimiya, S. *et al.* (1992) Generation of plasma kinin by three types of protease isolated from *Porphyromonas gingivalis* 381. *Archives of Oral Biology* **37**, 859–861

Hönig, J., Rordorf-Adam, C., Siegmund, C. *et al.* (1989) Increased interleukin-1-beta (IL-1β) concentration in gingival tissue from periodontitis patients and healthy controls. *Journal of Periodontal Research* **24**, 362–367

Hopps, R.M. and Sisney-Durrant, H.J. (1991) Mechanisms of alveolar bone loss in periodontal disease. In *Periodontal Disease Pathogens and Host Immune Response* (S. Hamada, S.C. Holt and J.R. McGhee, eds), pp. 307–320. Tokyo: Quintessence Publishing Co. Ltd

Horowitz, A. and Folke, E.A. (1972) Hydrogen sulphide and periodontal disease. *Periodontal Abstracts* **2**, 59–62

Hussain, A., Kennett, C.N., Allaker, R. and Hughes, R.J. (1997) Stimulation of cathepsin B activity in cultured gingival fibroblasts by host and bacterial factors. *Journal of Dental Research* **76** Abstr. 235, 1048

Jansen, H.-J., Grenier, D. and Van der Hoeven, J.S. (1995) Characterization of immunoglobulin G-degrading proteases of *Prevotella intermedia* and *Prevotella nigrecens*. *Oral Microbiology and Immunology* **10**, 138–145

Johnson, P.W. and Tonzetich, J. (1979) Solubilization of acid-soluble collagen by H$_2$S. *Journal of Dental Research* **58** Abstr. 763, 283

Johnson, P.W. and Tonzetich, J. (1982) Effect of H$_2$S on protein synthesis by gingival fibroblasts. *Journal of Dental Research* **61** Abstr. 736, 260

Johnson, P.W., Ng, W. and Tonzetich, J. (1992a) Modulation of human gingival fibroblast cell metabolism by methyl mercaptan. *Journal of Periodontal Research* **27**, 476–483

Johnson, P.W., Yaegaki, K. and Tonzetich, J. (1992b) Effects of volatile sulphur compounds on protein metabolism by human gingival fibroblasts. *Journal of Periodontal Research* **27**, 553–561

Kamin, S., Harvey, W., Wilson, M. and Scutt, A. (1986) Inhibition of fibroblast proliferation and collagen synthesis by capsular material

from *Actinobacillus actinomycetemcomitans*. *Journal of Medical Biology* **22**, 245–249

Kato, T., Takahashi, N. and Kuramitsu, H. (1992) Sequence analysis and characterization of the *Porphyromonas gingivalis* ptrC gene, which expresses a novel collagenase activity. *Journal of Bacteriology* **174**, 3889–3895

Kay, H.M., Birss, A.J. and Smalley, J.W. (1989) Glycylprolyl dipeptidase activity of *Bacteroides gingivalis* W50 and the avirulent variant W50/DE1. *Microbiology Letters* **57**, 93–96

Kennett, C.N., Cox, S.W., Eley, B.M. and Osman, I.A.R.M. (1993) Comparative histochemical and biochemical studies of mast cell tryptase in human gingiva. *Journal of Periodontology* **64**, 870–877

Kennett, C.N., Cox, S.W. and Eley, B.M. (1994) Comparative histochemical, biochemical and immunocytochemical studies of cathepsin B in human gingiva. *Journal of Periodontal Research* **29**, 870–877

Kennett, C.N., Cox, S.W. and Eley, B.M. (1995) Localization of active and inactive elastase, alpha-1-proteinase inhibitor and alpha-2-macroglobulin in human gingiva. *Journal of Dental Research* **74**, 667–674

Kennett, C.N., Cox, S.W. and Eley, B.M. (1997a) Investigations into the cellular contribution to host tissue protease activity in gingival crevicular fluid. *Journal of Clinical Periodontology* **24**, 424–431

Kennett, C.N., Cox, S.W. and Eley, B.M. (1997b) Ultrastructural localization of cathepsin B in gingival tissue from chronic periodontitis patients. *Histochemical Journal* **29**, 727–734

Kennett, C.N., Hussain, A., Allaker, R. and Hughes, R.J. (1997c) Stimulation of DPP IV activity in cultured gingival fibroblasts by host and bacterial factors. *Journal of Dental Research* **76** Abstr. 235, 1048

Kilian, M. (1981) Degradation of immunoglobulins A1, A2 and G by suspected principal periodontal pathogens. *Infection and Immunity* **34**, 757–765

Kirby, A.C., Meghji, S., Nair, S.P. *et al.* (1995) The potent bone-resorbing mediator of *Actinobacillus actinomycetemcomitans* is homologous to the molecular chaperone GroEL. *Journal of Clinical Investigation* **96**, 1185–1194

Kleinberg, I. and Westbay, G. (1992) Salivary and metabolic factors involved in oral malodour formation. *Journal of Periodontology* **63**, 768–775

L'Allemain, G., Franchi, A., Gragoe, E. and Pouyssegur, J. (1984) Blockage of the Na$^+$/H$^+$ antiport abolishes growth factor-induced DNA synthesis in fibroblasts. *Journal of Biological Chemistry* **259**, 4313–4319

Lancero, H., Niu, J. and Johnson, P.W. (1996) Exposure of periodontal ligament cells to methyl mercaptan. *Journal of Dental Research* **75**, 1994–2002

Lantz, M.S., Allen, R.D., Vail, T.A. *et al.* (1991a) Specific cell components of *Bacteroides gingivalis* mediate binding and degradation of human fibrinogen. *Journal of Bacteriology* **173**, 495–504

Lantz, M.S., Allen, R.D., Duck, R.D. *et al.* (1991b) *Porphyromonas gingivalis* surface components bind and degrade connective tissue proteins. *Journal of Periodontal Research* **26**, 283–285

Lantz, M.S., Allen, R.D., Chiorowski, P. and Holt, C.S. (1993) Purification and immunolocalization of a cysteine protease from *Porphyromonas gingivalis*. *Journal of Periodontal Research* **28**, 467–469

Larjava, H., Uitto, V.-J., Haapasalo, M. *et al.* (1987) Fibronectin fragmentation induced by dental plaque and *Bacteroides gingivalis*. *Scandinavian Journal of Dental Research* **95**, 308–314

Larjava, H., Hökkinen, L. and Rahemtulla, F. (1992) A biochemical analysis of human periodontal tissue proteoglycans. *Biochemical Journal* **284**, 267–274

Lasfargues, J.J. and Saffir, J.L. (1983) Effect of indomethacin on bone destruction during experimental periodontal disease on the hamster. *Journal of Periodontal Research* **18**, 110–117

Laughton, B.E., Syed, S.A. and Loesche, W.J. (1982a) API ZYM system for the identification of *Bacteroides* spp., *Capnocytophaga* spp. and spirochaetes of oral origin. *Journal of Clinical Microbiology* **15**, 97–102

Laughton, B.E., Syed, S.A. and Loesche, W.J. (1982b) The rapid identification of *Bacteroides gingivalis*. *Journal of Clinical Microbiology* **15**, 345–346

Lawson, D.A. and Meyer, T.F. (1992) Biochemical characterization of *Porphyromonas (Bacteroides) gingivalis* collagenase. *Infection and Immunity* **60**, 1524–1529

Lee, W., Aitken, S., Sodek, J. and McCullock, G. (1995) Evidence for a direct relationship between neutrophil collagenase activity and periodontal disease destruction *in vivo*; the role of active enzyme in human periodontitis. *Journal of Periodontal Research* **30**, 23–33

Lensgraf, E.J., Greenblatt, J.J. and Bowden, J.W. (1979) Effect of group A streptococcal peptidoglycan and group A streptococcal cell wall on bone in tissue culture. *Archives of Oral Biology* **24**, 495–498

Liakoni, H., Barber, P. and Newman, H.N. (1987) Bacterial penetration of pocket soft tissues in chronic adult and juvenile periodontitis cases. An ultrastructural study. *Journal of Clinical Periodontology* **14**, 22–28

Loesche, W.J., Syed, S.A., Schmidt, E. and Morrison, E.C. (1985) Bacterial profiles of subgingival plaques in periodontitis. *Journal of Periodontology* **56**, 447–456

Löwick, C.W.G.M., van der Pluijm, G., Bloys, H. *et al.* (1989) Parathyroid hormone (PTH) and PTH-like protein (PLP) stimulate interleukin-6 production by osteogenic cells: a possible role of interleukin-6 in osteoclastogenesis. *Biochemical and Biophysical Research Communications* **162**, 1546–1552

Mäkinen, K.K., Syed, S.A., Mäkinen, P.-L. and Loesche, W.J. (1986) Benzylarginine peptidase and immunopeptidase profiles of *Treponema denticola* strains isolated from the human periodontal pocket. *Current Microbiology* **14**, 85–89

Mäkinen, K.K., Syed, S.A., Mäkinen, P.-L. and Loesche, W.J. (1987) Dominance of immunopeptidase activity in the human oral bacterium *Treponema denticola* ATCC 35405. *Current Microbiology* **14**, 341–346

Mäkinen, K.K., Syed, S.A., Loesche, W.J. and Mäkinen, P.-L. (1988) Proteolytic profile of *Treponema denticola* ATCC 35580 with special reference to collagenolytic and arginine aminopeptidase activity. *Oral Microbiology and Immunology* **3**, 121–128

Manor, A., Lebendiger, M., Shiffer, A. and Torvel, H. (1984) Bacterial invasion of the periodontal tissues in advanced periodontitis in humans. *Journal of Periodontology* **55**, 567–573

Masada, M.P., Persson, R., Kenney, J.S. *et al.* (1990) Measurement of interleukin-1α and 1β in gingival crevicular fluid: implications for the pathogenesis of periodontal disease. *Journal of Periodontal Research* **25**, 156–163

McDermid, A.S., McKee, A.S. and Marsh, P.D. (1988) Effect of pH on enzyme activity and growth of *Bacteroides gingivalis* W50. *Infection and Immunity* **56**, 1096–1100

Meghji, S. (1992) Bone remodelling. *British Dental Journal* **172**, 235–242

Meghji, S., Sandy, J.R., Scutt, A.M. and Harvey, W. (1988) Stimulation of bone resorption by lipo-oxygenase metabolites of arachidonic acid. *Prostaglandins* **36**, 139–149

Meghji, S., Henderson, B., Nair, S. and Wilson, M. (1992) Inhibition of bone DNA and collagen production by surface-associated material from bacteria implicated in the pathology of periodontal disease. *Journal of Periodontology* **63**, 736–742

Meghji, S., Wilson, M., Henderson, B. and Kinane, D. (1992) Antiproliferative and cytotoxic activity of surface associated material from periodontopathic bacteria. *Archives of Oral Biology* **37**, 637–644

Meghji, S., Henderson, B. and Wilson, M. (1993) High titre antisera from patients with periodontal disease inhibit bacterial capsule-induced bone breakdown. *Journal of Periodontal Research* **28**, 115–121

Meghji, S., Barber, P., Wilson, M. and Henderson, B. (1994) Bone resorbing activity of surface-associated material from *Actinobacillus actinomycetemcomitans* and *Eikenella corrodens*. *Journal of Medical Microbiology* **41**, 197–203

Meikle, M.C., Heath, J.K. and Reynolds, J.J. (1986) Advances in understanding cell interactions in tissue resorption. Relevance to the pathogenesis of periodontal diseases and a new hypothesis. *Journal of Oral Pathology* **15**, 239–250

Mikx, F.H. and De Jong, M.H. (1987) Keratinolytic activity of cutaneous and oral bacteria. *Infection and Immunity* **55**, 621–625

Millar, S.J., Goldstein, E.J., Levine, M.J. and Hausmann, E. (1986) Lipoprotein: a Gram negative cell wall component that stimulates bone resorption. *Journal of Periodontal Research* **21**, 256–259

Miller, W.D. (1890) *The Micro-organisms of the Human Mouth. The Local and General Diseases which are Caused by Them.* Philadelphia: S.S. White Dental Manufacturing

Minhas, T. and Greenman, J. (1989) Production of cell-bound and vesicle-associated trypsin-like protease, alkaline phosphatase and N-acetyl-beta-glucosaminidase by *Bacteroides gingivalis* W50. *Journal of General Microbiology* **135**, 547–564

Miyaki, H., Sakao, S., Katoh, Y. and Takehara, T. (1995) Correlation between volatile sulphur compounds and certain oral health measurements in the general population. *Journal of Periodontology* **66**, 679–684

Moncla, B.L., Braham, P. and Hillier, S.L. (1990) Sialidase (neuraminidase) activity among Gram negative anaerobic and capnophilic bacteria. *Journal of Clinical Microbiology* **28**, 422–425

Moore, J., Wilson, M. and Kieser, J.B. (1986) The distribution of bacterial lipopolysaccharide (endotoxin) in relation to periodontally involved root surfaces. *Journal of Clinical Periodontology* **13**, 748–751

Mortensen, S.B. and Kilian, M. (1984) Purification and characterization of immunoglobulin A1 protease from *Bacteroides melaninogenicus*. *Infection and Immunity* **45**, 550–557

Moseley, R., Waddington, R.J., Evans, P. *et al.* (1995) The chemical moderation of glycosaminoglycan structure by oxygen-derived species *in vitro*. *Biochimica et Biophysica Acta* **1244**, 245–252

Nair, S.P., Meghji, S., Wilson, M. *et al.* (1996) Bacterially induced bone destruction: mechanisms and misconceptions. *Infection and Immunity* **64**, 2371–2380

Nakamura, M. and Slots, J. (1982) Aminopeptidases of *Capnocytophaga*. *Journal of Periodontal Research* **17**, 597–603

Nakamura, R., Hinode, D., Terai, H. and Morioka, M. (1991) Extracellular enzymes of *Porphyromonas (Bacteroides) gingivalis* in relation to periodontal destruction. In *Periodontal Disease: Pathogens and Host Immune Responses* (S. Hamada, S.C. Holt and J.R. McGhee, eds), pp. 129–141. Tokyo: Quintessence Publishing Co. Ltd

Nakaya, H., Oates, T.W., Hoany, H.M. *et al.* (1997) Effects of interleukin-1β on matrix metalloproteinase-3 levels in human periodontal ligament cells. *Journal of Periodontology* **68**, 517–533

Nara, F. (1977) The relationship between halitosis and the oral conditions of the periodontal patients. *Journal of the Japanese Association of Periodontology* **19**, 100–108

Ng, W. and Tonzetich, J. (1984) Effect of H$_2$S and CH$_3$SH on permeability of oral mucosa. *Journal of Dental Research* **63**, 994–997

Nilsson, T., Carlsson, J. and Sundqvist, G. (1985) Inactivation of key factors of the plasma proteinase cascade systems by *Bacteroides gingivalis*. *Infection and Immunity* **50**, 467–471

Nyman, S., Schroeder, H. and Lindhe, J. (1979) Suppression of inflammation and bone resorption by indomethacin during experimental periodontitis in dogs. *Journal of Periodontology* **50**, 450–461

Offenbacher, S., Odle, B.M., Gray, R.C. and van Dyke, T.E. (1984) Crevicular fluid prostaglandin E levels as a measure of periodontal disease status of adult and juvenile periodontitis patients. *Journal of Periodontal Research* **19**, 1–13

Offenbacher, S., Odle, B.M. and van Dyke, T.E. (1986) The use of crevicular fluid prostaglandin E2 levels as a predictor of periodontal attachment loss. *Journal of Periodontal Research* **25**, 101–112

Ohm, K., Albers, von H.-K. and Lisboa, B.P. (1984) Measurement of 8 prostaglandins in human gingival and periodontal disease using high pressure liquid chromatography and radioimmunoassay. *Journal of Periodontal Research* **19**, 301–311

Ohta, K., Mäkinen, K. and Loesche, W.G. (1986) Purification and characterization of an enzyme produced by *Treponema denticola* capable of hydrolysing synthetic trypsin substrates. *Infection and Immunity* **53**, 213–220

Otsuka, M., Endo, J., Hinode, D. *et al.* (1987) Isolation and characterization of a protease from culture supernatant of *Bacteroides gingivalis*. *Journal of Periodontal Research* **22**, 491–498

Page, P.C. and Schroeder, H.E. (1976) Pathogenesis of inflammatory periodontal disease. A summary of current work. *Laboratory Investigation* **33**, 235–249

Papapanou, P.N., Sandros, J., Lindberg, K. *et al.* (1994) *Porphyromonas gingivalis* may multiply and advance within stratified human junctional epithelium. *Journal of Periodontal Research* **29**, 374–375

Pearson, C.H. and Pringle, G.A. (1986) Chemical and immunochemical characteristics of proteoglycans in bovine gingiva and dental pulp. *Archives of Oral Biology* **31**, 541–548

Pekovic, D.D. and Fillery, E.D. (1984) Identification of bacteria in immunopathological mechanisms of human periodontal diseases. *Journal of Periodontal Research* **19**, 329–351

Persson, S. Claesson, R. and Carlsson, J. (1989) The capacity of the subgingival microbiota to produce volatile sulphur compounds in human serum. *Oral Microbiology and Immunology* **4**, 169–172

Persson, S., Edlund, M.B., Claesson, R. and Carlsson, J. (1990) The formation of H_2S and CH_3SH by oral bacteria. *Oral Microbiology and Immunology* **5**, 195–201

Pertuiset, J.H., Saglie, F.R., Lofthus, J. *et al.* (1987) Recurrent periodontal disease and bacterial presence in the gingiva. *Journal of Periodontology* **58**, 553–558

Pianotti, R., Lachette, S. and Dill, S. (1986) Desulphuration of cysteine and methionin by *Fusobacterium nucleatum*. *Journal of Dental Research* **65**, 913–917

Pike, R., McGraw, W., Potempa, J. and Travis, J. (1994) Lysine- and arginine-specific proteinases from *Porphyromonas gingivalis*. Isolation, characterization and evidence for the existence of complexes with hemagglutinins. *Journal of Biological Chemistry* **269**, 406–411

Purvis, J.A., Embery, G. and Oliver, W.M. (1984) Molecular size distribution of proteoglycans in human inflamed gingival tissue. *Archives of Oral Biology* **29**, 573–579

Que, X.-C. and Kuramitsu, H.U. (1990) Isolation and characterization of the *Treponema denticola* prtA gene coding for chymotrypsin-like protease activity and detection of a closely linked gene encoding Pz-PLGPA-hydrolysing activity. *Infection and Immunity* **58**, 4099–4105

Rangarajan, M., Aduse-Opoku, J., Slaney, J.M. *et al.* (1997) The prpR1 and prpR2 arginine-specific protease genes of *Porphyromonas gingivalis* W50 produces five biochemically distinct enzymes. *Molecular Microbiology* **23**, 955–965

Ratkay, L.G., Waterfield, J.D. and Tonzetich, J. (1995) Stimulation of enzyme and cytokine production by CH_3SH in human gingival fibroblast and monocyte cell cultures. *Archives of Oral Biology* **40**, 337–344

Reddi, K., Henderson, B., Meghji, S. *et al.* (1995a) Interleukin-6 production by lipopolysaccharide-stimulated fibroblasts is potentially inhibited by napthoquinone (vitamin K) components. *Cytokine* **7**, 287–290

Reddi, K., Meghji, S., Wilson, M. and Henderson, B. (1995b) Comparison of the osteolytic activity of surface-associated proteins of bacteria

implicated in periodontal disease. *Oral Diseases* **1**, 26–31

Reddi, K., Wilson, M., Poole, S., *et al.* (1995c) Relative cytokine-stimulating activities of surface components of the oral periodontopathic bacterium, *Actinobacillus actinomycetemcomitans*. *Cytokine* **7**, 534–541

Reddi, K., Wilson, M., Nair, S. *et al.* (1996a) Comparison of the pro-inflammatory cytokine-stimulating activity of surface-associated proteins of periodontopathic bacteria. *Journal of Periodontal Research* **31**, 120–130

Reddi, K., Nair, S., White, P.A. *et al.* (1996b) Surface-associated material from the bacterium, *Actinobacillus actinomycetemcomitans*, contains a peptide which in contrast to lipopolysaccharide, directly stimulates interleukin-6 gene transcription. *European Journal of Biochemistry* **236**, 871–876

Reynolds, J.J. (1996) Collagenases and tissue inhibitors of metalloproteinases; a functional balance in tissue degradation. *Oral Diseases* **2**, 70–76

Reynolds, J.J., Hembry, R.M. and Meikle, M.C. (1994) Connective tissue degradation in health and periodontal disease and the roles of matrix metalloproteinases and their inhibitors. *Advances in Dental Research* **8**, 312–319

Robertson, P.B., Lantz, P.T., Marucha, K.S. *et al.* (1982) Collagenolytic activity associated with *Bacteroides* species and *Actinobacillus actinomycetemcomitans*. *Journal of Periodontal Research* **17**, 275–283

Rosen, G., Naor, R., Rahamin, E. *et al.* (1995) Proteases of *Treponema denticola* outer sheath and extracellular vesicles. *Infection and Immunity* **63**, 3973–3979

Rossomando, E.F., Kennedy, J.E. and Hadjimichael, J. (1990) Tumour necrosis factor alpha in gingival crevicular fluid as a possible indicator of periodontal disease in humans. *Archives of Oral Biology* **35**, 431–434

Rozanis, J. and Slots, J. (1982) Collagenolytic activity of *Actinobacillus actinomycetemcomitans* and black-pigmented *Bacteroides*. *Journal of Dental Research* **61**, 275

Rozanis, J., Van Wart, H.E., Bond, M.B. and Slots, J. (1983) Further studies on collagenase of *Actinobacillus actinomycetemcomitans*. *Journal of Dental Research* **62**, 300

Ryan, M.E., Ramamurthy, S. and Golub, L.M. (1996) Matrix metalloproteinases and their inhibition in periodontal treatment. *Current Opinion in Periodontology* **3**, 85–96

Saglie, F.R., Carranza, F.A. Jnr, Newman, M.G. *et al.* (1982a) Identification of tissue-invading bacteria in human periodontal diseases. *Journal of Periodontal Research* **17**, 452–455

Saglie, F.R., Newman, M.J., Carranza, F.A. Jnr and Pattison, G.L. (1982b) Bacterial invasion of gingiva in advanced periodontitis in humans. *Journal of Periodontology* **53**, 217–222

Saglie, F.R., Carranza, F.A. Jnr and Newman, M.J. (1985) The presence of bacteria within the oral epithelium of human periodontal disease. I. A scanning and transmission electron microscopic study. *Journal of Periodontology* **56**, 618–624

Saglie, F.R., Rezende, J.H., Pertuiset, J. *et al.* (1986) The presence of bacteria within the oral epithelium in periodontal disease. II. Immunochemical identification of bacteria. *Journal of Periodontology* **57**, 492–500

Saglie, F.R., Rezende, J.H., Pertuiset, J. *et al.* (1987) Bacterial invasion during disease activity as determined by significant attachment loss. *Journal of Periodontology* **58**, 837–846

Saglie, F.R., Cheng, I. and Sadighi, R. (1988a) Detection of *Mycoplasma pneumoniae* DNA within diseased gingiva by *in situ* hybridization using a biotin labelled probe. *Journal of Periodontology* **59**, 121–123

Saglie, F.R., Pertuiset, J., Rezende, J.H. *et al.* (1988b) *In situ* correlative immuno-identification of mononuclear infiltrates and invasive bacteria in diseased gingiva. *Journal of Periodontology* **59**, 688–696

Saglie, F.R., Marfany, A. and Camargo, P. (1988c) Intragingival occurrence of *Actinobacillus actinomycetemcomitans* and *Bacteroides gingivalis* in active destructive periodontal lesions. *Journal of Periodontology* 59, 259–265

Sandros, J., Papapanou, P.N., Nannmark, U. and Dahlén, G. (1994) *Porphyromonas gingivalis* invades the human pocket epithelium *in vitro*. *Journal of Periodontal Research* 28, 219–226

Sato, M., Otsuka, M., Maehara, R. *et al.* (1987) Degradation of human secretory immunoglobulin A by a protease isolated from the anaerobic periodontopathic bacteria *Bacteroides gingivalis*. *Archives of Oral Biology* 32, 235–238

Savani, F., Listgarten, M.A., Boyd, F. *et al.* (1985) The colonization and establishment of invading bacteria in the periodontium of ligature-treated immunosuppressed rats. *Journal of Periodontology* 56, 273–280

Sawyer, S.J., MacDonald, J.B. and Gibbons, R.J. (1962) Biochemical characteristics of *Bacteriodes melaninogenicus*. *Archives of Oral Biology* 7, 685–691

Schenkein, H.A. (1988) The effect of proteolytic *Bacteroides* species on the proteins of the human complement system. *Journal of Periodontal Research* 23, 187–192

Schenker, B.J. (1987) Immunologic dysfunction in the pathogenesis of periodontal disease. *Journal of Clinical Periodontology* 14, 489–498

Scott, C.F., Whitaker, E.J., Hammond, B.F. and Colman, R.W. (1993) Purification and characterization of a potent 70-kDa thiol lysyl-proteinase (Lys-gingivian) that cleaves kininogens and fibrinogen. *Journal of Biological Chemistry* 268, 7935–7942

Scully, C., Elmaaytah, M., Porter, S.R. and Greenman, J. (1997) Breath odour: aetiopathogenesis, assessment and management. *European Journal of Oral Science* 105, 287–293

Seddon, S.V. and Shah, H.N. (1989) The distribution of hydrolytic enzymes among Gram negative bacteria associated with periodontitis. *Microbial Ecology in Health and Disease* 2, 181–190

Seymour, R.A. and Heasman, P.A. (1988) Drugs and the periodontium. *Journal of Clinical Periodontology* 15, 1–16

Shah, H.N., Garbia, S.E., Kowlessur, D. *et al.* (1991) Gingivian; a cysteine proteinase isolated from *Porphyromonas gingivalis*. *Microbial Ecology in Health and Disease* 4, 319–328

Sharp, L., Poole, S., Reddie, K. *et al.* (1998) A lipid A-associated protein of *Porphyromonas gingivalis*, derived from the haemagluttinating domain of the R1 protease family, is a potent stimulator of interleukin-6 synthesis. *Microbiology* 144, 3109–3023

Sighagen, B., Hamberg, M. and Fredholm, B.B. (1982) Formation of 12L-hydroxyeicosatetraenoic acid (12 HETE) by gingival tissue. *Journal of Dental Research* 61, 761–763

Simchowitz, I. and Cragoe, E. (1986) Regulation of human neutrophil chemotaxis by intracellular pH. *Journal of Biological Chemistry* 261, 6492–6500

Slots, J. (1981) Enzymatic characterization of some oral and non-oral Gram negative bacteria with the API ZYM system. *Journal of Clinical Microbiology* 14, 288–294

Slots, J. and Genco, R.J. (1984) Black-pigmented *Bacteroides* species, *Capnocytophaga* species and *Actinobacillus actinomycetemcomitans* in human periodontal disease: virulence factors in colonization, survival and tissue destruction. *Journal of Dental Research* 63, 412–421

Smalley, J.W. and Birss, A.J. (1987) Trypsin-like enzyme activity of the extracellular membrane vesicles of *Bacteroides gingivalis* W50. *Journal of General Microbiology* 133, 2883–2894

Smalley, J.W., Birss, A.J. and Suttleworth, C.A. (1988a) Degradation of type I collagen and human plasma fibrinogen by trypsin-like enzyme and extracellular membrane vesicles of *Bacteroides gingivalis* W50. *Archives of Oral Biology* 33, 323–329

Smalley, J.W., Birss, A.J. and Suttleworth, C.A. (1988b) Effect of the outer membrane fraction of *Bacteroides gingivalis* W50 on the glycosaminoglycan metabolism by human fibroblasts. *Archives of Oral Biology* 33, 547–553

Söderling, E., Mäkinen, P.L., Syed, S.A. and Mäkinen, K.K. (1991) Biochemical comparison of proteolytic enzymes present in rough- and smooth-surfaced *Capnocytophaga* isolated from the subgingival plaque of periodontitis patients. *Journal of Periodontal Research* 26, 17–23

Sojar, H.T., Lee, J.-Y., Bedi, G.S. and Genco, R.J. (1993) Purification and characterization of a protease from *Porphyromonas gingivalis* capable of degrading salt-solubilized collagen. *Infection and Immunity* 61, 2369–2376

Sorsa, T., Uitto, V.J., Suomalainen, K. *et al.* (1987) A trypsin-like protease from *Bacteroides gingivalis*. Partial purification and characterization. *Journal of Periodontal Research* 22, 375–380

Sorsa, T., Ingman, T., Suomalainen, K. *et al.* (1992) Identification of proteases from periodontopathic bacteria as activators of latent human neutrophil and fibroblast type interstitial collagenases. *Infection and Immunity* 60, 4491–4495

Steffan, E.K. and Hengtes, D.J. (1981) Hydrolytic enzymes of anaerobic bacteria isolated from human infections. *Journal of Clinical Microbiology* 14, 153–156

Suido, H., Nakamura, M., Mashimo, P.A. *et al.* (1986) Arylaminopeptidase activities of oral bacteria. *Journal of Dental Research* 65, 1335–1340

Suido, H., Neiders, M.E., Barua, P.K. *et al.* (1987) Characterization of the N-CBz-glycyl-glycyl-arginyl peptidase and glycyl-prolyl peptidase of *Bacteroides gingivalis*. *Journal of Periodontal Research* 22, 412–418

Suido, H., Eguchi, T. and Nakamura, M. (1988a) Investigation of periodontopathic bacteria based upon their peptidase activities. *Advances in Dental Research* 2, 304–309

Suido, H., Zambon, J.J., Mashimo, P.A. *et al.* (1988b) Correlations between gingival crevicular fluid enzymes and the subgingival microflora. *Journal of Dental Research* 67, 1070–1074

Sundqvist, G., Carlsson, J., Herrmann, B. and Tarnvik, A. (1985) Degradation of human immunoglobulins G and M and complement factors C3 and C5 by black-pigmenting *Bacteroides*. *Journal of Medical Microbiology* 19, 85–94

Sundqvist, G., Carlsson, J. and Hänström, L. (1987) Collagenolytic activity of black-pigmented *Bacteroides* species. *Journal of Periodontal Research* 22, 300–306

Takahashi, A. and Earnshaw, W. (1996) ICE-related proteases in apoptosis. *Current Opinions in Genetic Development* 6, 50–55

Takeuchi, H., Sumitani, M., Tsubakimoto, K. and Tsutsui, M. (1974) Oral organisms in the gingiva of individuals with periodontal disease. *Journal of Dental Research* 53, 132–136

Tashjian, A.H., Hohmann, E.L., Antoniades, H.N. and Levine, L. (1982) Platelet derived growth factor stimulates bone resorption via a prostaglandin-mediated mechanism. *Endocrinology* 111, 118–124

Tashjian, A.H., Voelkel, E.F., Lazzaro, M. *et al.* (1985) α and β human transforming growth factors stimulate prostaglandin production and bone resorption in cultured mouse calvaria. *Proceedings of the National Academy of Science, USA* 82, 4535–4538

Taubman, M.A., Haffajee, A.D., Socransky, S.S. *et al.* (1992) Longitudinal monitoring of humoral antibodies in subjects with destructive periodontal disease. *Journal of Periodontal Research* 27, 511–521

Tipler, L.S. and Embery, G. (1985) Glycosoaminoglycan depolymerizing enzymes produced by anaerobic bacteria isolated from the human mouth. *Archives of Oral Biology* 30, 391–396

Toda, K., Otsuka, M., Ishikawa, Y. *et al.* (1984) Thiol-dependent collagenolytic activity in culture media of *Bacteroides gingivalis*. *Journal of Periodontal Research* 19, 372–381

Tonzetich, J. (1971) Direct gas chromatographic analysis of sulphur compounds in mouth air in man. *Archives of Oral Biology* 16, 587–597

Tonzetich, J. (1977) Production and origin of oral malodour. A review of mechanisms and methods of analysis. *Journal of Periodontology* **48**, 13–20

Tonzetich, J. (1978) Oral malodour: an indicator of health status and oral cleanliness. *International Dental Journal* **28**, 309–319

Tonzetich, J. and Carpenter, P.A.W. (1971) Production of volatile sulphur compounds from cystine, cysteine and methionine by human dental plaque. *Archives of Oral Biology* **16**, 599–607

Tonzetich, J. and Catherall, D.M. (1976) Metabolism of thiosulphate and thiocyanate by human saliva and dental plaque. *Archives of Oral Biology* **22**, 125–131

Tonzetich, J. and Kesterbaum, R.G. (1969) Odour production by human salivary fractions and plaque. *Archives of Oral Biology* **14**, 815–821

Tonzetich, J. and Lo, K.K.C. (1978) Reaction of H_2S with proteins associated with the human mouth. *Archives of Oral Biology* **23**, 875–880

Tonzetich, J. and McBride, B.C. (1981) Characterization of volatile sulphur production by pathogenic and non-pathogenic strains of oral *Bacteroides*. *Archives of Oral Biology* **26**, 963–969

Travis, J., Pike, R., Imamura, T. and Potempa, J. (1997) *Porphyromonas gingivalis* proteinases as virulence factors in the development of chronic periodontitis. *Journal of Periodontal Research* **32**, 120–125

Tsai, C.C., McArthur, W.P., Baehni, P.C. *et al.* (1979) Extraction and partial characterization of a leukotoxin from plaque-derived Gram negative microorganisms. *Infection and Immunity* **25**, 427–439

Tsutsui, H., Kinouchi, T., Wakano, Y. and Ohnishi, Y. (1987) Purification and characterization of a protease from *Bacteroides gingivalis*. *Infection and Immunity* **55**, 420–427

Uitto, V.-J., Chan, E.C.S. and Chin Quee, T. (1986) Initial characterization of neutral proteinases from oral spirochaetes. *Journal of Periodontal Research* **21**, 95–100

Uitto, V.-J., Grenier, D., Chan, E.C.S. and McBride, B.C. (1988a) Isolation of a chymotrypsin-like enzyme from *Treponema denticola*. *Infection and Immunity* **56**, 2717–2722

Uitto, V.-J., Haapasalo, M, Laakso, T. and Salo, T. (1988b) Degradation of basement membrane collagen by proteases from some anaerobic oral microorganisms. *Oral Microbiology and Immunology* **3**, 97–102

Uitto, V.-J., Grenier, D. and McBride, B.C. (1989a) Effect of *Treponema denticola* on periodontal epithelial cells. *Journal of Dental Research* **68** Abstr. 223, 894

Uitto, V.-J., Larjava, H., Heino, J. and Sorsa, T. (1989b) A protease of *Bacteroides gingivalis* degrades cell surface and matrix glycoproteins of cultured gingival fibroblasts and induces secretion of collagenase and plasminogen activator. *Infection and Immunity* **57**, 213–218

Umemoto, T., Watanabe, K., Kumada, H. and Yamaji, Y. (1991) The role of motile rods in periodontal disease. In *Periodontal Disease: Pathogens and Host Immune Responses* (S. Hamada, S.C. Holt and J.R. McGhee, eds), pp. 65–76. Tokyo: Quintessence Publishing Co. Ltd

Vaes, G. (1988) Cellular biology and biochemical mechanism of bone resorption. *Clinical Orthopaedics and Related Research* **23**, 239–271

Vernillo, A., Ramamurthy, N., Golub, L. and Rifkin, B. (1994) The non-antimicrobial properties of tetracyclines for the treatment of periodontal disease. *Current Opinions in Periodontology* **2**, 111–118

Waddington, R.J. and Embery, G. (1991) Structural characterization of human alveolar bone proteoglycans. *Archives of Oral Biology* **36**, 859–866

Watanabe, H., Marsh, P.D. and Ivanyi, L. (1989) Antigens of *Actinobacillus actinomycetemcomitans* identified by immunoblotting with sera from patients with localized human juvenile periodontitis and generalized severe periodontitis. *Archives of Oral Biology* **34**, 649–656

Weakes-Dybvig, M., Sanavi, F., Zander, H. and Rifkin, B.R. (1982) The effect of indomethacin on alveolar bone loss in experimental periodontitis. *Journal of Periodontal Research* **17**, 90–100

White, P.A., Wilson, M., Nair, S.P. *et al.* (1995) Characterization of an anti-proliferative surface-associated protein from *Actinobacillus actinomycetemcomitans* which can be neutralized by sera from a portion of patients with localized juvenile periodontitis. *Infection and Immunity* **63**, 2612–2618

Wikström, M. and Lindhe, A. (1986) Ability of oral bacteria to degrade fibronectin. *Infection and Immunity* **51**, 707–711

Williams, R.C., Jeffcoat, M.K., Howell, T.C. *et al.* (1988) Ibuprofen: an inhibitor of alveolar bone resorption in beagles. *Journal of Periodontal Research* **23**, 225–229

Wilson, M. (1995) Bacterial activities of lipopolysaccharides from oral bacteria and their relevance to the pathogenesis of chronic periodontitis. *Scientific Progress* **78**, 19–34

Wilson, M. and Henderson, B. (1995) Virulence factors of *Actinobacillus actinomycetemcomitans* relevant to the pathogenesis of inflammatory periodontal diseases. *Microbiological Reviews* **17**, 365–379

Wilson, M., Kamin, S. and Harvey, W. (1985) Bone resorbing activity from purified capsular material from *Actinobacillus actinomycetemcomitans*. *Journal of Periodontal Research* **20**, 484–491

Wilson, M., Meghji, S. and Harvey, W. (1988) Effect of capsular material from *H. actinomycetemcomitans* on bone collagen synthesis *in vitro*. *Microbios* **54**, 181–185

Wilson, M., Meghji, S., Barber, P. and Henderson, B. (1993) Biological activities of surface associated material from *Porphyromonas gingivalis*. *Immunology and Medical Microbiology* **6**, 147–155

Wilson, M., Reddi, K. and Henderson, D. (1996) Cytokine-inducing components of periodontopathic bacteria. *Journal of Periodontal Research* **31**, 393–407

Winkler, J.R., Grassi, M. and Murray, P.A. (1988) Clinical description and aetiology of HIV-associated periodontal diseases. In *Oral Manifestations of AIDS* (P.B. Robertson and J.S. Greenspan, eds), pp. 49–70. Littleton, MA: PSG Publishing Company

Wolinsky, L.E., Saglie, F.R., Carranza, F.A. Jnr and Newman, M.J. (1987) The identification of *Treponema vincentii* in the gingival tissue of humans with adult periodontitis. *Journal of Periodontology* **58**, 337

Yoshimura, F., Nishikata, M., Suzuki, T. *et al.* (1984) Characterization of a trypsin-like protease from the bacterium *Bacteroides gingivalis* isolated from human dental plaque. *Archives of Oral Biology* **29**, 559–564

6

The effect of systemic factors on the periodontal tissues

The systemic conditions that can potentially affect the periodontal tissues are numerous, and will be described under the following headings:

1. Physiological changes
2. Systemic diseases
3. Infections
4. Drug reactions
5. Dietary and nutritional factors.

Physiological changes

The sex hormones

Oestrogens and progesterone are the predominant female sex hormones and are controlled by the ovary. Oestrogens produce the physiological changes in women at puberty, and progesterone prepares the female reproductive tract for fertilization. The androgen testosterone is the predominant male hormone, which produces the male characteristics at puberty and also promotes protein synthesis. Synthetic hormones that mimic the effects of the endogenous female hormones are used as oral contraceptives.

These hormones can affect the periodontal tissues. Oestrogens can promote keratinization and increase the mucopolysaccharide content of the connective tissue. Progesterone can increase the permeability of gingival blood vessels. Changes in the periodontal tissues may become clinically apparent, principally at puberty, during pregnancy and during the use of oral contraceptives, when there may be an exaggerated response to plaque products.

Puberty

The increasing levels of the sex hormones in the circulation at puberty have been linked to the increased prevalence and severity of gingivitis at this time (Sutcliffe,

1972), and this is supported by the observation that gingivitis peaks earlier in girls (11–13 years) than boys (13–14 years). However, a 6-year longitudinal study (Yanover and Ellen, 1986) failed to show any increase in gingivitis at puberty in 18 hormonally stable girls, and a significant increase of gingivitis was seen in girls experiencing precocious puberty.

It would appear that a small amount of plaque, which at a different age might cause minimal gingival inflammation, produces in puberty an obvious inflammation with gingival swelling and bleeding. When puberty is passed the inflammation tends to subside, but does not disappear until adequate plaque control is achieved.

Menstruation

With pre-existing gingivitis, gingival crevicular exudate increases at the time of ovulation in the menstrual cycle owing to the increased production of oestrogens and progesterone (Lindhe and Attström, 1967). However, no such increase was seen in healthy tissues (Holm-Pedersen and Löe, 1967). This may explain why, in a few women, a deterioration of a pre-existing gingivitis may occur at this time in their menstrual cycle.

Pregnancy

Folklore has always associated pregnancy with gingivitis and tooth loss, but where the mouth is clean gingivitis does not occur in pregnancy. However, as in puberty an otherwise low-grade plaque-induced inflammation will become more severe in pregnancy (*Figure 6.1*).

The incidence of gingivitis in pregnancy has been reported as between 30 and 100% (Löe, 1965; Adam *et al.*, 1973). The changes usually start about the third month of gestation and the severity of the inflammation gradually increases during pregnancy, with partial or complete resolution after parturition (Löe and Silness, 1963; Silness

Figure 6.1 Gingival inflammation caused by poor oral hygiene, the tissue response exaggerated by hormonal changes associated with pregnancy

Figure 6.2 Pyogenic granuloma ('pregnancy tumour') in a pregnant patient. (Courtesy Professor C Scully)

and Löe, 1964; Hugoson, 1970; Samant *et al.*, 1976). Gingivitis has also been reported to peak at 6 months' gestation and then resolve slightly in the third trimester (Cohen *et al.*, 1971). The gingivae may become bright red, swollen, sensitive and bleed spontaneously. There is also an increase in gingival exudate and tooth mobility.

It is believed that increasing levels of progesterone produce an increase in vascularity with alterations in the walls of the gingival vessels, which makes them more permeable. It has also been shown that the numbers of black-pigmented anaerobic bacteria in the subgingival flora increase as pregnancy progresses (Kornman and Loesche, 1980). This appears to be associated with raised levels of oestrogen and progesterone as the bacteria demonstrate an increased steroid uptake in pregnancy. This may relate to oestrogen becoming a substitute for methadione, which is a growth requirement for these bacteria.

To control gingivitis in the pregnant patient or in the adolescent it is important to explain the nature of the condition and the special care that needs to be taken during this period. Regular scaling and instruction in home care are essential; at the same time, all plaque retentive factors should be eliminated.

Pregnancy epulis (pyogenic granuloma of pregnancy)

The pregnancy epulis is a soft pedunculated granuloma, which usually arises from an inflamed gingival papilla. It is usually deep red in colour and bleeds easily, and may cause the patient great concern (*Figure 6.2*). It may arise from any gingival site, but tends to be most prevalent on the labial aspect of the anterior part of the mouth. It may appear at any time during pregnancy, but is most common about the third month, and usually grows slowly but can sometimes become quite large. It generally regresses partially or completely after parturition. It is usually associated not only with plaque deposits but also with an

additional factor, such as a carious cavity, poor tooth contact or overhanging filling.

Histologically, it resembles a pyogenic granuloma. It is composed of numerous, wide-spaced and thin-walled blood vessels within a delicate connective tissue stroma, which can intensify with age. A moderate to dense inflammatory infiltrate is present, with numerous PMNs. The covering epithelium is thin, and in areas of ulceration a thin fibrin exudate covers the surface.

An epulis should only be removed surgically in pregnancy if it is being traumatized by opposing teeth or a restoration, causing bleeding. The lesion can bleed profusely when excised, and electrocautery of the base of the lesion may be necessary to control this. The excised lesion should be placed in formal saline and sent for histological examination to confirm the diagnosis. Any secondary irritating factor associated with the lesion should also be corrected. There is a high recurrence rate of these lesions and, for this reason, removal should be delayed until after parturition whenever possible. At this stage the lesion usually regresses considerably and becomes more fibrous. It is therefore easier to remove the remnant lesion at this time, and the return of hormone levels to normal means that recurrence is rare.

Oral contraceptives

The hormonal oral contraceptive pill contains progesterone, often combined with an oestrogen. Many studies have shown that these produce a greater flow of gingival fluid and a higher prevalence of gingival inflammation (Chevallier, 1970). The degree of inflammation seems to be related to the length of time the woman is taking 'the pill'. As with pregnancy, these changes do not affect healthy tissues in a clean mouth, and the effect is to exaggerate a pre-existing gingivitis secondary to irritation from plaque. The exogenous hormones can also enhance the development of an anaerobic plaque in which black-pigmented anaerobic rods predominate (Jensen *et al.*, 1981).

As with the pregnant patient, special care with oral hygiene should be advised and this, combined with any necessary periodontal treatment, brings about a resolution of the condition (Pearlman, 1974).

Systemic diseases

Endocrines

Diabetes mellitus

Diabetes mellitus is a metabolic disorder characterized by glucose intolerance. It can be classified into two major categories, Type I or insulin dependent diabetes mellitus (IDDM), and type II or non-insulin dependent diabetes.

IDDM has a sudden onset and occurs usually before the age of 25 years. Symptoms include thirst, polyuria, hunger and weight loss, and it is controlled by daily injections of insulin. It is a primary disease of the cells of the islets of Langerhans.

Type II has a gradual onset and mainly affects obese middle-aged people. It is controlled by diet and hypoglycaemic drugs.

IDDM produces atherosclerotic changes in the arterioles, capillaries and venules in a wide range of organs, and renal, retinal and neural changes can occur.

The precise aetiology of IDDM is unclear, but it appears to involve genetic factors relating to the HLA system and has some features of an auto-immune condition. A large number of IDDM patients have antibodies to Coxsackie 6B virus, and it has been suggested that peptide sequences from viral proteins mimic those in certain protein antigens in the islet cells, such as glutamic acid dehydrogenase (GAD). T-cell immunity directed against these antigens would then damage or kill the islet cells. This would probably only occur in a group of susceptible individuals with the appropriate HLA (MHC) antigens, which would present the appropriate peptide sequence from the virus (Chapter 3). Approximately 2% of the population have IDDM, and the numbers are increasing.

Although scientific evidence is not clear cut, uncontrolled IDDM does appear to alter the periodontal tissues' response to plaque, especially in longstanding and severe cases. Diabetic children have more severe gingivitis than healthy children (Bernick *et al.*, 1975). However, opinion is somewhat divided with regard to adult diabetics' susceptibility to periodontitis. The studies fall into two categories; those that investigated a mixed group of type I and II diabetics, and those that just included IDDM cases. In both categories, some studies showed no relationship between diabetes and periodontal progression (Tervonen and Knuuttila, 1986; Goteiner *et al*, 1986), some showed slightly increased susceptibility (Glavind *et al.*, 1968; Cohen *et al.*, 1970), and some showed a marked increase

in susceptibility (Sznajder *et al.*, 1978; Cianciola *et al.*, 1982; Rylander *et al.*, 1986). A full list of studies can be seen in Seymour and Heasman (1992).

The consensus from these studies would seem to be that the well-controlled diabetic is at no greater risk from periodontal destruction than the normal population. However, several studies have shown that longstanding diabetics, and particularly those who show systemic complications, do appear to have greater rates of periodontal progression than age-matched healthy people. Diabetic patients with advanced periodontal disease also seem to suffer more frequently with complications such as lateral abscesses.

The possible reasons for their increased susceptibility could be the vascular changes and changes in polymorphonuclear leucocyte (PMN) function in IDDM.

The underlying mechanism of the vascular changes relates to the lack of heparin sulphate in basement membranes. The changes in the capillary basement membranes could have an inhibitory effect on the transport of oxygen, white blood cells, immune factors and waste products, all of which could affect the defence mechanism and tissue repair and regeneration. These vascular changes have been reported in the gingival tissues from IDDM patients (Lin *et al.*, 1975).

Impairment of PMN function is a feature of IDDM, and this includes reduced phagocytosis, intracellular killing and adherence (Saadoun, 1980). Diabetic patients and their relatives also have an impaired PMN chemotactic response (Clark, 1978). In addition, impairment of the chemotactic response of PMNs from the gingival crevice has been demonstrated in diabetic patients with severe periodontitis (Manouchehr-Pour *et al.*, 1981) and in families with a history of diabetes (McMullen *et al.*, 1981). It has been suggested that the defect is at the cellular level and may involve inhibition of the glycolytic pathway, abnormal cyclic nucleotide metabolism, which disrupts the organization of microtubules and microfilaments, or a reduction in leucocyte membrane receptors (Seymour and Heasman, 1992).

Nearly all diabetic patients respond to conventional periodontal treatment and benefit from regular monitoring and maintenance. If periodontal problems are to be avoided, a high standard of oral hygiene must be established and maintained. Diabetic patients are susceptible to infections, and these can disturb their metabolic control. It is therefore important that periodontal infections such as acute ulcerative necrotizing gingivitis (AUNG) or lateral periodontal abscesses should be promptly treated with the appropriate antibiotic. Also, if a diabetic requires periodontal surgery, then it is advisable to carry this out under antibiotic cover.

Genetic conditions

A number of conditions of genetic origin can affect the periodontal tissues, and these are listed below:

- Down's syndrome
- Hypophosphatasia
- Papillon–Lefèvre syndrome
- Ehlers–Danlos syndrome
- Hereditary gingival fibromatosis
- Mucopolysaccharidoses
- Hyperoxaluria
- Cyclic neutropenia
- Familial neutropenias
- Chediak–Higashi syndrome.

Down's syndrome

Down's syndrome results from trisomy of chromosome 21 caused by non-dysjunction during oogenesis. A few cases of the syndrome have a normal number of 46 chromosomes but have a reciprocal translocation of chromosome groups 13–15 and groups 21–22. The overall incidence of Down's syndrome is about 1 in 700 births, but increases to 1 : 100 if the mother is 45 or over. People with the syndrome have a variable degree of mental handicap and typical mongoloid facial features.

Orally, they typically have a Class III occlusion, an anterior open bite, a large tongue and a lack of lip seal. They are prone to infections, and their incidence of leukaemia is 20 times greater than the normal population. This is probably related to the presence on chromosome 21 of the genes for leucocyte development.

If living at home with their family or in a well-ordered community they usually have a very happy and trusting personality, and if they receive an appropriate education they can develop reasonable skill levels.

It is now well established by a large number of epidemiological studies that Down's syndrome cases are much more prone to destructive periodontitis than either the normal population or other mentally handicapped cases (Reuland-Bosma and Van Dijk, 1986; Seymour and Heasman, 1992). The overall incidence of periodontitis is in excess of 90%, but tends to be less in those living at home rather than in institutions. The distribution of disease is uneven, with the lower permanent incisors most commonly involved, and these teeth often have short conical roots. These are followed by the upper incisors and first molars, and the deciduous molars, premolars and canines. The commonest clinical presentation is mobility of the lower incisors with radiographical evidence of advanced alveolar bone loss (*Figure 6.3*). They also have an increased susceptibility to AUNG. In this regard, numerous black-pigmented anaerobic rods and spirochaetes can be frequently isolated from the subgingival flora of Down's cases (Brown, 1973).

The susceptibility to periodontitis is probably related to systemic disorders that are a feature of the syndrome, particularly those relating to the immune system. Many abnormalities have been reported in PMN from Down's cases. Their numbers in the peripheral blood are normal, but many cells are immature, possibly relating to a high rate of cell turnover (Kahn *et al.*, 1975). Impaired chemotaxis (Barkin *et al.*, 1980a), reduced phagocytosis (Rosner *et al.*, 1973) and intracellular killing (Kretschmer *et al.*, 1974) have been reported. This last feature may be related to disturbances in the intracellular oxidative metabolism in PMNs. Monocyte function is also impaired, but less so than PMNs (Barkin *et al.*, 1980b). However, monocyte sensitivity to interferon is three times higher than normal, and this may prevent their maturation to macrophages (Epstein *et al.*, 1980). B-lymphocytes display abnormalities in the form of capping of their immunoglobulin surface receptors (Naeim and Walford, 1980). This phenomenon also occurs in old age in normal people, suggesting that there may be a premature ageing of B-lymphocytes in Down's syndrome. T-lymphocyte function is profoundly affected in Down's syndrome, and the numbers of these cells in the circulation are low. There also

Figure 6.3 Radiograph showing advanced alveolar bone loss around the lower incisors of a 14-year-old boy with Down's syndrome

appears to be impaired maturation of these cells, possibly due to a defect in thymic processing (Levin *et al.*, 1979). Abnormalities have been seen in the thymus gland, and these include calcifications of Hassall bodies and a depletion of lymphocytes in the gland's cortex. In addition, there is a reduced T-lymphocyte response to mitogenic stimulation (Nishida *et al.*, 1981), and the response decreases further with age.

There are also some vascular changes in people with Down's syndrome, who suffer from circulatory problems due to abnormally thin and narrow peripheral arterioles and capillaries (Dallapiccola *et al.*, 1971). Capillary fragility is high in comparison to normal children or children with other forms of mental retardation. This could be due either to a connective tissue disorder or to diminished platelet activity. These vascular changes could lead to local tissue anoxia.

Patients with Down's syndrome need special care if dental problems are to be avoided or kept under control. They need frequent monitoring, with prompt treatment of any problem. Good plaque control must be established to combat periodontal problems, and scaling needs to be carried out frequently. Patient co-operation and acceptance of treatment and the support of the family and carers are of paramount importance. If the patient lacks the dexterity necessary for immaculate oral hygiene then these functions will need to be carried out by relatives or carers, and they will need to be trained in this function and informed about dental disease, its control and the increased susceptibility in Down's syndrome. These functions are considerably more difficult to carry out in an institution than in the home environment.

Hypophosphatasia

Hypophosphatasia is a rare condition with an autosomal recessive mode of inheritance. There is a deficiency of the enzyme alkaline phosphatase and a urinary excretion of phosphoethanolamine. It is characterized by abnormal mineralization of bones and dental tissues. In the infantile form, which appears at birth, there is softening of bones, fever, anaemia, hypocalcaemia and vomiting, which leads to death in infancy of more than half of the cases. The juvenile form, where the signs become apparent around 6 months of age, is less severe.

Several reports have appeared describing the dental and periodontal manifestations (Seymour and Heasman, 1992). These are fairly specific to the condition, and include premature exfoliation of the deciduous teeth, absence of gingival inflammation, presence of 'shell' teeth, and loss of alveolar bone, which is usually limited to the deciduous incisors and canines (Baer *et al.*, 1964). Microscopically, these teeth show either complete absence of cementum or isolated areas of abnormal cementum (Bruckner *et al.*, 1962). The loss of the deciduous teeth seems to result from the bone and cementum changes. The permanent dentition does not appear to be affected.

Papillon–Lefèvre syndrome

Papillon–Lefèvre syndrome is an autosomal recessive inherited disease characterized by a diffuse palmar–plantar keratosis and premature loss of both deciduous and permanent dentitions (Papillon and Lefèvre, 1924). Haneke (1979) reviewed 111 cases; 45 of these cases were from 22 families, and consanguinity of the parents was found in about a third of the cases. Males and females are equally affected. The condition is very rare, with an incidence of 1–4 per million, although 2–4 persons per 1000 are heterozygous (Gorlin *et al.*, 1964).

The characteristic skin lesions are diffuse erythematous, keratotic areas on the palms of the hand and soles of the feet. Ectopic calcifications of the falx cerebri and choroid plexus have also been reported in some cases. In the review of 111 cases (Haneke, 1979), 26 cases showed an increased susceptibility to infections. The dental condition affects the primary and permanent dentitions. The primary teeth are affected from the second year, are all prematurely exfoliated by the sixth year, and are lost in order of eruption (Baer and Benjamin, 1974). The tissues then heal and the permanent teeth erupt early. A similar destructive rapidly progressive periodontitis affects these teeth, and results in progressive bone loss and exfoliation. The clinical signs resemble those of an advanced adult periodontitis with severe gingival inflammation. The prognosis of the teeth is very poor, and most subjects are edentulous by the age of 16 years.

Periodontal treatment is usually unsuccessful (Haneke, 1979; Glenwright and Rock, 1990). Recently, some clinicians have suggested extraction of the primary teeth at 3 years with systemic antimicrobial therapy (tetracycline 250–500 mg per day) for 10 days during the period of the eruption of permanent teeth (Preus and Gjermo, 1987; Preus, 1988). A very high standard of oral hygiene is necessary for this treatment, and regular monitoring and treatment is required thereafter.

Ehlers–Danlos syndrome

Ehlers–Danlos syndrome is an inherited condition affecting the connective tissues, and is a disorder in collagen molecular biology. The main effects are excessive joint mobility, skin hyperextensibility, easy bruising and peculiar scarring after skin wounds. Ten variants of this condition have been described (Seymour and Heasman, 1992); the mode of inheritance of four types is autosomal dominant (I, II, III, VIII), three types are autosomal recessive (IV, VI, VII), and the other three types are X-linked (V, IX, X). The precise nature of the defect is unknown for most types, but in Type IV the defect in collagen is due to reduced lysyl hydroxylation of the molecule. Also in Type IV there is a deficiency in the synthesis, structure and secretion of Type III collagen and a deficiency of the enzyme procollagen peptidase.

The oral mucosa, gingival tissue, periodontium, teeth and temporomandibular joint are all affected. The oral mucosa is fragile and is susceptible to bruising. The gingival tissues bleed easily, particularly after brushing, and post-extraction haemorrhage may be a problem. The teeth are fragile and fracture easily, and recurrent subluxation of the temporomandibular joint can occur.

Patients with Type VIII Ehlers–Danlos syndrome have been reported to be susceptible to a rapidly progressive periodontitis (Stewart *et al.*, 1977), but this does not appear to be a feature of other variants (Barabas and Barabas, 1967).

Conventional periodontal treatment is difficult because of the oral mucosal and gingival fragility. This can give rise to serious complications if root planning or surgery is attempted. The tissues split under the slightest provocation and are very difficult to suture. Extractions are complicated by haemorrhage. Periodontal treatment should be as atraumatic as possible, and very careful, atraumatic oral hygiene techniques should be taught using a soft toothbrush.

Hereditary gingival fibromatosis

Hereditary gingival fibromatosis may occur singly or in association with other inherited syndromes. It is inherited as an autosomal dominant trait (Witkop, 1971), and has an incidence of 1:350 000. The condition does not become manifest until after the eruption of the teeth, and is most commonly seen associated with the permanent teeth. The hyperplasia is due to excessive production of collagen in the gingival corium. The enlarged gingival tissues (*Figure 6.4*) appear firm and pink with exaggerated stippling (Becker *et al.*, 1967). The tissue often completely covers the crowns of the teeth, and may interfere with speech and mastication. It may delay the eruption of teeth. The gingival hyperplasia may be generalized or localized, and local involvement mainly affects the maxillary tuberosities and lingual surfaces of the lower molars.

Figure 6.4 Hereditary gingival fibrous hyperplasia in a girl of 15 years. Regrowth of tissue has followed gingivectomy on three occasions. The fibrous overgrowth is associated with incomplete eruption of posterior teeth

Histologically, the tissues show a vast excess of collagen in an avascular corium with overlying parakeratinized epithelium.

The condition may occur with a number of other rare inherited syndromes, when it may be associated with some of the following: hypertrichosis, hypopigmentation, mental deficiency, epilepsy, optic and auditory defects, cartilage and nail defects and dentigerous cysts (see Seymour and Heasman, 1992).

It has recently been shown (Tipton *et al.*, 1997) that all the gingival fibroblasts in the gingival tissues of patients with this syndrome appear to have the characteristics of permanently activated fibroblasts. When compared with normal gingival fibroblasts, they have increased proliferation rates and show increased production of collagen and fibronectin.

Mucopolysaccharidoses

The mucopolysaccharidoses (MPS) are a group of inherited disorders characterized by disturbances of mucopolysaccharide metabolism, resulting in increased storage of these substances in various tissues. They include Hurler's syndrome (MPS I), Hunter's syndrome (MPS II), I-cell disease and MPS III, IV, V and VI. Hurler's syndrome is inherited as an autosomal recessive trait, whilst Hunter's syndrome is an X-linked recessive trait and I-cell disease probably represents the homozygous state of a recessive mutation (McKusick, 1969). Hurler's syndrome manifests in early childhood, and children usually die before the age of 10 years from respiratory infection or cardiac disease consequent on deposition of mucopolysaccharides in the heart valves and intima of the coronary arteries. The main clinical features of this syndrome are mental retardation, dwarfism, hernia, deformed head, typical facies, short neck and spinal deformities (Gardiner, 1971). Hunter's syndrome is less severe and the survival rate is greater. In both syndromes there are increased levels of chondroitin sulphate B and heparitin sulphate in the urine.

The teeth in these conditions are small and widely spaced, and exhibit delayed eruption (Cawson, 1962). Gingival enlargement may occur, and the tissue is nodular, fibrotic, oedematous and haemorrhagic (Cawson, 1962; Gardiner, 1971). The gingival tissues often contain the characteristic Hunter cells within the lamina propria. They are probably macrophages, and they contain large amounts of metachromatic material in their cytoplasm (Gardiner, 1968).

Hyperoxaluria and oxalosis

Primary hyperoxaluria is a rare autosomal recessive inherited disease of glycoxalate metabolism, and is due to an enzyme deficiency. It results in the deposition of calcium oxalate in various tissues throughout the body. Its clinical features are nephrolithiasis, nephrocalcinosis, acute arthritis, heart block and peripheral neuropathy. The life expectancy is poor, and death is usually due to renal failure. Secondary hyperoxaluria can also occur in chronic renal failure where oxalate deposits in the kidney, possibly due to recurrent dialysis failing to remove all the calcium oxalate.

The main oral changes of oxalosis are root resorption, both external and internal, and histologically these areas show deposits of calcium oxalate crystals and granulomatous foreign body reaction (Wysocki *et al.*, 1982). Pain may arise from an inflammatory reaction in the pulp and periodontal ligament to calcium oxalate crystal deposition. These crystals may also deposit in the gingiva and periodontal ligament, where they again evoke a chronic inflammatory response (Moskow, 1989). The crystals become surrounded by macrophages, multinucleated giant cells (macrophage polykaryons), lymphocytes and plasma cells. This reaction in the periodontal ligament or pulp may be the cause of root resorption (Fantasia *et al.*, 1982).

The only effective treatment of the root resorption appears to be extraction of the grossly involved teeth.

Granulomatous conditions

Crohn's disease

Crohn's disease (or regional enteritis) is a chronic inflammatory condition, primarily of the terminal ileum, and was first described by Crohn *et al.* (1932). It affects the submucosa of the gastrointestinal tract, and produces stenosis, necrotic breakdown and scarring of the mucosa. All areas of the tract including the mouth can be affected, but the initial lesion is in the terminal ileum. Symptoms include abdominal pain, pyrexia, intermittent diarrhoea, joint pains and generalized malaise. The overall incidence is about 15 per 100 000, but is higher in Jews and in the siblings of affected patients (Sandler and Golden, 1986).

The aetiology is unknown, but intolerance to certain foods (particularly those containing gluten) may be an important factor, and there is a familial tendency, although no genetic pattern has been established. A gluten-free diet is recommended for these subjects.

The oral manifestations of Crohn's disease are aphthous-like ulceration and a cobblestone appearance of the oral mucosa (*Figure 6.5*), labial and buccal gingival swellings, mucosal tags, fissuring of the midline of the lip and angular cheilitis (Bernstein and McDonald, 1978).

The characteristic gingival lesion is diffuse, erythematous, granular enlargement of the attached gingiva. The cobblestone appearance of the oral mucosa is mainly confined to the buccal mucosa, and the lesions are lobulated, oedematous and fissured, and ulceration may be present. The tag-like lesions in the mucobuccal fold resemble denture granulomata (Seymour and Heasman, 1992).

Severe periodontitis has been seen in patients with this condition (Lampster *et al.*, 1978, 1982; Engel *et al.*, 1988). Patients with active bowel disease have been reported to have high levels of circulating immune com-

Figure 6.5 Appearance of gingivae in Crohn's disease. (Courtesy Professor C Scully)

plexes and metabolically active PMNs compared to healthy controls (Lampster *et al.*, 1982). It has also been found that the PMNs from these patients had elevated levels of alkaline phosphatase, which is an indication of early release of these cells from the marrow (Koldjaer *et al.*, 1977). In addition, it has been found that these patients had low circulating B-lymphocyte numbers and high numbers of T-lymphocytes (Engel *et al.*, 1988). All of these factors could exacerbate an existing periodontal condition or accelerate its progress.

These patients usually respond well to conventional periodontal treatment.

Sarcoidosis

Sarcoidosis is a granulomatous condition of uncertain aetiology that may affect the lymph nodes, lungs, liver, spleen, skin, eyes, phalangeal bones and parotid glands. The worldwide prevalence is 20 per 100 000, with higher levels in blacks than in whites. Its prognosis is good with most cases showing spontaneous healing, which can be accelerated by the administration of corticosteroids.

Oral lesions rarely occur, with swelling of the parotid glands and cervical lymph nodes most common and gingival involvement least common. It may also affect the minor salivary glands. The histopathology is a collection of monocyte-derived epithelioid cells with T-lymphocytes and occasional plasma cells (Gold and Sager, 1976). Several cases of sarcoid gingivitis have been reported (see Seymour and Heasman, 1992). The gingivae have a hyperplastic, granulomatous appearance, and may have superficial ulceration. Histologically, there is an infiltration of macrophages and their polykaryons.

Scleroderma

Scleroderma or systemic sclerosis is a connective tissue disorder of uncertain aetiology. It produces inflammatory, vascular and fibrotic changes in the skin and other organs and structures. The changes may be limited to the skin or generalized, and in the latter form the prognosis is poor, particularly if there is involvement of the lungs, heart and kidneys.

The main change in the periodontium brought about by this condition is widening of the periodontal ligament space at the expense of alveolar bone. The changes affect the posterior teeth more than the anterior teeth. The teeth remain firm, and the apical level of the junctional epithelium is unaffected. There is a proportional increase in collagen and oxytalin fibres, and the fibrous tissue contains areas of degeneration with sclerosis and hyalinization (Wood and Lee, 1988).

Haematological conditions (blood diseases)

Blood diseases do not appear to cause gingivitis, but they do bring about tissue changes that alter the tissue response to plaque. The dentist has a special responsibility in relation to these diseases, as severe gingival bleeding is a common feature of acute leukaemia and the dentist may be the first person to examine the patient. Delay in the control of such a disease could be fatal.

Red blood cell (RBC) disorders

Anaemia

Anaemia is defined as a reduction in the concentration of haemoglobin in the blood below the normal level. The normal level is usually accepted as being 12.5–18.0 g/dl for males and 12.0–16.5 g/dl for females. There are a large number of causes of anaemia, including haemorrhage, chemical damage and disease, but the most common form is iron-deficiency anaemia, which is found in about 10% of the female population. Anaemia lowers the oxygen-carrying capacity of the blood so that the patient may feel tired and faint and may have difficulty in breathing and tingling of the fingers and toes. The skin may be pale, but this is frequently not the case; pallor of the tissue beneath the fingernails and of the oral mucosa, including the gingiva, is a more reliable sign, but even this may only occur when the anaemia is severe. The tongue may lose its normally rough papillated surface and become smooth. There may be recurrent aphthous ulcers and angular cheilitis in some cases. If anaemia is suspected, blood examination is necessary.

Aplastic anaemia

Aplastic anaemia can be caused by drugs, chemicals, radiation, infections or neoplasia. The resultant anaemia, leucopenia and thrombocytopenia produce weakness, fatigue, recurrent infections, pyrexia, epistaxis and retinal haemorrhage. The main oral effects are gingival bleeding and infections.

A rare autosomal recessive inherited form of aplastic anaemia with a poor prognosis is called Fanconi's anaemia. Orally, it produces a rapidly progressive destructive periodontitis with early tooth loss (Opinya *et al.*, 1988).

Acatalasia

This is a rare inherited disease caused by the absence of the enzyme catalase in RBCs and WBCs. Catalase converts hydrogen peroxide to oxygen and water. Plaque bacteria can produce hydrogen peroxide, which will oxidize haemoglobin in the deficient RBCs. This results in hypoxia and necrosis of gingival tissue. A case report of two siblings with this condition described gingival necrosis and severe destructive periodontitis (Delago and Calderon, 1979).

White blood cell (WBC) disorders

Neutrophils (PMNs) and monocytes are essential cells in the defence system of the periodontium. Reductions in their numbers or their function can have a profound effect on the periodontal tissues. The term leucopenia means an absolute reduction in numbers of WBCs, and neutropenia means a reduction in the number of PMNs. The leukaemias are a group of neoplastic conditions in which there is uncontrolled proliferation of the affected group of WBCs.

Neutropenia

Neutropenia may be genetic, familial, idiopathic or secondary to viral, bacterial or protozoan infections or systemic disease. All forms of neutropenia profoundly affect periodontal health. The main primary neutropenias are:

- Cyclic neutropenia
- Chronic benign neutropenia
- Familial neutropenias
- Chronic idiopathic neutropenia.

Cyclic neutropenia

This is a rare autosomal dominant inherited condition. It produces a cyclical depression of PMNs in the peripheral blood at intervals varying from 15 to 55 days, with occasional longer periods of neutropenia lasting 1–2 months (Page and Good, 1957). The main clinical manifestations are pyrexia, oral ulceration and skin infections. The condition appears to be due to periodic stem cell failure in the bone marrow related to a disorder of haemopoietic feedback control (Zucker-Franklin *et al.*, 1977).

The main oral and periodontal features of this condition are oral ulceration, severe gingivitis and rapid periodontal breakdown and alveolar bone loss. In the permanent dentition, the bone loss is most obvious around the teeth that erupt first, the first molars and lower incisors (Spencer and Fleming, 1985). Patients with this condition require regular periodontal maintenance for careful supra- and subgingival scaling, and meticulous oral hygiene should be encouraged. Antibiotic therapy will be necessary to control acute episodes, and antiseptic mouthwashes will help when oral ulceration is present.

Chronic benign neutropenia of childhood

The onset of this condition is usually between the ages of 6 and 20 months. There is a moderate neutropenia with an absolute lymphocytosis and monocytosis. The bone marrow appears normal, and the neutropenia may be due to increased peripheral destruction.

Pyogenic infections of the skin and mucous membranes are a feature of this condition. However, the increased numbers of monocytes can compensate for the neutropenia and may provide a reasonable resistance to infections (Biggar *et al.*, 1974).

Several case reports of the oral and periodontal features of this condition have appeared (Seymour and Heasman, 1992), and most of these relate to boys aged 4–12 years. There is a bright red, hyperplastic, oedematous gingivitis, which affects the free and attached gingivae, and the gingivae bleed easily. There appears to be premature loss of primary teeth due to bone loss. Some older children show a rapidly progressive periodontitis in the permanent dentition, with generalized bone loss. In most reports attempts to control the condition with periodontal treatment have been unsuccessful, and early loss of primary and permanent teeth seems difficult to prevent.

Familial neutropenias

Benign familial neutropenia is an autosomal dominant inherited condition. There is a moderate neutropenia and an accompanying monocytosis. The bone marrow appears normal, and the condition may be due to an anomaly in the marrow release mechanism (Mintz and Sachs, 1973).

The only case report of oral and periodontal changes in a 14-year-old boy with this condition (Deasy *et al.*, 1980) described a bright red, hyperplastic, oedematous gingivitis; the tissues bled profusely. There was also marked bone loss around the first molars, suggesting a rapidly progressive periodontitis. The treatment was plaque control, scaling and antiseptic mouthwashes, but no long-term follow-up of the patient's condition was reported.

Severe familial neutropenia is more severe than the benign form, and is inherited as an autosomal dominant trait. There is a more marked neutropenia and some monocytosis. Children are susceptible to repeated infections. The oral and periodontal changes are similar to those described above but more severe, and the prognosis is poor.

Chronic idiopathic neutropenia

Chronic idiopathic neutropenia was first described by Kyle and Linman (1968), and appears to occur mainly in females. There is a persistent neutropenia from birth, which is not cyclical, and there is no family history of the condition. There are persistent recurrent infections throughout the life of the sufferers. The cause of the condition is uncertain, but there does appear to be a maturation abnormality of granulocytes in the bone marrow, which could be related to an auto-immune disorder.

The periodontal features have been reported in two case reports (Kyle and Linman, 1970; Kalkwark and Gatz, 1981). There is a severe, oedematous, hyperplastic gingivitis with early bone loss, and the condition does not respond well to treatment.

Leukaemia

Leukaemias are malignant neoplastic disease of the white blood cell-forming tissues. They usually result in an increased number of leucocytes in the circulation, including developing blast cells, and an infiltration of leukaemic cells into other tissues, particularly lymph nodes. The condition may affect granulocytes (myeloid), monocytes (monocytic) or lymphocytes (lymphocytic), and can be either chronic or acute. In acute forms, large numbers of neoplastic primitive stem and blast cells proliferate in the marrow and enter the circulation. The acute forms of leukaemia are more common in children and young adults, and the chronic forms in adults over 40 years of age.

The clinical signs and symptoms are due to reduced numbers of other marrow cells such as red cells and megakaryocytes, which are crowded out by the proliferation of neoplastic cells, and the lack of normal function from the leukaemic cells themselves. Early symptoms include: tiredness, lethargy and fatigue due to anaemia; malaise, sore throat, oral ulceration and skin infections due to reduced white cell function; and enlargement of the lymph nodes, spleen and liver due to leukaemic infiltration. Chronic leukaemias have a slow, insidious onset, with tiredness, weight loss, fatigue, pyrexia and splenic enlargement being the main features.

The oral and periodontal features may reflect both the condition and its treatment with radiotherapy and chemotherapy. They include oral ulceration, petechiae and ecchymoses, gingival enlargement, gingival bleeding and bacterial, viral and fungal infections. Oropharyngeal lesions may be the initial complaint in over 10% of acute leukaemias (Scully and Cawson, 1987). The gingival enlargement (*Figure 6.6*) is due to infiltration of leukaemic cells (Barrett, 1986), and is most common in monocytic leukaemia. Gingival bleeding is secondary to the accompanying thrombocytopenia, and may present as oozing or frank bleeding. It is most marked when the platelet count drops below 10 000 per ml.

Infections may be due either to exacerbation of an existing condition or to susceptibility to a range of bacterial, viral and fungal infections. Existing periodontitis can be exacerbated by the leukaemia or by chemotherapy. A variety of infections can occur for similar reasons, and include acute ulcerative necrotizing gingivitis (AUNG), acute herpetic gingivostomatitis and fungal infections such as candidiasis (Barrett, 1984).

Leukaemic patients need careful hygiene care during acute episodes of the disease or during treatment with radiotherapy and chemotherapy. Regular gentle profes-

Figure 6.6 Gingival inflammation and swelling in a patient with myeloid leukaemia. (Courtesy Professor C Scully)

sional cleaning and swabbing with chlorhexidine can be very beneficial.

Every effort should be made to treat any periodontal condition during remission phases of the disease and, during this time, to encourage immaculate plaque control. Oral and periodontal infections may need to be treated with the appropriate antibiotic. The patient's physician should always be consulted before any treatment is carried out so that an appropriate regimen can be discussed and agreed.

Disorders of white cell function

These conditions affect the ability of PMNs to phagocytose and destroy bacteria intracellularly. Primary functional disturbances that affect the periodontal tissues are the Chediak–Higashi syndrome and the lazy leucocyte syndrome.

Chediak–Higashi syndrome

Chediak–Higashi syndrome is a rare autosomal recessive inherited disease. Clinical features include albinism with photophobia and nystagmus, and frequent pyogenic infections and ferbrile illnesses. Later, a lymphoma-like condition develops, with accompanying neutropenia, anaemia and thrombocytopenia. Death usually results from infection or haemorrhage. Circulating leucocytes have large abnormal lysosomes in their cytoplasm, and show defective migration and phagocytic degranulation and grossly diminished intracellular killing (Dale *et al.*, 1972).

The disease gives rise to a very severe gingivitis and periodontitis, and premature loss of the primary and permanent teeth. The condition does not appear to respond well to periodontal treatment.

Lazy leucocyte syndrome

Lazy leucocyte syndrome was first described by Miller *et al.* (1971). There is a defect in PMN chemotaxis and

random mobility. A severe gingivitis has been described in two children with this condition.

Chronic granulomatous disease

Chronic granulomatous disease is an inherited condition, transmitted as an autosomal recessive trait in females and as an X-linked recessive trait in males. It is characterized by the inability of phagocytes to destroy certain infective bacteria. The PMNs of subjects with this condition are unable to generate hydrogen peroxide, possibly because of the absence of the enzyme NADPH oxidase. A granulomatous response to inflammation occurs, and involves the lymph nodes, spleen, liver, skin and lungs. People with this condition are very prone to osteomyelitis, liver abscesses and pneumonia, and their prognosis is poor.

Case reports (Allan and Straton, 1983) have described a severe and diffuse gingivitis with ulceration, which spreads on to the buccal mucosa. This may respond to antibiotic therapy.

Immunological conditions

Hypogammaglobulinaemia

This can rarely occur as a X-linked recessive inherited disease. More commonly, it is secondary to chronic lymphatic leukaemia and myeloma. Patients are highly susceptible to infection, particularly of the respiratory tract. There have been some reports of severe destructive periodontitis (Roberts and Walker, 1976), but other reports have suggested that patients with primary immunodeficiencies suffer less gingivitis and caries than controls (Robertson *et al.*, 1978), although this could be associated with the extensive use of antibiotics in these cases.

Multiple myeloma

This is a multifocal malignant neoplasm of plasma cells. Deposits can occur in the mandible and maxilla. Lesions have also been reported involving the periodontium and gingiva (Petit and Ripamonti, 1990). The oral lesions described are gingival ulceration and bleeding, and the condition may produce a rapidly growing, retromolar myelomatous mass with multiple foci of alveolar bone destruction.

Immunosuppressive drugs

Immunosuppressive drugs are often given to combat autoimmune disease or to prevent rejection of transplants. They include corticosteroids, azathioprine and cyclosporin. Corticosteroids and azathioprine reduce the inflammatory response and may reduce gingivitis. Cyclosporin may produce gingival fibrous hyperplasia (see below).

Dermatoses

A number of skin diseases have oral manifestations that can occur on the gingivae. Some of these diseases are moderately common, such as lichen planus and some are extremely rare, such as pemphigus vulgaris.

Lichen planus

This disease is estimated to occur in 1% of the population. It is an inflammatory disease of doubtful aetiology that occurs in the skin and mucous membranes. It is more frequently observed in conjunction with diseases of immunity, e.g. ulcerative colitis, myasthenia gravis and hypogammaglobulinaemia, and there is increasing evidence that lichen planus is immunologically mediated. Lichen planus can occur in families, and there is an increasing frequency of HLA-B7 in the MHC (see Chapter 3). The oral lesion can occur either in the absence of skin lesions or with minimal or widespread skin lesions, and there is no difference in the oral lesion with or without skin involvement. The disease may be manifest in various forms (Shklar and McCarthy, 1961).

The reticulated form is the most common, and consists of an interlacing network of white lines found frequently on the cheeks, vestibule and gingiva (*Figure 6.7*). In other forms, milky white patches, eroded areas or papules are present on the mucosa, especially the tongue and cheeks. Erosive or reticular lesions can occur on the gingivae, and it is the most common cause of erosive (desquamative) gingivitis. The lesion may be symptomless or painful and sore, the latter being more common with the erosive form. The lesions are sensitive to spicy and acid foods.

Some recent reports have suggested that some cases of oral lichenoid lesions in contact with amalgam restorations (contact lesions) may be caused or aggravated by an allergy to mercury from the amalgam (Eley, 1993). Mercury deposits have been found in lysosomes of fibroblasts and macrophages from contact lesions (Bolewska *et al.*, 1990). Some of these cases show remission following the replacement of amalgam restorations with alternative restorative materials, and this may support the theory that mercury allergy may be a causative or aggravating factor in certain cases of localised oral lichenoid lesions.

Treatment of lichen planus is symptomatic, and topical applications of triamcinolone paste (Adcortyl A in Orabase) two to four times per day may alleviate symptoms.

Benign mucous membrane pemphigoid

This is a disease of the mucous membranes caused by an immunological disorder. Usually it occurs in older adults. The lesion is a bulla (*Figure 6.8*), which breaks down quickly to form an ulcer with an inflamed background that heals to form scarring (Shklar and McCarthy, 1959). It is most often seen in women at the menopause or after, but is not confined to women.

The disease may affect the gingivae, and it is an uncommon cause of erosive gingivitis. There is a diffuse erythema of the gingivae with grey patches of desquamated epithelium. The involved areas are very sensitive, and patients complain of soreness aggravated by spicy foods. The condition is chronic, with periods of remission.

Treatment is symptomatic. Irritant foods or drinks or mouthwashes should be avoided. Topical applications of triamcinolone paste (Adcortyl A in Orabase) may help, but Orabase alone is often just as effective. The patient needs to be reassured that the condition is benign, unless there is ocular involvement, when scarring may impair vision.

Figure 6.7 Lichen planus. Reticulated lesion in the cheek of a 50-year-old woman

Figure 6.8 Benign mucous membrane pemphigoid. Intact bullae on gingivae. (Courtesy Dr W R Tyldesley)

Pemphigus vulgaris

This is an auto-immune disease in which antibody and T-lymphocytes react with cells of mucous membranes, thus destroying the cells. If widespread involvement occurs the disease may be fatal and, as the oral lesions often occur before skin lesions appear, the dentist has a special diagnostic responsibility. Most cases develop in middle age, often in patients of Jewish or Italian extraction.

The disease is characterized by the formation of bullae (large vesicles or blisters) in any part of the oral mucosa, including the gingivae (*Figure 6.9*). The bullae break down rapidly to form ragged ulcers, which may heal slowly. There is pain and swelling and, if the lesions involve the palate and throat, swallowing is difficult.

Sometimes it is possible to make a diagnosis by using the 'Nikolsky sign', in which sliding pressure with the finger over apparently intact mucosa dislodges the mucosa. Definitive diagnosis is made by histological examination of biopsy specimens. If pemphigus is suspected, immediate referral to a physician is essential. The condition may be controlled by systemic corticosteroids.

Infections

Localized or generalized infections may involve the oral mucosa or periodontal tissues. Localized infections include acute necrotizing ulcerative gingivitis (Chapter 22) and acute lateral periodontal abscess (Chapter 19). Generalized infections include herpes simplex infections, herpes varicella/zoster infections, measles, tuberculosis, syphilis, *Candida albicans* infections (Chapter 21) and acquired immune deficiency syndrome (AIDS) (Chapter 7).

Drug reactions

In recent years it has been established that drugs that alter the haemopoietic system or the immune system, either to decrease or to enhance its activity, alter the response of the gingivae to plaque. As stated in Chapter 3, these findings support the idea of the involvement of the immune system in the pathogenesis of periodontal disease. It seems possible that, in the future, the influence of other drugs (e.g. antibiotics, analgesics, barbiturates, etc.) that are capable of producing a hypersensitivity response with skin eruptions and oral lesions may be revealed. However, the most common response of the gingiva to drugs is gingival hyperplasia, described below.

Drug-related gingival hyperplasia

The anticonvulsant drug phenytoin (Epanutin, Dilantin, DPH), given to epileptics, the immunosuppressive drug cyclosporin (Savage *et al.*, 1987) and the calcium channel blocking drug nifedipine (Barak *et al.*, 1987), given to treat cardiac angina, arrhythmias and hypertension, can produce fibrous hyperplasia of the gingiva.

Some degree of gingival enlargement occurs in a large percentage of epileptics taking phenytoin, especially those under 40 years of age. The condition is less common in patients on cyclosporin, but when it occurs it may be very severe. Nifedipine hyperplasia is less firm than the other two, and contains a higher proportion of ground substance.

The gingivae on the labial surface of the anterior teeth are usually more severely affected than the posterior teeth. The swelling is made up mainly of fibrous tissue and, unless inflammatory changes have supervened, is therefore firm, pink and lobulated (*Figure 6.10*). The swelling does not appear to be severe if oral hygiene is good, but once inflammatory changes have been provoked by plaque these appear to enhance the activity of fibroblasts so that they increase in number and produce more collagen

Figure 6.9 Pemphigus vulgaris. (Courtesy Dr W R Tyldesley)

Figure 6.10 Gingival hyperplasia in an epileptic patient on Epanutin

fibres and proteoglycans appear. However, the size of the swelling does not appear to be related directly to drug dosage.

With superimposed inflammation, the gingival swelling can become soft and red and bleed when provoked. The gingival enlargement can almost cover the teeth, and the condition may add to the social handicap that the epileptic patient may suffer.

Phenytoin is known to produce immunosuppression, folic acid depletion and possible suppression of adreno-cortical trophic hormone (ACTH). It also produces its effect of stabilizing the neuronal cell membrane by decreasing its permeability to calcium (Seymour and Heasman, 1992). Cyclosporin also causes immunosuppression, and nifedipine affects cell membrane calcium transport. All of these factors could influence fibroblast function.

Both inflammation and the effects of the drugs on androgen metabolism seem to be important in the cause of the fibrous hyperplasia (Sooryamoorthy and Gower, 1989a). Testosterone is a C19 androgenic steroid responsible for male characteristics, but is also found in the tissues of both sexes. Testosterone is converted by 5α-reductase into 5α-dihydrotestosterone (DHT), which is its main biologically active metabolite. Specific cell surface receptors for DHT are present in the gingivae (Southren et al., 1978), and these increase in number two- to three-fold in inflamed and hyperplastic gingival tissue. These DHT receptors are located on gingival epithelial cells and fibroblasts (Hernandez et al., 1981), and phenytoin has been found to stimulate 5α-reductase activity in fibroblasts from inflamed gingival tissue (Sooryamoorthy and Gower, 1989b). DHT stimulates gingival fibroblasts to produce and secrete collagen and proteoglycan. Because of its sexual function there is much more testosterone available in male tissues, and in healthy gingival tissue it is metabolized mainly by males. However, during inflammation gingival tissue metabolizes testosterone to the same extent in males and females (Ojanatoko et al., 1980). Phenytoin stimulates the biosynthesis of DHT from testosterone in gingival fibroblasts (Sooryamoorthy et al., 1988). Cyclosporin and nifedipine also carry out this function (Sooryamoorthy et al., 1990).

These drugs, probably as a result of the production of DHT, may also select a subpopulation of fibroblasts that produce large amounts of collagen with the production of an inactive form of collagenase (Hassell, 1978, 1982). This would produce an imbalance between the production and removal of collagen and proteoglycan, thus causing an overgrowth. This subgroup of cells may be more responsive to DHT stimulation.

It has also been found (McGaw and Porter, 1988; Hall and Squier, 1992) that fibrosis-inducing agents such as phenytoin and cyclosporin decrease the amount of phago-cytosed collagen with fibroblasts (see Chapter 1). In vitro experiments (McCulloch and Knowles, 1993) have also shown that phenytoin and cyclosporin inhibit the phagocytosis of collagen-coated beads by fibroblasts. Thus, in this way, these drugs could directly or indirectly decrease the amount of intracellular collagen degradation and

therefore contribute to the fibrosis associated with their use (Everts et al., 1996).

Changing the drug is rarely possible with epileptics, and never possible with patients taking the other two drugs. Treatment therefore must be restricted to oral hygiene instruction and supra- and subgingival scaling. Local removal of hyperplastic tissue may be carried out by gingivectomy or inverse bevel gingivectomy in some cases. Recurrence of hyperplasia is common, but may be reduced if immaculate oral hygiene can be maintained.

A regression of nifedipine-induced gingival hyperplasia has been shown to occur when patients have been switched onto other drugs in the same class of calcium channel blockers (Westbrook et al., 1997). They found that 60% of patients placed on the alternative calcium channel blocker, Isradiprine, had regression of their nifedipine-induced gingival hyperplasia. Furthermore, no patients placed primarily on Isradiprine developed gingival hyperplasia.

Dietary and nutritional factors

Theoretically, a deficiency of any essential nutrient might affect the status of the periodontal tissues and their resistance to plaque irritation; however, because of the delicately balanced interdependence of dietary elements, it is extremely difficult in human beings to define the consequences of a specific deficiency. Epidemiological studies demonstrated that, at any given age level, there is more severe periodontal disease in African and Asian populations than in Europeans. This could be due either to nutritional deficiency or to poor oral hygiene, both of which reflect socio-economic status. In Nigeria, well-fed children have better gingival health than badly-nourished children, irrespective of oral hygiene standards. Waerhaug (1967) found a correlation between the severity of periodontal destruction and the deficiency of vitamin B in a Sri Lankan population, but in general the effects of nutritional deficiency appear to be non-specific, i.e. the results of deficiency in several nutritional factors (Russell et al., 1965). In severe nutritional deficiency, usually accompanied by extremely poor oral hygiene, there is rapid destruction of the periodontal tissues and early tooth loss. The prevalence of acute necrotizing ulcerative gingivitis is also increased, and this may develop into a destructive and even fatal cancrum oris.

Severe periodontal destruction has long been associated with scurvy. Vitamin C is essential for collagen production, and therefore for normal turnover and repair, but experimental vitamin C deficiency has not produced a clear demonstration of gingival change. It seems likely that some plaque-induced inflammation is needed for gingival changes to take place in scurvy. There is no evidence to support the supplementation of an already balanced diet with extra vitamins in the treatment of periodontal disease.

References

Adam, D., Carney, J.S. and Dicks, D.A. (1973) Pregnancy gingivitis: a survey of 100 antenatal patients. *Journal of Dentistry* **2**, 106–110

Allan, D. and Straton, A.G. (1983) Chronic granulomatous disease with associated oral lesions. *British Dental Journal* **154**, 110–112

Baer, P.N. and Benjamin, S.D. (1974) In *Periodontal Disease in Children and Adolescents*, pp. 206–209. Philadelphia: Lippincott

Baer, P.N., Brown, N.C. and Hammer, J.E. (1964) Hypophosphatasia: report of two cases with dental findings. *Periodontics* **2**, 209–215

Barabas, G.M. and Barabas, A.P. (1967) Ehlers–Danlos syndrome. A report of the oral and haematological findings in nine cases. *British Dental Journal* **123**, 473–479

Barak, S., Engelberg, I.S. and Hiss, J. (1987) Gingival hyperplasia caused by nifedipine. *Journal of Periodontology* **58**, 639–642

Barkin, R.M., Weston, W.L., Humbert, J.R. and Marie, F. (1980a) Phagocytic function in Down's syndrome. I. Chemotaxis. *Journal of Mental Deficiency Research* **24**, 243–249

Barkin, R.M., Weston, W.L., Humbert, J.R and Sunada, K. (1980b) Phagocytic function in Down's syndrome. II. Bactericidal activity and phagocytosis. *Journal of Mental Deficiency Research* **24**, 251–256

Barrett, A.P. (1984) Gingival lesions in leukaemia: a classification. *Journal of Periodontology* **55**, 585–588

Barrett, A.P. (1986) Leukaemic cell infiltration of the gingiva. *Journal of Periodontology* **57**, 579–581

Becker, W., Colins, C.K., Zimmerman, E.R. *et al.* (1967) Hereditary gingival fibromatosis. *Oral Surgery, Oral Medicine, Oral Pathology* **24**, 313–318

Bernick, S.M., Cohen, D.W., Baker, I. and Laster I. (1975) Dental diseases in children with diabetes mellitus. *Journal of Periodontology* **46**, 241–245

Bernstein, M.L. and McDonald, J.S. (1978) Oral lesions in Crohn's disease: report of two cases and update of literature. *Oral Surgery, Oral Medicine, Oral Pathology* **46**, 234–245

Biggar, W.D., Holmes, B., Page, A.R. *et al.* (1974) Metabolic and functional studies of monocytes in congenital neutropenia. *British Journal of Haematology* **28**, 233–234

Bolewska, J., Holmstrup, P., Møller-Madsen, B. *et al.* (1990) Amalgam associated accumulations in normal oral mucosa, mucosal lesions of lichen planus and contact lesions associated with amalgam. *Journal of Oral Pathology and Medicine* **19**, 39–42

Brown, R.H. (1973) Necrotizing ulcerative gingivitis in mongoloid and non-mongoloid retarded and normal individuals. *Journal of Periodontal Research* **6**, 140–145

Bruckner, R.J., Rickles, N.H. and Porter, D.R. (1962) Hypophosphatasia with premature shedding of teeth and aplasia of cementum. *Oral Surgery, Oral Medicine and Oral Pathology* **15**, 1352–1369

Cawson, R.A. (1962) The oral changes in gargoylism. *Proceedings of the Royal Society of Medicine* **55**, 1066–1070

Chevallier, M.E. (1970) Mouth manifestations and oral contraceptives. *Revue Odonto-Stomatologie du Midi de la France* **28**, 96–103

Cianciola, L.J., Park, B.H., Bruck, E. *et al.* (1982) Prevalence of periodontal disease in insulin dependent diabetes mellitus (juvenile·diabetes). *Journal of the American Dental Association* **104**, 653–660

Clark, R. (1978) Disorders of granulocyte chemotaxis. In *Leukocyte Chemotaxis* (J. Gallin and P. Quie, eds), pp. 329–352. New York: Raven Press

Cohen, D., Friedman, L., Shapiro, J. *et al.* (1970) Diabetes mellitus and periodontal disease: 2-year longitudinal observations. Part I. *Journal of Periodontology* **41**, 709–712

Cohen, D., Shapiro, J., Firedman, L. *et al.* (1971) A longitudinal investigation of the periodontal changes during pregnancy and 15 months post-partum. Part II. *Journal of Periodontology* **42**, 653–657

Crohn, B.B., Ginzburg, L. and Oppenheimer, G.D. (1932) Regional ileitis, a pathological and clinical entity. *Journal of the American Medical Association* **99**, 1323–1329

Dale, D.C., Clark, R.A., Root, R.K. and Kimball, H.R. (1972) The Chediak–Higashi syndrome: studies of host defences. *Annals of Internal Medicine* **76**, 293–306

Dallapiccola, B., Alboni, P. and Ballerini, G. (1971) Capillary fragility in Down's syndrome. *Coagulation* **4**, 217–220

Deasy, M.J., Vogel, R., Macedo-Sobrinho, B. *et al.* (1980) Familial benign chronic neutropenia associated with periodontal disease – a case report. *Journal of Periodontology* **51**, 206–210

Delago, W. and Calderon, R. (1979) Acatalasia in two Peruvian siblings. *Journal of Oral Pathology* **8**, 358–368

Eley, B.M. (1993) *Dental Amalgam: A Review of Safety*, pp. 49–51. London: British Dental Association

Engel, L.D., Pasquinelli, K.L., Leone, S.A. *et al.* (1988) Abnormal lymphocyte profiles and leukotriene B4 status in a patient with Crohn's disease and severe periodontitis. *Journal of Periodontology* **59**, 841–847

Epstein, L.B., Lee, S.H.S. and Epstein, C.J. (1980) Enhanced sensitivity of trisomy 21 monocytes to the maturation-inhibiting effect of interferon. *Cellular Immunology* **50**, 191–194

Everts, V., Van der Zee, E., Creemers, L. and Beertsen, W. (1996) Phagocytosis and intracellular digestion of collagen, its role in turnover and remodelling. *Histochemical Journal* **28**, 229–245

Fantasia, J.E., Miller, A.S., Chen, S.-Y. and Foster, W.B. (1982) Calcium oxalate deposition in the periodontium secondary to chronic renal failure. *Oral Surgery, Oral Medicine, Oral Pathology* **53**, 273–279

Gardiner, B. (1968) Metachromatic cells in the gingiva in Hurler's syndrome. *Oral Surgery, Oral Medicine, Oral Pathology* **26**, 782–789

Gardiner, D. (1971) The oral manifestations of Hurler's syndrome. *Oral Surgery, Oral Medicine, Oral Pathology* **32**, 46–57

Glavind, L., Lund, B. and Löe, H. (1968) The relationship between periodontal status and diabetes duration, insulin dosage and retinal changes. *Journal of Periodontology* **39**, 341–347

Glenwright, H.D. and Rock, W.P. (1990) Papillon–Lefèvre syndrome. A discussion of aetiology and a case report. *British Dental Journal* **168**, 27–29

Gold, R.S. and Sager, E. (1976) Oral sarcoidosis: review of the literature. *Journal of Oral Surgery* **34**, 237–244

Gorlin, R.J., Sedano, H. and Andersen, V.E. (1964) A syndrome of palmar–plantar hyperkeratosis and premature periodontal destruction of the teeth. *Journal of Paediatrics* **65**, 895–908

Goteiner, D., Vogel, R., Goteiner, C. and Deasy, M. (1986) Periodontal and caries experience in insulin dependent diabetes mellitus. *Journal of the American Dental Association* **113**, 277–279

Hall, B.K. and Squier, C.A. (1992) Ultrastructural quantification of connective tissue changes in phenytoin-induced gingival overgrowth in the ferret. *Journal of Dental Research* **61**, 942–952

Haneke, E. (1979) The Papillon–Lefèvre syndrome. Keratosis palmoplantaris with periodontopathy. *Human Genetics* **51**, 1–35

Hassell, T.M. (1978) *In vivo* and *in vitro* studies of the pathogenesis of phenytoin-induced connective tissue alterations in the gingiva. Dissertation, University of Washington, Seattle

Hassell, T.M. (1982) Evidence for the production of an inactive collagenase by fibroblasts from phenytoin enlarged gingiva. *Journal of Oral Pathology* **11**, 310–317

Hernandez, M.R., Wenk, E.J., Southren, A.L. *et al.* (1981) Localization of 3H-androgens in human gingiva by radioautography. *Journal of Dental Research* **60**, 607–611

Holm-Pedersen, P. and Löe, H. (1967) Flow of gingival exudate as related to menstruation and pregnancy. *Journal of Periodontal Research* **2**, 13–20

Hugoson, A. (1970) Gingival inflammation and female sex hormones. *Journal of Periodontal Research* (Suppl.) **5**, 1–18

Jensen, J., Liljemark, W. and Bloomquist, C. (1981) The effect of female sex hormones on subgingival plaque. *Journal of Periodontology* **52**, 588–602

Kahn, A.J., Evans, H.E., Glass, L. *et al.* (1975) Defective neutrophil chemotaxis in patients with Down's syndrome. *Journal of Paediatrics* **87**, 87–89

Kalkwark, K.L. and Gatz, D.P. (1981) Periodontal changes associated with chronic idiopathic neutropenia. *Paediatric Dentistry* **3**, 189–195

Koldjaer, O., Klitgaard, N.A. and Schmitt, K.G. (1977) Indices of granulocyte activity in ulcerative colitis and Crohn's disease. *Danish Medical Bulletin* **24**, 72–76

Kornman, K.S. and Loesche, W.J. (1980) The subgingival microflora during pregnancy. *Journal of Periodontal Research* **15**, 111–122

Kretschmer, R.R., Lopez-Osuna, M., de la Rosa, L. and Armendares, S. (1974) Leucocyte function in Down's syndrome: quantitative NBT reduction and bactericidal capacity. *Clinical Immunology and Immunopathology* **2**, 449–455

Kyle, R.A. and Linman, J.W. (1968) Chronic idiopathic neutropenia: a newly recognized entity. *New England Journal of Medicine* **279**, 1015–1019

Kyle, R.A. and Linman, J.W. (1970) Gingivitis and chronic idiopathic neutropenia: a report of two cases. *Mayo Clinic Proceedings* **45**, 494–504

Lampster, I.B., Rodrick, M.L., Sonis, S.T. and Falchuk, Z.M. (1982) An analysis of peripheral blood and salivary polymorphonuclear leukocyte function, circulating immune complex levels and oral status in patients with inflammatory bowel disease. *Journal of Periodontology* **53**, 231–238

Lampster, I.B., Sonis, S.T., Hannigan, A. and Koldin, A. (1978) An association between Crohn's disease, periodontal disease and enhanced neutrophil function. *Journal of Periodontology* **49**, 475–479

Levin, S., Schesinger, M., Handzel, Z. *et al.* (1979) Thymic deficiency in Down's syndrome. *Paediatrics* **63**, 80–87

Lin, J., Duffy, J. and Roginsky, M. (1975) Microcirculation in diabetes mellitus: a study of gingival biopsies. *Human Pathology* **6**, 77–97

Lindhe, J. and Attström, R. (1967) Gingival exudation during the menstrual cycle. *Journal of Periodontal Research* **2**, 194–198

Löe, H. (1965) Periodontal changes in pregnancy. *Journal of Periodontology* **36**, 209–216

Löe, H. and Silness, J. (1963) Periodontal disease in pregnancy. I. Prevalence and severity. *Acta Odontologica Scandinavica* **21**, 533–551

Manouchehr-Pour, M., Spagnuolo, P.J., Rodman, H.M. and Bissada, N.F. (1981) Comparison of neutrophil chemotactic response in diabetic patients with mild and severe periodontal disease. *Journal of Periodontology* **52**, 410–415

McCulloch, C.A.G. and Knowles, G.C. (1993) Deficiencies in collagen phagocytosis by human fibroblasts *in vitro*: a mechanism for fibrosis. *Journal of Cell Physiology* **155**, 461–471

McGaw, T. and Porter, H. (1988) Cyclosporin-induced gingival overgrowth: an ultrastructural stereological study. *Oral Surgery, Oral Pathology and Oral Medicine* **65**, 187–190

McMullen, J.A., Van Dyke, T.E., Horoszewicz, H.U. and Genco, R.J. (1981) Neutrophil chemotaxis in individuals with advanced periodontal disease and a genetic predisposition to diabetes mellitus. *Journal of Periodontology* **52**, 167–173

McKusick, V.A. (1969) The nosology of the mucopolysaccharidoses. *American Journal of Medicine* **47**, 730–747

Miller, M.E., Oski, F.A. and Harris, M.B. (1971) Lazy leukocyte syndrome: a new disorder of leukocyte function. *Lancet* **1**, 665–669

Mintz, U. and Sachs, L. (1973) Normal granulocyte colony forming cells in the bone marrow of Yemenite Jews with genetic neutropenia. *Blood* **41**, 745–751

Moskow, E.B. (1989) Periodontal manifestations of hyperoxaluria and oxalosis. *Journal of Periodontology* **60**, 271–278

Naeim, F. and Walford, R.L. (1980) Disturbance of redistribution of surface membrane receptors on peripheral mononuclear cells of patients with Down's and aged individuals. *Journal of Gerontology* **35**, 650–655

Nishida, Y., Akaoka, I., Suzuki, T. *et al.* (1981) Serum lymphocytotoxins and lymphocyte responses to mitogens of Down's syndrome persons. *American Journal of Mental Deficiency* **85**, 596–600

Ojanotko, A., Neinstedt, W. and Harri, P. (1980) Metabolism of testosterone by human healthy and inflamed gingiva (*in vitro*). *Archives of Oral Biology* **25**, 481–484

Opinya, G.N., Kaimenyi, J.T. and Meme, J.S. (1988) Oral findings in Fanconi's anaemia. *Journal of Periodontology* **33**, 266–269

Page, A.R. and Good, R.A. (1957) Studies on cyclic neutropenia. A clinical and experimental investigation. *American Journal of Diseases in Children* **94**, 623–661

Papillon, M.M. and Lefèvre, P. (1924) Deux cas de keratodermie palmaire et plantaire symmétrique familiale (maladie de Meteda) chez le frère et la soeur. Coexistence dans les deux cas d'altérations dentaire grave. *Bulletin de la Societé Française de Dermatologie et de Syphilgraphie* **31**, 82–87

Pearlman, B.A. (1974) An oral contraceptive drug and gingival enlargement; the relationship between oral and systemic factors. *Journal of Periodontology* **36**, 209–216

Petit, J.C. and Ripamonti, U. (1990) Multiple myeloma of the periodontium. A case report. *Journal of Periodontology* **61**, 132–137

Preus, H. (1988) Treatment of rapidly destructive periodontitis in Papillon–Lefèvre syndrome. Laboratory and clinical observations. *Journal of Clinical Periodontology* **15**, 639–643

Preus, H. and Gjermo, P. (1987) Clinical management of prepubertal periodontitis in two siblings with Papillon–Lefèvre syndrome. *Journal of Clinical Periodontology* **14**, 156–160

Reuland-Bosma, W. and Van Dijk, J. (1986) Periodontal disease in Down's syndrome: a review. *Journal of Clinical Periodontology* **13**, 294–300

Roberts, W.R. and Walker, D.M. (1976) The periodontal management of a patient with a profound immunodeficiency disorder. *Journal of Clinical Periodontology* **3**, 186–192

Robertson, P.B., Wright, T.E., Mackler, B.F. *et al.* (1978) Periodontal status of patients with abnormalities of the immune system. *Journal of Periodontal Research* **13**, 37–45

Rosner, F., Kozinn, P.J. and Jervis, G.A. (1973) Leukocyte function and serum immunoglobulins in Down's syndrome. *New York State Journal of Medicine* **73**, 672–675

Russell, A.L., Leatherwood, E.C. and Consolazio, C.F. (1965) Periodontal disease and nutrition in South Vietnam. *Journal of Dental Research* **44**, 775–782

Rylander, H., Ramberg, P., Blohme, G., and Lindhe, J. (1986) Prevalence of periodontal disease in young diabetics. *Journal of Clinical Periodontology* **14**, 38–43

Saadoun, A. (1980) Diabetes and periodontal disease: a review and update. *Journal of the Western Society of Periodontology* **28**, 116–139

Samant, A., Malik, C.P., Chabra, S.K. and Devi, P.K. (1976) Gingivitis and periodontal disease in pregnancy. *Journal of Periodontology* **47**, 415–418

Sandler, R.S. and Golden, A.L. (1986) Epidemiology of Crohn's disease. *Journal of Clinical Gastroenterology* **8**, 160–165

Savage, N.W., Seymour, G.J. and Robinson, M.F. (1987) Cyclosporin A-induced gingival enlargement – a case report. *Journal of Periodontology* **58**, 475–480

Scully, C. and Cawson, R.A. (1987) *Medical Problems in Dentistry*, 2nd Edn, p. 119. Bristol: Wright

Seymour, R.A. and Heasman, P.A. (1992) In *Drugs, Diseases and the Periodontium*, pp. 19–54. Oxford: Oxford University Press

Shklar, G. and McCarthy, P.L. (1959) Oral manifestations of benign mucous membrane pemphigus (mucous membrane pemphigoid). *Oral Surgery, Oral Medicine, Oral Pathology* **12**, 950–966

Shklar, G. and McCarthy, P.L. (1961) The oral lesions of lichen planus. *Oral Surgery, Oral Medicine, Oral Pathology* **14**, 164–171

Silness, J. and Löe, H. (1964) Periodontal disease in pregnancy. II. Correlation with oral hygiene and periodontal condition. *Acta Odontologica Scandinavica* **22**, 121–135

Sooriyamoorthy, M. and Gower, D.B. (1989a) Hormonal influence on gingival tissue: relationship to periodontal disease. *Journal of Clinical Periodontology* **16**, 201–208

Sooriyamoorthy, M. and Gower, D.B. (1989b) Phenytoin stimulation of 5α-reductase activity in inflamed gingival fibroblasts. *Medical Science Research* **17**, 989–990

Sooriyamoorthy, M., Harvey, W. and Gower, D.B. (1988) The use of human gingival fibroblasts in culture for studying the effects of phenytoin on testosterone metabolism. *Archives of Oral Biology* **33**, 353–359

Sooriyamoorthy, M., Gower, D.B. and Eley, B.M. (1990) Androgen metabolism in gingival hyperplasia induced by nifedipine and cyclosporin. *Journal of Periodontal Research* **25**, 25–30

Southren, A.L., Rappaport, S.C., Gordon, C.G. and Vittek, J. (1978) Specific 5 alpha-dihydrotestosterone receptors in human gingiva. *Journal of Clinical Endocrinology and Metabolism* **47**, 1378–1382

Spencer, P. and Fleming, J.E. (1985) Cyclic neutropenia: a literature review and report of a case. *Journal of Dentistry for Children* **52**, 108–113

Stewart, R.E., Hollister, D.W. and Rimoin, D.L. (1977) A new variant of Ehlers–Danlos syndrome: an autosomal dominant disorder of fragile skin, abnormal scarring and generalized periodontitis. *Birth Defects* **13**, 85–93

Sutcliffe, P. (1972) A longitudinal study of gingivitis and puberty. *Journal of Periodontal Research* **7**, 52–58

Sznajder, N., Carraro, J.J., Rugna, S. and Seraday, M. (1978) Periodontal findings in diabetic and non-diabetic patients. *Journal of Periodontology* **49**, 445–448

Tervonen, T. and Knuuttila, M. (1986) Relation of diabetes control to periodontal pocketing and alveolar bone level. *Oral Surgery, Oral Medicine, Oral Pathology* **61**, 346–349

Tipton, D.A., Howell, K.J. and Dabbous, M. Kh. (1997) Increased proliferation, collagen and fibronectin production by hereditary gingival fibromatosis fibroblasts. *Journal of Periodontology* **68**, 524–530

Waerhaug, J. (1967). Prevalence of periodontal disease in Ceylon. Association with age, sex, oral hygiene, socio-economic factors, vitamin deficiencies, malnutrition, betel and tobacco consumption and ethnic group. Final report. *Acta Odontologica Scandinavica* **25**, 205–231

Westbrook, P., Bednarczyk, E.M., Carlson, M. *et al.* (1997) Regression of nifedipine-induced gingival hyperplasia following switch to same class calcium channel blocker, Isradipine. *Journal of Periodontology* **68**, 645–650

Witkop, C.J. (1971) Heterogeneity in gingival fibromatosis. *Birth Defects* **7**, 210–221

Wood, R.E. and Lee, P. (1988) Analysis of the oral manifestations of systemic sclerosis (scleroderma). *Oral Surgery, Oral Medicine, Oral Pathology* **65**, 172–178

Wysocki, G.P., Fay, W.P., Ulrichsen, R.F. and Ilan, R.A. (1982) Oral findings in primary hyperoxaluria and oxalosis. *Oral Surgery, Oral Medicine, Oral Pathology* **53**, 267–272

Yanover, L. and Ellen, R.P. (1986) A clinical and microbiological examination of gingival disease in parapubescent females. *Journal of Periodontology* **57**, 562–567

Zucker-Franklin, L'Esperance, P. and Good, R.A. (1977) Congenital neutropenia: an intrinsic cell defect demonstrated by electron microscopy of soft agar colonies. *Blood* **49**, 425–436

7

Acquired immunodeficiency syndrome (AIDS)

The acquired immunodeficiency syndrome (AIDS) is one of the principal threats to health worldwide; the number infected with the human immunodeficiency virus (HIV) is about 19.5 million, and the great majority of these will probably ultimately die of this condition.

The human immunodeficiency virus

The HIV is a retrovirus that is roughly spherical and is 0.0001 mm across. Its outer coat or envelope consists of a double layer of lipid molecules, and this is studded with proteins (*Figure 7.1*). One of these appears like a spike in electron microscope (EM) photographs, and is a glycoprotein (gp). The outer part is known as gp 120 (the number stands for the mass of the protein in daltons) and the inner part embedded in the membrane as gp 41. Below this is a matrix protein (p17), which surrounds the core or capsid, made of another protein (p24) in the shape of a hollow cone. This holds the genetic material in the form of RNA of about 9200 nucleotide bases. Molecules of the enzyme reverse transcriptase, which transcribes the RNA to DNA once the virus enters the cell, lie on the surface of the

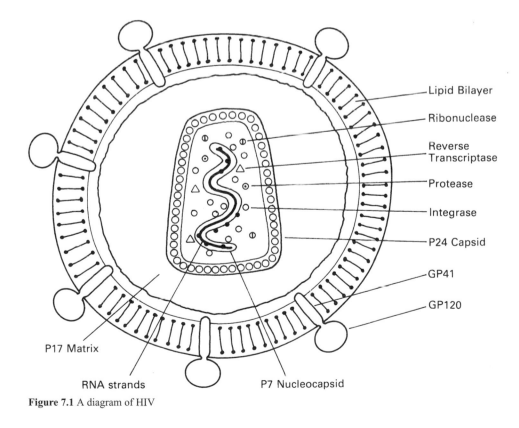

Lipid Bilayer

Ribonuclease

Reverse Transcriptase

Protease

Integrase

P24 Capsid

GP41

GP120

P17 Matrix

RNA strands

P7 Nucleocapsid

Figure 7.1 A diagram of HIV

strands. Also present within the capsid are integrase, protease and ribonuclease enzyme proteins.

The gp 120 protein can bind tightly to CD4 molecules present on several types of immune cells (*Figure 7.2*). When the virus binds to the cell the membranes fuse, a process governed by the gp 41 envelope protein, and the virus core and its contents are brought into the cell. The viral core then partially disintegrates, releasing the RNA. The reverse transcriptase then transcribes a DNA copy with the aid of the other viral enzymes. When activated the viral integrated DNA can code for viral RNA, which leaves the nucleus, codes for structural and other proteins, and buds new virus from the cell surface to infect other cells.

Pathogenesis of HIV infection and AIDS

Some CD4 bearing cells, known as dendritic cells, are present throughout the body's mucosal surfaces, and it is possible that these are the first cells infected in sexual transmission (Greene, 1993). Macrophages and monocytes also carry the CD4 molecule and are similarly vulnerable. They may carry HIV to other parts of the body, including the lymphoid organs and brain. The principal targets of the HIV virus are CD4 bearing T-helper lymphocytes, which help to activate other parts of the immune system, including the T4-effector cells, the T8-killer cells and the B cells.

An infected person mounts a vigorous defence when first infected. As a result of this, B cells produce antibodies to neutralize virus and killer T cells multiply and destroy the virus-infected cells. Although it is possible that the immune system may successfully fight off HIV at a very early stage, by the time antibodies to the virus have appeared in the blood, the infection is generally permanent. The clinical picture is firstly a mild flu-like illness with fever and muscle aches lasting no more than a few

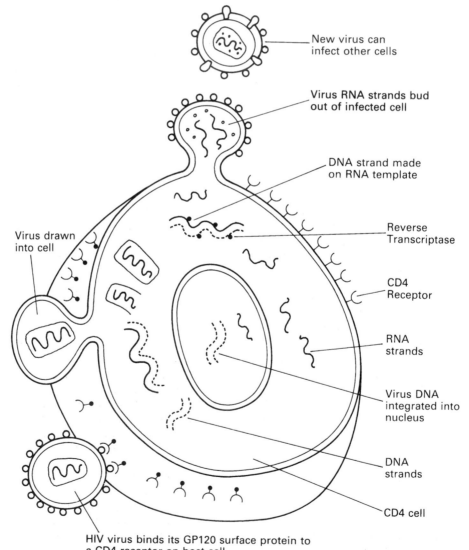

New virus can infect other cells

Virus RNA strands bud out of infected cell

DNA strand made on RNA template

Reverse Transcriptase

CD4 Receptor

RNA strands

Virus DNA integrated into nucleus

DNA strands

CD4 cell

Virus drawn into cell

HIV virus binds its GP120 surface protein to a CD4 receptor on host cell

Figure 7.2 The life cycle of HIV

weeks, and throughout this stage large amounts of virus are present in the bloodstream and transmission is easy. The immune system mounts its response, and begins to eliminate infected cells and circulating virus. However, a proportion of infected cells remains by eluding these defences, and the virus continues to replicate in low numbers for as long as a decade. For most of this period of chronic infection, the patient is quite well. It is only after several years, when the virus has significantly damaged the immune system, that opportunist infections and malignancies begin to appear.

At first it was thought that the damage to the immune system was due to the progressive decline in the numbers of T4 cells in the blood as a result of the killing of these cells by the virus. In support of this is evidence that the numbers of these cells decline from 1000 per mm^3 to 100 or less per mm^3 during the long subclinical phase of the illness. However, even in the late stages of the disease when there are very low numbers of T4 cells in the blood, the proportion of these cells producing virus is only 1 in 40 cells. In fact, in the early stages of the disease, only about 1 in 1000 T4 cells in the blood produce virus. One reason for the decline in T4 cells could be that the unaffected T8-killer cells could progressively destroy infected cells. Another possibility is that antibodies recognizing the viral gp 120 and gp 41 proteins on the viral envelope might also interfere with the MHC on healthy cells. A further theory, supported by experimental evidence, is that HIV might precipitate a widespread apoptosis (programmed death) of healthy immune cells.

Recent experimental evidence suggests that the most likely reason is that HIV infection gradually and progressively destroys the lymphoid organs, particularly the lymph nodes. There is evidence that in the long chronic asymptomatic phase HIV replicates mainly in the lymph nodes, and this gradually increases the body burden of infected cells in these organs. Thus, it seems that in the lymph nodes the viral burden is substantial and increases steadily throughout the chronic phase. The abrupt rise in the blood levels of the virus in the late stages of the disease is probably due to the burning out of the lymph nodes. Loss of follicular dendritic, T4-helper and memory cells probably leads to a rapid loss of immune function, and the virus spills out into the blood. The patient, now with a paralysed immune system, dies from recurrent opportunistic infections and neoplasms.

Clinical features of AIDS

General

The main clinical features of AIDS are lymphadenopathy, weight loss, unexplained diarrhoea, opportunistic infections and neoplasms. The infections include:

- Oral and pharyngeal candidiasis
- Mucocutaneous herpes simplex
- *Pneumocystis carinii* pneumonia
- *Mycobacterium tuberculosis*
- Atypical mycobacterial infections
- Salmonellosis
- Cryptococcal meningitis
- Cryptosporidiosis
- Toxoplasma encephalitis
- Cytomegalovirus disease.

The neoplasms include:

- Kaposi's sarcoma
- B-cell lymphoma
- Hodgkin's lymphoma.

Oral

AIDS has a variety of oral manifestations, and these have been classified by Pindborg (1989). The commonest of these are candidiasis, hairy leukoplakia, Kaposi's sarcomata and periodontal infections, and subjects with these lesions are likely to be HIV seropositive. However, a variety of oral lesions can occur, and these include the following:

1. *Fungal infections*
   - Candidiasis
   - Histoplasmosis
   - Cryptococcus
   - Goetrichosis
2. Bacterial infections
   - Acute necrotizing ulcerative gingivitis (ANUG)
   - Rapid periodontal destruction
   - *Mycobacterium avium intracellulare*
   - Actinomycosis
   - Cat-scratch disease
   - *Klebsiella pneumoniae*
   - *Enterobacteriacea*
   - *Escherichia coli*
   - Exacerbation of chronic abscesses
   - Sinusitis
   - Submandibular cellulitis
3. *Viral infections*
   - Herpes simplex stomatitis
   - Cytomegalovirus
   - Epstein–Barr (EB) virus
   - Varicella-zoster virus
   - Papillomavirus
4. *Neoplasms*
   - Kaposi's sarcoma
   - Non-Hodgkin's lymphoma
   - Squamous cell carcinoma
5. *Neurological disturbances*
   - Trigeminal neuropathy
   - Facial palsy

6.   *Unknown causes*
   • Recurrent aphthous ulceration
   • Progressive necrotizing ulceration
   • Toxic epidermolysis (Lyell's syndrome)
   • Delayed wound healing
   • Idiopathic thrombocytopenia
   • Salivary gland enlargement
   • Xerostomia
   • Oral mucosa hypopigmentation.

If a subject has two or more of these oral lesions, then they are 5.7 times more likely to be HIV seropositive (Melnick *et al.*, 1989).

Periodontal

The main periodontal infections associated with AIDS are ANUG and rapidly progressive atypical periodontitis. Two types of periodontal disease, HIV gingivitis (HIV-G) and HIV periodontitis (HIV-P) have been described in HIV patients by Winkler and Murray (1987).

HIV related ANUG

Localized ANUG can occur in HIV infected individuals, but is more common in full-blown AIDS. It has all the usual features of this condition, but may be more widespread and may expose bone (Winkler *et al.*, 1988). It also has the same association with smoking as is seen with non-HIV related ANUG (Swango *et al.*, 1991).

HIV gingivitis (HIV-G)

HIV-G manifests as a distinct erythema of the free and attached gingiva and, sometimes, the alveolar mucosa. It bleeds easily on toothbrushing and gentle probing. The gingival margins often show a well-circumscribed band of erythema. It may fail to respond to conventional treatment such as plaque control and scaling if the CD4 cell levels are low (see below).

HIV periodontitis (HIV-P)

HIV-P involves extensive soft tissue necrosis and marked loss of periodontal attachment. Soft tissue destruction can be rapid and is often accompanied by interdental necrosis and ulceration, which can expose bone. Unlike chronic periodontitis, there is no deep pocket formation, but rather marked recession, ulceration and exposure and, sometimes, sequestration of bone. Localized pain is a feature of this condition (Winkler *et al.*, 1988), and it is deeper-seated than that associated with ANUG.

The microbiology of HIV-G and HIV-P

The microbiology of subgingival HIV-G and HIV-P has been investigated by indirect immunofluorescence and culture techniques (Murray *et al.*, 1988). The findings were compared between a group of HIV seropositive subjects and HIV seronegative controls. Sites from the HIV-G and HIV-P subjects contained significantly more *Candida albicans* than controls. *Porphyromonas gingivalis, Prevotella intermedia, Fusobacterium nucleatum, Actinobacillus actinomycetemcomitans, Eikenella corrodens* and *Wolinella recta* were more prevalent in HIV-G and HIV-P sites than control sites. Serum antibody levels to these bacteria were higher in HIV-G and HIV-P subjects than controls. However, apart from *Candida albicans*, the distribution of bacterial species in HIV-G and HIV-P was similar to that seen with chronic periodontitis. It seems that a fall in the levels of CD4-lymphocytes may lead to a progression from HIV-G to HIV-P (Winkler and Murray, 1987).

Changes in defence mechanisms of AIDs patients

Often, HIV patients with normal levels of CD4-lymphocytes and good oral hygiene have healthy gingiva and do not differ from normal patients in their response to plaque. Thus it would seem that it is the disruption of immune function by HIV infection that increases the pathogenicity of subgingival bacteria. It has also been shown (Steinsvoll *et al.*, 1997) that HIV positive subjects with chronic periodontitis have significantly lower serum IgG antibody levels to putative periodontal pathogens than HIV-negative chronic periodontitis patients.

PMNs harvested from HIV-positive patients have been shown to have increased phagocytosis, oxidative bursts and F-actin formation when compared with those from normal controls (Ryder *et al.*, 1988). This would seem to suggest that PMNs from HIV patients show increased activity, and this is in contrast to the decrease in activity of these cells seen in rapidly progressing periodontitis. In chronic periodontitis the PMNs form the first line of defence and, as the disease progresses, they are increasingly replaced by macrophages and lymphocytes. In HIV subjects with low levels of CD4-lymphocytes this change is unlikely to occur, and thus the PMNs have a more important role in protecting the tissues in these subjects.

PMNs from AIDs patients are possibly primed because of their prolonged exposure to opportunistic fungal and bacterial infections and the failure of CD4-lymphocyte and macrophage response. They could also be primed as the result of the transient bacteraemia that can occur from chewing in the presence of periodontal disease. These hyperactive PMNs could produce local tissue damage.

Thus, the main factors that contribute to severe periodontal destruction seen in HIV patients would seem to be:

• Primed or hyperactive PMNs
• Failure of the CD4-lymphocyte and macrophage response

- Increased pathogenicity of bacteria species in the subgingival flora due to immunodeficiency.

Treatment of HIV-G and HIV-P

Very careful cross-infection control must be used with all these patients, as all periodontal procedures produce blood in the mouth.

Patients are normally treated by conventional periodontal therapy, i.e. plaque control, scaling and root planing. This may be supplemented by the use of chlorhexidine mouthwashes or local irrigation. The treatment is usually very successful in HIV infection, but not in AIDS.

Three treatment approaches have been evaluated in HIV-associated periodontitis (Grassi *et al.*, 1988). These were:

1. Conventional therapy, i.e. plaque control, scaling and subgingival scaling and root planing
2. Conventional therapy supplemented with a local irrigation of a 10% povidone iodine (Betidine)
3. Conventional therapy plus rinsing twice a day with a 0.12% chlorhexidine solution.

All patients were assessed at 1 and 3 months after scaling and root planing. Patients treated with conventional therapy and 0.12% chlorhexidine solution showed significant improvements in the clinical measurements, i.e. plaque index, gingival index and pocket depth, and complete resolution of spontaneous gingival bleeding. Patients using the 10% povidone iodine solution appeared to benefit from its topical anaesthetic effects.

Response to treatment in motivated HIV patients with good oral hygiene is usually good when the CD4 cell levels are good. However, the response to treatment is likely to fall as the CD4 cell levels decrease. Thus a failure to respond to treatment and the presence of opportunistic infections, such as candidiasis and hairy leukoplakia, may be indicative of a progression to AIDS.

HIV-related ANUG

The incidence of ANUG is higher in HIV patients than in the rest of the population (Pindborg and Holmstrup, 1987). The microbiology of this condition in HIV subjects is the same as that seen in non-infected subjects, and thus its severity appears to be due to the decreased immunocompetence. The condition becomes more prevalent and more resistant to treatment as the CD4 cell levels decrease.

The condition is treated in a similar way to ANUG in normal subjects. Thus, oxygenating mouthwashes such as Bocasan can be used to supplement local swabbing and scaling. The infection is treated by the appropriate antimicrobials, such as metronidazole or amoxycillin.

Other HIV-associated lesions on the gingiva

Other HIV-associated lesions may occur on the gingiva, and these include herpetic gingivostomatitis, candidiasis, human papillomavirus (HPV) causing multiple condylomas of the gingival margin and gingival ulceration due to infection with *Mycobacterium avium intracellulare* (Volpe *et al.*, 1985). Kaposi's sarcoma is the commonest oral tumour (Lozada *et al.*, 1983), and it can involve the gingival margin. Non-Hodgkin's lymphoma has been found in AIDS patients, and may appear as a diffuse gingival swelling, epulis or nodule (Phelan *et al.*, 1987).

References

Grassi, M., Williams, C.A., Winkler, J.R. and Murray, P.A. (1988) Management of HIV-associated periodontal diseases. In *Oral manifestations of AIDS* (P.R. Robertson and J.S. Greenspan, eds), pp. 119–130. Littleton MA: PSG Publishing Company

Greene, W.C. (1993) AIDS and the immune system. *Scientific American* (Sept.) pp. 67–73

Lozada, F., Silverman, S., Migliorati, C.A. *et al.* (1983) Oral manifestations of tumour and opportunistic infections in the acquired immunodeficiency syndrome (AIDS): finding in 53 homosexual men with Kaposi's sarcoma. *Oral Surgery, Oral Medicine, Oral Pathology* **56**, 491–494

Melnick S.L., Engel, D., Truelove, E. *et al.* (1989) Oral mucosal lesions: association with the presence of antibodies to the human immunodeficiency virus. *Oral Surgery, Oral Medicine, Oral Pathology* **68**, 37–43

Murray, P.A., Winkler, J.R., Sadkowski, L. *et al.* (1988) Microbiology of HIV-associated gingivitis and periodontitis. In *Oral manifestations of AIDS* (P.R. Robertson and J.S. Greenspan, eds), pp. 105–118. Littleton MA: PSG Publishing Company

Phelan, J.S., Saltzman, B.R., Friedland, G.H. and Klein, R.S. (1987) Oral findings in patients with acquired immunodeficiency syndrome. *Oral Surgery, Oral Medicine, Oral Pathology* **64**, 50–56

Pindborg, J.J. (1989) Classification of oral lesions associated with HIV infection. *Oral Surgery, Oral Medicine, Oral Pathology* **67**, 292–295

Pindborg, J.J. and Holmstrup, P. (1987) Necrotizing gingivitis related to human immunodeficiency virus (HIV) infection. *African Dental Journal* **1**, 5–8

Ryder, M.I., Winkler, J.R. and Weintrub, P.S. (1988) Elevated phagocytosis, oxidative bursts and F-actin formation in PMNs from individuals with intra-oral manifestations of HIV infection. *Journal of Acquired Immunodeficiency Syndrome* **1**, 346–356

Steinsvoll, S., Myint, M., Odden, K. *et al.* (1997) Reduced serum IgG reactivities with bacteria in dental plaque in HIV-infected individuals with periodontitis. *Journal of Clinical Periodontology* **24**, 823–829

Swango, P.A., Kleinman, D.V. and Konzelman, J.L. (1991) HIV and periodontal health. A study of military personnel with HIV. *Journal of the American Dental Association* **122**, 49–54

Volpe, F., Schwimmer, A. and Barr, C. (1985) Oral manifestations of disseminated *Mycobacterium avium intracellulare* in a patient with AIDS. *Oral Surgery, Oral Medicine, Oral Pathology* **60**, 567–570

Winkler, J.R. and Murray, P.A. (1987) Periodontal disease – a potential intra-oral expression of AIDS may be rapidly progressive periodontitis. *Journal of the Californian Dental Association* **15**, 20–24

Winkler, J.R., Grassi, M. and Murray, P.A. (1988) Clinical description and aetiology of HIV-associated periodontal diseases. In *Oral manifestations of AIDS* (P.R. Robertson and J.S. Greenspan, eds), pp. 49–70. Littleton MA: PSG Publishing Company

8

The natural history of periodontal disease

In health, the gingivae are firm, pink and knife-edged, and do not bleed on probing. There is a shallow gingival crevice or sulcus, and the junctional epithelium is attached to the enamel. The gingival fibre system is well organized. A few PMNs are present in the junctional epithelium as they pass through from the gingival vessels into the gingival crevice and the mouth. In the subjacent connective tissue, isolated inflammatory cells, mainly lymphocytes with the occasional plasma cell and macrophage, may also be seen. The picture manifests the quiet but dynamic balance of health.

Gingivitis

Because plaque accumulation is greatest in the sheltered interdental region, gingival inflammation tends to start in the interdental papilla and spread from there around the neck of the tooth.

The histopathology of chronic gingivitis has been described chronologically by Page and Schroeder (1976) in a number of stages: the initial lesion at 2–4 days, followed by an early gingivitis, which at 2–3 weeks becomes an established gingivitis. These changes were described by examining biopsies of experimental gingivitis lesions at different time intervals.

The initial lesion

The first observed change occurs around the small gingival blood vessels apical to the junctional epithelium. These vessels begin to leak and perivascular collagen disappears, to be replaced by a few inflammatory cells, plasma cells and lymphocytes (mainly T-lymphocytes), tissue fluid and serum protein. There is increased migration of leucocytes through the junctional epithelium, and exudation of tissue fluid from the gingival crevice. Other than the increased flow of fluid exudate and PMNs, there may be no clinical signs of tissue change at this stage.

Early gingivitis

If plaque deposition persists the initial inflammatory changes continue, with an increased flow of gingival fluid and migration of PMNs. Changes occur in both the junctional and crevicular epithelia, where there are signs of cell separation and some proliferation of basal cells. Fibroblasts begin to degenerate, and the collagen bundles of the dentogingival fibre groups break up so that the seal of the marginal cuff of gingiva is weakened. There is a small increase in the number of inflammatory cells, 75% of which are lymphocytes. There are also a few plasma cells and macrophages. The clinical signs at this stage are few, and the gingivae often appear clinically healthy. This is because the lesion, which has become more 'chronic' in nature, occupies a very small area of the gingiva. Also, the signs of acute inflammation reduce as the lesion becomes chronic. This stage is probably classed as gingival health in clinical dentistry.

Established gingivitis

If satisfactory oral hygiene is not re-established, clinically obvious gingivitis becomes established within 7–14 days. Clinical signs of inflammation appear, and the interdental papillae may become swollen and bleed on probing (*Figure 8.1*). The number of lymphocytes increases, and B-lymphocytes become more dominant. Many of these cells mature and develop into plasma cells, which manufacture specific antibodies to the many plaque antigens. Some macrophages appear, but there is a secondary stimulation of acute inflammation produced by complement activation. This results in the emigration of PMNs from blood vessels, and many of these also migrate through the junctional epithelium into the gingival cre-

Figure 8.1 The first clinical signs of gingival inflammation: swelling of interdental papilla and involvement of gingival margin

vice. The flow of gingival crevicular fluid (GCF), an inflammatory exudate, increases. Immunoglobulins, mainly IgG, are found in the gingival connective tissue and GCF. Mast cells are also found in the gingival connective tissue and junctional epithelium. These changes result in clinical gingival inflammation, and the gingivae are red, swollen and bleed easily (*Figure 8.2*). The lesion increases in size and occupies a larger volume within the gingival connective tissue.

With the increased destruction of collagen and inflammatory swelling the gingival margin can be separated easily from the tooth surface, giving rise to gingival or 'false' pocketing (*Figure 8.3b*). If there is considerable inflammatory oedema and gingival swelling, the gingival pocket can be quite deep. There is now degeneration of the cells of the junctional epithelium and some proliferation of its basal layers into the underlying connective tissue, but at this stage there is no significant migration of epithelial cells onto the root surface.

Figure 8.2 Established gingival inflammation with papillary swelling

Figure 8.3 Diagram to show the various forms of periodontal pathology: *(a)* gingival health and shallow gingival crevice; *(b)* gingival swelling with production of a 'false' or gingival pocket; *(c)* 'true' or periodontal pocket with apical migration of crevicular epithelium and associated resorption of alveolar crest to form a 'suprabony' pocket; *(d)* a suprabony pocket plus gingival hyperplasia producing a deep pocket but little bone loss; *(e)* an 'infrabony' pocket where the epithelial attachment is apical to the alveolar crest; *(f)* gingival recession, i.e. equal apical movement of gingival margin and alveolar crest

As the inflammation spreads along the trans-septal fibres, there may be some resorption of the alveolar crest. This is reversible on resolution of the inflammation.

One interesting feature of the disease is that no bacteria are found either in the epithelium or in the connective tissue.

As fibrous tissue is destroyed within the site of active inflammation, at more distant sites there is some proliferation of fibrous tissue and formation of new blood vessels. This productive or repair activity is a very important characteristic of the chronic lesion, and where the irritation and inflammation are longstanding the fibrous tissue element can become the predominant component of the tissue change.

Thus destruction and repair continue side by side, and the proportion of each affects the colour and shape of the gingivae. If the inflammation dominates, the tissues are red, soft and bleed easily; if fibrous tissue production dominates, the gingivae can be firm and pink, although swollen, and there may be little or no bleeding.

The systemic factors that determine the tissue response to plaque irritation are discussed in Chapter 6.

Effective treatment of gingivitis will remove the cause of irritation and the condition will resolve and turn back into a small lesion resembling the 'early' lesion, with a small number of lymphocytes occupying a small area of gingival connective tissue subjacent to the junctional epithelium. The gingiva then appears clinically healthy.

The lesions described so far have been described as 'contained', because they are limited to the gingiva and are largely reversible on removal of the plaque. They may remain contained for many years; on the other hand, an established gingivitis lesion may spread into the deeper tissues to become a destructive chronic periodontitis. This progression is not inevitable, and some longitudinal studies indicate that the incidence of conversion to periodontitis is very low (Albander *et al.*, 1986; Listgarten, 1988). There is considerable debate as to whether this progression is determined by the nature of the bacterial plaque, by host factors, or by both. Plasma cells appear to be related to more aggressive lesions, and it is possible that the proliferation of plasma cells may be provoked by particular plaque constituents.

Chronic periodontitis

With continuing plaque irritation and inflammation, the integrity of the junctional epithelium is increasingly damaged. The epithelial cells degenerate and separate, and the attachment to the tooth completely breaks down. At the same time the junctional epithelium proliferates into the connective tissue and down the root surface as the dento-gingival fibres and alveolar crest fibres are destroyed. Apical migration of the junctional epithelium continues and, as this epithelium separates from the root surface, a periodontal or 'true' pocket is formed (*Figure 8.3c*). This seems to be an irreversible change.

Once a true pocket is formed, plaque is in contact with the cementum. The connective tissue is oedematous, vessels are dilated and thrombosed and vessel walls break down, with haemorrhage into the surrounding tissues. There is a massive inflammatory infiltrate of plasma cells, lymphocytes and macrophages. IgG is the predominant immunoglobulin, but some IgM and IgA are present. The epithelium of the pocket wall may be intact or ulcerated. This appears to make no difference, as plaque products diffuse through the epithelium. The flow of GCF and migration of PMNs continues, and it is likely that the fluid flow helps to promote the deposition of subgingival calculus.

Extension of the inflammation into the alveolar crest is marked by the infiltration of some inflammatory cells into trabecular spaces, and these may increase in size. Bone resorption tends to be compensated for by deposition further away from the inflammatory zone, so the bone is remodelled but shows a net loss. Bone resorption usually starts interproximally, so where the table of interproximal bone is broad (as it is between molars) an interdental crater is formed and then, as the resorption process spreads laterally, the entire alveolar crest is resorbed (*Figure 8.4*).

The periodontal lesion also appears to be 'contained' because, as it advances and connective tissue is destroyed, the trans-septal fibres are continually reformed and seem to separate the main inflammatory infiltrate from the underlying bone.

The progression of the lesion is not continuous, periods of advance and remission take place and fibrosis is a constant feature, especially in the latter phase.

With destruction of periodontal ligament and alveolar crest resorption, the pocket deepens. At a later stage in the disease there may be varying degrees of suppuration and abscess formation. Finally, the teeth become loose, migrate and are lost.

Disease progression

At one time it was believed that periodontitis, once established, progresses continuously and inevitably, with a simple straight-line age correlation. This led to the notion that tooth-loss was part of the ageing process. So strong was this belief that many dentists recommended full extractions in middle age, when the patient was still 'adaptable' to dentures, rather than waiting until a time when the elderly person, having lost most or all the teeth, would find such adaptation difficult or impossible.

This belief about the pattern of disease progression was supported by clinical studies which reduced measurements of pocket depth or alveolar bone loss to average values for a given mouth, thus eliminating intra-oral variation and obscuring both sites of little or no disease and sites of worst disease. Epidemiological studies on various populations also used average values for age groups, and these findings too supported the belief in a straightforward age-correlated linear progression. In this way, ideas about longitudinal change were derived from the compilation of misleading findings from cross-sectional studies.

However, detailed measurement of loss of attachment at specific sites over time, i.e. a valid longitudinal study,

(a)

(b)

Figure 8.4 *(a)* Early resorption of interproximal alveolar crest. Note image of subgingival calculus on mesial of 2|. *(b)* More advanced and more generalized bone loss

contradicts the idea of continuous and inevitable disease progression, and indicates that:

1. As stated above, gingivitis, even when persistent and untreated, does not inevitably progress to periodontitis
2. Even when established, periodontal destruction is not continuous but progresses in an episodic manner, with 'bursts' of destructive activity alternating with periods of quiescence and, possibly, repair

3. There is great individual variation in the pattern of destruction, which also varies over time in the same individual.

Some research workers believe that the bursts of activity occur at random (Goodson *et al.*, 1982; Socransky, 1984), and that a past history of persistent and severe gingivitis or of periodontal destruction does not indicate future destructive activity. Thus, progress is unpredictable. Other workers find that progress is not random, and that there is a correlation between the initial degree of bone loss and the subsequent rate of bone loss (Papapanou *et al.*, 1989; Albander, 1990). Thus progression is, to some extent, predictable. Others have suggested that prognosis is affected by the site of disease, i.e. whether related to incisors, to molars, or distributed generally.

Many studies show that, once initiated, the average rate of bone loss is very slow; 0.05–0.1 mm per year (Suomi *et al.*, 1971; Sheiham *et al.*, 1986; Albander, 1990). However, this is not always the case; in some people rapid bone loss occurs early in life, and in others rapid bone loss may follow years of little or very slow tissue destruction.

It must be recognized that the amount of probing attachment loss (PAL) that can be reliably measured depends upon the threshold for the probing method used (see Chapter 12). Most of the clinical longitudinal studies that led to the development of the 'burst' theory of periodontal progression (Goodson *et al.*, 1982; Lindhe *et al.*, 1983; Haffajee and Socransky, 1986) used manual probing, which cannot reliably measure changes in PAL of less than 2.5–3 mm. They would therefore only detect rapidly progressive attachment loss (RAL) losing this amount or more, and would not detect gradual attachment loss (GAL) losing much smaller amounts, possibly over a longer time period. This therefore led to the notion that all periodontal progression occurs in bursts of activity over short time periods.

More recently electronic probes have been developed, which will measure PAL more reliably and accurately and have thresholds of 0.3–0.8 mm (see Chapter 12). Using an electronic probe that detects and measures from the cement–enamel junction (CEJ) with a threshold of 0.25 mm, Jeffcoat and Reddy (1991) monitored 30 patients with moderate to advanced chronic periodontitis for 6 months. Using a threshold of 0.4 mm they found 29% of sites with attachment loss (AL), and using a threshold of 2.4 mm they found AL at only 2% of sites. This latter figure is similar to the percentage in the studies above, which used manual probing. This indicated that, when using large thresholds, only RAL will be detected, whilst using smaller thresholds will detect both RAL and GAL, with a higher proportion of GAL sites. Thus it appears that both RAL, progressing by 'bursts', and GAL occur during the progression of chronic periodontitis. GAL could either result from small 'mini-bursts' of activity producing AL of less than 0.5 mm, or from slow progressive AL, or from both. It is likely that patients susceptible to periodontal disease will tend to progress more by bursts of RAL, whilst those with lesser susceptibilities would progress more slowly and gradually.

It has also been shown that, in patients with moderate chronic periodontitis, further attachment loss mostly occurred at sites with previous probing depths greater than 5 mm (Gribic and Lamster, 1991, 1992).

At present, we are handicapped in making precise diagnoses and prognoses by two important limitations:

1. We have no reliable markers for present disease activity (see Chapter 13)
2. We have no reliable criteria for identifying the 'at-risk' individual.

Bone defects

The pattern of alveolar resorption can vary from one tooth to the next, and on different aspects of the same tooth.

It is believed that inflammation spreads from the gingiva into the deeper tissues along three pathways; through the alveolar bone, the attached gingiva and the periodontal ligament. The primary pathway appears to be through the alveolar bone, in which inflammation tracks via perivascular and perineural channels into trabecular spaces. It may then travel laterally from bone into periodontal ligament and attached gingiva. If resorption of the alveolar crest is even, the base of the pocket remains coronal to the crest of the bone and a simple 'suprabony' pocket is formed, i.e. a pocket entirely surrounded by soft tissue (*Figure 8.3c*). If resorption of the alveolar crest proceeds more rapidly in one part than another, the base of the pocket becomes apical to the crest of the bone. This is known as an 'infrabony' pocket (*Figures 8.3e and 8.5*).

As cancellous bone is more vascular and less dense than cortical bone, it is likely that, as stated above, the central cancellous part of a broad alveolar septum will resorb more rapidly than the lateral parts made up of cortical bone, so that an infrabony pocket is formed in relation to an interdental 'crater'.

The variety of bone defects is infinite, but for purposes of description the defects have been classified according to their morphology as marginal defects, intra-alveolar defects, fenestration and furcation defects. These are very rough groupings, with considerable overlap. In chronic inflammation the formative bone response may more than compensate for the bone resorption, so that a thickened or bulbous alveolar margin is formed. Intra-alveolar defects, i.e. defects within the alveolar process, are commonly classified according to the number of bone walls, that is, one- two- or three-walled (*Figure 8.6*). This group also includes interdental craters and hemisepta.

Furcation defects have been classified according to the degree of bone loss in the furcation measured in a horizontal plane (*Figure 8.7*). An early or Class 1 defect is one that penetrates less than 2 mm into the furcation; a Class 2 defect is one where the bone loss is greater than

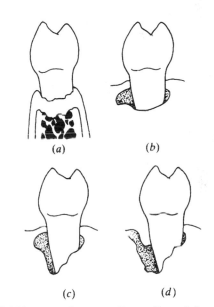

Figure 8.6 Diagram to show some forms of bone defect: *(a)* interdental crater; *(b)* three-walled defect; *(c)* two-walled defect; *(d)* one-walled defect or hemisepta

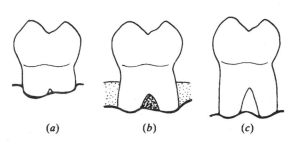

Figure 8.7 Diagram to show furcation defects: *(a)* Class 1; *(b)* Class 2; *(c)* Class 3

Figure 8.5 Radiographic appearance of bone defect associated with infrabony pocket mesial to|6. The bone defect is frequently described as an 'intrabony' defect. Note early alveolar crest resorption in other areas that are related to suprabony pockets

2 mm into the inter-radicular area but does not go completely through the furcation, so that one aspect of the bone is intact; in a Class 3 defect, so much inter-radicular bone has been lost that a probe can be passed between the roots from one side to the other (*Figure 8.8*).

There has been much speculation about the factors that might determine the pattern of bone resorption. Two factors appear to play an important role; the original morphology of the bone and excessive occlusal stress. Variations in original bone morphology must influence the type of bone defects in disease. A thin alveolar plate of bone is more likely to be completely resorbed than a thick plate of bone; a thin interdental septum between incisors may be completely destroyed, while an interdental crater will form in the septum between molars. A split or dehiscence may be formed where bone coronal to a developmental defect, a perforation or fenestration is resorbed by progressive inflammation.

Occlusal trauma

Considerable debate has centred on the role of occlusal forces in the development and progress of periodontal disease, as well as on the influence of these forces on the rate and form of alveolar bone destruction. Functional stresses on all parts of the skeleton tend to strengthen, while lack of function tends to weaken the tissues. Experimental rats fed on a coarse diet have thicker and heavier jaws than those fed on a soft diet, and the periodontal ligament is composed of more and thicker collagen bundles in the former group than in the latter.

Many experiments have been carried out on animals to determine the results of overloading teeth. A basic problem in such studies is to distinguish the effects of plaque-induced inflammation from those produced by occlusal stresses, and great care must be taken to maintain a high standard of oral hygiene in the experimental animals. A number of experiments demonstrate the kind of tissue changes produced in the tooth-supporting tissues

Figure 8.8 Radiographic appearance of trifurcation Class 3 defect

when overloaded, e.g. when pressures are applied to teeth by different types of appliance or when a high restoration is placed so that it interferes with the occlusion.

The pattern of changes in the periodontium depends on whether the forces applied to the teeth are uni- or multi-directional. The reactions of the tissues to both of these are described below.

Orthodontic-type trauma

This is brought about by single directional forces applied to a normal periodontium, such as occurs in orthodontic tooth movement. This type of trauma has been investigated in animal studies by histological examination of blocks of teeth and periodontium after varying time periods (Reitan, 1951; Mühlemann and Herzog, 1961; Ewan and Stahl, 1962; Warhaug and Hansen, 1966; Karing *et al.*, 1982). The crown of the tooth is tilted in the direction of the force and the tooth moves about its fulcrum at the apical third of the root, producing pressure and tension zones within the marginal and apical parts of the periodontium. On the pressure side the tissues become crushed, and this produces disruption and disorganization of the periodontal fibres, leading to hyaline degeneration and necrosis of connective tissues. The blood vessels are damaged, and haemorrhage and thrombosis is present. If the magnitude of the forces is within certain limits, the periodontal ligament cells remain vital and osteoclasts appear on the adjacent bone surface, leading to bone resorption. This is known as direct bone resorption. However, if the force is greater, then damage to the ligament cells prevents this from occurring. In this situation osteoclasts develop in the marrow spaces below the bone surface, leading to undermining or indirect bone resorption. This bone is resorbed until it reaches the hyalinized periodontium, when the tooth is able to move away from the pressure force. Macrophages and osteoclasts remove the damaged tissues, after which the area becomes revascularized, allowing new periodontal tissues to form. Bone deposition then occurs in the tension zones to compensate for the increased width of the periodontium in this area. Once the tooth has moved the pressure is nullified, and the full healing of the periodontal tissues takes place in both the pressure and tension zones.

Bodily movement of the teeth with fixed orthodontic appliances produces the same changes, except that the pressure and tension zones are more extended in the apical–coronal direction. If excessive forces are used, root cementum and dentine may also be resorbed.

These changes affect only the intra-alveolar periodontal ligament, and do not involve the supra-alveolar connective tissues. They therefore cannot affect the marginal periodontal tissues.

Jiggling-type trauma

The kind of stress that is transmitted to the tooth in occlusal trauma is not unidirectional but, rather, multi-directional. Cuspal interference imposes intermittent loading on opposing teeth, and this is usually resisted by soft tissue forces or secondary cuspal contacts. This produces alternating or 'jiggling' forces on the teeth. These have been investigated by a number of animal studies that have sought to reproduce these 'jiggling' forces (Wentz *et al.*, 1958; Glickman and Smulow, 1968; Svanberg and Lindhe, 1973; Meitner, 1975; Ericsson and Lindhe, 1982). The forces produce alternating pressure and tension zones within the intra-alveolar periodontium, which exhibit the same changes described above for the pressure zones in unidirectional forces. The direct or indirect bone resorption associated with this process leads to a generalized widening of the periodontal ligament space and, as a result of this, the tooth or teeth involved display progressive increasing mobility. When the effect of the forces is compensated by the increased width of the ligament space, the damaged tissues are removed and the widened periodontium heals. The tooth remains mobile within this widened periodontium.

As with unidirectional forces, these changes affect only the intra-alveolar periodontal ligament and do not involve the supra-alveolar connective tissues. Therefore, they cannot affect the marginal periodontal tissues.

Jiggling-type trauma applied to a reduced periodontium

The effects of these forces on a reduced but healthy periodontium have been studied in dogs by Ericsson and Lindhe (1977). The same changes as have been described above were produced around the whole intra-alveolar periodontium, which increased in width. The affected teeth became progressively mobile over several weeks, after which the enlarged space compensated for the forces. The bone resorption then ceased, and the periodontal tissues in the enlarged space healed. The teeth remained hypermobile but were surrounded by periodontal tissues, which had adapted to the increased functional forces. The supra-alveolar connective tissues and marginal periodontium were again unaffected by the changes.

Jiggling-type trauma superimposed on inflammatory chronic periodontitis

Older studies

The relationship between occlusal trauma and inflammatory periodontal disease has often been discussed in connection with human case reports and autopsy material. On the basis of this, Glickman (1964, 1965, 1967, 1971) claimed that the path along which the plaque-associated inflammatory lesion spread was affected by the presence of occlusal trauma. In this connection, it was suggested that occlusal trauma changed the vascular pattern so that the inflammatory lesion passed into the periodontal ligament space rather than into the alveolar crest (Macapanpan and Weinmann, 1954). Glickman and Smulow (1962, 1965, 1968) claimed from the results of human autopsy

and animal experiments that occlusal trauma imposed on inflammatory periodontitis produced angular bone resorption and infrabony pocketing. However, Warhaug (1979) examined human autopsy material and reported that angular bony defects and infrabony pockets usually occurred in areas unaffected by occlusal trauma. His findings supported the observations of Prichard (1965) and Manson (1976), which showed that the pattern of alveolar bone loss resulted from an interplay between the form of the alveolar bone and the apical extension of the subgingival plaque on the root surface. Furthermore, these findings did not support the concept of Glickman (1964, 1971), which described a zone of co-destruction within the periodontium that could be affected by the combined effects of marginal inflammation and occlusal trauma. These matters have now been largely resolved by the later studies described below.

Later studies

Experiments on humans and other animals described in the previous sections have shown that trauma from occlusion cannot induce changes in the supra-alveolar marginal tissues. The effects of jiggling trauma superimposed on progressive destructive periodontitis have been studied by a number of research groups (Lindhe and Svanberg, 1974; Meitner, 1975; Nyman *et al.*, 1978; Ericsson and Lindhe, 1982). In these experiments destructive periodontitis was first initiated in dogs or monkeys, and the teeth were then subject to jiggling trauma. The periodontal tissues in the combined pressure/tension zones were damaged as described previously. The intra-alveolar periodontium showed signs of inflammation, with hyperaemia, exudation, thrombosis and migration of inflammatory cells. Numerous osteoclasts differentiated on the adjacent bone surface, and bone was resorbed. This process gradually increased the width of the periodontal ligament space and, as a result, the teeth became increasingly mobile. Angular bone resorption could be seen on radiographs of the affected area. The forces became nullified by the increased width of the periodontal ligament space, and at this point the bone resorption ceased. The periodontium regenerated its normal tissues, and within this enlarged space the tooth mobility stopped increasing. The angular bone resorption persisted, but histological examination revealed that no further apical migration of the junctional epithelium had resulted from the imposition of occlusal trauma. This indicates that occlusal forces that allow adaptive alterations within the ligament will not aggravate inflammatory periodontal disease.

However, if this jiggling occlusal trauma generated greater forces and these were maintained for long time periods so that the periodontium could not become adapted, then the injury persisted and, in some cases, became permanent (Lindhe and Svanberg, 1974). In these cases, the pressure/tension zones displayed persisting inflammation and damage over several months. The osteoclasts residing in the alveolar wall continued producing continuing bone resorption, and the angular bone defects remained. These changes produced gradual progressive widening of the periodontal ligament space and progressively increased tooth mobility. Under these circumstances, the marginal inflammatory lesion merged with the 'trauma' lesion in the periodontium. The junctional epithelium proliferated apically, and the destructive periodontal disease was aggravated.

In another set of experiments in the dog (Ericsson and Lindhe, 1982), prolonged jiggling forces were applied for 10 months to some teeth with established chronic periodontitis, and these were compared with control teeth in the same dog, also with established chronic periodontitis, which were not jiggled. The traumatized teeth showed an increased rate of progression compared with control teeth.

Conclusion

Unidirectional or jiggling forces applied to the healthy periodontium will not result in loss of attachment, as trauma from occlusion cannot affect the marginal tissues. It does, however, produce tooth mobility within an adapted, widened periodontium. These changes are reversible on the removal of the trauma.

However, in teeth with established chronic periodontitis, superimposed prolonged and severe jiggling trauma may cause persistent damage within the periodontium such that adaptive changes are prevented. Under these circumstances the marginal periodontal and intraalveolar 'trauma' lesions may merge, and this can enhance the rate of periodontal disease progression.

The causes of excessive occlusal stress are discussed in Chapter 24. Loads can become excessive in two situations:

1. Where this is an actual alteration in occlusal load
2. Where there is a reduced capacity of the tooth-supporting tissues to absorb stress.

Tissue damage caused by applying excessive occlusal loads to a previously healthy periodontium has been called *primary occlusal trauma*. Damage caused by normal functional stress applied to an impaired periodontium has been called *secondary occlusal trauma*. The division into primary and secondary trauma is rather artificial as, more often than not, excessive loads are applied to an already impaired periodontium. However, it remains a useful conceptual distinction, as primary trauma is completely reversible (as in orthodontic treatment), while the tissue changes associated with secondary trauma may be only partly reversible.

Gingival recession (Figure 8.9)

Gingival atrophy results in apical movement of the gingival margin to produce gingival recession and exposure of the root of the tooth. Recession involves some destruction of the periodontal tissues and it may accompany chronic periodontitis, but it is not necessarily a feature of that disease. Gingival recession is one of those tissue changes

(a)

(b)

Figure 8.9 Gingival recession associated with *(a)* traumatic toothbrushing technique, which has also produced tooth abrasion (note associated area of gingival irritation over the premolars) and *(b)* a divergent palatal root

usually caused by the wear and tear of use, and which lies between health and active pathology. Like tooth attrition, gingival recession represents a departure from normal anatomy, which is not necessarily a sign of disease. It is extremely common, and frequently the cause of patients' concern.

A number of factors acting singly or in combination produce or affect gingival recession, and these are described below.

Physical abuse

Both healthy gingiva and the gingival wall of a periodontal pocket can atrophy under the stress of toothbrush friction, especially when an overzealous horizontal brushing technique is used. The sheltered interdental gingiva may escape this treatment so that the recession is restricted to labial tooth surfaces, which may also suffer abrasion. The maxillary canines and first premolars that form the corner of the arch receive the brunt of this form of aggression, and usually display the worst recession. The interdental gingiva may not escape the enthusiastic use of various interdental oral hygiene aids; some patients use wood sticks and floss like a hacksaw and, although gingiva and the underlying bone are remarkably resilient, they will atrophy in the face of determined attack.

Physical damage can also result from a variety of dental procedures – the carelessly applied matrix band or temporary crown, uncontrolled condensation of an inter-proximal or cervical restoration, pressure from a badly designed denture clasp or denture ('gum stripping') – or from strange habits, such as pressing a pencil into the gum!

Another physical factor is that associated with deep overbite, where the incisal edge of an upper incisor impinges on the lower labial gingiva or where a lower incisor strikes the palatal tissue.

Figure 8.10 Large frenum and healthy gingivae in 40-year-old man

Alveolar defects

The presence of an underlying alveolar margin defect, e.g. dehiscence, means that the overlying gingiva is unsupported and less able to withstand irritation. The Northern European skull is often dolicocephalic, i.e. long-headed, the jaws narrow and overcrowded and alveolar plates thin; developmental defects, dehiscence and fenestration are common, especially on the labial surface of canines, lower incisors and first molars. Defects of alveolar plates are frequently related to tooth position and root morphology.

Tooth position

The position of the tooth in the arch is a determinant of the thickness of bone overlying the root. A displaced tooth may be accompanied by some compensating thickness of overlying bone, but there is a limit to such accommodation and where teeth are placed in, say, a labial position, the labial alveolar margin is displaced apically or is deficient (dehiscence).

Furthermore, teeth can be moved through the alveolar bone by uncontrolled orthodontic forces and excessive occlusal stress, with resultant bone perforation and gingival recession.

Root morphology

Where roots diverge, which occurs especially on first upper molars or where the root is markedly convex (as it also may be on both upper and lower canines), the overlying bone may be very thin or deficient. This may not manifest in health, but where some tissue destruction has taken place a divergent palatal root of an upper first molar can be related to gross recession (*Figure 8.9b*).

Soft-tissue attachment

The presence of a frenum or muscle attachment does not influence healthy gingiva (*Figure 8.10*) but, in the pre-sence of inflammation and pocketing, tension from these anatomical structures may result in retraction of the gingiva and recession. This is often the case where the zone of attached gingiva is narrow or absent. However, the mere presence of a frenum never justifies surgical intervention; only when an anatomical feature is obviously related to progressive pathology is surgical modification indicated.

Disease

Acute necrotizing ulcerative gingivitis (see Chapter 22) can destroy gingival tissue, which may not be reformed when the disease has resolved.

If sufficient tissue is destroyed, recession results. In addition, the gingival wall of a periodontal pocket may move apically as the disease progresses or as inflammation subsides, producing root exposure.

Recession also follows pocket reduction surgery for the treatment of chronic periodontitis.

The treatment of all forms of gingival recession and its complications is considered in Chapter 18.

References

Albander, J.M. (1990) A 6-year study on the pattern of periodontal disease progression. *Journal of Periodontology* **17**, 467–471

Albander, J.M., Rise, J., Gjermo, P. and Johansen, R.J. (1986) Radiographic quantification of alveolar bone level changes. *Journal of Clinical Periodontology* **13**, 195–200

Ericsson, I. and Lindhe, J. (1977) Lack of effect of trauma from occlusion on the recurrence of experimental periodontitis. *Journal of Clinical Periodontology* **4**, 115–127

Ericsson, I. and Lindhe, J. (1982) The effect of longstanding jiggling on experimental marginal periodontitis in the beagle dog. *Journal of Clinical Periodontology* **9**, 497–503

Ewan, S.J. and Stahl, S.S. (1962) The response of the periodontium to chronic gingival irritation and long-term tilting forces in adult dogs.

Oral Surgery, Oral Medicine and Oral Pathology **15**, 1426–1433

Glickman, I. (1964) Trauma from occlusion in the etiology of periodontal disease. In *Clinical Periodontology*, 3rd Edn, pp. 286–299. Philadelphia, W.B. Saunders

Glickman, I. (1965) Clinical significance of trauma from occlusion. *Journal of American Dental Association* **70**, 607–618

Glickman, I. (1967) Occlusion and the periodontium. *Journal of Dental Research* **49** (Suppl. 1), 5

Glickman, I. (1971) Role of occlusion in the etiology and treatment in periodontal disease. *Journal of Dental Research* **50**, 199–204

Glickman, I. and Smulow, J.B. (1962) Alterations in the pathway of gingival inflammation into the underlying tissues induced by excessive occlusal forces. *Journal of Periodontology* **33**, 7–13

Glickman, I. and Smulow, J.B. (1965) Effects of excessive occlusal forces upon the pathway of gingival inflammation in humans. *Journal of Periodontology* **36**, 141–147

Glickman, I. and Smulow, J.B. (1968) Adaptive alteration in the periodontium of the Rhesus monkey in chronic trauma from occlusion. *Journal of Periodontology* **39**, 101–105

Goodson, J.M., Tanner, A.C.R., Haffajee, A.D. *et al.* (1982) Patterns of progression and regression of advanced destructive periodontal disease. *Journal of Clinical Periodontology* **9**, 472–481

Gribic, J.T. and Lamster, I.B. (1991) Risk indicators for future clinical attachment loss in adult periodontitis. Patient variables. *Journal of Periodontology* **62**, 322–329

Gribic, J.T. and Lamster, I.B. (1992) Risk indicators for future clinical attachment loss in adult periodontitis. Tooth and site variables. *Journal of Periodontology* **63**, 262–269

Haffajee, A.D. and Socransky, S.S. (1986) Attachment level changes in destructive periodontal disease. *Journal of Clinical Periodontology* **13**, 461–472

Jeffcoat, M.K. and Reddy, M.S. (1991) Progression of probing attachment loss in adult periodontitis. *Journal of Periodontology* **62**, 185–189

Karing, T., Nyman, S., Thilander, B. and Magnusson, I. (1982) Bone regeneration in orthodontically produced alveolar bone dehiscences. *Journal of Periodontal Research* **17**, 309–315

Lindhe, J. and Svanberg, G. (1974) Influence of trauma from occlusion on progression of experimental periodontitis in the beagle dog. *Journal of Clinical Periodontology* **1**, 3–14

Lindhe, J., Haffajee, A.D. and Socransky, S.S. (1983) Progression of periodontal disease in adult subjects in the absence of periodontal therapy. *Journal of Clinical Periodontology* **10**, 433–442

Listgarten, M.A. (1988) Why do epidemiological data have no diagnostic value? In *Periodontology Today* (B. Guggenheim, ed.), pp. 59–67. Basel: S. Karger

Macapanpan, L.C. and Weinmann, J.P. (1954) The influence of injury to the periodontal membrane on the spread of gingival inflammation. *Journal of Dental Research* **33**, 263–272

Manson, J.D. (1976) Bone morphology and bone loss in periodontal disease. *Journal of Clinical Periodontology* **3**, 14–22

Meitner, S.W. (1975) Co-destructive Factors of Marginal Periodontitis and Repetitive Mechanical Injury. Thesis, Rochester, USA: Eastman Dental Center and The University of Rochester

Mühlemann, H.R. and Herzog, H. (1961) Tooth mobility and microscopic tissue changes produced by experimental occlusal trauma. *Helvetica Odontologica Acta* **5**, 33–39

Nyman, S., Lindhe, J. and Ericsson, I. (1978) The effect of progressive tooth mobility on destructive periodontitis in the dog. *Journal of Clinical Periodontology* **7**, 351–360

Page, R.C. and Schroeder, H.E. (1989) Pathogenesis of inflammatory periodontal disease. A summary of current work. *Laboratory Investigation* **3**, 235–249

Papapanou, P.N., Wennstrom, J.L. and Grondahl, K. (1989) A 10-year study of periodontal disease progression. *Journal of Clinical Periodontology* **16**, 403–411

Prichard, J.F. (1965) *Advances in Periodontal Disease*. Philadelphia: W.B. Saunders

Reitan, K. (1951) The initial tissue reaction incident to orthodontic tooth movement as related to the influence of function. *Acta Odontologica Scandinavica* **10** (Suppl.)

Sheiham, A., Smales, F.C., Cushing, A.M. and Cowell, C.R. (1986) Changes in periodontal health in a cohort of British workers over a 14-year period. *British Dental Journal* **160**, 125–127

Socransky, S.S., Haffajee, A.D., Goodson, J.M. and Lindhe, J. (1984) New concepts of destructive periodontal disease. *Journal of Clinical Periodontology* **11**, 21–32

Suomi, J.D., Greene, J.C., Vermillion, J.R. *et al.* (1971) The effect of controlled oral hygiene procedures on the progression of periodontal disease in adults: results after third and final year. *Journal of Periodontology* **42**, 152–160

Svanberg, G. and Lindhe, J. (1973) Experimental tooth hypermobility in the dog. A methodological study. *Odontologisk Revy* **24**, 269–282

Warhaug, J. (1979) The infrabony pocket and its relationship to trauma from occlusion and subgingival plaque. *Journal of Periodontology* **50**, 355–365

Warhaug, J. and Hansen, E.R. (1966) Periodontal changes incident to prolonged occlusal overload in monkeys. *Acta Odontologica Scandinavica* **24**, 91–105

Wentz, F.M., Jarabak, J. and Orban, B. (1958) Experimental occlusal trauma imitating cuspal interferences. *Journal of Periodontology* **29**, 117–127

9

Epidemiology of periodontal disease (the size of the problem)

In the past few years, as described in Chapter 8, there has been a radical change in our ideas about the natural history of periodontal diseases. There has also been a parallel reappraisal of their prevalence and the methods by which they are studied. Until recently periodontal disease was regarded as the main cause of tooth loss, and a WHO report of 1978 stated that 'almost all the adult population has experienced gingivitis, periodontitis or both'. These ideas are out-of-date and are now seen as the result of invalid methods of data collection and interpretation.

There has been a reduction in disease prevalence, and the reasons for the improvement in periodontal health that has taken place in the industrialized countries are probably related to better personal and oral hygiene, improved standards of living, reduction in cigarette smoking, decrease in the use and dosage of oral contraceptives, plus the effects of fluoride, fewer proximal restorations and overhanging margins (Sheiham, 1990).

In order to measure the prevalence of the disease, its severity, and its relationship to other factors, such as age, oral hygiene status, nutrition and so on, special indices have been that which attempt to provide an objective measure or to score specific identifiable features so that reliable comparisons can be made. Using these indices and applying the appropriate statistical tests should allow the interested observer to make a valid comparison of, for example, the periodontal condition of young adults in the USA with the periodontal condition of individuals of any age anywhere in the world. Also, if successful public health measures are to be implemented, and personnel trained and recruited, the character and size of the problems to be tackled need to be defined.

Indices

All indices should be appropriate to the nature of the investigation and the circumstances under which this is being undertaken. Thus, the assessment of the gingival condition and oral hygiene status of 10–12-year-old children in an inner city area in Britain will require a very different approach from a study of the periodontal status of an East African nomadic cattle-breeding tribe, such as the Masai or Dinka! The application of any particular index needs to meet several criteria:

1. It must be practical and acceptable to the subject. The method of examination must not be painful or more uncomfortable than the individual can reasonably tolerate, e.g. taking six pocket measurements on every tooth in a child's mouth is impractical. Any examination in the absence of adequate illumination or sterilization facilities is not acceptable.
2. It must reflect the reality of the situation; thus pocket measurements on the buccal aspects of teeth may be irrelevant and misleading when the main site of periodontal destruction is interproximal. Also, pocket depth is an indicator of past pathology, and cannot validly be used as an indicator of current disease activity.
3. It should be sufficiently standardized and reliable to allow comparison between different examiners, and between examinations at different times, as in longitudinal studies.
4. It should allow numerical quantification and therefore statistical analysis. Assessment of gingival inflammation by degree of redness is subjective and quantifiable only in the grossest terms.
5. It should be sufficiently sensitive to detect small changes. Thus, bleeding on probing the pocket may or may not indicate the presence of active disease, and does not tell us about the strength of that activity; biochemical assessment of crevicular fluid might be sufficiently sensitive for that purpose.

Indices of the gingival condition use colour, change of contour, readiness to bleed on gentle probing, bleeding time, measurement of gingival fluid exudate, counts of white cells in gingival fluid and gingival histology. Indices of periodontal destruction depend largely on probing depth and probing attachment level measurements. Some of the tests require special equipment and special skills, and are used therefore only in sophisticated laboratory studies. Conditions in the field usually do not permit other than the simplest tests to be used, especially where large numbers of individuals are inspected. The most commonly used indices of gingival inflammation are the gingival index (Löe and Silness, 1963) and the bleeding on probing index (Löe, 1967), which has a number of variations (Barnett *et al.*, 1980). The three periodontal indices to be described, the periodontal index (Russell, 1956), the periodontal disease index (Ramfjord, 1959) and the community periodontal index of treatment needs (CPITN; Ainamo, 1983), score both gingival inflammation and periodontal destruction.

Gingivitis indices

Gingival index (GI)

The severity of the condition is indicated on a scale of 0 to 3:

0   Normal gingivae
1   Mild inflammation, slight change in colour, slight oedema. No bleeding on probing
2   Moderate inflammation, redness, oedema and glazing. Bleeding on probing
3   Severe inflammation, marked redness and oedema, ulceration. Tendency to spontaneous bleeding.

The mesial, buccal, distal and lingual gingival units are scored separately. This index is particularly sensitive in the early stages of gingivitis.

The gingival index is reversible, as its values return to zero with the disappearance of the disease. By contrast, indices of chronic periodontitis measure the amount of periodontal destruction, which is irreversible. Furthermore, as the progress of chronic periodontitis tends to be phasic, a periodontal index does not measure active disease.

Bleeding on probing index

0   Normal gingivae
1   Signs of gingival inflammation but no bleeding on gentle probing
2   Bleeding on probing
3   Spontaneous gingival bleeding.

The mesial, buccal, distal and lingual gingival units are scored separately.

Periodontal destruction indices

Periodontal index (PI) (Russell, 1956)

All teeth are examined; the scores used in this index are as follows:

0   Negative: there is neither overt inflammation in the investing tissues nor loss of function due to destruction of supporting tissues
1   Mild gingivitis: there is an overt area of inflammation in the free gingivae, but this area does not circumscribe the tooth
2   Gingivitis: inflammation completely circumscribes the tooth, but there is no apparent break in the gingival attachment
6   Gingivitis with pocket formation: the epithelial attachment has been broken and there is a pocket (not merely a deepened crevice due to swelling in the free gingivae). There is no interference with normal masticatory function; the tooth is firm in its socket, and has not drifted
8   Advanced destruction with loss of masticatory function: the tooth may be loose, may have drifted, may sound dull on percussion with metallic instrument, may be depressible in its socket.

Rule: When in doubt, assign the lesser score.

This index has been applied with success to large population groups. Its limitation is that its score for periodontal destruction is so heavily weighted that it is not possible to distinguish the early stages of a chronic periodontitis.

Periodontal disease index (PDI) (Ramfjord, 1959)

The periodontal disease index introduced by Ramfjord is a development of the Russell index. The Ramfjord index is particularly designed for assessing the extent of pocket deepening below the cemento-enamel junction. Scoring is as follows:

0   Health
1   Mild to moderate inflammatory change, not extending all around tooth
2   Mild to moderate inflammatory change extending all around tooth
3   Severe gingivitis, characterized by marked redness, tendency to bleed, ulceration
4   3 mm apical extension of pocket base from enamel–cement junction
5   3–6 mm extension
6   Over 6 mm extension.

Another feature of the PDI is that only six teeth, 6|14, 41|6 are selected for examination and measurement. The data from these teeth have been found to be representative of the dentition as a whole, and their average score is the score of the patient.

Community periodontal index of treatment needs (CPITN)

If an attempt is made to provide an adequate dental service for a particular community, it is necessary to assess its treatment need. The CPITN (Ainamo, 1983) has become the most widely employed system for this purpose, and uses the following method:

1. A specially banded probe with a ball head (*Figure 9.1*) has been designed for use with the index. It is to be used as an extension of the examiner's fingers in the gentle manipulation of the gingivae. The sensing force should correspond to about 20 g or less, and pain during probing indicates that too much pressure is being applied. A pressure guided probe has been designed to produce a standard force, but it is difficult to see the relevance of such sensitive instrumentation in the context of CPITN.
2. The dentition is divided into six segments or sextants (four posterior and two anterior) in which there are two or more teeth present and not indicated for extraction. When only one tooth remains in a sextant, it is included in the adjacent sextant.
3. The scoring system is:
   Code 0   Health: no pocketing or gingival bleeding on probing
   Code 1   Gingival bleeding on probing
   Code 2   The presence of calculus or other plaque-retentive factors such as overhanging margins of restorations that can be seen or felt on probing
   Code 3   Pocketing of 4–5 mm; that is, when the gingival margin is on the black area of the probe
   Code 4   Pocketing of 6 mm or more; i.e. when the black area of the special probe is no longer visible

Code X   When only one tooth or no teeth are present in a sextant. Third molars are excluded unless they function in the place of second molars.

4. When used for epidemiological purposes (alternative 1), ten specific teeth are examined; these are $\overline{761|67}$, $\overline{76|167}$, and the worst of the two molar scores is recorded, thus making six scores. When used for treatment purposes (alternative 2), for children and adolescents six index teeth $\dfrac{61|6}{6|61}$ are examined, while for adults (20 years and older) all teeth are examined.
5. It is suggested that an appropriate treatment plan can be worked out on the following basis:
   Code 0 requires no treatment
   Code 1 requires improvement in home care
   Codes 2 and 3 require supra- and subgingival scaling and improvement in home care
   Code 4   requires more complicated treatment, i.e. supra- and subgingival scaling and root planing, improvement in home care and surgery.

The CPITN has proved to be a very useful broad screening tool, and as such has been usefully employed in very many WHO surveys throughout the world. A good example of its use is illustrated in *Figure 9.2*. This shows on a three-dimensional bar diagram the mean number of sextants according to CPITN scores of 2784 people in a 1986 Dutch National Dental Survey (reported in the FDI *Guidelines for Community Periodontal Care*, 1992). In a comparison of the periodontal index (PI) and CPITN, Cuttress *et al.* (1986) demonstrated that the CPITN index was more sensitive than PI.

However, the CPITN is too insensitive to be used to produce a detailed diagnosis, prognosis and treatment plan for the individual patient in practice, or to monitor the individual patient on a regular basis.

Indices assessing extent of disease

An index to measure the extent and severity of periodontitis has been proposed by Carlos *et al.* (1986), and has been called the extent and severity index.

Extent and severity index (ESI)

This has two components:

1. Extent – proportion of tooth sites in the subject with destructive periodontitis
2. Severity – mean value of attachment loss at the diseased sites.

An attachment loss threshold of >1 mm was set as the criteria to qualify as disease affected. By the use of this arbitrary figure it distinguishes the fraction of the dentition affected by disease and prevents non-affected sites from contributing to the subject mean attachment loss

Figure 9.1 The CPITN probe

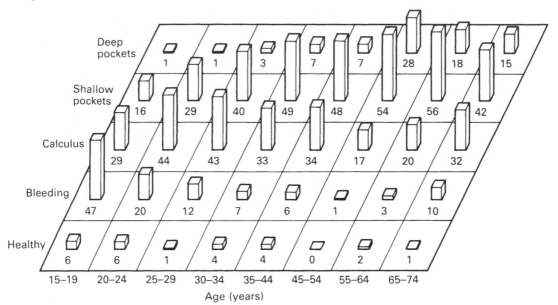

Figure 9.2 CPITN scores in Dutch National Survey. (Reproduced from *Guidelines for Community Periodontal Care*, by kind permission of FDI World Dental Press Ltd)

value. It obviously depends on the use of an accurate and reliable measurement of attachment loss from the cement–enamel junction, and this is difficult to attain. It is biphasic in expression, and gives a detailed description of attachment loss patterns. For example, an ESI of 90,2.5 indicates a generalized early periodontitis, whereas an ESI of 20,7.0 indicates a severe localized advanced periodontitis.

The same principles have been applied to the development of a partial index system based on radiographic assessment of alveolar bone loss (Papapanou *et al.*, 1991a, 1991b) suitable for radiographic surveys of chronic periodontitis.

Limitation of indices

All periodontal indices have the following limitations:

1. The criteria are subjective to some degree, and there is considerable variation in examiner assessment of degrees of inflammation and pocket depth or loss of attachment.
2. The scoring systems are arbitrary. Thus a lesion scoring Russell PI 6 is not actually three times as severe as a lesion scoring PI 2; indeed gingivitis and periodontitis cannot be compared numerically in this way.
3. Although a gingivitis score measures present inflammation, pocket measurement is a reflection of past disease. If we accept the well-established idea that periodontal breakdown is episodic, pocket depth gives us no indication of disease activity at the time of measurement. The production of bleeding on care-

ful probing of the pocket with a blunt probe has been regarded as an indicator of disease activity but, as Nevins *et al.* (1989) point out, 'At best, bleeding on probing has a predictive value of 30%'. In this regard, the absence of bleeding on probing appears to be a good indicator of periodontal stability, whereas bleeding on probing is a very poor indicator of disease activity (Lang *et al.*, 1990). It also seems more likely that the provocation of bleeding on probing is a factor of the enthusiasm or clumsiness of the examiner than of current disease activity. However, as the mechanisms involved in tissue destruction are clarified, parameters of current disease activity are being defined. Also, some indicators of those individuals at risk from advanced periodontal disease, e.g. juvenile periodontitis, are being unravelled (see Chapter 20).

Oral hygiene

The most commonly used indices of oral hygiene status are the oral hygiene index (Greene and Vermillion, 1960) and the plaque index (Silness and Löe, 1964).

Oral hygiene index

This is a composite index that scores debris and calculus deposition either on all or on selected tooth surfaces.

Oral debris is any soft foreign matter that is attached to the tooth. Oral debris and calculus are scored separately. The oral debris scoring is as follows:

0   No debris or stain present

1 Soft debris covering not more than one-third of the tooth surface
2 Soft debris covering more than one-third but not more than two-thirds of the tooth surface
3 Soft debris covering more than two-thirds of the tooth surface.

The calculus scores are assigned according to the same criteria, with the addition that individual flecks of subgingival calculus are given score 2 and a continuous heavy band of subgingival calculus is scored 3.

The debris and calculus scores are added and divided by the number of surfaces examined to give the Oral Hygiene Score.

Plaque index (PI)

Criteria for scoring are:

0 No plaque
1 Film of plaque visible only by removal on probe or by disclosing
2 Moderate accumulation of plaque which can be seen by the naked eye
3 Heavy accumulation of soft material filling the niche between the gingival margin and the tooth surface. The interdental region is filled with debris.

This index has been used with the gingival index to provide precise evidence of the causal relationship between plaque and gingival inflammation. Variations of these indices measure the amount of calculus and plaque retention factors such as overhanging margins of fillings.

Problems with accurately assessing the prevalence of periodontal disease

It is difficult to determine the prevalence, severity, extent and progression of periodontal disease because of poor correlation between the signs and symptoms of the disease and the disease process itself. Periodontal disease is a chronic inflammatory disease, induced by bacterial irritation, which is recognized by a number of signs and symptoms. These, in order of increasing severity, include visual inflammation, bleeding on probing, gingival enlargement, pocket formation, loss of periodontal attachment and alveolar bone, tooth mobility and tooth loss. Therefore, it is probable that disease definitions based on single or on combinations of several symptoms and signs will result in different prevalence estimates. Periodontal disease is site-specific and the number of sites involved varies from patient to patient, adding another quantitative variable to disease definition. Also, many of the measurements made to assess the severity of disease – such as probing depth, probing attachment loss and radiographic assessment of alveolar bone loss – are far

from reliably accurate and are subject to many technique variables (see Chapter 12). This makes precise disease level definitions difficult. This is particularly the case in epidemiological studies, where large numbers of patients are examined in short periods of time and often under far from ideal conditions. Furthermore, it is necessary to define what level of attachment loss is required to consider periodontitis as an important oral health problem, and whether this should this be uniform for the whole dentition or should depend on tooth type, root length or the age of the patient. These are all very important questions to consider in determining disease definition.

Both cross-sectional and longitudinal studies have used different diagnostic criteria and examination methodologies, and are therefore often difficult to compare. Finally, some studies have used partial mouth recording systems, and these may seriously underestimate the extent of disease present. They are, therefore, difficult to compare with studies using whole mouth recording.

Prevalence of gingivitis

The prevalence of gingival inflammation varies significantly with age.

The deciduous dentition

The gingivae around deciduous teeth appear to be remarkably resistant to plaque-induced inflammation. Even when toothbrushing is withdrawn for 3 weeks, there is a significant difference in tissue response to that in the adult. Early studies of American and English children under 5 years old recorded little or no gingival inflammation but, using more rigid criteria, Poulsen and Moller (1972) found a 25% prevalence in Danish 3-year-olds. In a study of 128 5–6-year-old Australian children, Spencer *et al.* (1983) found a high prevalence of mild inflammation around the deciduous teeth, little severe inflammation, and little correlation between the oral hygiene status and the severity of inflammation. It seems likely that this finding reflects a difference in the intensity of the immunological response in the young child, or in the microflora of the gingival crevice. The prevalence of spirochaetes and of *Bacteroides melaninogenicus* is lower at 3–7 years old than in the adult (de Araujo and MacDonald, 1964).

The transitional period

This period covers the mixed dentition from about the age of 5 or 6 years through to puberty. It is marked by tooth irregularity and hormonal changes. Chronic gingivitis has been found in 80% of children under 12 years of age and approaches 100% by the age of 14 years (WHO, 1978).

This high prevalence was also found in a UK study of 1015 11–12-year-old children, in which Addy *et al.* (1986) recorded that all the children had some inflammation as demonstrated by bleeding on probing, at one or more sites, with a good correlation between plaque and gingivitis scores.

In older studies, the prevalence of inflammation (i.e. the number of individuals in whose mouth some inflammation was present) was recorded, but not the fact that this was restricted to few teeth. Therefore, the figures greatly exaggerated the size of the problem.

After about 14 years of age there is a decrease in the severity of inflammation; a sexual difference also appears. Before 14, the severity of inflammation for girls is higher than for boys, the girls' scores peaking at about 12 years old; boys' scores peaked at 14 and were found to be higher than those for girls. This could be related to changing patterns in oral hygiene habits, but in fact in a study of the gingival status at puberty, Sutcliffe (1972) found that the increased severity of inflammation was not related to an increase in plaque deposition. One must conclude that, in puberty, the tissues react more vigorously to any given amount of plaque; after puberty, the severity of inflammation does diminish.

The adult

After the post-puberty decline in inflammation, prevalence appears to increase and has been recorded as high as 100% of young men aged 17–22 years. However, as indicated above, such figures need to be interpreted with caution. A study of 15–19-year-olds in New Zealand (Cuttress *et al.*, 1983) showed that, although 79% of mouths had some gingival inflammation, only 34% of tooth sites were inflamed, and in this group only 1% showed some periodontal breakdown. In a detailed analysis of data obtained in 1981 from the examination of 7078 people aged 19 years and older in 48 states of the USA (therefore regarded as representative of 147 million Americans), Brown *et al.* (1989) found that 15% were free of any kind of periodontal disease, and that gingivitis without periodontitis occurred in 50% of the remaining people. The prevalence of gingivitis declined from 54% in the group aged 19–44 years to 44% at 45–64 years, and to 36% in people of 65 years. In most people the gingivitis was restricted to a few teeth.

There is evidence that the transition from chronic gingivitis to chronic periodontitis takes place at an earlier age in Asiatic people than in Europeans or people of European origin. Although it is possible that genetic factors influence tissue vulnerability to plaque products (as appears to be the case in juvenile periodontitis), it is more likely that this difference may be explained by differences in oral hygiene habits, which relate to educational and income levels. The role of nutrition in the gingival condition is uncertain, but it is likely that, in the well-nourished people of developed countries, nutritional factors play little or no part (Chapter 6).

Acute ulcerative gingivitis has a very low prevalence in rich countries and a higher one in poorer countries, often affecting malnourished children (Chapter 22).

Prevalence of periodontitis

Children and adolescents

Periodontal breakdown in children is often associated with some fault in host response (as in Down's syndrome, hypophosphatasia, juvenile diabetes, etc.; see Chapter 6), but early destructive periodontal disease, i.e. juvenile periodontitis (JP) (see Chapter 20), has been reported by Cogen *et al.* (1992) in healthy Alabama children. This radiographic study of 4757 children (3172 black and 1585 white) under the age of 15 years revealed a prevalence of juvenile periodontitis of 1.5% in black children and 0.3% in white children. Amongst the black children the male : female ratio with JP was almost equal, while among the white children it was 1 : 4. A further finding was that, in 71.4% of the black children with JP, previous radiographs also revealed bone loss around deciduous teeth.

The results of more than 100 WHO surveys in over 60 countries of adolescents, i.e. 15–19-year-olds, using the CPITN have been reported by Miyazaki *et al.* (1991a). The most frequently observed condition was score 2 (calculus with or without gingival bleeding), which was much more prevalent in non-industrialized countries than in industrialized countries. Some shallow pocketing of 4–5 mm was present in two-thirds of all populations observed, but it usually affected only a minority in the sample, and then only in one or two sextants. Some of this was probably due to false pockets caused by gingivitis and gingival oedematous or fibrous enlargement.

Adults

There is considerable palaeontological evidence of periodontal disease in early humans, and past epidemiological studies have emphasized the general prevalence of the disease. Hence the widespread belief that all adults would, at some time during their lifetime, experience deterioration of the periodontal tissues, and that a large proportion of edentulousness was due to periodontal disease. Indeed, many regarded periodontal breakdown as an inevitable part of the ageing process.

The earlier epidemiological surveys carried out in between 1950 and 1970 mostly employed radiographical evidence of alveolar bone loss as a means of distinguishing between gingivitis and periodontitis. The influential study by Marshall-Day *et al.* (1955) involving 1187 dentate subjects was representative in demonstrating that, by the age of 40 years, 90% of adults had some periodontal disease. Findings from other epidemiological surveys of this period (Shour and Massler, 1948, Belting *et al*., 1953; Sandler and Stahl, 1954; Bossert and Marks, 1956; Russell, 1957; Shei *et al*., 1959; Gupta, 1962; Littleton, 1963; Johnson *et al*., 1965; Ramfjord *et al*., 1968; Sheiham and Hobdell, 1969), despite some differences in design, have also shown a very high prevalence of periodontitis in the adult population, with a clear increase in prevalence with age. In 1964, Sherp reviewed the epidemiological literature at that time and concluded that periodontal disease appears to be a major global health problem affecting the majority of the adult population after the age of 35–40 years. This work indicated that it appeared to start as gingivitis in youth which, if left untreated, progressed to periodontitis, with more than 90% of the variance of severity in the population explainable by age and oral hygiene.

Such findings set the tone of attitudes to the conservation of the dentition. The question, why go to all this trouble if I am going to lose my teeth? reflected many people's attitudes to restorative dentistry. As stated earlier in the text, such notions were based on imperfect methods of data collection and interpretation. As Pilot (1992) points out, 'we have been brain-washed by averages; reports on mean attachment loss per year do not show those sites that are breaking down at a much faster rate than average, nor are persons indicated who have many of those sites and are in fact in the high risk category of losing their teeth at an early stage. Persons and sites with no attachment loss at all are also obscured in mean figures' and, 'in the early epidemiological surveys on periodontal conditions, any deviation from the ideal was recorded and implicitly considered as disease'.

Epidemiological surveys in the 1980s provided a more thorough description of the high variation in the periodontal conditions between different populations and individuals. Hugoson and Jordon (1982) examined 600 randomly selected subjects in Sweden, aged 20–70 years, by clinical and radiological means. Reporting on data relating to 1973 they found that, in the age groups of 30 and 40 years, 96% and 85% respectively of the subjects had no signs of alveolar bone loss. Severe periodontal destruction affected about 8% of subjects between 40 and 70 years. The same research group (Hugoson *et al*., 1992) reported on the data from 597 subjects of a similar age, examined 10 years later and relating to 1983. This showed that 98% of the 20-year-olds and 77% of the 30-year-olds were classifiable as either as periodontally healthy or as gingivitis patients. In the entire sample, a higher percentage of subjects (11%) were placed in the severe periodontitis group than in their previous study. However, this apparent increase was accompanied by retention of more teeth and a decrease in the percentage of edentulous subjects (16% vs. 12% in ages 40–60 years).

Recently, the same group (Hugoson *et al*., 1998) compared the distribution of periodontal disease in Swedish adults in 1973, 1983 and 1993, using their previous data and a new survey in 1993. The subjects were divided into five groups: healthy (group 1); gingivitis (group 2); moderate alveolar bone loss, i.e. up to one-third loss (group 3); severe alveolar bone loss, i.e. ranging from one-third to two-thirds loss (group 4); and angular bony defects and/or furcation defects (group 5). During these 20 years, the proportion of subjects in groups 1 and 2 increased from 49% in 1973 to 60% in 1993. In addition, there was a decrease in the proportion of subjects in group 3 with moderate periodontitis. The subjects with severe periodontitis in groups 4 and 5 comprised 13% of the population, and showed no change from 1983 to 1993. However, the subjects in these groups had more teeth than their counterparts in 1983. In 1973 the numbers in these groups were smaller, because greater numbers had become edentulous due to lack of suitable periodontal care at this time. In 1993, the subjects in groups 3–5 were also divided according to the percentage of surfaces with gingivitis only or periodontal pockets $\geq$ 4 mm. At this time, 20%, 42% and 67% of individuals in groups 3, 4 and 5 respectively were classified as in need of periodontal treatment, with more than 20% of sites bleeding on probing and more than 10% of sites with periodontal pockets $\geq$ 4 mm.

Thus, over this period there has been an increase in the number of individuals with no marginal bone loss, and a decrease in the number with moderate alveolar bone loss. Although the numbers of subjects in the severe disease group remained the same, the number of teeth retained by each individual increased.

Douglass *et al*. (1983) compared data on periodontal disease from the US National Center for Health Statistics for the years 1960–62 and 1971–74, and found a definite downward trend in the prevalence of both gingivitis and periodontitis in younger adults.

Data taken from the UK 1988 Adult Dental Health Survey shows that 75% of the UK population aged between 35 and 45 years at that time had shallow pockets, and 17% of the dentate population of 45 years and older had deep pockets. A similar pattern of prevalence was found in the large American survey reported by Brown *et al*. (1989) and cited above. The prevalence of periodontitis increased with age from 29% at age 19–44 years up to about 50% in people 45 years and older. Moderate periodontitis (i.e. at least one pocket of 4–6 mm deep) occurred in 28% of all people, while only 8% had advanced disease (i.e. at least one pocket greater than 6 mm), and only 10% had six or more teeth with pocketing of 4–6 mm. Pocketing over 6 mm deep was found in only one in twelve people, and then only around one or two teeth. The need for extraction was found in only 4%, while less than 20% of all absent teeth were listed as missing due to periodontal disease.

Baelum *et al*. (1986) carried out a cross-sectional study of plaque, calculus, gingivitis, periodontitis and tooth loss in a sample of adult Tanzanians aged 30–69 years, and reported a tooth site frequency of plaque of more than 90%, calculus of 50–65%, gingival bleeding of 30–40%, pockets deeper than 3 mm of less than 10%, attachment loss of ⩾ 4 mm of less than 35% and attachment loss > 6 mm of less than 10%. None of the subjects were edentulous, and very few had experienced any major loss of teeth. It was also shown that 75% of the tooth sites with attachment loss of ⩾ 7 mm were found in 31% of subjects. Thus, in this population attachment loss was found at a small number of tooth sites, and was often associated with gingival recession rather than pocketing. Furthermore, it was shown that a small subset of the population studied was responsible for most of the attachment loss found.

The same group (Baelum *et al.*, 1988) also reported a similar study on 1131 Kenyan subjects aged 15–65 years, which confirmed their previous findings. Poor oral hygiene in the subject group was reflected by high plaque, calculus and gingivitis scores. However, significant attachment loss showed a skewed distribution and was found in only a small proportion of individuals. Furthermore, in these individuals, significant attachment loss was found at less than 20% of their tooth sites. This suggests that, in these subjects, destructive periodontal disease was not an inevitable consequence of gingivitis but rather a feature of individual differences in susceptibility (Lembariti, 1983).

Yoneyama *et al.* (1988) described probing depth, probing attachment level and recession data from 319 randomly selected Japanese adults aged 20–79 years. The percentage of sites with deep pockets (⩾ 6 mm) was small, ranging from 0.2% at the age of 30–39 years to 1.2% at the age of 70–79 years. However, the percentage of sites with advanced attachment loss (⩾ 5 mm) ranged from 1% in the younger group to 12.4% in the older group, and this discrepancy was attributed to gingival recession. They also found that relatively small groups of individuals accounted for substantial amounts of the observable attachment loss, but the number of these individuals increased with age and markedly so after the age of 60 years. Therefore, destructive periodontitis was much more prevalent and widespread in a susceptible subgroup of older subjects. Furthermore, this study showed a similar pattern of destructive periodontitis to that found in Tanzania and Kenya by Baelum *et al.* (1986, 1988).

The results of the 1985–86 National Survey of Oral Health in the United States was published by Brown *et al.* (1990). The sample included 15 132 employed males and females aged 18–64 years, who were examined with respect to gingivitis, gingival recession and probing pocket depths at the mesial and buccal sites of all teeth in two randomly selected quadrants, one upper and one lower. The findings revealed that destructive periodontitis was very uncommon in the sample. Gingivitis was found in 44% of subjects, and occurred at an average of 2.7 sites per subject and less than 6% of the sites examined. Its frequency decreased slightly with age. Periodontal pockets of 4–6 mm were found at 1.3% of the sites assessed

and occurred in an average of 13.4% of the subjects, ranging from 6% at 18–24 years to 18% at 55–64 years. Pockets ⩾ 7 mm were only found at 0.03% of all sites, were observed in only 0.6% of all subjects and were most frequent in subjects of 55–64 years (1.1%). Gingival recession of ⩾ 3 mm occurred in 17% of subjects (range 3–46%), and when it occurred it was not extensive, affecting an average of between one and two sites per subject.

Much higher prevalence figures were reported by another study performed in the USA (Horning *et al.*, 1990), which employed full mouth circumferential probing in a sample of 1984 males and females, aged 13–84 years, at a military dental clinic. The prevalence of subjects with at least one 4 mm deep pocket was 63%, and with at least one ⩾ 7 mm deep pocket was 17%. Part of the discrepancy between the two American surveys may be because of population differences and the fact that a dental clinic population is more selective for subjects with disease than a random population sample. It could also have been affected by the use of partial recording methods by Brown *et al.* (1990), which may have underestimated the true prevalence.

Figures from the WHO Global Oral Dental Bank, based on CPITN data from over 50 countries, have been published (Miyazaki *et al.*, 1991b). Miyazaki *et al.* considered the age groups 35–44 and 45–74 years (*Figure 9.3*), and found that calculus and shallow pocketing were the most frequently observed conditions and, with a few exceptions, the percentages of persons (5–20%) and the mean number of sextants per person with deep pockets were small to very small, with a tendency to increase with age. The assumed differences between industrialized and non-industrialized countries with regard to the prevalence and severity of periodontal diseases were not reflected in the survey data examined. Marked differences between two groups of countries were only seen for the estimated national levels of edentulousness, which was very low for the non-industrialized countries (perhaps a reflection of a smaller dentist : population ratio?).

From these data it appears that the progress of periodontal disease with age is not shown by an increase in CPITN scores but an increasing number of missing teeth, which could be the result of factors other than periodontal disease. In the age group 65–74 years this results, on average, in almost half of all sextants being excluded. Of the remaining sextants, approximately half had both shallow and deep pockets.

All studies show that poor oral hygiene is an important factor affecting both the prevalence and severity of gingivitis, which may progress to periodontitis. Other factors already discussed in relation to gingivitis have, as expected, a similar relationship to chronic periodontitis.

Socio-economic factors, in particular educational level and economic status, bear a significant relationship to prevalence and severity. This could well explain some observed ethnic differences, but others are probably due

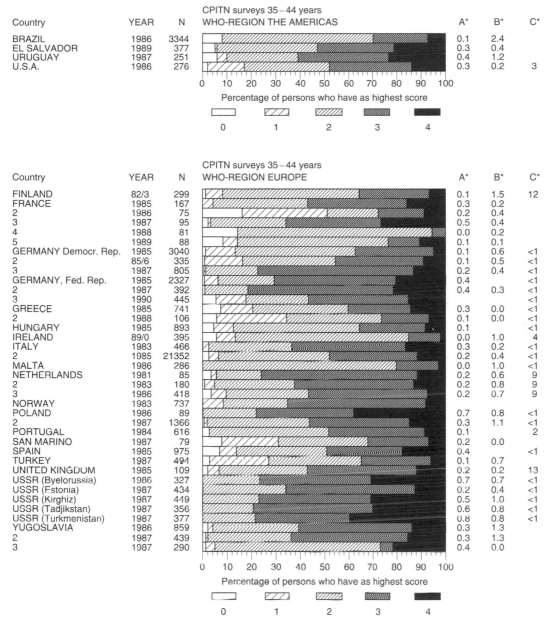

Figure 9.3 The observed periodontal conditions measured by the CPITN in America and Europe at age 35–44 years, from WHO Global Oral Data Bank, 1st August, 1990.
Column A*: mean number of sextants with CPITN score 4 = pockets ≥ 6 mm; Column B*: number of sextants with CPITN score X = sextant excluded, less than two teeth; Column C*: percentage edentulous.
From Miyazaki *et al.* (1991b). (©Butterworth-Heinemann for Fédération Dentaire Internationale)

to genetic variation. If equal age groups in Asian and European populations are compared (Löe *et al.*, 1978), the transition from gingivitis to periodontitis appears to be earlier and the severity of destruction greater in the Asian group than in the European group. Both oral hygiene habits and nutritional status were better in the latter group, and this probably reflected educational and income levels. If one compares different ethnic groups with equivalent income and educational levels, the disease profile is very similar.

The onset of periodontal destruction, when it occurs, appears to take place most commonly in the young adult, and then both prevalence and severity may increase with age, becoming clinically significant in the fourth decade of life. However, for the large majority of most of the observed populations the progress of periodontal diseases seems to be compatible with the retention of the natural dentition into older age.

Recent epidemiological studies seem to indicate that progression from gingivitis to periodontitis appears to take place in a much smaller proportion of individuals than was previously believed (Papapanou, 1994). Unfortunately, we cannot yet predict which individuals will progress from gingivitis to periodontitis, and much current research is directed to trying to define the person who is 'at risk'. A great deal of epidemiological and clinical research in the past decade has also highlighted considerable variation in clinical features and rates of disease progression of chronic periodontitis (Papapanou, 1994).

Natural history of periodontal disease as shown by longitudinal studies of disease progression

An accurate assessment of the natural history of any disease requires extensive knowledge of its aetiology and pathology, the population's attitudes towards the disease, the availability of a healthcare system and the effect of preventive and therapeutic measures, and this is a complicated matter. Furthermore, the assessment of the natural history and progression of chronic periodontitis requires a longitudinal study over many years. The studies suitable for this purpose are longitudinal studies of periodontal disease progression in which the periodontal conditions of subjects exposed to little or no therapeutic intervention are monitored for relatively long periods.

Lindhe *et al.* (1983) studied the progression of periodontal disease in the absence of treatment in two subject groups consisting of 64 Swedish and 36 American subjects. The Swedish group included subjects with moderate periodontal attachment loss at entry, and was monitored for attachment level changes at baseline, 3 months and 6 years. The American group consisted of subjects with advanced periodontitis at entry, and was monitored at baseline and 1 year. Of 4101 tooth sites examined at baseline and 3 years in the Swedish group, only 158 sites (3.9%) showed attachment loss of more than 2 mm. Of 4097 sites examined at baseline and 6 years, 523 sites (11.6%) showed progressive attachment loss of the same magnitude. Approximately half the sites that showed no measurable change in the first 3-year period showed loss in the second 3-year period, while two-thirds of the sites with disease progression between baseline and the 3-year examination were stable during the second monitoring period.

In the American group, 102 out of 3210 sites (3.2%) showed attachment loss of 2 mm or more during 1 year of monitoring. When the association between initial and progressive attachment loss was examined by linear regression analysis, the hypothesis that sites with advanced attachment loss were more prone to exhibit disease progress than sites with less initial loss could not be supported.

Based on the results of this and other studies, the same research group challenged the concept of slow, continuous progressive attachment loss until treatment or tooth loss, and suggested instead that periodontal disease progressed in recurrent acute episodes (Socransky *et al.*, 1984). They further suggested that these bursts of activity occurred in short periods of time at individual sites, and were followed by relatively long periods of remission. Once a burst has occurred, certain sites may show no further activity, while others may experience several additional bursts at later time periods. It was also suggested (Haffajee and Socransky, 1986) that the random nature of the burst hypothesis should not be interpreted to suggest that episodes of disease activity may occur irrespective of microbiological, anatomical, clinical or other conditions of the particular site, but rather as random with respect to time.

The possible three models of periodontal progression (see also Chapters 8 and 12), namely constant slow progression, instantaneous increments of progression (random burst) and variable non-instantaneous progression (asynchronous multiple burst), have been mathematically modelled so that longitudinal data can be loaded into a computer program to see which model it best fits (Sterne *et al.*, 1992). Using available longitudinal data, they found a better fit for the burst models over the continuous model, but were unable to distinguish between the random burst and asynchronous multiple burst models.

However, it is apparent that the ability to reliably measure small amounts of attachment loss (such as would occur in the constant slow progression model) is not possible at present, so it is quite possible that all three types of progression may occur in different patients and in different situations in the same patient (see Chapter 8). There is some evidence to support this concept, with the development of electronic probes that will measure probing attachment level more reliably and accurately. One such probe (Jeffcoat and Reddy, 1991), which detects and measures the attachment level from the cement–enamel junction, has been claimed to have a threshold ranging from 0.3–0.8 mm (see Chapter 12). Using this probe, Jeffcoat and Reddy (1991) monitored 30 patients with moderate to advanced chronic periodontitis for 6 months. Using a threshold of 0.4 mm they found 29% of sites with attachment loss, and using one of 2.4 mm they found attachment loss at only 2% of sites. This indicated that, when using large thresholds, only rapid attachment loss (either random burst or asynchronous multiple burst) will be detected, whilst using smaller thresholds will detect both rapid and slow constant attachment loss with a higher proportion of slow constant attachment loss sites.

One of the few longitudinal studies to investigate the initiation, rate of progression of periodontal disease and consequent tooth loss in a population never exposed to any dental treatment or preventive programmes is that carried out in Sri Lanka by Löe *et al.* (1986). They examined 480 male tea labourers in Sri Lanka aged between 14 and 30 years, initially in 1970, with respect to plaque, calculus, gingivitis and attachment loss at the mesial and buccal aspects of all their teeth. Five subsequent examinations were carried out up to 1985, when the study was terminated. At this stage, 161 individuals from the initial examination remained. The subjects did not practise any conventional oral hygiene measures and had uniformly large aggregates of plaque and calculus, and inflammation was present at virtually every gingival site. Based on the measured rates of attachment loss and tooth loss, three subgroups of subjects were identified: individuals with rapid progression (RP) of periodontitis (8% of the sample); those with moderate progression (MP) (81%); and those with no progression (NP) (11%). At 35 years of age, subjects in the RP group showed a mean attachment loss of 9 mm, the subjects in the MP group an average of 4 mm and subjects in the NP group less than 1 mm. At 45 years, there was a mean loss of 13 mm in the RP group in comparison to 7 mm in the MP group. The annual progression rate in the RP group ranged between 0.1 and 1 mm, in the MP group between 0.05 and 0.5 mm and in the NP group between 0.04 and 0.09 mm. Since these subjects were entirely caries free, all missing teeth were lost due to periodontal disease. There was an average loss of 12 teeth at age 35 years and 20 teeth at age 40 years in the RP group, while in the MP group an average of only seven teeth was lost at age 45 years. The NP group showed no tooth loss.

In a later publication (Löe *et al.*, 1992) this group reanalysed this data in respect of gingival recession, and reported that more than 30% of the subjects exhibited gingival recession before the age of 20 years whilst gingival recession was present in 100% of subjects aged over 40 years, affecting 70% or more of the buccal surfaces, 50% or more of the lingual surfaces and 40% of the interproximal surfaces.

The overall rates of progression in this study are higher than those found in populations practising oral hygiene, due to the much higher levels of plaque and calculus. However, the study also clearly shows different levels of susceptibility in this population, which are very similar in percentage terms to those found in other population groups. It also shows that gingival recession is a major reflector of attachment loss in these subjects. It is important to realize that gingival recession as a reflector of attachment loss will not show up in some methods of data collection, such as the CPITN, and this could severely limit its usefulness.

Papapanou *et al.* (1989) reported on the progression of periodontitis, assessed radiographically over 10 years, in a group of 201 Swedish subjects aged 25–70 years. Tooth loss (expressed as a percentage of the number of teeth present at the initial examination) varied between 3 and 28%, and was highest in the subjects initially over 50 years old. The mean annual bone loss varied between 0.07 and 0.14 mm in ages from 25 to 65 years, but was twice as high (0.28 mm) in individuals of 75 years at the completion of the study. A mean bone loss of $\geqslant 0.5$ mm was found in 75% of the subjects, while 7% showed a loss of $\geqslant 3$ mm. The same pattern was found on a tooth site level, with the majority of the sites showing small degrees

of bone loss but relatively few sites showing greater magnitudes of bone loss. In this regard, about 15% of patients accounted for half of the observed sites with advanced bone loss ($\geqslant 6$ mm). While the subjects most affected by bone loss at entry were the ones most prone to develop further disease progression, the same trend could not be found at the tooth site level.

Ismail *et al.* (1990) reported on a longitudinal study carried out between 1959 and 1987 in Michigan, USA. Out of an initial sample of 526 subjects who participated in the baseline examination, 167 dentate subjects remained at the completion of the study. Over the 28-year period, 11% of the teeth initially present in these subjects were lost. Twenty-two subjects (13%) showed an average attachment loss of $\geqslant 2$ mm, five subjects (3%) of $\geqslant 3$ mm and two subjects (1.2%) of $\geqslant 4$ mm.

Thus, all the longitudinal studies reported appear to show that there is a small subgroup of patients who have high susceptibility to periodontitis and a small subgroup of patients who are resistant to this condition, and this holds true irrespective of plaque levels.

Summary

Worldwide epidemiological studies have shown that gingival inflammation is present in most populations, but that the more severe stages of periodontal disease, whilst not as prevalent as previously believed, are still of significant magnitude, affecting up to 15–20% of most populations over the age of 35 years. Although gingivitis is very common, it does not inevitably progress to periodontitis. Oral hygiene, and therefore periodontal health, is improving in the majority of people in industrialized countries.

References

Addy, M., Dummer, P.M.H., Griffiths, G. *et al.* (1986) Prevalence of plaque, gingivitis and caries in 11–12-year-old children in South Wales. *Community Dentistry and Oral Epidemiology* **14**, 115–118

Ainamo, J. (1983) Assessment of periodontal treatment needs. Adaptation of the WHO community periodontal index of treatment needs (CPITN) to European conditions. In *Public Health Aspects of Periodontal Disease in Europe* (A. Frandsen, ed.). Berlin: Quintessence Verlag

Baelum, V., Fejerskov, O. and Karring, T. (1986) Oral hygiene, gingivitis and periodontal breakdown in adult Tanzanians. *Journal of Periodontal Research* **21**, 221–232

Baelum, V., Fejerskov, O. and Manji, F. (1988) Periodontal diseases in adult Kenyans. *Journal of Clinical Periodontology* **15**, 445–452

Barnett, M.I., Ciancio, S.G. and Mather, M.L. (1980) The modified papillary bleeding index during the resolution of gingivitis. *Journal of Preventive Dentistry* **6**, 135–138

Belting, C.M., Massler, M. and Schour, I. (1953) Prevalence and incidence of alveolar bone disease in men. *Journal of the American Dental Association* **17**, 190–197

Bossert, W.A. and Marks, H.H. (1956) Prevalence and characteristics of periodontal disease in 1200 persons under periodic dental observation. *Journal of the American Dental Association* **53**, 429–442

Brown, L.J., Oliver, R.C. and Löe, H. (1989) Periodontal diseases in the US in 1981: Prevalence, severity, extent and role in tooth mortality. *Journal of Periodontology* **60**, 363–380

Brown, L.J., Oliver, R.C. and Löe, H. (1990) Evaluating periodontal status of US employed adults. *Journal of the American Dental Association* **121**, 226–232

Carlos, J.P., Wolfe, M.D. and Kingman, A. (1986) The extent and severity index: a simple method for use in epidemiological studies of periodontal disease. *Journal of Clinical Periodontology* **13**, 500–505

Cogen, R.B., Wright, T. and Tate, A.L. (1992) Destructive periodontal disease in healthy children. *Journal of Periodontology* **63**, 761–765

Cuttress, T.W., Hunter, P.B.V. and Hoskins, D.I.H. (1983) Adult oral health in New Zealand 1976–1982. Dental Research Unit, Medical Research Council of New Zealand, Wellington, N.Z.

Cuttress, T.W., Hunter, P.B.V. and Hoskins, D.I.H. (1986) Comparison of the periodontal index (PI) and community periodontal index of treatment needs (CPITN). *Community Dentistry and Oral Epidemiology* **14**, 39–42

de Araujo, W.C. and MacDonald, J.B. (1964) Gingival crevice microbiota of pre-school children. *Archives of Oral Biology* **9**, 227–228

Douglass, C., Gillings, D., Solecito, W. and Gammon, M. (1983) The potential for increase in the periodontal needs of the aged population. *Journal of Periodontology* **54**, 721–730

Greene, J.C. and Vermillion, J.R. (1960) The oral hygiene index. A method for classifying oral hygiene status. *Journal of the American Dental Association* **61**, 172–179

Gupta, O.P. (1962) Epidemiological studies of dental disease in the state of Kerala. I. Prevalence and severity of periodontal disease. *Journal of the All India Dental Association* **34**, 45–50

Haffajee, A.D and Socransky, S.S. (1986) Attachment level changes in destructive periodontal diseases. *Journal of Clinical Periodontology* **13**, 461–472

Horning, G.M., Hatch, C.L. and Lutskus, J. (1990) The prevalence of periodontitis in a military treatment population. *Journal of the American Dental Association* **121**, 616–622

Hugoson, A. and Jordon, T. (1982) Frequency distribution of individuals aged 20–70 years according to severity of periodontal disease. *Community Dentistry and Oral Epidemiology* **10**, 187–192

Hugoson, A., Laurell, L. and Lundgren, D. (1992) Frequency distribution of individuals aged 20–70 years according to severity of periodontal disease experience in 1973 and 1983. *Journal of Clinical Periodontology* **19**, 227–232

Hugoson, A., Norderyd, O., Slotte, C. and Thorstennsson, H. (1998) Distribution of periodontal disease in a Swedish adult population in 1973, 1983 and 1993. *Journal of Clinical Periodontology* **25**, 542–548

Ismail, A.I., Morrison, E.C., Burt, B.A. *et al.* (1990) Natural history of periodontal disease in adults: findings from the Tecumseh periodontal disease study, 1959–87. *Journal of Dental Research* **69**, 430–435

Jeffcoat, M.K. and Reddy, M.S. (1991) Progression of probing attachment loss in adult periodontitis. *Journal of Periodontology* **62**, 185–189

Johnson, E.S., Kelly, J.E. and Van Kirk, L.E. (1965) Selected dental findings in adults by age, race and sex. United States 1960–62. *U.S. Department of Health Education and Welfare, National Center for Health Statistics* Series 11, No. 7, 1

Lang, N.P., Alder, R., Joss, A. and Nyman, S. (1990) Absence of bleeding on probing. An indicator of periodontal stability. *Journal of Clinical Periodontology* **17**, 714–721

Lembariti, B.S. (1983) *Periodontal Diseases in Urban and Rural Populations in Tanzania.* Tanzania: Dar es Salaam University Press

Lindhe, J., Haffajee, A.D. and Socransky, S.S. (1983) Progression of periodontal disease in adult subjects in the absence of periodontal therapy. *Journal of Clinical Periodontology* **10**, 433–442

Littleton, N.W. (1963) Caries and periodontal disease among Ethiopean civilians. *Dental Abstracts* **8**, 763–764

Löe, H. (1967) The gingival index, the plaque index and the retention index systems. *Journal of Periodontology* **38**, 610–616

Löe, H. and Silness, J. (1963) Periodontal disease in pregnancy. I. Prevalence and severity. *Acta Odontologica Scandinavica* **21**, 532–551

Löe, H., Anerud, A., Boysen, H. and Smith, M. (1978) The natural history of periodontal disease in man. The rate of periodontal destruction before 40 years of age. *Journal of Periodontology* **49**, 607–620

Löe, H., Anerud, A., Boysen, H. and Morrison, E. (1986) The natural history of periodontal disease in man. Rapid, moderate and no loss of attachment in Sri Lankan laborers 14 to 46 years of age. *Journal of Clinical Periodontology* **13**, 431–440

Löe, H., Anerud, A. and Boysen, H. (1992) The natural history of periodontal disease in man: prevalence, severity and extent of gingival recession. *Journal of Periodontology* **63**, 489–495

Marshall-Day, C.D., Stephens, R.G. and Quigley, L.F. (1955) Periodontal disease: Prevalence and incidence. *Journal of Periodontology* **26**, 185–191

Miyazaki, H., Pilot, T., Leclercq, M.-H. and Barmes, D.E. (1991a) Profiles of periodontal conditions in adolescents measured by CPITN. *International Dental Journal* **41**, 67–73

Miyazaki, H., Pilot, T., Leclercq, M.-H. and Barmes, D.E. (1991b) Profiles of periodontal conditions in adults measured by CPITN. *International Dental Journal* **41**, 74–80

Nevins, M., Becker, W. and Korman, K. (1989) *Proceedings of the World Workshop in Clinical Periodontics*, pp. 1–24. Princeton, NJ: American Academy of Periodontology

Papapanou, P.N. (1994) Epidemiology and natural history of periodontal disease. In *Proceedings of the 1st European Workshop on Periodontology* (N.P. Lang and T. Karring, eds), pp. 23–41. London: Quintessence Publishing Co. Ltd

Papapanou, P.N., Wennström, J.L. and Gröndahl, K. (1989) A 10-year retrospective study of periodontal disease progression. *Journal of Clinical Periodontology* **16**, 403–411

Papapanou, P.N., Wennström, J.L. and Johnsson, T. (1991a) Extent and severity index based on assessments of radiographic bone loss. *Community Dentistry and Oral Epidemiology* **19**, 313–317

Papapanou, P.N., Wennström, J.L. and Johnsson, T. (1991b) Evaluation of a radiographic partial recording system assessing the extent and severity of periodontal destruction. *Community Dentistry and Oral Epidemiology* **19**, 318–320

Pilot, T. (1992) Implications of the high-risk strategy and of improved diagnostic methods for health screening and public health planning in periodontal diseases. In *Risk Makers for Oral Diseases Vol. 3. Periodontal Diseases* (N.W. Johnson, ed.), pp. 441–453. Cambridge, Cambridge University Press

Poulsen, S. and Moller, I.J. (1972) The prevalence of dental caries, plaque and gingivitis in 3-year-old Danish children. *Scandinavian Journal of Dental Research* **80**, 94–103

Ramfjord, S.P. (1959) Indices for prevalence and incidence of periodontal disease. *Journal of Periodontology* **30**, 51–59

Ramfjord, S.P., Emslie, R.D., Greene, J.C. *et al.* (1968) Epidemiological studies of periodontal diseases. *American Journal of Public Health* **58**, 1713–1722

Russell, A.L. (1956) A system of classification and scoring for prevalence surveys of periodontal disease. *Journal of Dental Research* **35**, 350–359

Russell, A.L. (1957) Some epidemiological characteristics in a series of urban populations. *Journal of Periodontology* **28**, 286–293

Sandler, H.C, and Stahl, S.S. (1954) The influence of generalized diseases on clinical manifestation of periodontal disease. *Journal of the American Dental Association* **49**, 656–667

Schour, I. and Massler, M. (1948) Prevalence of gingivitis in young adults. *Journal of Dental Research* **27**, 733–738

Shei, O., Waerhaug, J., Lövidal, A. and Arno, A. (1959) Alveolar bone loss as related to oral hygiene and age. *Journal of Periodontology* **30**, 7–16

Sheiham, A. (1990) Public Health Approaches to the Promotion of Periodontal Health, p. 2. In Monograph Series No. 3. Joint Department of Community Dental Health and Dental Practice. University College London

Sheiham, A. and Hobdell, M.H. (1969) Decayed, missing and filled teeth in a British adult population. *British Dental Journal* **126**, 401–404

Sherp, H.W. (1964) Current concepts in periodontal disease research: epidemiological contributions. *Journal of the American Dental Association* **68**, 667–675

Silness, J. and Löe, H. (1964) Periodontal disease in pregnancy. II. Correlation between oral hygiene and periodontal condition. *Acta Odontologica Scandinavica* **22**, 121–135

Socransky, S.S., Haffajee, A.D., Goodson, J.M. and Lindhe, J. (1984) New concepts of destructive periodontal disease. *Journal of Clinical Periodontology* **11**, 21–32

Spencer, A.J., Beighton, D. and Higgins, T.J. (1983) Periodontal disease in 5- and 6-year-old children. *Journal of Periodontology* **54**, 19–22

Sterne, J.A.C., Kingman, A. and Löe, H. (1992) Assessing the nature of periodontal disease progression – an application of covariance structure estimation. *Applied Statistics* **41**, 539–552

Sutcliffe, P. (1972) A longitudinal study of gingivitis and puberty. *Journal of Periodontal Research* **7**, 52–58

WHO (1978) *Epidemiology, Etiology and Prevention of Periodontal Diseases.* Technical Report Series No. 621. Geneva: World Health Organization

Yoneyama, T., Okamoto, H., Lindhe, J. *et al.* (1988) Probing depth, attachment loss and gingival recession. Findings from a clinical examination in Urhiku, Japan. *Journal of Clinical Periodontology* **15**, 581–591

10

Prevention of periodontal disease

The essential requirement for the prevention of a disease is an understanding of its cause. Chapter 4 describes the cause of chronic periodontal disease, but the prevalence of the disease bears sad witness to our inability to apply that knowledge to the full. Many factors, social and economic, are beyond the influence of the dental profession, but the profession has certain undeniable obligations. These are to educate the patient in good oral hygiene habits, to attempt to motivate the patient to apply advice given, to provide a regular service for professional cleaning, to apply fluoride to young teeth and, if disease occurs, to practise sound dentistry that does not potentiate disease.

These ideas are also discussed in the treatment of chronic gingivitis (see Chapter 14), but patients without disease represent a different starting point from the patient with established disease. Both the patient and the practitioner are faced with a slightly different psychological situation, and unfortunately it is one with which few dentists by training or experience are properly equipped to deal. Conversion to the philosophy of prevention involves nothing less than a revolutionary reorientation of thoughts and attitudes of every dentist.

Patient education and motivation cannot be a once-and-for-all process, but must involve a continuing commitment to the patient. Such a commitment can be fulfilled only when dental personnel are organized to that end (Sims, 1968). A preventive service can be provided in a general dental practice, which is largely devoted to treatment, but it is possible that better results are obtained when both therapist and patient are freed from the constraints of the conventional dental surgery situation. In a therapeutic situation the patient adopts a passive attitude in the face of professional authority. In providing a preventive service the patient's active participation is essential; indeed, even the word 'patient' seems inappropriate in this situation – perhaps 'pupil' would be better.

In situations where patients have to take responsibility for their own welfare, as in the control of diabetes or periodontal disease, they are accountable for both the success and, of great importance, the failure of what they do. In the latter case, people used to being passive and putting the burden on the professional person have only themselves to blame.

At the same time, the professional person may find him or herself in an ambiguous situation. There is a conflict between the professional as expert and authority, which reflects the traditional patient–professional relationship, and the professional person as teacher and counsellor. In the preventive situation the professional sets out to help patients help themselves, and needs to recognize from the outset that he or she is separated from the patient in a number of respects, the most important of which are knowledge, values and language.

Many professional people – not just doctors and dentists, but lawyers, accountants, etc. – seem to overlook the fact that they possess special knowledge, particular attitudes to the problems of their patients or clients and an exclusive vocabulary that they have learned and take for granted. These factors create a gap that must be bridged so that a creative dialogue can be pursued. The values and attitudes of the dentist do not necessarily coincide with those of the patient; the latter wants to eat in comfort and look nice, while the dentist wants a plaque score of zero and a balanced occlusion. These different levels of aspiration need to be approximated, and two factors become essential. The first is the provision of information in language the patient can understand, and the second is the generation of motivation, i.e. an explanation of the real advantages that will result from taking the professional advice, as well as the disadvantages of ignoring it.

Unfortunately, many dentists do not feel they can give the time to this, or are ill-equipped to deal with these challenges, and become impatient and even patronizing. The problem can be solved by having someone in an ancillary capacity, the practice nurse or hygienist, who has the time, the training and the personal motivation to take on the responsibility of undertaking the preventive programme.

The provision of information and instruction in home care can take place inside or outside the dental surgery: it may be applied to an individual or a group; it can be carried out by an informed patient or schoolteacher as well as by dental personnel. Information can be given through a variety of media; films, slides, lectures and printed material. The one-to-one relationship between therapist and patient is likely to be the most effective system but, where this is not possible, group instruction is better than no instruction at all. Ancillary personnel, in particular the dental hygienist, have an extremely valuable role to play in prevention. Hygienist training includes a much greater emphasis on prevention than does the conventional dental undergraduate course, and in the patient's mind the hygienist is often associated with this aspect of dentistry.

Certain groups are more receptive to information and instruction than others: adolescents with a developing awareness of self and interest in their general appearance and well-being; expectant and nursing mothers; young couples whose sense of responsibility is sharpened by new parenthood. This is not to imply that the older person is beyond reach; the message that teeth can and should last for life is a powerful incentive to a mature person who has knowledge of the problems suffered by less fortunate members of his or her peer group.

Regular guidance and encouragement are essential and, for the young patients, the application of topical fluorides can be included in the periodic checks. The long-term studies in Sweden by Axelsson and Lindhe (1974, 1978, 1981, 1986) provide overwhelming evidence of the benefits of an organized programme of regular professional care.

Prior to instituting a preventive programme, one must establish that disease is not already present. One cannot take it for granted in any individual that periodontal disease is not present; careful examination of every mouth is essential. Health is the starting point of a preventive programme, the aim of which is the maintenance of that state by the control of plaque deposition. By far the major part in plaque control must be played by the individual. The responsibilities of professional personnel are:

1. To provide information about dental health
2. To provide information and guidance about the techniques of plaque control
3. To attempt to change the individual's evaluation of dental health; in jargon terms, to motivate the patient.

Providing information

Providing a patient with the necessary information takes time and some insight into the limitations of the patient's understanding. It also requires the ability to express oneself in simple language. As stated, too often dentists do not have the time to provide patients with sufficient information, and sometimes patients do not appreciate the value of time spent in giving advice. Too frequently adequate knowledge is taken for granted, and when a description is provided it is expressed in technical terms quite incomprehensible to the patient. It is useless to tell a patient that 'bacterial plaque in proximity to the dentogingival junction provokes gingival inflammation'. The patient may not know what plaque or the dentogingival junction is, that the mouth is full of bacteria or that gingiva means gum!

In addition, information provided in abstract may be only partly understood and quickly forgotten. Information needs to be given by demonstration in the patient's own mouth, and before any treatment is carried out. It is useful to give the patient a hand-mirror so that he or she can follow some of the examination; plaque and calculus are pointed out, and the relationship to disease explained. At this time it is demonstrated that the principal cause of disease, the bacterial plaque, is almost invisible, but can be revealed by using a disclosing agent. This is a completely harmless dye, e.g. 4% Erythrosine, usually pink or blue, which is absorbed by the bacterial plaque (*Figure 10.1*). To emphasize the harmful nature of the plaque, a little of the stained deposit can be scraped off the tooth

(a)

(b)

Figure 10.1 Deposits of bacterial plaque *(a)* before and *(b)* after staining with a disclosing agent, which makes the presence of plaque obvious to the patient with a probe and shown to the patient with some remark about its bacterial content.

The patient is then given a toothbrush (if his or her own, so much the better) and told to attempt to remove all the stained plaque. At this stage no attempt should be made to instruct the patient in any particular brushing technique. The difficulties of the operation become apparent to the patient right away, who is thus more receptive to advice and instruction. Once the patient is aware of the problems in removing all the plaque, he or she may be allowed to develop a personal technique, but initially it is a good idea to demonstrate a formal technique as a basis for developing the necessary skill.

In starting treatment, it is very important to avoid confusing the patient with too much detail about toothbrushes and other oral hygiene aids, or to make the whole exercise seem too difficult or time consuming. Overenthusiasm at this stage can be counterproductive, but it must be made quite clear that the job of cleaning the mouth needs to be carried out methodically section by section and that frantic activity with the toothbrush is likely to do more harm to the gingiva than good.

Mechanical methods of plaque removal

Toothbrushing techniques

A large number of toothbrushing techniques have been advised, but the requirements of a satisfactory method are few:

1. The technique should clean all tooth surfaces, in particular the area of the gingival crevice and the interdental region. A scrubbing technique will clean the tooth convexities well and yet leave plaque in more sheltered places.
2. The movement of the brush should not injure the soft or hard tissues. Vertical and horizontal scrubbing methods can produce gingival recession and tooth abrasion.
3. The technique should be simple and easy to learn. A technique that one person finds easy to use may be difficult for someone else; therefore each person needs individual guidance.
4. The method must be well organized so that each part of the dentition is brushed in turn and no area overlooked. The mouth can be divided into a number of sections depending on the size of the dental arch and the size of the toothbrush.

Toothbrushing techniques can be demonstrated both on a model and in the patient's mouth.

The roll technique (*Figure 10.2a*)

This is a relatively gentle technique, which was once popular. The side of the toothbrush is placed against the side of the tooth with the bristles pointing apically and parallel to the axis of the tooth; the back of the brush is at

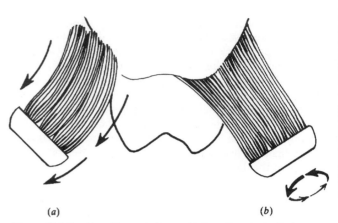

(a)   **(b)**

Figure 10.2 Toothbrushing techniques: *(a)* the roll method; *(b)* the Bass technique

the level of the occlusal surface of the teeth. The brush is then rotated deliberately down in the upper jaw and up in the lower jaw so that bristles sweep across the gum and tooth. About 10 strokes are given to each section, and the brush is moved in turn from one section to the next. If the arch in anterior segments is narrow, the brush can be used vertically. When all buccal and lingual surfaces have been brushed, the biting surfaces can be brushed with a rotary movement. This technique is no longer recommended for general use because it fails to clean the most important areas of the tooth – i.e. the junction of the tooth with the gingival margin and the gingival crevice – and it has been superseded by the Bass technique below.

The Bass technique (*Figure 10.2b*)

This brushing technique aims to clean the gingival crevice, and to this end the brush is held so that the bristles are about 45° to the axis of the teeth, the end of the bristles pointing into the gingival crevice (*Figure 10.3*). The brush is pressed towards the gingiva and moved with a small circular motion so that the bristles go into the

Figure 10.3 A toothbrush positioned for lingual cleaning using the Bass technique

crevice and are also forced between the teeth. This may be uncomfortable if the tissues are inflamed and sensitive, and thus will alert patients to this situation. It has been shown to be a most effective method for the removal of plaque, particularly from the gingival area of the tooth and gingival crevice. Therefore, it can be recommended as the method of choice for general use. It must be carried out with a suitable soft toothbrush, i.e. one with soft, flexible, rounded bristles in its brush head, which can penetrate into the gingival crevice without causing trauma.

Requirements of a satisfactory toothbrush

There are now on the market a large number of toothbrushes of different sizes and shapes, with bristles of various materials, textures, length and density. Overwhelmed by available choices, the man in the street is as likely to choose a brush that matches the bathroom tiles as one that will work well. Even a dentist may well be confused on this issue, since a great many studies have been carried out on the specifications of a satisfactory toothbrush (see Fransden, 1972), with contradictory results on almost every characteristic examined.

The bristles of toothbrushes are usually arranged in about 40 tufts in three or four rows (*Figure 10.4*). Hard brushes should never be recommended, as they can lacerate the gingiva, encourage gingival recession and cause tooth abrasion, particularly of exposed root surfaces. Furthermore, the bristle diameter of hard brushes is too large to penetrate into the gingival crevice. Soft toothbrushes should be recommended for all patients, since they minimize gingival and tooth abrasion and maximize the efficiency of cleaning procedures, particularly around the gingival margin and into the gingival crevice. Toothbrushes for children should be smaller and should relate to the mouth size at various ages. The bristles of children's toothbrushes should always be soft (0.1 mm–0.15 mm).

Certain basic requirements need to be met:

1. The brush head should be small enough to be manipulated effectively everywhere in the mouth, yet not be so small that it has to be used with extreme care in order to obtain complete coverage of the dentition. A length of about 2.5 cm is satisfactory for an adult; about 1.5 cm is suitable for a child.
2. The bristles should be of even length so that they function simultaneously. A convex or concave brush with bristles of different lengths will not clean a flat surface without undue pressure on some bristles. Short bristles will fail to reach interdental sites, and may also be so rigid that they injure the tissues.
3. The texture should allow effective use without causing damage to either soft or hard tissues. Stiffness depends on the diameter and length of the filament and its elasticity. It also depends on whether the brush is used wet or dry, and on the temperature of the

(a)

(b)

Figure 10.4 A toothbrush head *(a)* viewed from the side and *(b)* viewed from above, showing its upper surface

water. The bristles should be capable of penetrating into the gingival crevice without causing trauma.
4. The brush should be easy to keep clean. Densely packed tufts tend to retain debris and toothpaste at the base of the bristle. Modern synthetic fibre filaments are much more hygienic than natural bristle.

5. The toothbrush handle must rest comfortably and securely in the hand. It should be broad and thick enough to allow a firm grip and good control.

The main requirements of a satisfactory toothbrush are best summarized as:

- Having good cleaning ability
- Causing minimal damage to soft and hard dental tissues
- Having a reasonable lifespan (i.e. good wear characteristics)
- Being hygienic
- Being non-toxic.

User performance is a huge variable, and a balance must be achieved between this and requirements 1, 2 and 3 above. However, many of the factors involved in the brush head design can be defined reasonably precisely.

The handle

This is made of a variety of materials, such as acrylic and polypropylene. Its flexibility, size and shape must be convenient for manual use in the mouth, but details are more often a matter of styling rather than utility.

The toothbrush handle must rest comfortably and securely in the hand. It should be thick enough to allow a firm grip and good control. As the stiffness of the handle is one of the factors affecting the force applied to the teeth and gingiva during use, toothbrushes are now also made with flexible (stress breaking) handles (Ko *et al.*, 1995).

The brush head (*Figure 10.4*)

The shape of the brush head may have a utility aspect, but is often the result of styling. It should be small enough to be manipulated effectively everywhere in the mouth, yet not so small that it has to be used with extreme care to obtain complete coverage of the dentition. A length of about 2.5 cm is satisfactory for an adult; about 1.5 cm is suitable for a child.

The filaments (bristles)

Today, toothbrush bristles are either polyester or nylon. In 1938 DuPont created nylon, and its first application was the toothbrush bristle, gradually replacing pig bristle. Initially Nylon 66 (Exon) was used, but this was first replaced by Nylon 610 and then Nylon 612 (Tynex). Polyester and nylon are polymers with good chemical resistance and are inert, so they will pass through the body unchanged if swallowed. Nylon is said to wear less rapidly than polyester and, because of its antistatic properties, is more hygienic.

The diameter of the filaments varies considerably from 0.064–1.524 mm, but those used for toothbrushes fall into three categories:

1. Soft – 0.15–0.18 mm (0.006–0.007 in)
2. Medium – 0.18–0.23 mm (0.007–0.009 in)
3. Hard/extra hard – 0.23–0.28 mm (0.009–0.011 in).

Bristle stiffness also depends upon the length of the filament, its elasticity, whether the brush is used wet or dry, and the temperature of the water. In general, nylon loses 30% of stiffness when wet.

The bristles of children's brushes should always be soft (0.1–0.15 mm). Hard brushes should never be recommended, as they can lacerate the gingiva, encourage gingival recession and cause tooth abrasion. Furthermore, the bristle diameter of hard bristles is too large to reach into the gingival crevice; soft brushes, if used properly, can clean effectively around the gingival margin and into the crevice and minimize gingival and tooth abrasion.

Bristles should be of even length so that they function simultaneously. A convex or concave brush with bristles of different lengths will not clean a flat surface without undue pressure on some bristles. Short bristles will fail to reach into interdental sites and are also more rigid, causing gingival and tooth abrasion. Bristles in an adult's toothbrush are usually about 10–11 mm long (*Figure 10.4a*).

To be as non-abrasive as possible, the end of the bristle should be round. It is essential that this applies to at least 90% of the bristles.

The tufts (*Figure 10.4*)

The toothbrush bristle density is the number of bristles divided by the brush head area and there is some evidence that the greater this is, the better the plaque removing ability (Pretara-Spanedda *et al.*, 1989). However, forcing too many filaments into the tuft hole stresses the filaments against the tuft-hole wall so that the filaments curl over in the direction of the stress. On the other hand, too few bristles in the tuft-hole leaves them free to work loose. Many factors contribute to the balance between effectiveness, lack of tissue damage and wear, and these are as follows:

- *Hole pattern in the brush head.* Wisdom® brushes lay the hole pattern from centre to centre at a minimum spacing of 2.3 mm lengthwise by 2.1 mm widthwise. Closer spacing than this tends to weaken the handle. The hole pattern is spread out in the brushes specifically designed for interdental penetration.
- *Tuft-hole diameter.* This is usually about 1.6–1.7 mm, but can be as high as 2.0 mm.
- *Number of tufts in the brush head.* This varies greatly. Wisdom brushes use 42–45, and some larger American brushes use 60. These are arranged in three or four rows (*Figure 10.4b*).
- *The density of the filaments in the tuft.* This varies widely, but 18–26 filaments per tuft appears to provide good wear performance. The brush should be easy to keep clean, and densely packed tufts tend to retain debris and toothpaste at the base of the bristle.
- *Tuft length.* This is usually about 10 mm (*Figure*

10.4a). Wear performance deteriorates as tuft length increases.

- *Optimal packing factor.* Optimal wear performance is controlled by putting the right number of filaments in the tuft-hole to produce the correct packing factor. This is the ratio of the filament cross-section area minus the anchor wire area. The optimal packing factor is 0.63–0.74. The chosen dimensions of the diameters of the tuft-hole and the filament are not arrived at arbitrarily, but need to produce this packing factor.
- *Anchor wire thickness.* The anchor wire is the metal clip that holds the tuft of bristles in the tuft-hole, and this usually has a thickness of 0.20–0.35 mm.
- *Tuft knot retention.* According to the BSI standard, this must exceed 17 Newtons. Many European manufacturers do not use a minimum standard.
- *Single strand filament retention.* According to the BSI this must exceed 1 Newton.

The automatic toothbrush

The automatic toothbrush is now a well-accepted part of the home care armamentarium. There are a number of designs available, with different forms of movement: arcuating, vibrating and reciprocating.

There have been many studies comparing the effectiveness of the hand and automatic brush, and the results indicate that the subject's control is more important than the appliance. These studies can be divided into two groups: those that have shown no added benefit of electric brushes over manual ones in respect of plaque levels and gingival health (Niemi, 1987; Murray *et al.*, 1989, Walsh *et al.*, 1989; Ainamo *et al.*, 1991; Van der Weijden *et al.*, 1991), and those that have (Killoy *et al.*, 1989; Van der Weijden *et al.*, 1993, 1994; Stoltz and Bay, 1994; Ainamo *et al.*, 1997), and in some cases the same research group has produced both results at different times. Some studies have also suggested that some electric toothbrushes produce less gingival abrasion than manual ones (Niemi *et al.*, 1986; Niemi, 1987).

Properly used, the manual brush and automatic brush can both remove plaque effectively. As many people do not use the conventional brush properly, the automatic brush may be beneficial in their hands. For the uninstructed patient the automatic brush is as effective if not more so than the manual brush. The small head allows access to difficult areas, and many people find the sensation of the moving brush very pleasant.

The automatic brush is especially useful to the handicapped person; indeed it may be the only oral hygiene aid that can be used with a fair degree of success either by the individual or by a parent, careworker or nurse.

Interdental cleaning

As the interdental region is the most common site of plaque retention and the most inaccessible to the tooth-brush, special methods of cleaning are needed. These include the use of floss, tape, dental woodsticks, the interspace brush and the miniature interproximal brush. Once again it needs to be stated that, during the first stages of instruction in home care, the technique advised must be fairly easy for the patient to carry out. If it is not easy, discouragement will soon set in. The point of the exercise is the removal of plaque without injuring the soft tissues, and the use of woodsticks or floss where inappropriate may be harmful.

A further word of caution needs to be given about supplying the patient with too many gadgets; two implements at the most, e.g. a toothbrush and floss or interproximal brush, will suffice to start with.

Dental floss

Dental floss, either waxed or unwaxed, can be very effective in removing interproximal plaque. To be effective, the floss should be pulled around the tooth curvature so that close contact with the tooth surface is made. It needs to be used with control so that the gingiva is not cut *(Figure 10.5)*; many people find it difficult to use in posterior segments. A floss-threader is necessary to clean bridge abutments. As with all oral hygiene aids, the use of floss must be demonstrated in the patient's mouth, after which the patient repeats the performance under supervision. Comprehensive flossing should be carried out once a day.

A number of different designs of floss holder are available on the market, some of which allow floss to be applied in the recommended way *(Figure 10.6)*. Suitably designed floss-holders may make the task easier and quicker for some people, and thus make it more likely to be carried out every day.

Figure 10.5 Handling dental floss so that it can be used with control when being placed against an interproximal tooth surface. Note that the floss is wound round the fingers to prevent slipping

Figure 10.6 A floss-holder in use. The floss has been applied to the mesial surface of the first premolar and can be used in the conventional way to clean the gingival crevice and the proximal surface

The interspace brush

This is a single-tuft brush designed for cleaning areas difficult to access with a normal toothbrush, such as around irregular teeth, in a space where a tooth is missing, and around bridge abutments and pontics. The automatic rotating brush has also proved to be very effective in these situations, as well as for general interproximal cleaning.

Interproximal brush

The interproximal brush is an important device for cleaning between molar teeth and furca, particularly after surgery. The proximal furrow in the root is not adequately cleaned by floss or woodsticks, but will accommodate an interproximal brush well.

The dental woodstick

Once upon a time it was believed that bacterial invasion was better resisted by well-keratinized gingivae, and therefore that regular gingival massage was beneficial. The definition of the junctional epithelium as the portal of entry of bacterial products has undermined the rationale for this kind of exercise. The woodstick is used not to keratinize the gingivae, but to clean the interdental dentogingival junction. There must be an adequate interdental space to use a woodstick effectively and without damaging the tissues. If a woodstick is rubbed on inflamed gingiva, it is more likely to stimulate the inflammation than aid its resolution.

Irrigating devices (Water–Pik)

An irrigating device can be a useful supplement to the toothbrush, particularly where there is fixed bridgework;

however, it needs to be made clear to the patient that irrigation can remove food debris but cannot remove plaque. In the immediate postoperative phase following periodontal surgery, irrigation with warm or even a fairly hot and weak saline solution can be very soothing. It is unlikely that the addition of antiseptics, e.g. chlorhexidine, to the irrigating fluid is of much benefit, because the solution will be too dilute to affect the oral flora. On the other hand, if the taste is pleasant it might encourage the patient to use the device frequently and therefore help to make the home care process more enjoyable and less of a chore. Using the device on full strength may be hazardous. It is possible for the impact of the fluid to drive pocket bacteria into the tissues and produce a periodontal abscess.

Frequency of brushing

Theoretically, one could clean the teeth once every other day and prevent plaque from accumulating to the point where it would provoke some gingival inflammation. However, few people clean their teeth so well at one time that all the plaque is removed; therefore, more frequent brushing is essential. In addition, the presence of food debris or plaque build-up on the teeth is unpleasant, especially to people who are sensitive to the state of their mouth.

It has become the convention to clean teeth morning and night, and certainly the establishment of regular oral hygiene habits is essential; however, the rush to start the day or the fatigue of day's end do not provide the best climate for effective home care. In advising patients about the pattern of home care, it seems wise to take into account the kind of life they lead. Many people do have both the time and energy, as well as access to a washbasin, to spend time on cleaning their teeth in the middle of the day. These days many people work in places with good toilet facilities, and the habit of keeping a toothbrush at the place of work is to be encouraged.

The essential requirement is the acquisition of an awareness of the state of the mouth. Once an individual knows what a clean mouth feels like, a dirty mouth becomes intolerable and the need to use a toothbrush is encouraged. Splaying of the bristles is the most obvious sign of toothbrush wear. This is influenced more by the quality, i.e. resilience of the bristle, than by small differences in toothbrush design. Renewal of a toothbrush is usually recommended after three months' use. Market research indicates that women change their brushes more frequently than men.

Toothpaste

Essentially, toothpastes contain mild abrasives, which enhance the efficiency of the toothbrush in removing plaque deposits, as well as antibacterial agents, which may help retard the regrowth of plaque deposits (De La

Rosa *et al.*, 1979). Many contain fluoride to retard enamel demineralization and promote remineralization, and thus help to prevent and reduce caries. Some also contain chemicals to help to desensitize exposed and sensitive dentine.

There is a large variety of toothpaste formulations, which can be very complicated. Typical constituents are as follows:

- Abrasives, e.g. calcium carbonate, calcium pyrophosphate, aluminium silicate, diatomacious earth, etc.
- Antibacterial agents, e.g. sodium lauryl sulphate, zinc citrate trihydrate, triclosan, metal ions, etc.
- Anti-caries agents, e.g. sodium monofluorophosphate, sodium fluoride, stannous fluoride
- Desensitizing agents, e.g. strontium salts, sodium fluoride, formalin, etc.
- Fillers and thickeners, e.g. sodium carboxymethyl cellulose
- Humectants to keep the paste moist, e.g. glycerine
- Detergents, e.g. sodium lauryl sulphate
- Flavouring agents, often mint
- Colouring agents
- Sweeteners, e.g. sodium saccharin.

In the De La Rosa study (*ibid*), after prophylaxis, subjects brushed their teeth for 2 minutes with and without toothpaste over a 28-day period. Plaque levels were measured immediately after brushing and then after 24 hours. After each brushing, about 40% of the plaque was removed, leaving 60% to promote plaque regrowth. The regrowth rate for the group brushing with toothpaste was 27% lower than that for the group brushing without toothpaste. In subsequent studies, Rustogi *et al.* (1984) compared the effects of brushing with tap water for 1 minute with that of brushing with various abrasives, including silicon dioxide and sodium bicarbonate, and found that brushing with the abrasives removed 59–69% of 48-hour-old plaque compared with only 27–33% after brushing with tap water.

Other chemotherapeutic agents are discussed in Chapter 15.

Chemical control of plaque deposition

Mechanical methods of plaque removal require time and manual dexterity, and therefore a high level of patient motivation. These problems have stimulated the research for a chemical cleaner to supplement or replace mechanical cleaning. The central difficulty has been to find a substance that is both effective and harmless to the tissue.

Chemical control may be achieved in a number of ways:

1. Suppression of the oral flora
2. Inhibition of bacterial colonization of the tooth surface
3. Inhibition of plaque-forming factors, e.g. binding carbohydrates such as dextran
4. Dissolution of established plaque
5. Prevention of mineralization of plaque.

These are discussed more fully in Chapter 15.

Mouthwashes

Mouthwashes have been used for a number of purposes: to clear the mouth of food debris; as carriers of antibacterial agents to prevent or reduce plaque accumulation; containing anti-caries fluorides; and to reduce the activity of odour-producing micro-organisms.

The simplest and most frequently used mouth rinse has been a dilute saline solution, and when warm this is especially useful in postoperative care. However, much more complicated formulations are now available to achieve the above objectives.

Mouthwashes are commonly mixtures of:

- An antibacterial agent; 0.2% chlorhexidine gluconate appears to be the most effective, but its powerful taste and tendency to stain teeth are disadvantages. Quaternary ammonium salts, e.g. cetylpyridinium chloride, are frequently used
- Alcohol to enhance antibacterial activity and taste, and to help keep flavouring agents in solution
- A humectant, e.g. sorbitol, to prevent drying-out
- A surfactant, to help keep ingredients in solution
- Flavourings, colouring agents and preservatives, and water as the vehicle.

There is evidence that the activity of the antibacterial agent is prolonged by absorption to the hydroxyapatite of tooth enamel (Jensen, 1978).

It is usually recommended that the mouthwash is used for about 30 seconds twice a day, before or after toothbrushing or independently of brushing. However, the evidence of many studies (Lobene *et al.*, 1979; Ashley *et al.*, 1984) supports the use of mouthwashes in conjunction with regular toothbrushing. Binney *et al.* (1993) tested five commercial mouthwashes as pre-brushing rinses, and found that they were of no greater use than water, nor did they enhance the efficiency of subsequent toothbrushing; however, the benefits of their use as adjuncts to normal hygiene procedures has been demonstrated in some studies.

Problems to be overcome

Satisfactory plaque control is not easy. If practitioners are to guide patients towards this goal, they must be aware of all the problems that the patients might encounter.

Manual dexterity

By training and experience dentists achieve a high level of manual skill, and it may be difficult for them to understand that many individuals are not so well endowed. Manual dexterity does not necessarily go with intellect, and some of the brightest patients prove to be extremely clumsy. The extent of the patient's difficulty can be recognized by witnessing the patient's performance, and efforts must be directed with patience and tact. It is necessary to find out which technique the patient can best perform. It is useless to insist on a technique that the patient finds difficult. The scrubbing technique is probably the easiest to perform, and if it is the only technique the patient can command, so be it, at least initially, but some effective form of interdental cleaning must also be taught. Given time and persistence, skills do come to most people, even the least dextrous. Positive encouragement is essential: criticism can be counterproductive.

Oral perception

Visual, oral and olfactory faculties vary from one person to another, and there is also considerable variation in tactile sensibility in the mouth. Just as some people are tone deaf or cannot smell the difference between curry and garlic, so some people can have a very dirty mouth without being aware of the condition, while others are sensitive to the presence of the smallest foreign body. However, sensibility can be developed, although in some people it can be a slow process. The tongue is the most powerful instrument of oral tactile sensation, and the patient can be instructed to run the tongue over the teeth before and after brushing and to recognize the glass-like feeling of clean teeth.

Tooth position

Malalignment is one of the most common causes of difficulty. Where teeth have been extracted and neighbouring teeth have tilted a triangular space forms, which can be difficult to clean. Areas of crowding can produce special problems, as any form of interdental cleaning, even with floss, may be difficult and even harmful. Areas of special difficulty should be defined and techniques devised for those areas.

The form of tooth contact

The contact point or area takes many forms depending on tooth shapes and relationships. The smaller the area of contact, the easier it is to clean. As attrition and interdental wear take place, the contact area increases in size. If the teeth are rectangular in shape, the contact area can be extremely wide. If the related embrasure space is filled by healthy gingiva, interdental cleaning may not be necessary; however, if inflammation is present interdental cleaning is essential, and floss or tape may be the only effective aid.

Restorative and prosthetic dentistry

As emphasized in the text, badly executed restorative dentistry is an extremely common cause of plaque retention. The overhanging margin of the interproximal restoration creates a zone of plaque retention that is totally inaccessible to the patient's best efforts, and if possible should be removed before subgingival scaling is undertaken. Badly designed contact areas, overcontoured crowns, subgingival crown margins, badly designed bridge pontics, especially the ridge-lap pontic, extracoronal precision attachments placed too close to the gingiva, etc., create problems of plaque control that can be extremely difficult to correct. It is in these latter cases that chemical cleaning can be beneficial in the short term.

It is obviously much more satisfactory to avoid creating these problems in the first place, and all restorative and prosthetic work must be undertaken with its effect on the periodontium in mind.

Diet

Few health topics exercise people's concern as much as their diet. More myths and more neuroses attend the subject of nutrition than most other topics, and its relation to dental health is no exception. 'How does diet affect my gums?' is a constant question, and a satisfactory answer should cover two aspects of this subject:

1. Nutritional deficiencies do not cause gum disease. However, if plaque-induced disease is already present, nutritional deficiency might affect its development; therefore a balanced diet is necessary.
2. Both the chemical composition and the physical character of food are important. Although some tooth surfaces can be cleaned by using hard and fibrous foods, it has been clearly demonstrated that such foods as apples, carrots, celery, etc. have no effect on plaque deposits in the sheltered gingival crevice, especially in the interdental regions. On the other hand, hard fibrous foods do not encourage the deposition of plaque and are therefore beneficial as substitutes for soft, sticky foods, which do encourage plaque deposition. The consumption of sugar in any form is to be discouraged, particularly between meals.

For the concerned person, a simple 5-day diet analysis can be extremely revealing. All food and drinks, including between-meals snacks, are recorded, and in going through the list with the patient all refined carbohydrate is underlined. Even a superficial analysis of this sort can shed light on the idiosyncrasies and limitations of the individual's diet, and seeing their total consumption in black and white can be a salutary experience. In dealing with young people, the co-operation of the parents is essential and even the help of teachers is useful.

Unfortunately there are pressures from all sides to promote the consumption of refined carbohydrate and sugar. The weight of convention and the pressure of advertising tend to limit the effectiveness of diet control advice, and basic changes should not be anticipated or aimed for in the short term. Control of between-meals snacks can be achieved and can effect significant benefits.

Such an exercise must be an uphill task, but in one regard dental personnel should be successful; that is in setting an example by their own performance and their own dental health.

Smoking

The prevalence and severity of chronic periodontitis and acute ulcerative necrotizing gingivitis is greater in current smokers when compared to patients who have never smoked and patients who have quit smoking (Haber and Kent, 1992; Bolin *et al.*, 1993; Haber *et al.*, 1993; Grossi *et al.*, 1994, 1995). This implies that quitting smoking may slow down or halt the progress of periodontal disease. Periodontists in the USA, UK and other countries are more likely to give advice regarding stopping smoking than either other specialists or general dentists (Telivuo *et al.*, 1992). They also found that 'healthy' smokers are more likely to visit their dentist than their physician. Thus, anti-smoking advice from the dentist may be beneficial to the smoking patient from a number of different health aspects.

Another concern is that 90% of regular smokers start smoking before the age of 18 years (MacKenzie *et al.*, 1994). Dentists can give advice to this young population on all aspects of its effects, including those on periodontal disease.

One recent study (MacGregor, 1996) has shown that dental hospital periodontal patients given advice regarding the dangers of smoking were much more likely to cease smoking or reduce the number of cigarettes smoked than patients who had expressed a wish to reduce tobacco consumption but were given periodontal treatment without this advice. After being told that smoking was a major risk factor in periodontal disease and a factor likely to prevent a good response to treatment, subjects were asked to set a target for their daily cigarette consumption, and this was recorded. They also kept a record of their actual consumption. They were followed up for periods ranging from 3 months to 1 year. In the group given the anti-smoking advice, 65% had reduced their smoking up to 50% and 13% had quit smoking. In the control group not given the advice, the proportions were 30% and 5% respectively. All the subjects in both groups had expressed a desire to stop smoking, and of all of the patients interviewed for participation in the study only 8% did not want to stop or cut down their smoking. Thus it seems good practice routinely to provide dental patients with anti-smoking advice.

Anti-smoking advice should cover all the well-known medical risks from tobacco products as well as the strong link between smoking and periodontal disease. It should also inform patients of the various available aids to quitting smoking, and outline a reasonable regimen to undertake. Such a regimen of quitting smoking should only be suggested to patients who have expressed a desire to do so.

Patient motivation

In motivating a patient to good home care, one has to bring about change – change in knowledge and understanding, change in attitude and, thus, change in habit.

In the provision of any form of treatment some explanation of the patient's problem is essential, and this is especially the case in the control of periodontal disease, where the patient must take on the responsibility for his or her own well-being. In this respect the periodontal patient is similar to the diabetic patient – both must look after themselves if the disease is to be controlled, and that control is likely to be effective if the patient has a clear understanding of the rationale behind the discipline.

In providing an explanation of the patient's problem, as already stated certain rules must be followed:

1. Do not take any prior knowledge for granted; assume that the patient knows very little about dental matters and that what information he or she may have garnered is likely to be a compound of gossip, old wives' tales and pseudo-science. For example, few patients realize that teeth are held in bone and that the gum is simply a cover for the bone; many people believe that plaque is degraded food.
2. Give information in simple everyday language and avoid jargon. To say 'You have a plaque-induced gingival infection exacerbated by iatrogenic retention factors' will be meaningless to most patients. Thus, use the word 'bacteria' not 'micro-organism', 'gum' instead of 'gingiva', 'stick' instead of 'adhere', 'swollen' rather than 'hyperplastic', etc.
3. Do not give too much information at one time, and repeat everything that you have said. When the light dawns, it may dawn very slowly.

Change in attitude to dental health

Periodontal health is important; teeth are worth keeping for life. The patients must believe this; otherwise any change in habit as an immediate response to the dentist's admonitions will be short-lived.

Several arguments may be employed, and the experienced practitioner can tailor these to the patient's perceived needs. Adolescents and adults may respond to different arguments:

1. *Impaired function.* No appliance can function as efficiently as the natural and healthy dentition, and full dentures may be an extremely poor substitute for

the patient's own teeth.

2. *Personal hygiene*. These days most people are concerned about personal cleanliness, and yet there may be a marked contrast between patients' general appearance and the state of their mouth. This usually represents a lack of awareness of oral hygiene and when the true state of affairs is demonstrated, individuals who are truly concerned about personal hygiene will be ready to change their habits. Patients should be given a hand-mirror to witness the examination of the mouth, and deposits of plaque and calculus can be pointed out. The use of a disclosing agent is valuable.

3. *Social handicap*. Periodontal disease produces halitosis; dirty teeth and inflamed gums are unsightly. The idea of possessing offensive breath or an ugly smile is often sufficient incentive for patients to improve their home care. Today's television and screen heroes and heroines usually provide a good example to be cited if the dentist feels this is appropriate.

4. *General health*. Although there is little evidence that gingival disease can have an adverse effect on general health, it is possible that, where other pathology exists – e.g. gastric ulcer – oral sepsis can aggravate the condition. A healthy mouth in a healthy body could be a good maxim.

As stated earlier, the dentist and dental staff should set an example and be seen to practise what they preach.

Preventive programmes

Prevention in children

Studies by Axelsson and Lindhe (1974) and Axelsson *et al*. (1976) have shown the effect of regular plaque control on periodontal disease in children. Their programmes included fortnightly attendance for dental health education and instruction in oral hygiene (IOH). The test participants were given information and IOH. At each of the fortnightly visits these children received mechanical tooth cleaning, including approximal plaque removal using dental floss and special polishing tips, combined with topical application of monofluorophosphate. Control group children brushed their teeth at school under supervision each month using 0.2% sodium fluoride solution, but received no instruction or professional prophylaxis. During the first 2 years of the studies, the test regimen resulted in reduction of disease to almost negligible levels with regard to plaque, gingivitis and caries, whereas the control group showed continuing or more severe levels of disease during this period. Similar results have been reported by Hamp *et al*. (1978).

The preventive programmes reported by other workers, e.g. Ashley and Sainsbury (1981), have achieved less success in comparison with the above studies, perhaps because the Scandinavian group were more highly motivated and disciplined.

Prevention in adults

Several studies have investigated the effectiveness of plaque control regimens on adult subjects. Lovdal *et al*. (1961) carried out a 5-year study on 1428 subjects who received IOH and scaling every 6 months. They found that plaque levels were reduced most in those subjects with initially good oral hygiene. Subjects with poor oral hygiene initially demonstrated minor reductions in deposits. Lightner *et al*. (1971) investigated the influence of the frequency of IOH on the response of the patient. The study lasted 46 months and involved 470 subjects. They found that the subjects who received IOH showed decreased plaque and inflammation. They also showed the least loss of attachment.

A 3-year study by Suomi *et al*. (1973) involved 326 subjects divided into a group who received scaling and IOH at 2–4 monthly intervals, and a control group who received no treatment. At the end of the study the oral hygiene score was more than four times greater in the control group than for the experimental subjects. Gingival inflammation scores were greater in the control group; there was also $3\frac{1}{2}$ times greater loss of epithelial attachment and greater loss (by 0.18 mm) of alveolar bone.

These studies have been reinforced by the work of Axelsson and Lindhe (1978, 1981). In a 3-year study, subsequently extended to 6 years, involving 375 test and 180 control subjects, the test group received scaling and IOH every 2–3 months. This stimulated individuals to adopt effective oral hygiene habits, with resulting resolution of inflammation, and prevented further clinical attachment loss (CAL) and caries. In contrast, the control patients showed plaque retention, gingivitis, CAL and caries.

In another Swedish study by Wennström *et al*. (1993) 225 patients aged 18–65 years were monitored over 12 years in a community clinic. Between 1978 and 1990 all patients received regular care, and it was found that there were fewer tooth sites with inflammation in 1990 (4%) than in 1978 (15%). The mean attachment loss over the 12 years was 0.5 mm, and radiographs showed only 0.2–0.4 mm alveolar loss. Over this period, patients of 30–53 years showed a definite improvement in periodontal health, while older patients demonstrated stability rather than improvement.

The variation in the degree of success achieved by these studies emphasizes the need to design preventive programmes based on established educational methods and planned for the special needs of the individual. Techniques that have attempted to motivate individuals by arousing fear of tooth loss to persuade them to participate in preventive procedures have met with limited success; it has been found that better results have been achieved by methods using persuasion and encouragement.

Self-assessment

As previously stated, awareness of the nature of the problem is central to any preventive programme, and methods of self-assessment can form a powerful tool to self-awareness. Most methods of self-assessment of oral hygiene improvement and motivation have been directed to plaque control, but in recent years checks on gingival colour and gingival bleeding have been used as methods of monitoring their gingival status and oral hygiene regimen (Glavind and Attstrom, 1979).

In a US study of about 500 14–15-year-olds with gingivitis, one group received instruction in oral hygiene techniques, and a second group received in addition instruction in the self-assessment of gingival bleeding. After 2 years both groups demonstrated very positive benefits with indications of additional benefit in the children assessing their gingival bleeding. A similar finding was demonstrated in a study of Finnish army conscripts (Kallio *et al.*, 1990).

References

Ainamo, J., Hormia, M., Kaunisaho, K. *et al.* (1991) Effect of manual versus powered toothbrushes. *Journal of Dental Research* **70**, 557

Ainamo, J., Xia, Q., Ainamo, A. and Kallio, P. (1997) Assessment of the effect of an oscillating/rotating electric toothbrush on oral health. A 12-month longitudinal study. *Journal of Clinical Periodontology* **24**, 28–33

Ashley, F.P. and Sainsbury, R.H. (1981) The effect of a school-based plaque control programme on caries and gingivitis. A 3-year study in 11 to 14-year-old girls. *British Dental Journal* **150**, 41–45

Ashley, F.P., Skinner, A., Jackson, P. *et al.* (1984) The effect of a 0.1% cetylpyridinium chloride mouthrinse on plaque and gingivitis in adult subjects. *British Dental Journal* **157**, 191–196

Axelsson, P. and Lindhe, J. (1974) The effect of a preventive programme on dental plaque, gingivitis and caries in schoolchildren. Results after 1 and 2 years. *Journal of Clinical Periodontology* **1**, 126–138

Axelsson, P. and Lindhe, J. (1978) The effect of controlled oral hygiene procedures on caries and periodontal disease in adults. *Journal of Clinical Periodontology* **5**, 133–151

Axelsson, P. and Lindhe, J. (1981) The significance of maintenance care in the treatment of periodontal disease. *Journal of Clinical Periodontology* **8**, 281–295

Axelsson, P. and Lindhe, J. (1986) The effect of controlled oral hygiene procedures on caries and periodontal diseases in adults. Results after 6 years. *Journal of Clinical Periodontology* **8**, 239–248

Axelsson, P., Lindhe, J. and Waseby, J. (1976) The effect of various plaque control measures on gingivitis and caries in schoolchildren. *Community Dentistry and Oral Epidemiology* **4**, 232–239

Binney, A., Addy, M. and Newcombe, R.G. (1993) The plaque removal effects of single rinsings and brushings. *Journal of Periodontology* **64**, 181–185

Bolin, A., Eklund, G., Frithiof, L. and Lavsted, S. (1993) The effects of changed smoking habits on marginal alveolar bone loss. *Swedish Dental Journal* **17**, 211–216

De La Rosa, M., Guerra, J.Z., Johnston, D.A. and Radike, A.W. (1979) Plaque regrowth and removal with daily toothbrushing. *Journal of Periodontology* **50**, 661–664

Frandsen, A. (ed.) (1972) *Oral Hygiene.* Report of a symposium held at Malmo, Sweden, May 1971. Copenhagen, Munksgaard

Glavind, L. and Attstrom, R. (1979) Periodontal self-examination, a motivational tool in periodontics. *Journal of Clinical Periodontology*, 238–251

Grossi, S.G., Zambon, J.J., Ho, A.W. *et al.* (1994) Assessment of risk for periodontal disease. I. Risk indicators for attachment loss. *Journal of Periodontology*, **65**, 260–267

Grossi, S.G., Genco, R.J., Machtei, E.E. *et al.* (1995) Assessment of risk for periodontal disease. I. Risk indicators for alveolar bone loss. *Journal of Periodontology* **66**, 23–29

Haber, J. and Kent, R.L. (1992) Cigarette smoking in periodontal practice. *Journal of Periodontology* **63**, 100–106

Haber, J., Wattles, J., Crowley, M. *et al.* (1993) Evidence for cigarette smoking as a major risk factor for periodontitis. *Journal of Periodontology* **64**, 16–23

Hamp, S.E., Lindhe, J. and Fornell, J. (1978) Effect of a field program based on systematic plaque control on caries and gingivitis in schoolchildren after 3 years. *Community Dentistry and Oral Epidemiology* **6**, 17–23

Jensen, J.E. (1978) Binding of dyes to hydroxyapatite treated with cetylpyridinium chloride or cetrimonium bromide. *Scandinavian Journal of Dental Research* **86**, 87–92

Kallio, P., Ainamo, J. and Dusadeepan, A. (1990) Self-assessment of gingival bleeding. *International Dental Journal* **40**, 231–236

Killoy, W.J., Love, J.W., Love, J. *et al.* (1989) Effectiveness of a counter-rotary action powered toothbrush and a conventional toothbrush on plaque removal and gingival bleeding. *Journal of Periodontology* **60**, 473–477

Ko, C.C., Douglas, W.H., Versluis, A. *et al.* (1995) The relationship between brush stiffness and brushing forces. *Journal of Dental Research* **74** Abstr. 1872, 245

Lightner, L.M., O'Leary, T.J., Drake, R.B. *et al.* (1971) Preventive periodontic treatment procedures: results after 46 months. *Journal of Periodontology* **42**, 555–561

Lobene, R.R., Kashket, S., Spoarkar, P.M. *et al.* (1979) The effect of cetylpyridinium chloride on human plaque bacteria and gingivitis. *Pharmacology and Therapeutics in Dentistry* **4**, 33–47

Lovdal, A., Arno, A., Schei, O. and Waerhaug, J. (1961) Combined effect of subgingival scaling and controlled oral hygiene on the incidence of gingivitis. *Acta Odontologica Scandinavica* **19**, 537–555

MacGregor, I.D.M. (1996) Efficiency of dental health advice as an aid to reducing cigarette smoking. *British Dental Journal* **180**, 292–296

MacKenzie, T.D., Bartecchi, C.E. and Schrier, R.W. (1994) The human costs of tobacco use. *New England Journal of Medicine* **331**, 975–980

Murray, P.A., Boyde, R.L. and Robertson, P.B. (1989) Effect on periodontal status of rotary electric toothbrush versus manual toothbrushes during periodontal maintenance. II. Microbiological results. *Journal of Periodontology* **60**, 396–401

Niemi, M.-L. (1987) Gingival abrasion and plaque removal after brushing with an electric and a manual toothbrush. *Acta Odontologica Scandinavica* **45**, 367–370

Niemi, M.-L., Ainamo, J. and Etemadzadeh, H. (1986) Gingival abrasion and plaque removal with manual brushing versus electric toothbrushing. *Journal of Clinical Periodontology* **13**, 709–713

Pretara-Spanedda, P., Grossman, E., Curro, F.A. and Generallo, C. (1989) Toothbrush bristle density: relationship to plaque removal. *American Journal of Dentistry* **2**, 345–348

Rustogi, K.N., Volpe, A.R., Fishman, S. *et al.* (1984) Removal of 48-hour plaque by either brushing with dentifrices or water. *Journal of Dental Research* **63** Abstr. 1273, 312

Sims, W. (1968) Preventive dentistry for the dental practitioner. *Dental Practitioner* **18**, 309–314

Stoltz, K. and Bay, L. (1994) Comparison of a manual and a new electric toothbrush for controlling plaque and gingivitis. *Journal of Clinical*

Periodontology **21**, 86–90

Suomi, J.D., Smith, L.W., Chang, J.J. and Barbano, J.P. (1973) Study on the effect of different prophylaxis frequencies on the periodontium of young adults. *Journal of Periodontology* **44**, 406–410

Telivuo, M., Murtomaa, H. and Lahtinen, A. (1992) Observations and concepts of the oral health consequences of tobacco use of Finnish periodontists and dentists. *Journal of Clinical Periodontology* **19**, 15–18

Van der Weijden, G.A., Danser, M.M., Nijboer, A. *et al.* (1991) The plaque removing efficiency of a resiproque rotating toothbrush. *Journal of Dental Research* **70**, 557

Van der Weijden, G.A., Danser, M.M., Nijboer, A. *et al.* (1993) The plaque removing efficiency of an oscillating/rotating toothbrush. A short-term study. *Journal of Clinical Periodontology* **20**, 273–278

Van der Weijden, G.A., Timmerman, M.F., Reijerse, E. *et al.* (1994) The long-term effect of of an oscillating/rotating toothbrush on gingivitis: an 8-month study. *Journal of Clinical Periodontology* **21**, 139–145

Walsh, M., Heckman, B., Leggott, P. *et al.* (1989) Comparison of a manual and powered toothbrushing with and without adjunctive oral irrigation for controlling plaque and gingivitis. *Journal of Clinical Periodontology* **16**, 419–427

Wennström, J.L., Serino, G., Lindhe, J. *et al.* (1993) Periodontal conditions of adult regular care attendants. A 12-year longitudinal study. *Journal of Clinical Periodontology* **20**, 714–722

11

Clinical features of chronic periodontal disease

Chronic gingivitis

The manifestations of gingival inflammation vary considerably between individuals and from one part of the mouth to another. This variation reflects the aetiological factors at work and the tissue response to these factors. The response is essentially a mixture of inflammation and fibrous tissue repair. When the former predominates, signs and symptoms are more obvious; when the fibrous tissue component predominates, clinical manifestations can be much more subtle and recognized only by careful examination.

In making a diagnosis it is important to keep in mind the appearance of health, departures from which may indicate disease. Clinical features are:

1. Altered gingival appearance
2. Gingival bleeding
3. Discomfort and pain
4. Unpleasant taste
5. Halitosis.

Figure 11.1 Signs of a relatively early chronic gingivitis. Gingival papillae and margins are swollen and red and bleed on probing

Altered gingival appearance

Changes in appearance are usually described according to colour, shape, size, consistency and surface characteristics.

Healthy gingivae are pale pink and the margin is knife-edged and scalloped; a streamlined papilla is often grooved by a sluice-way and the attached gingiva is stippled.

Because the interdental embrasure is the site of greatest plaque stagnation, gingival inflammation usually starts in the interdental papilla and spreads around the margin. As the blood vessels dilate, the tissue becomes red and swollen with inflammatory exudate. The knife-edged margin becomes rounded, the interdental sluice-way is lost and the surface of the gingiva becomes smooth and glossy (*Figure 11.1*). As the gingival fibre bundles are broken up by the inflammatory process, the gingival cuff loses tone and comes away from the tooth surface so that a shallow pocket is formed. If the inflammation becomes more diffuse and spreads into the attached gingiva, the stippling disappears. If inflammation is severe it can spread across the attached gingiva to the alveolar mucosa and so obliterate the normally well-defined mucogingival junction.

Usually the most pronounced inflammatory swelling is seen in adolescents and young adults, so that 'false pocketing' is formed. It is called 'false' as opposed to 'real' or periodontal pocketing, which is formed by apical migration of the crevicular epithelium as the periodontal ligament is destroyed by inflammation. Where several aetiological factors combine, e.g. plaque deposition plus lack of lip-seal plus the endocrinal changes of puberty, gingival swelling, especially papillary swelling, can be pronounced.

If plaque irritation is longstanding and low grade, the main tissue reaction will be fibrous tissue production so that the gingiva may remain firm and pink but become thickened and lose its streamlined shape.

Gingival bleeding

Gingival bleeding is probably the most frequent patient complaint. Unfortunately, gingival bleeding is so common that people may not take it seriously and even believe it to be normal; however, unless bleeding obviously follows an episode of acute trauma, bleeding is always a sign of pathology. It occurs most frequently on toothbrushing. Bleeding may be provoked by eating hard food such as apples, toast, etc., as well as by probing the gingival crevice or pocket on periodontal examination. 'Bleeding on probing' has been used as a sign of disease activity but, as stated earlier, this is an unreliable indicator of disease activity and may be the result of injudicious examination. When gingivae are extremely soft and spongy, bleeding can occur spontaneously.

Blood may be tasted by the patient and may be smelt on the patient's breath.

If the tissue response is fibrous overgrowth, there is no bleeding even with vigorous toothbrushing.

Discomfort and pain

These are uncommon features of chronic gingivitis, and this is probably the main reason for the disease being overlooked. The gingivae may feel sore when the patient brushes the teeth, and because of this he or she brushes more lightly and less frequently, so that plaque accumulates and the condition is perpetuated.

This relative absence of pain is one of the symptoms that differentiates a chronic gingivitis from an acute ulcerative gingivitis.

Unpleasant taste

Patients may notice the taste of blood, particularly if they suck at an interdental space. However, the senses are quickly blunted and a disagreeable taste is a relatively infrequent complaint.

Halitosis

'Bad breath' frequently accompanies gingival disease, and is a common cause of a visit to the dentist. The smell derives from blood and poor oral hygiene, and must be distinguished from smells from different sources.

Halitosis has a number of causes, both intra- and extra-oral. Oral disease and residual food deposits, especially those of a volatile nature such as peppermint, garlic, curry, etc., represent the most common cause of halitosis. Pathology of the respiratory tract, nose, sinuses, tonsils and lungs can cause an embarrassing smell, as can diseases of the digestive tract. Some items of diet, e.g. garlic, are absorbed by the intestines, taken into the intestinal bloodstream and finally exhaled by the lungs, so they can be smelt a long time after they have been eaten. Mouth odour is common on waking and between meals, when it is associated with food stagnation and reduced salivary flow. Metabolic diseases, diabetes and uraemia give characteristic smells to the breath. Halitosis can increase with age.

Chronic periodontitis

The clinical features of chronic periodontitis are:

1. Gingival inflammation and bleeding
2. Pocketing
3. Gingival recession
4. Tooth mobility
5. Tooth migration
6. Discomfort
7. Alveolar bone loss
8. Halitosis and offensive taste.

Of these, only pocketing and alveolar bone loss are essential features of chronic periodontitis.

Gingival inflammation and bleeding

Although gingival inflammation is a necessary precursor to periodontitis, obvious manifestations of inflammation become less apparent with the progress of periodontitis. Frequently, the gingivae are pink and firm, the contours may be almost normal, there may be no bleeding on careful probing and the patient may not complain of bleeding on brushing. It is as though, with the development of the pocket, the disease has gone underground.

The presence and severity of gingival inflammation depend upon oral hygiene status; where this is poor, gingival inflammation is evident and bleeding or brushing, or even spontaneous bleeding, is noticed by the patient. When the patient's toothbrushing is good enough to control plaque but where subgingival deposits, because of inadequate scaling, persist, the presence of periodontal disease may not be apparent on superficial examination. If a careful history is taken, many such patients report a history of past bleeding that stopped when their toothbrushing technique improved. Periodontal destruction in the average adult is the product of past neglect, not the result of present oral hygiene habits.

Pocketing

Pocket measurement is an essential part of periodontal diagnosis, but must be interpreted together with gingival inflammation and swelling, and radiographic evidence of alveolar bone loss. Theoretically, if there is no gingival swelling, a pocket over 2 mm deep indicates some apical migration of crevicular epithelium. However, inflammatory swelling is so common, especially in the younger individual, that pocketing of 3–4 mm may be entirely gingival, or 'false'. Pocketing of 4 mm is likely to indicate an early chronic periodontitis (*Figure 11.2*).

The precise measurement of pockets is difficult because:

1. Probing the pocket can be uncomfortable and even painful if there is frank inflammation.
2. Pocket depth is extremely variable around a tooth. Interproximal pocketing is usually deepest because that is the site of greatest plaque accumulation, while pocketing on the facial aspect of the tooth is usually most shallow as this is where the toothbrush makes the greatest impact and may even produce gingival recession. This means that six measurements may be required on each tooth to give an accurate picture.
3. Where present oral hygiene is good, the gingival cuff may be so tight around the neck of the tooth as to resist the insertion of an ordinary periodontal probe without causing pain. The measurement of pockets in anaesthetized tissue often produces quite different results from previous measurement made in sentient tissue.
4. Tooth contour and angulation, subgingival calculus or restorations, as well as carious cavities, may impede the insertion of the probe. The deepest aspect of interproximal pockets usually lie below the contact area. Therefore the probe has to be inclined inwards to reach this point in molar or premolar teeth. Compensation should be made for the effect of this angulation on the probing depth measured, and it is usual to subtract 1 mm from the measurement value in these circumstances.

Figure 11.2 Pocket-measuring probe inserted into pocket as parallel to the axis of the tooth as possible

Other factors that affect the accuracy of the measurement of probing depth are discussed in Chapter 12.

There are many designs of pocket-measuring probe, some of which are too thick to provide accurate measurement and some of which are sharp so that the tissue is penetrated unless great care is taken. The special CPITN probe has been described in Chapter 9. There are also probes that can control the pressure of probing, and these are described in Chapter 12.

It has been shown that pockets of over 3 mm are measured with diminishing reliability, and it is unfortunate that much periodontal research is based upon such an unreliable criterion.

Sometimes a purulent discharge can be expressed from the pocket by pressure on the pocket wall.

Gingival recession

Gingival recession and root exposure may accompany chronic periodontitis, but are not necessarily a feature of the disease. Where recession occurs, pocket depth measurement is only a partial representation of the total amount of periodontal destruction. The other causes of gingival recession are discussed in Chapter 8.

Tooth mobility

Some tooth mobility in a labiolingual plane can be elicited in healthy single-rooted teeth, especially lower incisors, these being more mobile than multirooted teeth. Increasing tooth mobility is produced by:

* Increased width of periodontal ligament with no loss of alveolar bone or other supporting tissue
* Increased width of periodontal ligament plus loss of alveolar bone or other supporting tissue
* Loss of alveolar bone or other supporting tissue without an increased width of periodontal ligament.

These tissue changes may be produced by:

1. Spread of inflammation from the gingiva into the deeper tissues
2. Loss of supporting tissue
3. Occlusal trauma.

Mobility also increases after periodontal surgery and in pregnancy. In periodontal pathology, tissue destruction is always accompanied by inflammation and frequently by occlusal trauma. Mobility that is produced by inflammation and occlusal trauma is reversible, as demonstrated by the reduction in mobility following scaling and occlusal adjustment; mobility associated with destruction of supporting tissue is not reversible.

Assessment of mobility for research purposes can be made using special apparatus, but clinical assessment is usually subjective. It is elicited by exerting pressure on one side of the tooth under examination with an instrument or fingertip, while placing a finger of the other hand on the other side of the tooth and its neighbour, which is used as a fixed point so that relative movement can be discerned. Another way of eliciting mobility (although not assessing it) is to place fingers over the facial surfaces of the teeth while the patient grinds the teeth.

The degree of mobility may be graded as follows:

Grade 1   Just discernible, 0.2–1 mm in a horizontal direction

Grade 2   Easily discernible, and over 1 mm labiolingual displacement

Grade 3   Well-marked labiolingual displacement, mobility of the tooth up and down in an axial direction.

There is an element of subjectivity in this grading. No doubt sufficient determination can elicit mobility in perfectly secure teeth!

More refined methods of mobility assessment have been devised. Muhlemann (1954) invented the periodontometer, which measured tooth displacement when a small force was applied to the tooth. More recently, Schulte *et al.* (1992) have produced the Periotest, which is a refinement of the Muhlemann device. Essentially the Periotest is a horizontal rod, which taps the tooth at a known velocity; on impact the tooth is deflected, the rod decelerated and the contact time recorded. This ranges between 0.3–2.0 milliseconds, being shorter for stable than for mobile teeth.

Tooth migration

Movement of a tooth (or teeth) out of the original position in the arch is a common feature of periodontal disease, and one that alerts the patient to the problem. Tooth position in health is maintained by a balance of tongue, lip and occlusal forces. Once supporting tissue is lost, these forces determine the pattern of tooth migration. The incisors move most frequently in a labial direction, but teeth may move in any direction or become extruded (*Figure 11.3*). Once a tooth migrates the force on that tooth changes, and this may promote further stress and further migration. If an upper incisor migrates labially, the lower lip may come to lie lingual to the incisal edge of the tooth and produce further migration.

Discomfort

One of the most important features of chronic periodontitis is the almost total absence of discomfort or pain, unless acute inflammation supervenes. This is one of the main distinctions between periodontal and pulp disease. Discomfort or pain on percussion of the tooth indicates some active inflammation of the supporting tissues, which is at its most acute in abscess formation, when the tooth becomes exquisitely sensitive to touch. Sensitivity to hot and cold is sometimes present when there is gingival

Figure 11.3 Drifting of the upper incisors, which alerted the patient to the presence of disease

recession and root exposure. Indeed one common clinical experience is the appearance of sensitivity, especially to cold, when roots once covered in calculus are cleaned. On occasion pulp pathology may be a complication of advanced periodontal disease, and severe pain may then develop.

Alveolar bone loss

Resorption of alveolar bone and the associated destruction of periodontal ligament is the most important feature of chronic periodontitis, and the one that leads to tooth loss. There is considerable variation in both the form and rate of alveolar bone resorption, and in constructing a treatment plan the amount of bone loss, the rate at which resorption is progressing and the pattern of bone loss need to be accurately established. Radiographic examination is an essential part of periodontal diagnosis and, with certain limitations, provides evidence of the alveolar bone height, the form of bone destruction, the width of the periodontal ligament space and the density of cancellous trabeculation. Serial radiographs taken over a period of time can provide information about the rate of bone loss. However, radiographic examination without careful clinical examination can be very misleading. A periodontal diagnosis cannot be made from radiographs alone, as there is no way of distinguishing past bone destruction from current bone resorption on the radiograph.

Because the images of the facial and lingual plates of bone are largely obscured by the dense image of the tooth, diagnosis depends upon obtaining a clear image of the interdental bone. Careful angulation of the X-ray beam and a standardized routine of exposure and of processing the radiographic film is essential.

The first radiographic sign of periodontal destruction

is loss of density of the alveolar margin. This is most clearly seen between posterior teeth where in health the broad interdental septum projects a dense and well-defined image of the alveolar margin (*Figure 11.4*). The image of the narrow interdental septa between anterior teeth is less well-defined in health, and early pathological changes are less easy to see. With continuing bone resorption, the height of the alveolar bone is further reduced (*Figure 11.5*). Even correctly angulated, the radiographs may not disclose the true state of interdental resorption, e.g. an interdental crater between molars can be masked by the images of the facial and lingual walls of the defect.

Bone defects that lie over the facial or lingual aspects of the teeth, e.g. marginal gutters, may be completely obscured and are revealed only when flaps are raised at surgery. Moreover, distinguishing between facial and lingual defects may not be possible from radiographic evidence alone.

Two radiographs taken at slightly different angles often reveal defects undetected by one. This is especially true in the diagnosis of furcation defects. These are usually revealed by radiographic examination, but the exact form of the defect may not be discernible. The thick palatal root of an upper molar may mask a trifurcation defect. Widening of the periodontal space in the furcation provides evidence of an early lesion. Widening of the periodontal ligament space on one side or all around a tooth frequently indicates excessive occlusal stress. This is sometimes accompanied by widening or funnelling of the coronal aspect of the socket.

All departures from the normal radiographic appearance must be checked against other clinical features, in particular pocket depth and mobility patterns, and if these do not correspond, re-examination should be carried out. Clinical and radiographic features taken together should make a reasonable fit that sheds light on both the pathological condition and its aetiology. Thus, where radiographic examination of a mobile tooth reveals that the supporting bone is virtually intact, careful examination of the occlusion is essential. There must always be an identifiable reason for any pathological change.

The factors that affect the accuracy of radiographic detection of alveolar bone loss are discussed in Chapter 12.

Figure 11.4 Signs of early marginal bone loss shown on a bitewing radiograph. Most bone loss is around the upper molars, but note hollowing of septum at 6̄5̄|. The bite wing film is very useful for revealing early bone loss in posterior segments

Halitosis and offensive taste

The metabolism of many of the oral bacteria (in particular the Gram negative anaerobic bacteria in saliva, the gingival crevice and plaque), when acting on substrates in the mouth, e.g. food debris and plaque, can produce sulphur-bearing compounds such as hydrogen sulphide and methylmercaptan; these can impart an offensive smell to the mouth and exhaled breath.

An offensive taste and smell frequently accompany periodontal disease, especially when oral hygiene is poor. Acute inflammation with the production of pus, which exudes from pockets on pressure, also causes halitosis. A source of constant surprise is the lack of awareness of many affected individuals and their partners of the powerful fetor which, like a malignant wind, escapes from their mouths when they speak. Lack of sensibility and unconcern about dental health seem to go hand in hand, and as patient co-operation is essential to the success of periodontal treatment, this sensibility – or lack of it – can provide a clue to prognosis.

Figure 11.5 Fairly advanced bone loss in a 46-year-old woman. Note irregularity of bone margin with vertical defects distal to 7̄|and 5̄|

References

Muhlemann, H.R. (1954) Tooth mobility. The measuring method. Initial and secondary tooth mobility. *Journal of Periodontology* **25**, 22–29

Schulte, W., Hoedt, B., Lukas, D. *et al.* (1992) Periotest for measuring periodontal characteristics – correlation with periodontal bone loss. *Journal of Periodontal Research* **27**, 184–190

Further reading

Eley, B.M. and Cox, S.W. (1998) Advances in periodontal diagnosis. Part 1 Traditional clinical methods of diagnosis. *British Dental Journal* **184**, 4, 12–16

12

Diagnosis, prognosis and treatment plan

Making a diagnosis

The diagnosis should not be limited to giving a name to the condition. If periodontal disease is to be treated and its recurrence prevented, a diagnosis should include the identification of all aetiological factors, that is:

1. Those factors that predispose to plaque deposition and retention
2. Those factors, local or systemic, which influence adversely the behaviour of the tissues.

It should go without saying that you cannot remove or control factors that have not been identified, yet all too frequently treatment is reduced to the control of signs and symptoms and, inevitably, disease recurs.

At the time of the initial examination some attempt should be made to assess the patient's attitude to dental health. Patient co-operation is essential to the success of periodontal treatment, and it is this fact that makes the treatment of periodontal disease different from that of caries and other dental diseases, when the patient can take a more passive attitude.

Patient examination

The examination should be methodical and comprehensive, and should follow the standard pattern of the classic case history.

Present complaint and its history

A patient with periodontal disease may have no complaint at all and be oblivious to the presence of any disease in the mouth; indeed, the patient may be suspicious of any suggestion that disease is present! The most common complaints are bleeding gums, loose teeth, drifting of the teeth (usually the upper incisors), nasty taste, halitosis, swelling of the gums, discomfort and, occasionally, acute pain.

Few patients at the initial consultation provide concise and completely relevant information. All too often the necessary information has to be elicited by abstraction from a long and sometimes rambling account, which must be listened to with patience and close attention. In addition, pertinent questions should be asked:

- Are you in pain?
- Where is the pain?
- Is it a throbbing or a dull pain?
- Does the pain keep you awake?
- What brings on the pain – hot, cold, sweet, biting?
- Have you had pain in the past, or is this the first time?
- What treatment have you received for pain?
- Do your gums ever bleed
  When you brush your teeth?
  When you eat hard food?
- Did your gums bleed in the past?
- If so, what treatment did you receive?
- Do any of your teeth feel loose?
- Have you always had that space between your front teeth?
- Have you had any swelling in your mouth? Where, when, etc.?

Dental history

- Do you go to the dentist regularly?
- What was the last treatment you received?
- When did you last have a scaling, i.e. cleaning by your dentist?
- Do you have any dentures (false teeth that you can take out) – if so, how long have you had them?
- Have you any false teeth that are fixed in – if so, how long have you had them?

At this stage, questioning about home care can be a waste of time. Answers to such questions as 'How often do you clean your teeth?' are often suspect, as patients are likely to say what they imagine they are supposed to say – i.e. twice a day, night and morning. Even if this happens to be the truth, it gives no indication of the quality of the performance; only an examination of the mouth provides information about that.

At this time, some idea about habits should be gleaned, e.g. smoking, clenching, night-grinding, biting pencils and so on.

Medical history

Although a medical history may not seem relevant to some patients, it is essential to obtain one for a number of reasons:

1. The patient may be suffering from some condition, e.g. cardiovascular disease, renal disease, etc., which will require special precautions and/or modification of the treatment, and will necessitate communication with the patient's physician.
2. Systemic conditions, e.g. pregnancy, diabetes, will alter the way in which the periodontal tissues behave, and may demand medical attention before periodontal treatment can be carried out.
3. The mouth may be the site of some manifestation of a systemic condition, e.g. anaemia, which could affect any periodontal treatment.
4. The patient may be receiving medication, e.g. tricyclic antidepressants for depression, which may conflict with medication involved in the periodontal treatment, e.g. general anaesthetics.

A medical history should record any present illness and medication, any past serious illness and medication (e.g. steroids taken in the recent past), allergies (especially any history of penicillin sensitivity) and abnormal bleeding tendencies (in particular, excessive bleeding after injury or tooth extraction).

The use of a questionnaire may be helpful.

Where some systemic problem exists, communication with the patient's physician is essential.

Patient appraisal

While taking the history a general appraisal of the patient should be made, and such features as obesity, general posture, pallor, skin rash, heavy breathing and lip posture should be noted.

Oral examination

The examination of the mouth should be carried out in a methodical and thorough manner; this is the dentist's special area. Halitosis is noted as the mouth is opened, or even earlier, when the patient is giving a history. The following areas should be systematically examined.

The oral mucosa

Cheeks, lips, tongue, palate, floor of mouth and vestibules are examined for ulceration, vesicles, swelling, eroded patches, abnormal colour and white lines or patches. Tooth indentations in the margin of the tongue and interdental keratosis, i.e. a white line in the cheek at the level of the occlusion, often indicates a clenching or grinding habit.

Aphthous ulcers frequently occur in the labial or lingual vestibule or inside the lips. Lichen planus may be seen as fine, interlacing white lines on the cheeks or alveolar mucosa. Vesicles or eroded patches should be fully investigated.

A sinus on the alveolar mucosa, with or without the discharge of pus on pressure, indicates the presence of an alveolar abscess.

In the older individual, a squamous cell carcinoma may appear as a painless swelling, ulcer or eroded white patch in any part of the oral mucosa, but especially in the vestibules. Oral lesions of primary, secondary or tertiary syphilis may appear on the lips, tongue, palate and even the gingivae; widespread candida lesions in a young male could be indicative of HIV infection.

Any departure from the norm must be examined carefully and, if infection or malignant disease is suspected, an examination of the submandibular and cervical lymph nodes will help with a diagnosis. Immediate referral to the physician or appropriate specialist is essential.

Removable appliances

If these are present, they should be examined for their fit, design and relationship to any inflammation of the oral mucosa and gingiva.

Oral hygiene

Note presence and position of plaque, supragingival and subgingival calculus. Subgingival calculus can be detected with a probe such as a WHO probe or a Cross calculus probe, but may also be seen as a dark blue shadow in the gingival margin. The use of a disclosing agent will help to identify plaque and demonstrate its presence to the patient. Sometimes the location of plaque and calculus points to a predisposing factor, e.g. better oral hygiene on the left side is usually associated with right-handed toothbrushing; interproximal deposits and gingival inflammation may be caused by the overhanging margins of restorations or poor contact relations.

Teeth

Teeth are charted, and cavities, restorations and malalignments recorded. Attrition may indicate a grinding habit; abrasion, a vigorous and damaging toothbrushing technique.

Gingivae

The gingivae are examined for colour, shape, size and consistency, keeping in mind the picture of health – pink, knife-edged, streamlined and firm. Any departure from this could indicate pathology.

Periodontium

The various signs of attachment loss should be looked for, measured and recorded.

Periodontal charting should be carried out, and should include probing depth and gingival recession measurements on each tooth. In addition, furcation involvement and tooth mobility should be recorded when and where present. Probing depth and recession measurements should be usually made at six points around each tooth. Ideally, true mesial, distal, facial and lingual measurements are required, but this is possible only where teeth are missing so that unimpeded access to these surfaces is possible. Where proximal teeth are present, measurement is made at the line angles, and on facial and lingual surfaces. Taking six readings on each tooth is ideal, but may be very time-consuming. If diagnosis is made at a reasonably early stage in periodontal breakdown, four measurements may be sufficient, made at the mesiobuccal, mesiolingual, distobuccal and distolingual line angles. Where there appears to be furcation involvement of molars, or drifting of incisors, facial and lingual measurements on these teeth are essential.

A pocket-measuring probe must be fine enough to enter a narrow pocket, but must have a blunt end so that the tissue is not perforated. The sharp-ended probe used for the detection of caries should not be used. The pocket-measuring probe should be inserted into the pocket as near parallel to the axis of the tooth as possible (*Figure 12.1*). However, if adjacent teeth are present, parallel placement of the probe at interdental sites will not allow the area under the contact point to be reached, and this is the site where the pocket is deepest.

Parallel placement will therefore result in a significant underestimation of interproximal pockets. For this reason, it is necessary to slightly angulate the probe beneath the contact area on molar and premolar teeth to reach the

Figure 12.1 A periodontal probe inserted into the mesiobuccal pocket of the lower right first molar. It has been slightly angled lingually to pass under the contact area to reach the deepest part of the pocket. It is measuring a deep pocket, which would have been missed if the probe had been placed parallel to the tooth surface at the mesiobuccal line angle

base of the deepest interdental pockets (*Figure 12.1*); the effect of the angulation should be compensated for when recording the measurement. Great care has to be taken to manipulate the probe so that the true depth of the pocket is recorded. Delicate handling of the probe must be employed to negotiate subgingival deposits without impaction against the root surface. Vigorous probing is not only painful, but is likely to give an inaccurate reading; even gentle probing of inflamed gingivae can be painful. The problems of pocket measurement can be demonstrated by the fact that pocket measurements following local anaesthesia usually give greater readings than when taken in unanaesthetized tissue.

If a lot of supragingival calculus is present at the first visit, periodontal charting should be postponed until supragingival scaling has been carried out.

If infrabony pocketing is suspected in more advanced cases, this will usually not be detected by either probing or radiography alone. However, in this situation there is usually lack of agreement between the probing depth measurement and the apparent bone level on the radiograph, and further information may be gained by placing gutta-percha or silver points, which may be calibrated, to the base of the pocket in question during radiographic examination. This will then show the relationship of the pocket to the bone.

In addition to recording pocket depth, it is also important to record gingival recession at all sites where it is present so that the total amount of measured attachment loss can be meaningfully compared with bone levels on radiographs.

It is also important to try to assess the true probing attachment level, i.e. probing depths measured from the amelocemental junction (CEJ) or some other fixed point. This allows more meaningful serial comparisons to be made in order to monitor periodontal progression. Where there is considerable gingival hyperplasia, pocketing may be fairly deep (say 5–7 mm) but attachment loss may be small or nil. Where there has been considerable gingival recession, a shallow pocket may be associated with considerable destruction of the periodontal tissues. Therefore, in order to interpret pocket measurement one must also note:

1. The position of the gingival margin on the tooth surface
2. The position of the alveolar crest as seen on the radiograph.

The factors affecting the accuracy of periodontal probing are discussed further in the following section.

Radiographic examination

Radiographic examination will demonstrate the position of the alveolar margin and the condition of the alveolar bone. In a child or adolescent, radiographic examination may not be essential; however, if any doubt exists about the integrity of the alveolar margin, bite wing films of posterior teeth and periapical films of the incisors should provide adequate information. If there is evidence of established bone loss, further radiographic examination can then be undertaken.

In the adult, full mouth examination may be necessary. The long-cone paralleling technique provides the most reliable radiographic evidence (*Figure 12.2a*). The bisecting angle technique is more likely to give a distorted picture of the relationship of the alveolar margin to the CEJ. Rinn bite blocks, film holders and localization devices can be used to ensure that the X-rays pass perpendicular to the teeth and film, preventing any distortion of the bone/teeth relationships.

(a)

(b)

Figure 12.2 Radiographs taken to show alveolar bone loss: *(a)* A vertical bitewing radiograph of $\frac{654|}{765|}$ showing horizontal alveolar bone loss; *(b)* A paralleling technique radiograph of 654| showing horizontal alveolar bone loss

Using these devices can also help to make subsequent radiographs of the same site comparable. Vertical bite wing radiographs (*Figure 12.2b*) are useful for posterior teeth, and can be used for teeth with probing depths up to 6 mm; the orthopantomograph (OPG) provides an overall picture, but detail of the alveolar margin is frequently ill-defined. Repeat radiographs may be necessary, at intervals of not less than 3 years and determined by patient susceptibility, to show progression. Sophisticated techniques such as subtraction radiography and computer-assisted image analysis (see below) have been used as research tools to detect small changes in bone mass, but at present these have no place in clinical practice. However, the advent of digital radiography makes the use of such techniques more likely in the future.

It cannot be stressed too strongly that the traditional techniques of clinical radiography can provide a great deal of reliable information, but only if great care is taken in beam angulation, exposure and processing, and in interpretation of the radiographic image.

Occlusion

The examination of occlusion should include:

1. The angle's classification
2. Overbite and overjet
3. Tooth relation in protrusive and lateral positions and movements
4. Any deviation from the normal path of opening and closure
5. Any temporomandibular joint (TMJ) discomfort or clicking
6. Any spasm in the masticatory muscles
7. Any history of habits such as clenching or grinding the teeth.

The occlusion needs to be examined closely where:

- Teeth are mobile or sensitive
- There is discomfort, clicking, deviation of the mandible on opening and closing, or limitation of movement
- One or more of the masticatory muscles is tender to palpation
- Radiographs show widening of the periodontal spaces, i.e. possible signs of excessive occlusal stress.

Advances in diagnostic techniques

The methods described above are suitable for most clinical situations, but do suffer from a number of drawbacks. These are:

1. Clinical or radiological measurements of attachment loss are not precisely accurate and, if not carried out very carefully, can be misleading. This is particularly the case for periodontal probing, but also concerns oral radiography.

2. Full mouth recording is necessary because of the site-specific and episodic nature of much periodontal progression.

3. Individual susceptibility to periodontitis, as to all bacterial disease, varies over time, and this needs to be determined and taken into account.

4. All clinical diagnostic techniques give us retrospective information about past disease and are unable to diagnose disease activity.

5. If the periodontal examination is required for periodontal research purposes, much more accurate diagnostic techniques are necessary.

All of these issues are discussed below.

Factors affecting the accuracy of periodontal probing

The periodontal probing depth (PPD) is the distance from the gingival margin to the base of the periodontal pocket, and it is usually measured at six points around the tooth – i.e. mesial, buccal and distal from the buccal side, and mesial, lingual and distal from the lingual side (see Chapter 11). The mesial and distal measurements should be the same from both the buccal and lingual sides, but may not be because the access to them may be better from one side or the other. The amount of gingival recession, i.e. the distance from the cement–enamel junction (CEJ) to the base of the periodontal pocket should also be measured. These measurements are recorded onto a periodontal chart by the dental nurse during the recording process. If these measurements are to be related to future serial measurements in order to attempt to monitor disease progression, they must be made very carefully.

In controlled clinical studies, it is necessary to additionally record probing attachment levels (PAL). This is the distance from a fixed, reproducible point and the pocket base. The ideal fixed point is the CEJ, if it can be reliably located, but alternatives are the occlusal surface or a fixed point on a stent precisely located over the teeth to be recorded.

A periodontal probe must be fine enough to enter a narrow periodontal pocket, but must have a blunt end so that it reduces the likelihood of penetration of the tissues at the base of the pocket. Great care must be taken to manipulate the probe to reach the base of the deepest aspect of each pocket without penetrating its base. A number of factors can affect the accuracy of periodontal probing. These are:

- The size of the probe
- The angulation of the probe
- The contour of the tooth and root surface
- The probing force used
- The inflammatory state of the tissues.

A number of studies have shown that periodontal probing often fails to record the true pocket depth (Listgarten *et al.*, 1976; Van der Velden, 1979; Listgarten, 1980). These studies have shown a discrepancy between the actual position of the probe and the true base of the pocket in

histological sections of block dissections of animal and human cadaver tissue. The size of the probe and its angulation may be controlled, but errors resulting from alterations in probing force and the severity of inflammation in the tissues are more difficult to avoid.

With regard to probing force, it has been shown that the force used by different clinicians can vary from 3–130 g and may differ by more than twice as much for the same clinician from one examination to another (Gabathuler and Hassell, 1971; Hassell *et al.*, 1973). Generally, the greater the probing force the greater is the probing depth measured, since the probe penetrates deeper into the tissues at the base of the pocket. In order to limit errors due to differences in probing force, pressure sensitive probes have been developed (Van der Velden and de Vries, 1978; Vitek *et al.*, 1979; Polson *et al.*, 1980). These enable the dentist to probe with a predetermined force.

If the gingival tissues are inflamed, the marginal tissues may be swollen by oedema or hyperplasia. This alters the position of the gingival margin and produces an element of false pocketing. In addition, in untreated periodontal disease the connective tissue adjacent to the pocket epithelium is infiltrated with inflammatory fluid and cells, and the pocket epithelium is also infiltrated with inflammatory cells and thinned or ulcerated. In this situation these tissues are very easily penetrated by the periodontal probe, even with relatively light probing forces, and in some instances the probe penetrates as far as the bone margin. This obviously results in an overestimation of the true pocket depth (Armitage *et al.*, 1977; Robinson and Vitek, 1979; Polson *et al.*, 1980). Conversely, when the inflammatory infiltrate decreases following successful treatment and new collagen fibres are laid down in the connective tissue, the dentogingival tissues become more resistant to probing and the tip of the probe usually fails to reach the base of the pocket. Therefore, this often results in an underestimation of the true pocket depth. For these reasons, the difference between probing measurements and the histological 'true' pocket depth may vary by fractions of a millimetre to several millimetres (Listgarten, 1980). For these reasons, manual probing cannot reliably measure changes in PPD of less than 2.5–3 mm (Haffajee and Socransky, 1986).

From this discussion, it should be realized that the reductions in PPD that follow successful periodontal treatment are produced by the tissue changes outlined above and not by any true gain in connective tissue attachment. In spite of this, these post-treatment reductions in PPD are often reported as a 'gain in clinical attachment', which is very misleading since the changes result from a resolution of inflammation without any true gain in attachment.

The episodic nature of chronic periodontitis

A number of longitudinal clinical studies (Socransky *et al.*, 1984) have recorded clinical attachment loss at individual sites in different subjects over time periods ranging from 2 to 5 years. These have revealed that, despite the presence of inflammation, most sites showed no progression during the study period. Instead attachment loss occurred at only a few sites, and even at these sites was interspersed with long periods of stability or quiescence. This type of episodic, site-specific attachment loss has given rise to the burst theory of chronic periodontitis. It has further been proposed that these bursts might occur randomly throughout an individual's life (random burst), or there may be periods when bursts of periodontal breakdown in many sites are more likely (asynchronous multiple burst).

The implications of the burst theories are that:

1. Gingival inflammation at a site may not indicate that further periodontal breakdown is occurring or that it will occur at a later date.
2. Periodontal disease is site-specific, and may affect different teeth in the same mouth at different rates.
3. Full mouth periodontal charting on a regular basis is necessary to identify sites with attachment loss, to determine the pattern and rate of progression and the patient's susceptibility.
4. Each tooth must be considered separately for treatment.

In these studies, only fairly large changes (≥ 3 mm) of clinical attachment level could be reliably measured (see below), and smaller changes could not be detected. Therefore, although these studies show clearly that site-specific, episodic disease progression does occur, they do not preclude other patterns of progression, including slow regular progression, from also occurring. It seems most likely that episodic progression would predominate in susceptible patients with more rapid rates of progression.

Susceptible and resistant patients

Periodontal attachment loss has been found to be more marked in some patients than others, even when differences of oral hygiene are taken into account (Löe *et al.*, 1978). Studies from a number of different countries have suggested that about 10% of subjects appear to have a high risk of developing destructive periodontal disease and experience severe periodontal destruction with rapid progression and tooth loss (*Figure 12.3*). About 80% of subjects are susceptible to periodontitis that progresses rather slowly and rarely results in tooth loss. The remaining 10% appear to be relatively resistant to destructive periodontitis (See *Figure 4.5*, Chapter 4), despite the continued presence of gingivitis (Löe *et al.*, 1978; Page and Schroeder, 1986; Papapanou *et al.*, 1989). Identification of each patient's individual susceptibility to periodontitis is important, since this will determine the type and frequency of treatment required.

Advances in measurement of periodontal attachment loss

The main objective of periodontal diagnosis is to detect changes in periodontal attachment level. The traditional methods of recording this are the use of manual probing with a graduated periodontal probe, and radiographic examination. The accuracy of probing is affected by a number of factors, including the position and angulation of the probe, the probing pressure and the inflammatory state of the tissues. If probing measurements are to be used sequentially to detect progressive loss of attachment, these factors need to be controlled where possible and the measurements made from a fixed reproducible point. This cannot be the gingival margin, which can change its position as a result of inflammatory swelling or recession, and the ideal reference point is the CEJ. However, the CEJ is difficult to locate precisely because it usually lies subgingivally and it may be obscured by calculus or dental restorations. For these reasons, other points, such as the occlusal surface or a fixed point on a stent, are often used in clinical research studies.

Probing measurements, even with those controls, are not precisely reproducible between different clinicians, even when they standardize their procedures. In addition, replicate measurements of the same site at close time intervals are not always reproducible for the same clinician (Haffajee *et al.*, 1983).

To overcome these problems in clinical studies, they suggested the use of the *tolerance method* to determine the threshold for confirmed attachment loss based on probing. With this method, two replicate measurements of each site are made for each subject and their standard deviation (SD) is calculated. The differences between all duplicate measurements for all the test sites within each patient are then used to calculate the patient SD, and patient SDs are then averaged to produce a population SD. In a longitudinal clinical study of periodontal attachment loss, this method is generally used to confirm measured progressive attachment loss. With this method, if the mean of the second of a pair of attachment level measurements is to be considered significantly different from the mean of the first pair, then the attachment level change has to exceed:

- The site threshold, which is calculated as 3 site SDs
- The patient threshold, which is calculated as 3 patient SDs
- The population threshold, which is calculated as 2 population SDs.

The site measurement standard deviation has been calculated as 0.82 mm in the Haffajee studies, which makes the subject tolerance 2.46 mm. Thus, using this method, any change below 3 mm is considered to be unreliable, and this makes it impossible to measure small changes of attachment using manual probing. For this reason, the National Institute for Dental Research (NIDR) of the USA in 1979 requested the development of more sensitive methods (Parakkal, 1979). They wanted:

Figure 12.3 *(a)* A 15-year-old girl with severe gingival inflammation and advanced periodontitis with drifting of teeth. *(b)* Radiographs of the same girl showing marked generalized alveolar bone loss. She had already lost a lower incisor due to extreme mobility. Her mother had also lost all her teeth at a young age, and wore full dentures. No evidence for systemic disease was found; however, all such cases should always be investigated for any underlying systemic cause, such as a leucocyte dysfunction

1. A precision of ± 0.1 mm and a range of 10 mm
2. A constant probing force
3. Measurement from a fixed reproducible point
4. A guidance system to ensure a reproducible pathway
5. A non-invasive procedure
6. Digital output of data.

These criteria were met by the Florida research group (Gibbs *et al.*, 1988), who developed the Florida probe system. This incorporates:

- Constant probing force
- Precise electronic measurement
- Computer storage of data.

It eliminates errors of visual reading, which become more important with age! It consists of a probe handpiece, a digital readout, a foot switch and a computer interface and computer (Magnusson *et al.*, 1988a). It has been found to be significantly superior to manual probing (Magnusson *et al.*, 1988b). Two models have been devel-

oped, which differ in their fixed reference point. These are the stent and disc models. The probe of the stent model has a 1 mm metal collar that rests on a prepared ledge on a prefabricated vacuoform stent, while the disc model has an 11 mm disc that rests on the occlusal surface or incisal edge of the tooth (*Figure 12.4a*).

The reproducibility of both types of Florida probe have been compared with conventional manual probing (Low *et al.*, 1989; Osborn *et al.*, 1990). They were both significantly superior to manual probes, with a site standard deviation (SD) range of 0.21–0.28 mm. The calculated subject tolerance is 0.63–0.84 mm, meaning that changes in attachment of 1 mm can be reliably measured by this method.

The Florida probe can also read probing depths using an interchangeable pocket depth handpiece. This has a collar surrounding the probe, which is related to the gingival margin, and the distance from this to the base of the pocket is electronically recorded (*Figure 12.4b*).

All of this data, along with other readings such as

(a)

(b)

Figure 12.4 *(a)* A Florida electronic probe with attachment level disc on occlusal surface; *(b)* a Florida electronic probe with sleeve of pocket depth attachment at gingival margin

bleeding on probing, can be recorded and saved on a disk or printed on to special charts using a suitable compatible printer.

Other electronic probes have been developed, and these include:

- The Interprobe (Goodson and Kondon, 1988). This has an optical encoder transduction element.
- The Birek probe (Birek *et al.*, 1987). This works by constant air pressure, and uses the occlusal surface as its reference point. The site SD has been calculated as 0.46 mm and the subject threshold as 1.38 mm.
- The Jeffcoat probe (Jeffcoat *et al.*, 1986, 1989). This claims to detect the CEJ automatically, and has a

calculated site SD of 0.17 mm and a subject threshold of 0.51 mm. This appears to be the lowest subject threshold reported to date.

Radiographic examination

Transmission radiography can show the relationship between the alveolar bone margin and the CEJ, and changes in the distance from the bone margin to the CEJ, normally 1–2 mm, are indicative of alveolar bone loss. To achieve an accurate display of this distance, the rays must be perpendicular to the tooth and bone surfaces and the tube must also be at the correct antero-posterior angulation. Two types of view can be used in conventional radiography to achieve this:

1. Vertical bite wings (*Figure 12.2a*)
2. Long cone paralleling views (*Figure 12.2b*).

To detect serial changes in this relationship further controls are necessary, and these involve:

- A constant film position
- A constant tube geometry.

A constant film position can be achieved by the use of a stent, which can be in the form of an acrylic impression of the occlusal surfaces of the teeth on the bite block of the film holder. A mark can also be made to ensure that the film is always placed in the same position in the holder. By these means the holder is accurately located with respect to the teeth and the film with respect to the holder for each serial radiograph.

A constant tube geometry can be achieved by relating the tube to positioning devices attached to the film holder (Rinn system) or by the use of a cephalostat (Jeffcoat *et al.*, 1987).

Bone loss can also be expressed as a percentage of the root length to compensate for errors of foreshortening or elongation.

Computer-aided systems

Techniques have recently been developed to aid the detection of small serial changes in alveolar bone level. These rely on digitization of the radiographic image to allow computer processing and analysis. Two techniques have been developed mainly for research purposes, and these are:

1. Digital subtraction radiology
2. Computer-assisted linear radiography.

However, computer-aided techniques based on the principle of digitization of the image are beginning to be developed for clinical usage, and are likely to appear in the near future. These will allow a very low exposure time to radiation and also allow the image to be stored in the computer and printed out as many times as required.

Digital subtraction radiology

The best known computer-aided technique is digital subtraction radiology (Webber *et al.*, 1982; Gröndahl and Gröndahl, 1983; Jeffcoat *et al.*, 1987). The purpose of this technique is to subtract all unchanged structures from a pair of serial films and display only the areas of change. For periodontal films, this means subtraction of the teeth, cortical bone and trabecular pattern, leaving only bone loss or gain standing out against a neutral grey background.

The digitization process converts the analogue (nearly continuous grey level information) contained in the transmission radiograph to numbers that are proportional to the brightness of the radiograph at a particular location. This is done by taking a picture of the radiograph with a sensitive black and white video camera. The digitizer automatically superimposes a grid over this picture and converts the grey level of the radiograph within each box in the grid to a number ranging from zero (black) to 255 (white). The fineness of the grid determines the spatial resolution of the digitized image and usually a 512 × 480 picture element (pixel) grid is used.

This process does not increase the information on the radiograph, and in fact decreases it a little. It does, however, put the information in a form that the computer can use so that it can process it in a way which will aid the dentist or researcher to detect changes in bone level not visible to the unaided eye from the original radiograph. The computer subtracts all structures present in the first radiograph of the serial pair from those in the second radiograph, leaving only bone loss (dark) or bone gain (light). Location of bony change can be more readily seen by superimposing the subtracted image over the original radiograph. Subtracted images can also be colour coded by the computer to increase clarity. Bone loss is usually colour coded red and bone gain green.

If this technique were reliable and accurate, it could be useful in assessing the natural history of periodontal disease progression and in longitudinal studies of various types, including investigations of potential biomarkers of disease activity or proposed new treatment methods. However, the accuracy of digital subtraction radiography has been questioned by Benn (1990) on the basis of his own measurements using this technique. Subtraction radiography depends critically on the very precise registration of the two sequential radiographs. He created two identical digital images of a single radiograph to test the response of the system to small displacements of 0.1–0.42 mm in the X, Y, and XY directions before subtraction. He found that displacements of 0.1–0.14 mm in the Y or XY directions caused 20–25% of crestal pixels to vary by more than ± 2.5% of grey range (2.5% is the noise threshold used for this technique). Larger displacements of 0.3–0.42 mm caused 65% of crestal pixels to vary by more than ± 2.5% of grey range. Such small displacements would be hard to avoid when using this technique with serial radiographs, and so false crestal bone gain or loss could

regularly result from these causes. The use of a much higher noise threshold of about ± 8% would need to be used to avoid these critical errors.

Computer-assisted linear radiography

Benn (1992) has designed a computer-aided method for making linear measurements on serial radiographs using stored regions of interest. In this system, the radiographs are first calibrated and digitized as described above. Under the control of a computer program, regions of interest (ROI) of 7.5 mm × 7.5 mm, sufficient to cover the mesial and distal CEJ to alveolar crest margin regions of adjacent teeth, are chosen. The measuring process involves placing the cursor pixel point on the CEJ and clicking the mouse button, which records and marks this position. This is then repeated for the alveolar crest, after which the distance is calculated and stored by the computer. The ROI with its marked reference points is also stored. The process is then repeated for the first serial radiograph, and the ROI of the first measurement with its marked points is redisplayed close to the area to be measured. This reminds the operator of the chosen reference points, reducing the chances of error. The computer automatically calculates the distances, the average distances of the two readings and the difference between the two readings. This process is then repeated for the second serial radiograph, initially using prompts for the siting of reference points from the displayed ROI from the first radiograph. When the sites for the second radiograph image have been measured twice, the computer automatically calculates the differences between the two films and the confidence value attached to the measured change.

The accuracy and reliability of this system were tested with 28 examiners with minimal training (Benn, 1992). They each measured 14 different sites and repeated the process 4 weeks later; 13 out of 14 sites produced an intra-examiner SD threshold of ≤ 0.15 mm with the ROI method, but 0 out of 14 without. The inter-examiner threshold for 13 out of 14 sites was ≤ 0.22 mm using the ROI method and 0 out of 14 without. Therefore, this system would appear to be accurate to ≤ 0.22 mm and would seem to be useful for clinical research.

Special tests

If the severity of the inflammation or the degree of periodontal destruction appears to be out of proportion to the observed aetiological factors, or if general appraisal of the patient suggests that some systemic factor may be operating, then blood and urine examination or other special tests may be required. In such cases it is imperative to communicate with the patient's physician prior to the start of treatment.

Making a prognosis

A prognosis is a prediction of the way in which the tissues are likely to respond to treatment. Before a definitive treatment plan can be formulated, a prognosis must be made. This should allow one to establish not merely what treatment can be carried out but, more importantly, what treatment is justified in the attempt to achieve long-term periodontal stability. Frequently the patient will ask that such a prediction be made, and the more complicated the treatment, the more important making a prognosis becomes. Looking into the future can be a hazardous exercise, but a prediction of the way in which the periodontal tissues will behave can be made on the basis of an understanding of the way in which the tissues of that individual have behaved in the past in the face of disease-producing factors.

A number of parameters need to be considered:

1. The extent of periodontal destruction. This is represented by the amount of alveolar bone loss as seen on the radiograph; obviously, the greater the amount of bone loss, the poorer the prognosis.
2. The age of the patient. This, together with the extent of periodontal destruction, provides an idea of the rate at which destruction has taken place. The older the individual, the better the prognosis for any given degree of periodontal destruction.
3. The form of the bone loss. The presence of vertical bone defects must mean a less favourable prognosis than where bone loss is horizontal, for several reasons:
   (a) Because the level of attachment is frequently more apical
   (b) Because the possibility of fill-in of such defects is uncertain
   (c) Because the presence of vertical defects usually indicates that factors other than plaque-induced inflammation are operating. Furcation involvement can present home care problems, even after satisfactory periodontal treatment, and if the furcation lesion is related to pulp pathology, prognosis is compounded by any defects in endodontic treatment.
4. The possibility of removing aetiological factors. The control of aetiological factors is essential to the achievement of long-term health, but control can only be exercised after these factors have been identified. Without such identification, treatment becomes symptomatic. Careful examination and an understanding of clinical features is essential. It is always necessary to ask 'Why are these clinical features present?'
5. Patient co-operation. This is essential for satisfactory plaque control, but is also necessary for the control of predisposing and aggravating aetiological factors, e.g. the replacement of an ill-fitting partial denture. Patient co-operation is more likely to be forthcoming after the patient has been given information about the nature of the problem. Time spent in providing such information and in explaining the rationale behind the treatment plan will improve the chances of achieving a good prognosis.
6. The number, position and form of teeth present. The number of teeth and their position in the arch will determine the occlusal load on each tooth, whether a prosthesis is necessary, and the amount of tooth support for an appliance. In this context, the form of the appliance is extremely important; a removable appliance makes greater demands on the tooth supporting tissues than a fixed appliance. The symmetrical distribution of the teeth in the arch is likely to provide a better prognosis than where several teeth are placed on one side of the arch. The root base can be a crucial factor in the stability and usefulness of a tooth. An upper molar with widespread roots and therefore a large root base has a much better prognosis than a conical-rooted premolar or incisor with the same amount of bone loss.
7. General health. Although certain conditions do affect the periodontal tissue response, e.g. diabetes, Down's syndrome and agranulocytosis, the general health of the patient does not usually affect the periodontal condition directly, but any debility, physical or emotional, can interfere with the patient's oral hygiene regimen.
8. The immunological status in relation to plaque bacteria. The individual's response is critical to the development and progress of periodontal destruction, and is the subject of much recent research. As described in Chapter 20, a few young individuals appear to suffer some deficiency in the cell-mediated immune response to plaque antigens, which leads to an extremely poor prognosis. It seems likely that other variations in immune response will be identified in the future, and some laboratory tests may be developed which will provide a more objective guide to prognosis than is currently available.

All the factors outlined above must be taken together to provide a periodontal prognosis for that particular individual. This exercise has to be carried out with great care and thought. The assessment of prognosis provides an acid test of the operator's understanding of the biological forces operating in the mouth under examination. Furthermore, the limitations of our understanding of the disease process do handicap our ability to make absolute prognoses.

Periodontal diagnosis in general dental practice

Since the vast majority of dental patients are treated in dental practices, and some stage of periodontal disease affects practically all patients, a minimum standard of basic periodontal examination should be undertaken of all these patients. The following guidelines for this, outlined below, follow those recommended by the British Society of Periodontology (1986) and the Royal College of Surgeons of England, Faculty of Dental Surgery (1997).

Basic periodontal examination

All patients should be screened for the presence of periodontal diseases as part of their dental examination, and the basic periodontal examination (BPE) represents the minimum examination for this purpose. It consists of:

1. A clinical assessment using the community periodontal index of treatment needs (CPITN), as detailed in Chapter 9. In older individuals, recession and furcation involvement may be present, causing significant attachment to go unrecorded with this system and, for this reason, a modification is recommended. Where the total attachment loss exceeds 7 mm, or if a furcation can be probed, the sextant is scored by an asterisk (*) rather than the CPITN code.
2. Appropriate supportive dental radiography when indicated by the clinical examination (see below).

The BPE should be performed at the initial dental examination of all new patients, and patients with insignificant periodontal disease on the initial visit should be screened again at regular routine dental inspections with a frequency of a least every 12 months. In addition to routine screening, all patients being considered for advanced restorative or orthodontic treatment should be screened.

In view of the evidence of early periodontal breakdown in a few susceptible individuals (Alibander *et al.*, 1991), screening of children, adolescents and young adults is also advised. Problems arise with false pocketing in children, and this must be taken into account by attempting to locate the cement–enamel junction in sites where pocketing is suspected in these subjects. In patients under 19 years of age, only one tooth per sextant needs to be probed; these should be the first molars and the upper left central incisor and the lower right central incisor.

The BPE will need augmentation by detailed periodontal charting (*Figure 12.2*) when the screening has revealed significant disease in one or more sextants, i.e. with CPITN codings of 3, 4 or *. This must include:

- Pocket depths (six points per tooth)
- Recession (six points per tooth)

- Bleeding on probing
- Mobility
- Furcation involvement.

CPITN is not a suitable index to produce a site-related diagnosis, which is needed for patients with significant pocketing. It is also not suitable to monitor the response to treatment. In both of these situations, full periodontal charting is indicated.

All patients with identifiable disease at screening should be regularly monitored with further CPITN screening if the disease is early, i.e. codes 1, 2, or full periodontal charting in the case of codes 3, 4, *. Results from epidemiological studies show that, in the presence of plaque and calculus, periodontal disease may increase in severity with age. In addition, it has been shown that periodontal disease progresses at different rates in different sites in the mouth, and may at individual tooth sites undergo long periods of quiescence or short periods of progression (Lindhe *et al.*, 1983; Haffajee *et al.*, 1983). Therefore, there is a need to repeat full periodontal charting of patients with initial evidence of periodontitis at regular intervals.

Selection criteria for periodontal radiography

Radiographs should only be taken if their results are likely to affect the patient's treatment, and their need should be based on the results of the clinical examination. There is a lack of consensus as to which type of radiograph (i.e. bite wing, site-related periapicals or panoramic tomogram) is most appropriate. Osborne and Hemmings (1992) have shown that panoramic radiography is an acceptable alternative to full mouth periapicals on the basis of its diagnostic yield of unsuspected pathology. However, a large proportion of the disease identified by panoramic radiographs does not affect clinical care. Also, the accuracy and resolution of panoramic tomograms in detecting the landmarks for assessing bone loss are less than those achievable with properly aligned long cone, paralleling periapicals. For these reasons, there is little to support its use for routine screening of periodontal purposes (Valachovic *et al.*, 1986).

Radiographic selection criteria for periodontal disease should take into account the data obtained from a detailed periodontal examination, with particular reference to pocket depths, recession and the overall state of the

Table 12.1 Radiographic selection criteria for periodontal disease

Disease status	*Radiograph*
Uniform pocketing < 5 mm	Posterior bite wings
Uniform pocketing < 5 mm plus ectopic third molars	Panoramic radiograph
Uniform pocketing 5–6 mm plus otherwise sound dentition	Vertical bite wings of molars and premolars plus long cone periapicals of anterior teeth if indicated by pocket depths on these teeth
Irregular pocketing > 5 mm or multiple crowned and/or heavily restored teeth or history of endodontic treatment	Full mouth long cone periapicals or Panoramic radiograph plus additional long cone periapicals of key sites

If gingival recession is present then these criteria would need adjustment to account for it.

dentition. The selection criteria (*Table 12.1*) are based on those suggested by Hirschmann *et al.* (1994).

Radiographs should not be repeated unless serial periodontal charting indicates significant progression of disease at the site in question.

Treatment plan

The objectives of treatment are:

1. The elimination of disease
2. The restoration of efficient function
3. The production of a satisfactory appearance.

One might also add, a contented patient.

It should be evident from the above list that periodontal treatment is not primarily concerned with the conservation of individual teeth, but with the long-term preservation of a healthy dentition. Indeed, there are situations in which individual teeth have to be sacrificed to the greater good. This concept of treating the dentition as a functioning unit is in conflict with the traditional dental teaching, in which the tooth rather than the dentition is the focus of concern.

Because each patient presents an individual problem, one cannot prescribe a rigid pattern of treatment. Treatment is determined not only by the condition defined by the diagnosis, but also by the patient's age, general health, attitude and aspirations. Nevertheless, it is important that a well-ordered plan of action is designed at the outset, keeping in mind that departures from this plan may be required as treatment proceeds. No treatment, other than emergency treatment, should be started before a plan is established and explained to the patient.

The following outline should provide a guide to treatment management:

1. Emergency treatment
2. Extraction of teeth with poor prognosis
3. Patient information
4. Plaque control and scaling
5. Subgingival scaling and root planing
6. Initial occlusal adjustment
7. Reassessment
8. Surgery
9. Reconstruction
10. Maintenance.

Emergency treatment

The control of pain comes before any other treatment but, to be effective, requires accurate diagnosis. An alveolar abscess of pulpal origin can be misdiagnosed as a periodontal lesion, with consequent errors in treatment and persistence of pain.

Swelling, even without pain, requires immediate attention. Acute infection may require the prescription of anti-biotics before further treatment can be carried out, but the use of antibiotics is justified only where pain and infection can be controlled in no other way. A localized and pointing abscess should be treated by incision and drainage rather than by antibiotics.

Large, carious cavities and pulp disease should be treated. Endodontics may be necessary as an emergency measure where there is a pulpitis, apical abscess or a combined periapical–periodontal abscess.

Extremely mobile teeth that seriously interfere with function should be splinted or extracted.

Extraction of teeth with poor prognosis

A decision about extraction should be based not only on the condition of the individual tooth and its supporting tissues, but also upon the possible consequences of the extraction. Where periodontal breakdown is advanced, the extraction of weak teeth may create an insoluble prosthetic problem. Such developments need to be anticipated prior to extraction. The provision of removable prostheses may be necessary at this time, and care should be taken with their design, even if temporary.

Patient information

Some time should be allowed prior to definitive treatment to explain to the patient the nature of the problem and the kind of treatment needed. Where different lines of treatment are available, these options, with their advantages and disadvantages, should be explained. Frequently, decisions have to be made by the patient, and these can be made intelligently only on the basis of information.

Plaque control and scaling

Plaque control and scaling are the most important procedures in periodontal treatment. Where the condition is diagnosed and treated at an early stage, they are the only treatments required. They also provide a clue as to patient attitude, dexterity and level of co-operation. Where that level of co-operation is inadequate, any indicated surgical treatment or other complicated treatment is not justified. This phase of treatment should also include the correction of filling overhangs and the replacement of defective restorations. It is unrealistic and unjust to expect a high level of plaque control where conditions exist which make that impossible; therefore, all plaque retention factors should be corrected at this stage.

Subgingival scaling and root planing

Periodontal pockets require careful subgingival scaling to remove subgingival calculus and root planing to smooth the root surface and remove any necrotic cementum. This is by far the most important procedure in the treatment of chronic periodontitis. If this procedure is carried out successfully it will result in cessation of bleeding on probing, and if this sign persists then it is indicative of residual subgingival calculus. The procedure also results in a change in the subgingival flora (see Chapters 14 and 15), which itself brings about a resolution of gingival inflammation and a regeneration of junctional epithelium. These changes probably result from changes in the nutritional sources, particularly of protein, brought about by this procedure. They last for about 3 months, which is why these procedures need to be repeated 3-monthly.

Subgingival scaling and root planing is a time-consuming procedure which requires appropriate subgingival scalers, freshly sharpened instruments and considerable clinical skill (see Chapter 14).

Initial occlusal adjustment

This is necessary for repair of the periodontal lesion, and may be carried out alongside plaque control. Gross occlusal disharmonies should be eliminated and temporary splints applied to very mobile teeth. At this stage, any minor tooth movement necessary can be carried out. Such movement should be complete and any retention apparatus in place before surgery is carried out. A bite-guard may be provided in cases of definite bruxism.

Reassessment

A reassessment of the periodontal condition should be made at this stage. The tissue response to the treatment already provided may be better than anticipated, so that little or no surgery may be required. Pockets may shrink and mobile teeth become stable after the relatively simple procedures carried out so far. Dramatic stabilization of neighbouring teeth can follow the extraction of an infected tooth.

On the other hand, tissue response or patient co-operation may not be as satisfactory as anticipated, in which case a reappraisal of the case will be needed.

Surgery

The management of the surgical phase of treatment, when it is required, depends upon the size of the problem and the patient's domestic and work commitments and their physical and emotional status. Not every patient can cope with several surgical procedures under local anaesthesia over an extended period of time. Furthermore, some patients find it difficult to maintain a satisfactory level of plaque control with a surgical wound, sutures and dressings in their mouth. Therefore, any necessary surgery should be carried out in as few stages as possible over as short a time as possible. The options available, i.e. local anaesthesia, general anaesthesia or local anaesthesia plus intravenous

sedation, should be offered to the patient, with explanations of the obvious advantages and disadvantages, so that decisions can be made which meet their individual needs.

The immediate postoperative phase must be closely supervised for the first 2 months postoperatively, after which permanent reconstruction work can be started.

Reconstruction

This phase should include fine adjustment of the occlusion and the provision of permanent restorative and prosthetic work. In the design of restorations, subgingival preparation should be avoided, except perhaps (minimally) on the labial aspect of upper incisors, where appearance is important. Embrasure spaces, allowing easy interdental cleaning, are essential. A balanced occlusion should be constructed (Chapter 24).

Any temporary splints can be removed and the need for permanent splinting can be assessed at this stage (see Chapter 25).

If they have not already been made, bite-guards for persistent bruxism can be provided.

Maintenance

Eternal vigilance is the watchword of successful periodontal treatment and, in that sense, periodontal treatment is never complete. Patients require recall for inspection, oral hygiene monitoring and scaling at intervals of 3, 6, 9 or 12 months, depending on their previous disease experience and susceptibility. Individual radiographs may have to be repeated if pocket measurements show that disease is progressing.

One must avoid creating a situation where the patient is totally dependent upon professional care. Some individuals are happy to abdicate responsibility for the state of their mouth to the dentist or hygienist. It is essential to make it clear to the patient that, in the end, the patient must be responsible for his or her own dental health. It is only through a partnership that long-term dental health can be achieved.

References

Alibander, J.M., Barmes, D., Beagrie, G. *et al.* (1991) Destructive forms of periodontal disease in adolescents. A 3-year longitudinal study. *Journal of Periodontology* 62, 370–376

Armitage G.C., Svanberg G.K. and Löe H. (1977) Microscopic evaluation of clinical measurements of connective tissue attachment level. *Journal of Clinical Periodontology* 4, 173–190

Benn, D.K. (1990) Limitations of the digital image subtraction technique in assessing alveolar bone crest changes due to misalignment errors during image capture. *Dentomaxillofacial Radiology* 19, 97–104

Benn, D.K. (1992) A computer-assisted method for making linear radiographic measurements using stored regions of interest. *Journal of Clinical Periodontology* 19, 441–448

Birek, P., McCulloch, C.H. and Hardy, V. (1987) Gingival attachment level measurements with an automated periodontal probe. *Journal of Clinical Periodontology* **14**, 472–477

British Society of Periodontology (1986) *Periodontology in General Dental Practice in the United Kingdom. A First Policy Statement* (R.F. Mosedale, P.D. Floyd and F.C. Smales, eds). London: British Society of Periodontology

Gabathuler H. and Hassell T. (1971) A pressure-sensitive probe. *Helvetica Odontologica Acta* **15**,114–117

Gibbs, C.H., Hirschfield, J.W., Lee, J.G. *et al.* (1988) Description and clinical evaluation of a new computerized periodontal probe – the Florida probe. *Journal of Clinical Periodontology* **15**, 137–144

Goodson, J.M. and Kondon, N. (1988) Periodontal pocket depth measurements by fiber-optic technology. *Journal of Clinical Dentistry* **1**, 35–38

Gröndahl, H.-G. and Gröndahl, K. (1983) Subtraction radiology for the diagnosis of periodontal bone lesions. *Oral Surgery, Oral Medicine, Oral Pathology* **55**, 208–213

Haffajee, A.D. and Socransky, S.S. (1986) Attachment level changes in destructive periodontal disease. *Journal of Clinical Periodontology* **13**, 461–472

Haffajee, A.D., Socransky, S.S. and Goodson, J.M. (1983) Comparison of different data analysis for detecting changes in attachment level. *Journal of Clinical Periodontology* **10**, 298–310

Hassell, T.M., Germann, M.A. and Saxer, V.P. (1973) Periodontal probing: investigator discrepancies and correlations between probing force and probing depth. *Helvetica Odontologica Acta* **17**, 38–42

Hirschmann, P.N., Horner, K. and Rushton, V.E. (1994) Selection criteria for periodontal radiography. *British Dental Journal* **176**, 324–325

Jeffcoat, M.K., Jeffcoat, R.L., Jens, S.C. and Captain, K. (1986) A new periodontal probe with an automated cement–enamel junction detection. *Journal of Clinical Periodontology* **13**, 276–280

Jeffcoat, M.K., Reddy, M. and Webber, R.L. (1987) Extraoral control of geometry for digital subtraction radiology. *Journal of Periodontal Research* **22**, 396–402

Jeffcoat, M.K., Jeffcoat, R.L., Captain, K. *et al.* (1989) A new periodontal probe with an automated CEJ detection: clinical trials. *Journal of Dental Research* **68**, 236

Lindhe, J., Haffajee, A.D. and Socransky, S.S. (1983) Progression of periodontal disease in adult subjects in the absence of periodontal therapy. *Journal of Clinical Periodontology* **10**, 433–442

Listgarten, M.A. Periodontal probing: what does it mean? (1980) *Journal of Clinical Periodontology* **7**, 165–176

Listgarten, M.A., Mao, R. and Robinson, P.J. (1976) Periodontal probing and the relationship of the probe to the periodontal tissues. *Journal of Periodontology* **47**, 511–513

Löe, H., Anerud, A., Boysen, H. and Smith, M. (1978) The natural history of periodontal disease in Man. *Journal of Periodontology* **49**, 607–620

Low, S.B., Taylor, M., Marks, R.G. *et al.* (1989) Measuring attachment level with an electronic disc probe. *Journal of Dental Research* **68**, 359

Magnusson, I., Clark, W.B., Marks, R.G. *et al.* (1988a) Attachment level measurements with a constant force electronic probe. *Journal of Clinical Periodontology* **15**, 185–188

Magnusson, I., Fuller, W.W., Heins, P.J. *et al.* (1988b) Correlation between electronic and visual readings of pocket depth with a newly developed constant force probe. *Journal of Clinical Periodontology* **15**, 180–184

Osborn, J., Stoltenberg, J., Huso, B. *et al.* (1990) Comparison of measurement variability using a standard and constant force probe. *Journal of Periodontology* **61**, 497–503

Osborne, G.E. and Hemmings, K.W. (1992) A survey of disease changes observed on panoramic tomograms of patients attending a periodontal clinic. *British Dental Journal* **173**, 166–168

Page, R.C. and Schroeder, H.E. (1986) *Periodontitis in Man and Other Animals*. Basel: Karger

Papapanou, P.N., Wennström, J.J. and Gröndahl, K. (1989) A 10-year retrospective study of periodontal disease progression. *Journal of Clinical Periodontology* **16**, 403–411

Parakkal, P.F. (1979) Proceedings of the workshop on quantitative evaluation of periodontal diseases by physical measuring techniques. *Journal of Dental Research* **58**, 547–553

Polson A.M., Caton J.G., Yeaple R.N. and Zander H.A. (1980) Histological determination of probe tip penetration into gingival sulcus of humans using an electronic pressure-sensitive probe. *Journal of Clinical Periodontology* **7**, 479–488

Robinson P.J. and Vitek R.M. (1979) The relationship between gingival inflammation and resistance to probe penetration. *Journal of Periodontal Research* **14**, 239–243

Royal College of Surgeons of England, Faculty of Dental Surgery (1997) *National Clinical Guidelines. Screening of Patients to detect Periodontal Diseases*. London: Royal College of Surgeons

Socransky, S.S., Haffajee, A.D., Goodson, J.M. and Lindhe, J. (1984) New concepts of destructive periodontal disease. *Journal of Clinical Periodontology* **11**, 21–32

Valachovic, R.W., Douglass, C.W., Reiskin, A.B. *et al.* (1986) The use of panoramic radiography in the evaluation of asymptomatic dental patients. *Oral Surgery, Oral Medicine, Oral Pathology* **61**, 289–296

Van der Velden, U. (1979) Probing force and the relationship of the probe tip to the periodontal tissues. *Journal of Clinical Periodontology* **6**, 106–114

Van der Velden, U. and de Vries, J.H. (1978) Introduction of a new periodontal probe: the pressure probe. *Journal of Clinical Periodontology* **5**, 188–197

Vitek, R.M., Robinson, P.J. and Lautenschlager, E.P. (1979) Development of a force-controlled periodontal instrument. *Journal of Periodontal Research* **14**, 93–94

Webber, R.L., Ruttimann, U.E. and Gröndahl, H.-G. (1982) X-ray image subtraction as a basis for assessment of periodontal changes. *Journal of Periodontal Research* **17**, 509–511

Further reading

Eley, B.M. and Cox, S.W. (1998) Advances in periodontal diagnosis. 1. Traditional clinical methods of diagnosis. *British Dental Journal* **184**, 12–16

Eley, B.M. and Cox, S.W. (1998) Advances in periodontal diagnosis. 2. New clinical methods of diagnosis. *British Dental Journal* **184**, 71–74

13

Diagnostic tests of disease activity

The relationship of bacteria, saliva and gingival crevicular fluid components to periodontal disease and their possible use in diagnostic tests

One of the liveliest areas of current periodontal research is concerned with the search for diagnostic tests of periodontal disease activity. These tests have potential relevance to both diagnosis and treatment because current clinical diagnostic methods are not precisely accurate and only allow retrospective diagnosis of attachment loss. To improve on this, however, diagnostic tests would need to be predictive of disease activity rather than just correlate with its occurrence.

Potential biomarkers of disease activity would need to be involved in the disease process in some way and therefore need to undergo extensive and careful basic research investigation before undergoing clinical evaluation. Only when the source, precise nature and the role of the potential marker are known and understood can clinical evaluation be meaningful.

The process of developing a predictive diagnostic test

The first consideration is to determine from which source the potential marker should be obtained. Four potential sources are possible:

1. Blood or serum
2. Saliva
3. Subgingival plaque sample
4. Gingival crevicular fluid (GCF).

Markers from the first two sources relate to either the whole patient or the whole mouth. Markers from the latter two sources relate to the condition of the local periodontal site. The methods of obtaining these samples are described below.

Periodontal disease progression is site-specific and episodic in nature, and reflects individual patient susceptibility (see Chapter 12). Since factors in the blood relate to the whole patient, they are unlikely to be able to diagnose local site activity. Factors in saliva come from the salivary glands, the oral flora or from GCF, and relate to the whole mouth rather than a local site. They are therefore also very unlikely to be able to diagnose local periodontal activity. At best they could give some information on the patient's overall periodontal condition. Therefore, factors from subgingival plaque samples or GCF are most likely to give information on local site activity.

Development of a predictive test based on any of the factors discussed in this section requires a combination of basic and applied research over a long time-scale, and the stages are listed below:

1. *Basic research*
   - Separation and characterization
   - Investigation of tissue chemistry
   - Investigation of its sources in the periodontal tissue
   - Investigation of its role in the microbiology or pathology of chronic periodontitis
   - Development of a selective and sensitive assay system
   - If GCF samples are to be used, then verification is necessary that gingival tissue or bacterial components are the same as those found in GCF
2. *Applied clinical research*
   - Ligature induced periodontitis in animals
   - Experimental gingivitis in humans
   - Natural disease process.

Investigations on the natural disease process involve the following:

- Cross-sectional studies of its relationship to disease severity

- Study of the levels before and after successful periodontal treatment
- Longitudinal studies of its relation to attachment and bone loss
- Development of simplified test system for chairside use
- Comparison of this simplified system with full laboratory analysis
- Clinical trial using test system.

Each of these stages is detailed below.

Basic research

Separation and characterization

The factor under investigation must first be separated from the complex mixture of substances present in the sampled material, which may be either subgingival plaque, gingival crevicular fluid (GCF), saliva or blood. This usually involves a variety of chemical, biochemical, immunochemical or microbiological separation techniques.

Secondly, the precise nature of the factor must be determined. Tissue factors present in the periodontal tissues or GCF need to be characterized by biochemical or immunocytochemical techniques, whilst bacteria need to be speciated by biochemical, immunochemical or genetic techniques.

Thirdly, a number of other factors present in the collection medium may interfere with the detection of the factor under investigation, and these interfering factors must be identified and controlled. An example of this might be the presence of natural inhibitors to enzymes under investigation in GCF or blood, which may interfere with its detection. Another might be the fastidious growth requirements needed by most of the bacteria in subgingival plaque, which might interfere with their survival during collection, transport or culture.

Investigation of tissue chemistry

Many factors present in the gingival and periodontal tissues pass into GCF in the inflammatory exudate. Before these factors can be assessed, their precise biochemical functions in the tissues must be known. For instance, if the factor is an enzyme, its normal substrate(s) (i.e. the molecule(s) that the enzyme attacks and cleaves) must be investigated. Its precise mode of action and the precise site(s) of cleavage of the substrate need to be known. Also, its requirements for activity, i.e. its pH optimum and the need for co-factors or activators, must be studied. Finally, the normal control mechanisms for the enzyme (e.g. its natural inhibitors) need to be investigated.

Investigation of its sources in the periodontal tissue

The precise location of the factor in the periodontal tissues must be studied. For example, the cellular source(s) and precise intracellular location of enzymes in the periodontal tissues need to be determined.

Investigation of its role in the microbiology or pathology of chronic periodontitis

The possible role(s) of the potential marker in periodontal pathology need to be studied. Examples of this would be the association of particular subgingival bacteria with periodontal disease progression and investigations of the ways in which bacterial products could potentially damage the tissues. Another example would be an investigation of the possible role of potential tissue enzyme markers to degrade the various gingival and periodontal tissue components.

Development of a selective and sensitive assay system

The assay system developed to detect the marker in question must be sensitive, i.e. it must detect the factor in low concentrations in the source material. Also, it must be highly selective, i.e. it should detect the factor in question but should not detect any interfering factors in the source material. An example of this would occur in the detection of enzymes in GCF. A particular substrate used in the assay system might be cleaved by a number of enzymes including the one in question. In this situation, the assay system may be made selective by controlling the assay conditions by the inclusion of an appropriate buffer to control the pH, appropriate activators of the enzyme in question and selective inhibitors of the interfering enzymes.

Verification that gingival tissue or bacterial components are the same as those found in GCF or saliva

If GCF or saliva is used as the source material for the factor in question, then it must first be confirmed that the factor assayed in these sources is the same as that found in the periodontal tissues. This is usually done by careful biochemical investigations of the factor extracted from the periodontal tissues and identical investigations of the factor in GCF or saliva so that their characteristics can be compared.

Applied clinical research

All of these studies should be blind, i.e. the levels of the marker must be unknown to the clinician carrying out the clinical measurements and vice versa, and this must apply right up to the completion of the study. It is also preferable that the clinician carrying out the clinical measurements, usually in duplicate, should be unaware of the measurements recorded at each site. This can be arranged with the use of electronic probes, since the values are measured by the computer and displayed on the screen for recording. This screen can be turned away from the clinician and displayed only to the recording dental nurse. Alternatively, they can be stored in the computer's memory and printed out later.

Ligature induced periodontitis in animals

Periodontal pockets can be artificially produced in animals, usually dogs, by the placement of silk ligatures into the gingival crevice. The ligatures accumulate plaque, and plaque growth is promoted by giving the animal a plaque-promoting soft diet. The ligatures are forced down apically at 2-week intervals for 16–20 weeks. The ligatures detach the junctional epithelium from the tooth and promote inflammation. As a result of this process attachment is rapidly lost, and true periodontal pockets form and progressively deepen. Corresponding bone loss also occurs.

The procedure is usually performed on the molars and premolars on one side of the jaw and the other side is left alone to serve as the control side. Also, the control side is usually given oral hygiene to induce gingival health. The period for which the ligatures remain *in situ* is classified as the disease progression phase. After the planned period, usually 16–20 weeks, the ligatures are removed and scaling and root planing is performed to promote the resolution of inflammation. Oral hygiene is also given three times per week over the next 8 weeks, which is classified as the disease recovery phase.

This model is generally used for short longitudinal studies spanning the 16–20 weeks of disease progression and the 8 weeks of disease resolution. The levels of the marker are compared at test and control site both during the disease progression and the disease recovery phases. Pocket depths are measured by manual or electronic probing, and bone loss by radiographical techniques. Samples of GCF are collected on strips every 2 weeks before the ligatures are displaced further apically during the disease progression phase, and at 2-week intervals in the disease recovery phase.

Experimental gingivitis in humans

Experimental gingivitis is induced in subjects with perfect gingival and periodontal health. These subjects must have no signs of attachment loss, and gingival health is enhanced by intensive oral hygiene instruction and any necessary scaling prior to the short experimental period. The point at which full gingival health is obtained serves as the baseline. Gingivitis is then induced over a 10–21-day period by ceasing all oral hygiene procedures and allowing plaque to accumulate. After 10–21 days oral hygiene procedures are reinstated, and the gingivitis resolves over the next 7–10 days. Levels of the marker in GCF are compared at varying time periods from baseline both during the gingivitis promotion phase and the resolution phase.

Experimental gingivitis can also be induced locally by using an acrylic shield to cover the test teeth during oral hygiene procedures. Normal oral hygiene is then carried out with the shield in place, which prevents plaque removal in the test (covered) area. The levels of marker can then also be compared at test and control sites during the experimental period.

The natural disease process

Investigations on the natural disease process are described below. In these studies, samples of the marker are collected from gingival crevice sites in patients with varying stages of chronic periodontitis.

Cross-sectional studies of marker's relationship to disease severity

Subjects for these studies are usually patients with varying levels of chronic periodontitis, ranging from early to advanced stages. They need to have all of their teeth, or at least all their functional molar and premolar teeth. GCF or bacterial samples are taken from all the test sites at one time for each patient, and this time could be different for any of the other patients.

Levels of the marker (total amounts and concentrations in the case of GCF constituents) are then compared with measurements and indices of disease severity and tested for significance by appropriate statistical tests. The usual measurements of disease severity are probing depth, PD, probing attachment level, PAL (probing depth from a fixed reference point), and radiographical measurements of bone loss (see Chapter 12). Indices of gingivitis severity, gingival index (GI) (Löe, 1967) and gingival bleeding index (GBI) (Barnett *et al.*, 1980), and plaque levels, plaque index (PI) (Löe, 1967), are also often compared. Since these studies only relate to one point in time of the disease process, they can only relate to disease severity at that time and give no indication of disease progression. Twenty or more patients are required for these studies for statistical purposes.

Studies of marker levels before and after successful periodontal treatment

These studies usually require patients who have not recently had any periodontal treatment. They need to have varying levels of chronic periodontitis, ranging from early to advanced stages. The subjects need to have all or most of their teeth. Samples are taken at baseline before any measurements are made. The PD and PAL are then measured, and the GI, GBI and PI are scored. The patients then receive a full course of periodontal treatment consisting of oral hygiene instruction and supra- and subgingival scaling and root planing. Four to eight weeks after the completion of this treatment the samples are taken again and the measurements and indices are repeated.

The levels of the marker (total amounts and concentrations in the case of GCF constituents) are compared before and after treatment, and the success of the treatment is measured by similar comparisons of PD, PAL, GI,

GBI and PI. All the comparisons are tested for significance by an appropriate statistical test. Twenty or more patients are required for these studies for statistical purposes.

These studies give additional information to cross-sectional studies, as they indicate whether or not the levels of the marker reduce following disease resolution. They do not, however, relate the marker to disease progression, which is the function of longitudinal studies.

Longitudinal studies of marker's relation to attachment and bone loss

If a potential marker is to be of any use clinically then it must be capable of *predicting* future periodontal attachment loss, and this is definitely tested in a carefully constructed longitudinal study of chronic periodontitis patients. In these studies the level of a marker has to be shown to correlate with confirmed attachment loss, not only at the time that loss is recorded but also at a visit before this (i.e. the predictive time).

The number of patients taking part in such a study must be sufficient for meaningful statistical comparisons, and is usually between 25 and 75. They need to be carefully chosen with regard to the extent and distribution of their periodontal lesions. They should have all or most of their teeth, and a good distribution of moderate to advanced chronic periodontitis lesions. The test teeth are usually the molars and premolars, since the disease on these teeth is more likely to progress. The patients should be fit and well and should not be taking any medication, including antibiotics. They should preferably not smoke, and the patient group should be balanced for age and sex.

Patients in such a study receive standard periodontal treatment, i.e. oral hygiene instruction, supra- and sub-gingival scaling and root planing, prior to the baseline examination visit. At this visit, samples of the marker are first collected from gingival crevicular fluid (GCF) or subgingival plaque and then careful clinical measurements are taken of probing attachment level (PAL) from a fixed reproducible point and probing depth (PD) at the chosen sites of the test teeth. In addition, gingival and plaque indices are usually scored (Löe, 1967; Barnett *et al.*, 1980). Also, the first set of serial radiographs are usually taken to record the alveolar bone levels. In order for serial radiographs to be comparable, the film-to-tooth position and tube geometry must be carefully controlled. This will allow meaningful comparisons of serial films (see Chapter 12). Radiographs are usually taken at yearly intervals in a 2-year study.

The patients are then usually monitored every 3 months over the period of the study, which can be for anything from 6 months to 2 years. Longer studies give more useful results. At each of these visits, further samples of the marker are taken and the clinical measurements are repeated. The patients are monitored for significant changes in attachment and bone levels, and these need to be confirmed to be above the threshold for the method of measurement used.

Assessment of attachment loss

Attachment level change between two points in time is usually assessed retrospectively at the completion of the study by the tolerance method (Haffajee and Socransky, 1986). Duplicate measurements of PAL are taken at each time point to calculate examiner error. The standard deviation (SD) of the duplicate measurements at each site at the first and second time points are pooled to provide the site SD. The difference between all duplicate measurements for all the test sites within each patient are used to compute the patient SD. Patient SDs are then averaged to produce a population SD. For the mean of the second of a pair of attachment level measurements to be considered significantly different from the mean of the first pair, the attachment level change had to exceed:

1. The population threshold, which was 2 population SDs
2. The patient threshold, which was 3 patient SDs
3. The site threshold, which was 3 site SDs.

Measurements of PAL and PD in these studies are usually made with electronic constant pressure probes (see Chapter 12), which are capable of more reliable measurements. These probes have measurement thresholds of 0.3–0.8 mm, compared with 3 mm for manual periodontal probing.

Radiographical measurements

Assessment of progressive bone loss can be made from careful measurements of carefully controlled serial films using conventional radiography (see Chapter 12). A change of 1 mm or more is usually taken as significant. Alternatively, computer-aided systems such as digital subtraction radiology or computer-assisted linear radiography (see Chapter 12) may be used, which are capable of recording smaller changes.

Statistical comparisons

Two types of attachment loss have been identified (Jeffcoat and Reddy, 1991) (see Chapter 8), and these are:

1. Rapid, episodic attachment loss (RAL)
2. Gradual attachment loss (GAL).

Both types may be identified in longitudinal studies using electronic probes with small measurement thresholds, and in this case both types can be compared with the marker. Markers tend to produce better associations with RAL than GAL because of the nature of their temporal patterns.

The levels of the marker must be unknown to the researcher making the attachment level measurements so that the study is blind. Using electronic probes, the attachment level measurements may also be made blind to the clinician by recording them from the computer screen turned away from the clinician making the measurements.

Statistical comparisons are made at the end of the study at both site and patient levels using both total amounts and concentrations of the marker. Site level comparisons can be made between paired attachment loss and non-attachment loss sites. In this case, control and test teeth must be of the same type and must have very closely similar baseline clinical measurements. These comparisons are ideal, because the sites are paired in the same patient and are independent of patient level influences. The alternative is to pool the attachment loss sites and non-attachment loss sites separately and then to compare them with complex statistical techniques. This situation is fraught with difficulties in trying to compensate for huge numerical imbalances and for patient-related effects (Sterne *et al.*, 1990). Because of these factors they need to use multilayer analyses of variance, which are highly complicated. Also, in such a system it is impossible to know the degree of weighting to give to the various patient effects, and therefore this can never be precise. For these reasons, comparisons of test and control sites, paired in each patient, are to be preferred. The site comparisons must be made at both the time of attachment loss and the predictive time.

Both RAL and GAL sites can be compared in this way, but the determination of the predictive time is very difficult with GAL sites because of the long time-scale of slow progressive attachment loss. It is probably best to base the statistical comparisons with GAL sites on either the highest value at the GAL site during the study or on its mean level over the whole period of the study. Also, a critical value (CV) for diagnostic testing (see below) is much more difficult to assign for GAL sites, but could again be based either on an average of the highest values at these sites or an average of their mean levels over the time period of the study. However, it is doubtful if markers are as well suited to the detection of GAL lesions as they may be for RAL lesions.

In addition, the diagnostic efficiency of the marker needs to be tested using 2 × 2 contingency tables (*Figure 13.1*). First, a critical value (CV) for the marker has to

be determined, one for total amount of the marker and one for its concentration, as both need to be tested. They should also be tested at both the attachment loss time and the prediction time. The number of true positive (sites correctly diagnosed as RAL sites by the CV), false positive (sites incorrectly diagnosed as RAL sites by CV), true negative (sites correctly diagnosed as non-attachment loss sites by the CV) and false negative sites (sites incorrectly diagnosed as non-attachment loss sites by the CV) over the course of the study are determined using this value, and are entered into the 2 × 2 table. These data are then used to calculate the sensitivity, specificity and positive and negative prediction values, as shown in *Figure 13.1*.

All these values should be very high using CVs for both total amount and concentration of the marker, and this should be the case at both the attachment loss time and the prediction time for the marker to be clinically useful. However, it is the values at the prediction time that will determine whether or not the marker is capable of predicting periodontal disease activity.

The most importance values are the positive and negative prediction values, as they determine whether the CV for the marker can correctly distinguish between true RAL sites and true non-attachment loss sites. The positive prediction value represents the percentage of RAL sites correctly identified by the CV of the marker, and the negative prediction value the percentage of non-attachment sites correctly identified by the CV of the marker. Both need to be high, but the negative prediction value needs to be close to 100% since diagnosing a RAL site as a non-attachment site would result in under-treatment and hence progression of disease at this site. On the other hand, misdiagnosing a few non-attachment sites as RAL sites would result in slight over-treatment, which would not harm the patient.

In addition, patient level comparisons can back up these findings. In this regard, comparisons of the mean levels in attachment loss and non-attachment loss patients give some indication of patient level effects and also of patient susceptibility.

Development of simplified test system for chairside use

The potential markers are usually detected by laboratory assays in the cross-sectional and longitudinal studies used to assess their efficiency, and these need to be simplified and modified to make an assay system suitable for use in a dental surgery. This involves producing a test kit system, which involves no specialized equipment and is easy to read. In this last regard, colour detection systems are usually preferred.

If the sample is collected with a strip (e.g. GCF), it is preferable that this is uncontaminated by reaction chemicals, which could be irritant, toxic, carcinogenic or allergenic to the patient. Secondly, it is important that any chemicals used in the reaction are in clearly and simply labelled plastic containers from which it is easy to dispense the correct amount.

Most enzyme-linked immunosorbent assay (ELISA)

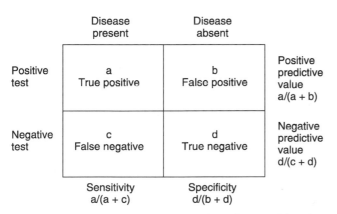

Figure 13.1 Diagnostic testing of critical values of a potential marker using 2 × 2 contingency tables

systems and biochemical and histochemical reactions utilizing simple substrates (see below) are easy to scale down to a simplified kit form, and most commercially available diagnostic kits involve one of these systems. More complicated assay systems are difficult or impossible to scale down, and this may preclude some potentially good markers from being used clinically. Some systems using molecular biological techniques such as DNA test kits for putative periodontal pathogens (see below) involve taking a subgingival plaque sample, transferring this to a transport medium and then mailing this to the laboratory for analysis. These are obviously not as convenient as chairside test systems.

The details of available commercial kit systems are provided in the relevant subsequent part of this series.

Comparison of simplified test system with the laboratory analysis

When the assay system is scaled down to a kit form it is usually only capable of semi-quantitative analysis, and it is necessary to compare the diagnostic accuracy of this system with the full laboratory quantitative analytical system in order to check that the results are closely similar.

Clinical trial

Potential markers that have produced good cross-sectional and longitudinal study results and appear to be capable of predicting periodontal disease activity in research at one centre usually progress to a multicentre trial at several independent centres to see whether their results are comparable. This may either be carried out with the full laboratory quantitative analytical system or with the kit form and semi-quantitative analysis. If the results of these trials are good, then the diagnostic kit may then be tested in the normal clinical environment with a controlled clinical trial in dental practice.

All of these factors should be taken into account in assessing the potential of a new marker system and should also be used in the assessment of the evidence for the potential markers described below.

The main candidates for biomarkers

The main candidates in the search for biomarkers have been:

1. Bacteria and their products
2. Inflammatory and immune products
3. Enzymes released from dead cells
4. Connective tissue degradation products
5. Products of bone resorption.

These will each be considered separately.

Microbiological markers

Bacterial plaque plays a primary role in the initiation and progression of periodontal diseases, but the composition of the subgingival flora is complex and may vary from patient to patient and site to site. Despite these differences and the complex interactions that exist between bacteria and the host, a number of possible pathogens have been suggested on the basis of their association with disease progression and animal pathogenicity, and their possession of virulence factors that could damage the tissues (Genco *et al.*, 1988; Listgarten, 1992; Socransky and Haffajee, 1992). The main bacteria are shown below, and this issue is discussed more fully in Chapters 2 and 4.

Bacteria associated with periodontal diseases

Porphyromonas gingivalis
Prevotella intermedia
Bacteroides forsythus
Actinobacillus actinomycetemcomitans
Capnocytophaga ochracea
Eikenella corrodens
Campylobacter (previously *Wollinella*) *recta*
Fusobacterium nucleatum
Treponema denticola.

These bacteria may be present in the gingival crevice or periodontal pocket, within saliva, or on the surface of the oral mucosa in various parts of the mouth.

There is no evidence for any one specific pathogen in chronic periodontitis, and therefore it may be considered as a non-specific bacterial disease (Theilade, 1986). The bacteria listed above tend to be present in higher numbers at active disease sites (Socransky and Haffajee, 1992), and in some cases produce products capable of damaging the tissues either directly or indirectly. However, they may also be present in healthy and inactive sites, and the composition of all these sites may vary between patients or even in the same patient. Furthermore, the composition of the pocket depends on many factors, including the presence of essential nutrients, the redox potential and the effects of the host defence mechanisms. These considerations may therefore limit the value of diagnostic tests based on bacteria.

Attempts to relate microbiological data to clinical events have proved difficult because of the variability and unreliability of clinical diagnostic methods. Another factor that complicates the quantitative and qualitative assessments of the subgingival flora is the technical difficulty associated with sampling and culturing processes.

Obtaining a bacterial sample

Samples from the oral mucosa or from saliva are usually obtained with sterile paper points or swabs and then transferred directly into an appropriate anaerobic transport medium.

In order to obtain a true sample of subgingival plaque it is first necessary to remove all traces of supragingival plaque, which would otherwise contaminate the sample. The subgingival sample can then be removed, either with a fresh, clean and sterile curette or with a sterile paper point. This is then rapidly transferred to the anaerobic transport medium. It is vitally important not to touch any other surface in making this transfer, since this would also contaminate the sample with unwanted bacteria. The wearing of a fresh mask is also necessary for the same reasons.

Virtually all the subgingival bacteria are anaerobic, and therefore exposure to the air should be minimal. The anaerobic environment of the transport medium is also necessary for this reason, and it should contain all the necessary nutrients for the particular bacteria in question. The nature of the investigation or test will dictate all the other details.

The relationship of bacteria to periodontal disease progression

A microbiologically based diagnostic system should identify one or more primary pathogens responsible for the disease (Listgarten, 1992). It is, however, impossible to determine which bacteria in the subgingival flora of a particular patient are causing periodontal disease, and it seems likely that many species may be involved at different stages of the disease. Nevertheless, certain bacterial species have been considered by some workers as markers of disease because of their association with sites with progressive attachment loss. However, it must be appreciated that these bacteria are not always present in all such sites, and may also be present at stable sites.

Most oral bacteria can be cultured from saliva including the putative periodontal pathogens, *A. actinomycetemcomitans*, *P. gingivalis*, *P. intermedia*, *P. nigrescens*, *C. reta*, *E. corrodens*, *F. nucleatum*, *Capnocytophaga* species and spirochaetes (Van Os *et al.*, 1986; Frisken *et al.*, 1987; Chen *et al.*, 1989; Asikainen *et al.*, 1991, Von Troil Linden *et al.*, 1995, 1997; Muller *et al.*, 1997; Timmerman *et al.*, 1998). One report states that their presence and numbers in saliva reflect their presence and numbers in periodontal pockets (Timmerman *et al.*, 1998), whilst another (Muller *et al.*, 1997) does not. The numbers of these bacteria in saliva increase with age, and are rare in children and healthy young adults and frequent in patients with chronic periodontitis (Matto *et al.*, 1996, 1998). In chronic periodontitis patients, the numbers of particular bacterial species in saliva have been show to correlate with clinical parameters of disease severity and to significantly decrease following periodontal treatment (Von Troil Linden *et al.*, 1995). Specific IgA and IgG antibodies to all these bacteria are found in saliva (Nieminen *et al.*, 1996).

There is accumulated evidence that the predominant microflora of the periodontal pocket at possible active sites, i.e. those that have shown significant attachment and bone loss within short time intervals, is characterized by the presence of *Porphyromonas gingivalis*, *Prevotella intermedia*, *Bacteroides forsythus*, *Peptostreptococcus micros*, *Campylobacter recta*, *Fusobacterium nucleatum* and *Actinobacillus actinomycetemcomitans* (Tanner *et al.*, 1984; Slots *et al.*, 1985, 1986; Dzink *et al.*, 1985, 1988; Moore *et al.*, 1991). Furthermore, retrospective studies (Slots *et al.*, 1986; Bragd *et al.*, 1987; Wennström *et al.*, 1987; Slots and Listgarten, 1988) have suggested that microbiological assays for critical levels of the target bacteria *A. actinomycetemcomitans*, *P. gingivalis* and *P. intermedia* at subgingival sites might be of diagnostic value. However, it should be noted that in these studies the samples were taken after breakdown had occurred, and although they showed an association between the number of these bacteria and previous attachment loss at the site, they were not shown to be predictive of future attachment loss. In another retrospective study (Schmidt *et al.*, 1988), a group of 23 untreated and 13 maintenance patients were monitored with the BANA test (see below). They reported selectivity and sensitivity values of 83% for negative and positive tests in untreated patients. However, the values were much lower on maintained patients and were not diagnostic. Although these studies showed the ability of the test to correctly identify sites pre-defined as healthy or diseased, they were not predictive of future periodontal breakdown.

The numbers of spirochaetes and motile bacteria have been shown to predict future periodontal attachment loss in a 1-year prospective study of patients on maintenance following treatment for periodontitis when no treatment was carried out in the test period (Listgarten and Levin, 1981). However, they were not predictive when patients were scaled every 3 months during a 3-year study (Listgarten *et al.*, 1986). Furthermore, when *A. actinomycetemcomitans*, *P. gingivalis* and *P. intermedia* were tested as predictors of future periodontal attachment loss in a similar 3-year study of patients on regular maintenance, they were not shown to have any diagnostic potential (Listgarten *et al.*, 1991).

Bacterial species numbers may be determined in a variety of ways, which vary in selectivity and sensitivity (Listgarten, 1992). These include the following methods.

Darkground or phase contrast microscopy

The main advantage of these techniques is the ability to count all the bacteria in the sample, and the main drawbacks are the inability to speciate micro-organisms or determine their relative susceptibility to antimicrobial agents. However, studies using these techniques have shown that in gingival health there is a scant subgingival flora of cocci and non-motile rods, whilst in gingivitis there is the appearance of motile rods and spirochaetes, and in periodontitis a vast increase in these morphotypes, with particularly large numbers of spirochaetes (Listgarten and Levin, 1981; Listgarten, 1986).

Culture techniques

These techniques are able to analyse the nature of the micro-organisms in a sample since they can be speciated with a variety of laboratory-based methods, including selective subcultures, biochemical tests, SDS PAGE, gene probes, ribotyping, DNA fingerprinting and cell wall long chain fatty acid analysis (Genco *et al.*, 1986; Greenstein, 1988). Their susceptibility to antimicrobials can also be tested. However, not all bacteria can be readily cultured, and the proportional recovery of cultivable species is unlikely to match their proportions in the periodontal pocket. Also, the use of selective media will restrict the species that are able to grow (Mandell and Socransky, 1981).

Immunological assays

The use of immunological techniques such as immuno-fluorescence (Zambon *et al.*, 1985b; Zambon *et al.*, 1986) or enzyme-linked immunosorbent assay, ELISA (Ebersole *et al.*, 1984), can detect individual bacterial species. These have proved useful to detect the presence and relative proportions of selected bacterial species. These techniques use specific antibodies that bind to the selected bacterial antigens and are then detected by labelling the primary antibody directly with a fluorescent marker (direct immunofluorescence) (*Figure 13.2a*) or with a fluorescent secondary antibody (indirect immuno-fluorescence) (*Figure 13.2b*). In the ELISA assay (*Figure 13.2c*) the primary antibody is detected through a colorimetric reaction, which is catalysed through an enzyme (usually horseradish peroxidase or alkaline phosphatase) linked to the antibody. These techniques are very specific if controls are used to check for non-specific reactions. They can only detect species for which an antibody is available.

DNA probes

In recent years, DNA probes have been developed to identify nucleotide sequences that are specific for bacteria believed to be of diagnostic significance (Highfield and Dougan, 1985), including suspected periodontal pathogens (French *et al.*, 1986; Savitt *et al.*, 1988; Loesche, 1992). These probes can detect as few as 103 cells in a sample, and provide information on the presence of selected species in the sample. However, they cannot provide reliable quantitative data and are limited by the availability of probes. They are totally specific, and it is possible for a species to be present in large numbers in the sample and not be detected because it was not specifically sought.

Enzyme-based assays

BANA assays

Another approach to the detection of selected bacterial species is to look for an enzyme that is unique to one or

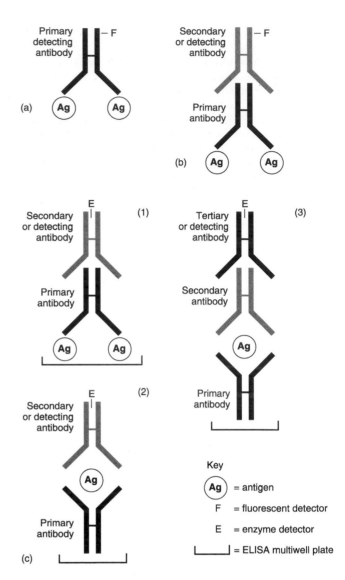

Figure 13.2 Diagrams showing the basis of: *(a)* direct immunofluorescence; *(b)* indirect immunofluorescence using a secondary antibody; *(c)* an enzyme-linked immunosorbent (ELISA) assay: (1) indirect ELISA, (2) sandwich ELISA with third detecting antibody (3). In ELISA techniques the detecting antibody is linked to an enzyme, usually horseradish peroxidase or alkaline phosphatase, which catalyses a chain reaction that generates colour

more of the relevant bacterial species. The plaque sample is exposed to a substrate that can only be hydrolysed by a specific enzyme. An example of this method is the detection of the trypsin-like protease. This protease is produced mainly by *Porphyromonas gingivalis* and to a much lesser extent by *Bacteroides forsythus* and *Treponema denticola*, and hydrolyses benzyl arginine naphthylamide, BANA (Loesche, 1986; Loesche *et al.*, 1990; Loesche, 1992). Since some of these species grow poorly in cultures and account for a significant proportion of the protease activity of the subgingival flora, these enzyme assays provide a rapid and inexpensive method of screening samples for these bacteria.

The main drawbacks are a lack of quantitative data and the inability to determine which of the three bacteria are responsible for the enzyme production. In most cases, however, this will be *Porphyromonas gingivalis*, since this produces much more of this protease than the two other bacteria combined (Gazi *et al.*, 1994; Gazi *et al.*, 1996). Also, the BANA system does not include inhibitors of host proteinases, which could cleave this substrate and could also contaminate the bacterial sample tested (Cox and Eley, 1989a, 1989b, 1989c).

Quantitative fluorescence polarization

Molecules tagged with a fluorescent label emit fluorescent light in the same polarized plane when excited with plane polarized light, provided that the molecule remains stationary throughout the excited state. Instruments (FPM-1™FP analyser, Jolley Consulting and Research Inc., Grayslake, IL) have been developed to measure this in real-time (Schade *et al.*, 1996; Jolley, 1996). Labelled proteins have enough mass to rotate only slightly, and the emitted light that is measured from them remains polarized. After addition of proteolytic enzymes the millipolarization value (mP) drops with time, since the labelled small molecules that result from degradation produce enough kinetic movement to depolarize the light and thus reduce the mP value. A fluorescent moiety 4,4'-difluoro-5,7-dimethyl-4-boro-3a,4a-diaza-s-indacene-3-propionic acid, succinimidyl ester (BODIPY FL C3-SE, Molecular Probes-Inc. – BODIPY®) has been linked to a protein substrate, bovine casein, to produce a suitable fluorescent substrate for this purpose (Schade *et al.*, 1996; Jolley, 1996) They have also shown that these assays can be carried out in the presence of whole bacteria.

This method has been used to detect *Mycobacterium bovis* extracellular protein (Lin *et al.*, 1996) and could be adapted to measure proteins or protease from plaque bacteria. It will thus measure protease activity from any of the plaque bacteria that produce enzymes that can cleave casein.

However, this technique might be difficult to scale down and simplify for use in dental practice.

Volatile sulphur compounds

Volatile sulphur compounds such as hydrogen sulphide, H_2S, methyl mercaptan, CH_3SH, dimethyl sulphide, $(CH_3)_2S$, and dimethyl disulphide, $(CH_3)_2S_2$, are all toxic by-products of Gram negative anaerobic bacterial metabolism of sulphur-containing amino acids (see Chapter 5). *Porphyromonas gingivalis*, *Prevotella intermedia*, *Prevotella melaninogenica*, *Bacteroides forsythus*, *Treponema denticola* and *Fusobacterium nucleatum* have all been shown to be capable of producing them through their metabolic pathways (Persson *et al.*, 1989a, 1990).

A recently developed commercially available instrument, Diamond Probe/Perio 2000 System® (Diamond General Development Corporation, Ann Arbor, USA), has been designed so that it combines the features of a periodontal probe with the detection of volatile sulphur compounds in the periodontal pocket.

In this regard, it has been found that the levels of volatile sulphur compounds in the periodontal pocket are higher in chronic periodontitis patients than healthy controls (Yaegaki and Sanda, 1992a, 1992b). A number of other studies have indicated that sulphide levels are higher in deeper pockets than in shallow ones, and decrease when pockets are surgically reduced (Horowitz and Folke, 1972; Yaegaki and Sanda, 1992a, 1992b). The sulphide readings of the probe have also been shown to relate to clinical parameters of disease severity (Polychronopoulou, 1998). However, clinical relevance of these results was hampered by the finding that the sensitivity of the probe was poor at both the low and high ranges of its scale. This resulted in the majority of the readings at both apparently healthy and diseased sites being zero. The sensitivity would need to be improved for this instrument to be suitable for clinical use. Furthermore, there are no longitudinal studies of the relationship of volatile sulphur compounds to periodontal disease progression and, therefore, its diagnostic potential is unknown.

Bacterial proteases in saliva and GCF

Saliva

Whole, non-stimulated saliva sample is required for the detection of bacterial enzymes in this situation.

A trypsin-like protease can be detected in saliva, and the levels of this enzyme correlates with clinical indices of disease severity and also reduces following periodontal treatment (Zambon *et al.*, 1985a; Nieminen *et al.*, 1993a). However, it has been shown (Ingman *et al.*, 1993) that this enzyme (or enzymes) does not have all the biochemical properties of the *P. gingivalis* trypsin-like protease, gingivain. The enzyme(s) detected in saliva could therefore either be of host origin or a mixture of host and bacterial derived enzymes.

GCF

Bacterial proteases are released into the pocket and can be detected in GCF (Cox *et al.*, 1989a). Selective biochemical assays have been developed for both bacterial dipeptidylpeptidase (DPP) and trypsin-like proteases, and can distinguish them from interfering tissue-derived proteases (Eley and Cox, 1994; Gazi *et al.*, 1995). The trypsin-like protease detected by this assay is a cysteine proteinase, and has the characteristics of the enzyme now called arg-gingivain or arg-gingipain (see Chapter 5). These enzymes correlate positively with clinical indices of disease severity, and reduce significantly following periodontal treatment (Eley and Cox, 1995a).

A 2-year longitudinal study of GCF bacterial DPP and arg-gingivain/arg-gingipain in 75 patients has recently been completed (Eley and Cox, 1996a). It used both site, patient and population thresholds for probing attachment loss measured with a Florida electronic probe and radiological measurements for confirmed progressive attachment loss. All clinical parameters and enzyme levels significantly reduced following basic periodontal treatment prior to baseline. Over the 2 years there were 124 sites in 49 patients with confirmed attachment loss, giving an annual rate of 5.17% of sites. Ninety-one of these sites in 36 patients were rapid episodic attachment loss (RAL), and 33 sites in 22 patients showed gradual progressive attachment loss over a longer time period (GAL).

Levels above critical values chosen for both bacterial DPP and arg-gingivain for total enzyme activities and enzyme concentrations were present at all RAL sites both at the time of attachment loss and 3 months previously (predictive time). They were all significantly higher than values at control sites in the same patients. These levels were also shown to be predictive of attachment loss in diagnostic testing. In this regard, the values for arg-gingivain were somewhat higher overall than those for bacterial DPP. The values for arg-gingivain were 100% (sensitivity) and 99.93% (specificity) for both total enzyme activity and enzyme concentration. The values for bacterial DPP were 100% (sensitivity) and 99.54% (specificity) for total enzyme activity, and 100% (sensitivity) and 99.57% (specificity) for enzyme concentration. The differences can be seen more clearly in the positive and negative predictive values calculated in these tests for the two bacterial proteases. The values were 93.81% (positive prediction) and 100% (negative prediction) for arg-gingivain, and 60.81% (positive prediction) and 100% (negative prediction) for bacterial DPP.

The mean levels over the 2 years and the highest recorded levels at GAL sites were also both above their respective critical values, and were statistically significantly higher than those values at control sites in the same patients for both enzymes. In addition, all comparisons of mean patient values in patients with or without attachment loss were highly statistically significant.

Thus, GCF arg-gingivain/arg-gingipain appears to be an excellent predictor and GCF DPP a moderately good predictor of future progressive attachment loss. A test system (see details in following section) suitable for chairside use has been developed (Cox *et al.*, 1990), and has been shown to produce similar results to the laboratory system.

Commercial diagnostic test kits

Diagnostic test kits based on some of these systems have already been marketed. However, some of them have been marketed before verifiable evidence of their predictive ability to detect periodontal attachment loss has been shown. They use either paper point or curette bacterial sampling from the pocket, and include the following.

Evalusite (Kodak)

This is a number of enzyme-linked immunosorbent assays (ELISA) (*Figure 13.2c*) using antibodies to detect antigens for *P. gingivalis*, *P. intermedius* and *A. actinomycetemcomitans*. The reactions are carried out in a simple chairside reaction kit. Subgingival plaque samples are reacted with the antibodies and detection substrate in a multiwell reaction dish.

Omnigene (OmniGene, Inc.) and BTD (Biotechnica Diagnostics, Inc.)

These are DNA probe systems for a number of subgingival bacteria. A paper point sample of subgingival plaque is placed in the container provided and mailed off to the company for assay. Probes are available for *A. actinomycetemcomitans*, *P. gingivalis*, *P. intermedius*, *E. corrodens*, *F. nucleatum*, *C. recta*, *T. denticola* and *T. pectinovorum*.

Perioscan (Oral-B Laboratories)

This is a chairside test kit system that utilizes the BANA (BzArgNA) test for bacterial trypsin-like proteases. These are mainly produced by *P. gingivalis*, but lesser amounts are also produced by *B. forsythus* and *T. denticola*. A subgingival plaque sample is reacted in the kit with the substrate linked to a colour detection system. The system is particularly simple to use.

Diamond Probe/Perio 2000 System® (Diamond General Development Corporation, Ann Arbor, USA)

A recently developed commercially available instrument, Diamond Probe/Perio 2000 System® (Diamond General Development Corporation, Ann Arbor, USA) has been designed so that it combines the features of a periodontal probe with the detection of volatile sulphur compounds in the periodontal pocket. However, since there are no longitudinal studies of the relationship of volatile sulphur compounds with progressive periodontitis, its diagnostic potential is unknown.

Potential diagnostic tests worthy of development

Bacterial proteases in GCF

A test system suitable for chairside use has been developed in the research laboratory of one of the authors, in conjunction with researchers from Enzyme System Products/Prototek, Dublin, California, USA (Cox *et al.*, 1990), and this can be used to detect the bacterial proteases arg-gingivain/gingipain and DPP in GCF. It is fully described in the section below on hydrolytic and proteolytic host enzymes.

The commercial firms owning these tests are constantly changing because some of them sell the rights to their products to others. For this reason, names of the firms cited as owning these tests may not remain accurate.

Advantages and disadvantages of diagnostic tests using bacteria and their products

Advantages

The possible advantages are listed and described below:

- Some markers appear to be predictive of disease activity in longitudinal studies, e.g. GCF bacterial proteases
- The commercial tests are simple to use
- Results of chairside test kits are available in a short time
- Chairside test kits produce a visual result, which can be shown to the patient.

All of the markers used in these test systems have been shown to be associated with active sites on a retrospective basis, and some (e.g. GCF bacterial proteases) appear to be predictive of disease activity in longitudinal studies. The chairside tests are simple to use, and their results are available within a relatively short time. They also produce a visual result, which can be shown to the patient and related to the site from which they were obtained.

Disadvantages

The main disadvantages are listed and described below:

- The polymicrobial nature of the disease makes diagnosis difficult
- Most tests are not predictive of disease activity
- It is necessary to know which site to sample
- The tests only detect the bacteria that you look for
- Some need to be sent away to a special laboratory
- Cost.

Polymicrobial nature of the disease

The subgingival flora is complex and may vary slightly from site to site and patient to patient, and no single pathogen can be shown to be the cause of chronic periodontitis (see above). The putative periodontal pathogens that have been shown to be associated with progressing sites on a retrospective basis vary in proportion at both active and stable sites. It is therefore difficult to choose the particular bacterial species to assay as a marker in any particular case.

Predictive ability of bacterial markers

Several putative periodontal pathogens have been shown to be associated with active sites (see above), but none have been shown to be predictive of periodontal disease activity. The BANA test for bacterial trypsin-like activity

has been tested for its predictive ability in a clinical setting in a multicentre trial (Loesche *et al.*, 1990). It has been shown to correlate well with ELISA test detection of *P. gingivalis*, *B. forsythus* and *T. denticola*, but it has relatively poor predictive abilities for periodontal disease activity.

The only bacterial factors that have so far been shown to have good predictive ability (Eley and Cox, 1996a) are GCF arg-gingivain/arg-gingipain and bacterial dipeptidyl peptidases (DPPs). In this respect, GCF arg-gingivain/arg-gingipain gave the best results in diagnostic testing (see above). A chairside diagnostic testing system has been designed for these bacterial enzymes (Cox *et al.*, 1990), but this is not yet commercially available.

Which site to sample

It is not possible to sample all the sites in the mouth with any diagnostic test system, and therefore the site(s) to be tested have to be preselected. This usually means testing sites that already show clinical signs of previous attachment loss. Whilst these sites are slightly more likely to progress than other sites, the pattern of progression of periodontitis is very irregular and unpredictable. This may make the choice of sites difficult.

Which bacteria to select as markers

All genetic and antibody detection systems are entirely specific, and will thus only detect the sequence or antigen against which they are directed. Therefore, all DNA probes (Highfield and Dougan, 1985; French *et al.*, 1986; Savitt *et al.*, 1988) and ELISA-based detection systems (Ebersole *et al.*, 1984) will only detect the specific bacterial species against which they are directed. One would therefore need to decide which specific bacterial species one wishes to detect before deciding on the test system to use. This choice is difficult, because there are 12 or more putative periodontal pathogens whose proportions may vary from site to site and from patient to each patient.

In this regard, the use of bacterial protease markers is less specific. The BANA test (Loesche *et al.*, 1990) detects proteases from *P. gingivalis*, *B. forsythus* and *T. denticola*, but the majority of this activity comes from *P. gingivalis*. In respect of GCF bacterial proteases (Cox and Eley, 1989a, 1989b, 1989c; Cox *et al.*, 1992a; Gazi *et al.*, 1993; Eley and Cox, 1995; Eley and Cox, 1996a; Gazi *et al.*, 1996), these are detected with selective assay systems and thus the situation is a little different. The trypsin-like protease (arg-gingivain) detected in the clinical studies (Eley and Cox, 1995b; Eley and Cox, 1996a) is specific for the enzyme from *P. gingivalis*. In contrast, the bacterial DPPs are produced by *P. gingivalis*, *P. intermedia* and *Capnocytophaga* species, and the assay system used detected all of these proteases.

Special laboratory required

Samples for DNA probe testing (Highfield and Dougan, 1985; French *et al.*, 1986; Savitt *et al.*, 1988) of bacterial species have to be sent away to a special laboratory, and this has two main disadvantages. First, samples may deteriorate during transit; to minimize this problem, the companies offering this service provide transport vessels and media. Secondly, the result is delayed and is not available to the dentist or patient on the day of the appointment.

Cost

All diagnostic test systems are expensive, and in this regard they cannot be used in NHS practice without incurring a financial loss. The cost of the kit and the time involved in taking, reacting and reading the sample would need to be added directly to the patient's bill. The costs are relatively high, because one is paying both for the manufacturing, service and profit costs and for the development costs of the system. With respect to the relative cost of each system, the DNA probe service is the most expensive and the ELISA and BANA systems the least expensive.

Inflammatory and immune markers

There is no doubt that the bacteria in dental plaque and the subgingival flora are the primary cause of periodontal disease (see Chapters 2 and 4). However, these bacteria also trigger inflammatory and immune host responses which, along with the direct effects of the bacteria, cause most of the tissue destruction (Genco, 1992). A number of substances are released from inflammatory and immune cells into the tissues, and many of these pass into gingival crevicular fluid (GCF) and are thus easily available for analysis (Page, 1992; Lamster, 1992). Samples of these substances can usually be obtained from paper strip GCF samples.

The substances released by inflammatory and immune cells during the disease process include antibodies (immunoglobulin, Ig), complement proteins, inflammatory mediators such as prostaglandin (PG), and the pro-inflammatory cytokines such as the various interleukins (IL) and tumour necrosis factor (TNF). Those of possible relevance to periodontal pathology are listed below.

Immune response	Antibody
	Total IgG and IgG subgroups
	Complement
Inflammatory mediators	Arachidonic acid
	derivatives, e.g. PGE_2
	Cytokines, e.g. IL-1, IL-6

Sampling of saliva

A whole non-stimulated saliva sample is usually required, since it will contain factors from the salivary glands, factors from oral bacteria growing within it and factors from the gingival crevicular fluid that flow into it. The sample can usually be spat into a suitable sterile container

and then processed according to the requirements of the potential marker of interest.

Sampling of gingival crevicular fluid

Gingival crevicular fluid (GCF) is an exudate that can be harvested from the gingival crevice or periodontal pocket using either filter paper strips (*Figure 13.3*) or micropipette tubes. As the fluid traverses the inflamed tissue it may pick up enzymes and other molecules that participate in the disease process. It can also pick up the products of cell and tissue degradation. Therefore, it offers great potential as a source of factors that may be associated with disease activity.

The exact placement of the sampling device and the collection time are of great importance, since they influence the composition of GCF collected (Curtis *et al.*, 1988; Page, 1992). Placement of a sampling device into the crevice or pocket induces a steady flow of exudate, whilst repeat sampling depletes GCF volume and harvested components per unit of time. Lengthy sampling periods, particularly with micropipette tubes, will sample mainly inflammatory exudate from vessels rather than the contents of the crevice. The procedure adopted varies for the particular components of interest and its method of analysis, but there is general agreement that the method of choice is the one that causes the least interference with the site and takes the shortest time to harvest fluid prior to sampling. Thus, sampling for 30 seconds or less by the placement of paper strips at the orifice of the site seems to be ideal, provided it ensures a sample of sufficient size to analyse with the technique used.

Correlation of host factors with disease

Subgingival temperature

The hyperaemia associated with inflammation increases the local temperature of the part affected and is one of the

Figure 13.3 Chromatography paper strips collecting gingival crevicular fluid (GCF) from the mesiobuccal surfaces of the lower right premolars and molars

cardinal signs of inflammation. A device called Perio-temp® (Abio Dent, Danvers, MA, USA) has been developed to measure small changes in the sublingual and subgingival temperature, and increased subgingival temperature has been positively correlated with increased pocket depths, decreased attachment levels, clinical parameters of gingival inflammation, higher proportions of putative periodontal pathogens and gingival crevicular fluid enzymes (Haffajee *et al.*, 1992a, 1992b, 1992c; Dinsdale *et al.*, 1997; Wolff *et al.*, 1997). Both the sublingual and subgingival temperatures have also been found to be significantly higher in smokers compared to non-smokers (Dinsdale *et al.*, 1997).

One longitudinal study of the relationship between subgingival temperature and progressive attachment loss has been carried out (Haffajee *et al.*, 1992a, 1992b, 1992c). Twenty-nine chronic periodontitis subjects had clinical parameters and subgingival temperature measured at six sites per tooth every 2 months. Differences between sublingual and subgingival temperatures were also recorded. Attachment loss greater than 2.5 mm occurred at one or more sites at 16 of the 49 subject visits. Elevated mean subgingival temperature was related to subsequent attachment loss, particularly in individuals who exhibited more than one progressive site. The odds ratio of a subject exhibiting new attachment loss at one site was 14.5, and at two or more sites was 64.0 if the subject's mean subgingival temperature exceeded 35.5°C. Subjects with high subgingival temperature and widespread previous attachment loss appeared to be at the greatest risk for new attachment loss. Using diagnostic testing, a sensitivity and specificity of 75% and 76% respectively was found.

Humoral immune response

Patients with various forms of periodontal disease produce antibodies to antigens from periodontopathic bacteria (Lamster, 1992; Page, 1992). These antibodies can be detected in serum, saliva, gingival tissue and GCF.

Secretory immunoglobulin A (sIgA) is actively secreted into saliva, and IgG and M pass into saliva mainly from GCF (Macotte and Lavoie, 1998). Levels of salivary IgG and IgA and specific antibody are very low in healthy patients, and there is an increase in salivary IgG in 34% of moderate and 57% of advanced periodontitis patients (Sandholm and Gronblad, 1984; Sandholm *et al.*, 1987). Specific IgA antibody to *Actinobacillus actinomycetemcomitans* is present in the saliva of refractory periodontitis patients (Nieminen *et al.*, 1993b, 1996). However, the level of this specific antibody has only been found to be raised in 19% of chronic periodontitis patients (Sandholm *et al.*, 1987). In addition, it has been shown that the serum and saliva concentrations of IgG and IgA reduce following periodontal treatment of chronic periodontitis patients, probably because of a reduction in the antigenic stimulus (Reiff, 1984). This reduction is more pronounced in early periodontitis than in more advanced cases.

In GCF, the total amount of immunoglobulin (Ig) positively correlates with that from adjacent gingival tissue. This shows that both serum and locally produced antibody contributes to that in GCF.

The relationship of GCF antibodies to periodontal status has been studied in various ways (Page, 1992). These include measuring the total amount of Ig, the relative amounts of IgG subclasses and specific antibody titres to antigens from various periodontal bacteria. These relationships are complex and difficult to interpret.

The total Ig in GCF does not correlate with disease severity or progression, and indeed may be lower at progressive sites (Page, 1992; Lamster, 1992). There has been one report (Reinhardt *et al.*, 1989) that compared IgG subclasses in GCF at progressive and stable sites. It found that the concentrations of IgG1 and IgG4 subclasses were significantly higher at progressive sites.

Numerous studies (Page, 1992; Lamster, 1992) have compared specific antibodies, titres to antigens from periodontal bacteria with periodontal disease status, but these have found no correlation between them. The relationship of specific antibodies in GCF to those in serum is also complex, with some being higher and some lower, with considerable variation from patient to patient and site to site in sequential measurement at the same site.

Thus, specific antibody or total Ig in GCF appears to be of no use in distinguishing between stable and active sites. Furthermore, some evidence suggests that a reduction in specific antibody in serum and consequently GCF in patients with existing disease can place them at risk for further disease progression (Lamster, 1992). This relationship has been demonstrated in juvenile periodontitis and acute necrotizing ulcerative gingivitis. Specific antibodies in the gingival tissues and serum are important in modulating the pathology of periodontal diseases but, with the present level of knowledge, do not offer a means of identifying patients at risk for active disease.

Complement

Complement is a battery of nine (or more) related proteins which join together sequentially in an enzyme-mediated cascade (*Figure 13.4*). The major components can be divided into a recognition unit, C1, in the classical pathway, an activation unit, C4, C2, C3, and the membrane units, C5 through to C9. The complement cascade is initiated by the combination of specific immunoglobulin and the first complement component, C1. It can also be activated by the alternative pathway by other factors, such as endotoxin (lipopolysaccharide, LPS) from the cell walls of Gram negative bacteria. The final product of the cascade is an esterase, which damages or lyses the cell walls of bacteria. Two intermediary products of the cascade, C3a and C5a, attach to receptor sites on mast cells and inflammatory cells. They release histamine and other pro-inflammatory substances from mast cells and prostaglandins from inflammatory cells. These released substances increase vascular permeability.

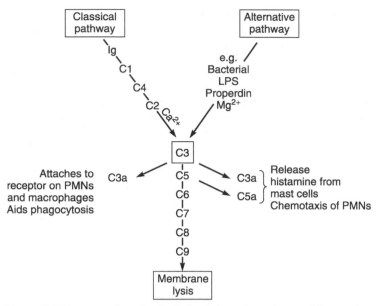

Figure 13.4 Diagram to show the classical and alternative pathways of the complement cascade

They are also chemotactic for polymorphonuclear neutrophil leucocytes (PMNs). C3a also aids phagocytosis by attaching the antigen to the phagocyte via the C3 receptor on the surface of PMNs, monocytes and macrophages.

Complement proteins are present in GCF from sites with inflammation, and the split fragments C3 and Factor B have been detected during experimental gingivitis (Patters *et al.*, 1989). However, none of these factors has been shown to be associated with disease activity.

Cellular immune response

As periodontal disease is a chronic condition, it is not surprising that activation of the cellular immune mechanism is a feature of periodontal pathology. Neopterin is a well-established marker of the immune system, and its concentrations in body fluids have been used as an indication of its degree of activation. In this regard it has been recently shown that neopterin concentrations in saliva significantly correlated with the number of teeth with deep pockets in the mouth. Also, when the patients were grouped according to the median number of diseased teeth, the group with 1–20 diseased teeth had significantly higher neopterin concentrations than the group with more than 20 (Vrecko *et al.*, 1997).

Cytokines

Cytokines are best described as cell-to-cell messengers or local hormones. They are all small proteins or peptides that are produced and released by one cell type so that they can link onto a specific receptor on the cell membrane of another cell(s) of either the same type or another type(s). Attachment to the receptor switches on a particular intracellular messenger system in the cell, which leads to a particular function. The best known examples of cytokines are the interleukins (IL), which pass messages between the leucocytes. However, cytokines are involved in the cell-to-cell communications of most if not all cells in the body and are present in all tissues and body fluids, including serum, saliva and GCF. The cell source, target cells and the main action(s) of the common cytokines of relevance to periodontal diseases are shown in Table 3.1 in Chapter 3.

Saliva

The only potential marker in this class investigated in saliva is platelet activation factor (PAF), which stimulates the activities and production of platelets. Salivary PAF levels have been found to be significantly higher in untreated chronic periodontitis patients compared to controls (Rasch *et al.*, 1995; Garito *et al.*, 1995). Its levels correlate with clinical indices of disease severity and the extent of disease, and also significantly reduce following periodontal treatment.

GCF

Interleukin (IL)-1 and tumour necrosis factor alpha (TNFα) are produced by activated macrophages and other cells and have pro-inflammatory effects of relevance to periodontal pathology, which include the stimulation of PGE$_2$ and collagenase production. Since monoclonal antibodies have been produced for these cytokines, they can be measured by ELISA and may therefore have potential for use in a clinical test system.

IL-1α and β are present in inflamed gingiva (Hönig *et al.*, 1989). They are also present in GCF from patients with periodontitis with extremely low concentrations at healthy sites (Masada *et al.*, 1990). Their levels are reduced following scaling and root planing, but did not correlate with probing depth measurements. The amount of IL-1β in GCF also correlated with messenger RNA in adjacent gingival tissue.

TNFα is also present in GCF, but does not correlate with probing depth or gingival inflammation, and its total amount was inversely related to tissue inflammation (Rossomando *et al.*, 1990).

The levels of IL-1 and IL-6 in refractory periodontitis have also been studied (Reinhardt *et al.*, 1993). There were no significant differences in the mean level of IL-1 in refractory or stable patients, but refractory sites produced significantly more IL-6.

A recent study (Lee *et al.*, 1995a) has measured the levels of of IL-1β, IL-2, IL-4, IL-6 and TNFα in GCF by ELISA assays. Their levels at active and inactive sites in 10 patients with refractory periodontitis were compared in a short 3-month longitudinal study. Active sites were defined as those sites that lost $\geqslant 2$ mm of attachment, measured with a Florida probe (see Chapter 12), over the 3 months of the study. According to these criteria there were 8 active and 12 inactive sites. The active sites had significantly higher levels of IL-2 and IL-6 than inactive sites at both baseline and the 3-month visit. This suggests that these cytokines might both predict and associate with progressive attachment loss. Also, the levels of IL-1β were significantly higher at active sites at 3 months, but not at baseline. This suggests that this cytokine might associate with but not predict progressive attachment loss.

The investigators also used subtraction radiology (see Chapter 12) to detect alveolar bone loss over the 3 months, and found that sites with bone loss had significantly higher levels of IL-1β and IL-2 than sites with no evidence of bone loss.

This study suggests that IL-2 and IL-6, and possibly IL-1β, may be predictive of future attachment loss in refractory periodontitis. However, the level of predictive ability of these cytokines is unclear because the numbers of true and false positive and negative sites were not calculated in this study and not related in a diagnostic test. This is probably because the small number of active and inactive sites in this study precludes the use of this method of analysis in a meaningful way. Thus the true relationship of these cytokines to periodontal disease activity will only become clearer with another longitudinal study over a longer time period and using greater numbers of chronic periodontitis patients.

Since this is the only longitudinal study to date of GCF cytokines, it is at present unclear as to whether they are of diagnostic use.

Prostaglandins

Prostaglandin E$_2$ (PGE$_2$) has pro-inflammatory and immunoregulatory effects, and its concentration in gingival tissue is sufficient to elicit significant effects on cell responses and functions (Offenbacher *et al.*, 1993). In bone organ culture (see Chapter 5) it stimulates osteoclastic bone resorption. It may thus play a significant role in periodontal pathology.

There is a great deal of evidence that correlates PGE$_2$ levels in the periodontal tissues and GCF to the severity of periodontal disease. PGE$_2$ levels are low in health and non-detectable at many sites (Offenbacher *et al.*, 1993). In naturally occurring gingivitis there is a modest rise in GCF PGE$_2$ levels to about 32 ng/ml, and a higher rise (about 53 ng/ml) in experimental gingivitis. Untreated periodontitis patients have significantly higher levels than gingivitis patients.

In one study, following scaling and root planing the periodontitis patients were divided into two groups, those that experienced no further attachment loss and those that experienced one or more sites of $\geqslant 3$ mm of attachment loss (Offenbacher *et al.*, 1986). At this time the group that experienced no further attachment loss in the study period had mean GCF PGE$_2$ levels that were significantly lower than the group with attachment loss, and were similar to those with untreated gingivitis. In contrast, the group that experienced significant attachment loss at one or more sites in the following 6 months had significantly higher mean GCF PGE$_2$ levels of 113 ng/ml. This observation is the basis of the claim that GCF PGE$_2$ is predictive for periodontal disease activity (Offenbacher *et al.*, 1986).

Levels greater than 66 ng/ml were found to be predictive of further possible loss of attachment, and this level was used as a cut-off value in a positive and negative screening test. This gave a sensitivity of 0.76, a specificity of 0.96 and an overall predictive value of 0.92–0.95 (Offenbacher *et al.*, 1993). This shows that it could be predictive of periodontal disease activity.

Although GCF PGE$_2$ has considerable potential as a screening test for periodontal activity, strangely no commercial efforts are currently underway to develop one.

Diagnostic tests

Commercial diagnostic tests

A commercial device, Periotemp® (Abio Dent, Danvers, MA, USA), has been developed to measure small changes in the subgingival temperature, and positive cross-sectional comparisons with clinical parameters have been found. One longitudinal study of the relationship between subgingival temperature and progressive attachment loss has also been carried out (Haffajee *et al.*, 1992a, 1992b, 1992c), and a positive relationship between them has been found.

Potential diagnostic tests worthy of development

Although GCF PGE$_2$ has considerable potential as a screening test for periodontal activity, no commercial efforts are currently underway to develop one. In this regard, it is now possible to assay GCF PGE$_2$ with an ELISA assay utilizing a monoclonal rabbit anti-PGE$_2$ antibody (Nakashima *et al.*, 1994). This technique could be simply modified to develop a diagnostic test system suitable for clinical use.

Cytokines are also assayed using ELISA techniques, which could be developed into chairside kits. However, at present the predictive ability of these markers is still in doubt. Thus, the most likely diagnostic marker of the inflammatory and immune factors described above is GCF PGE$_2$.

Advantages and disadvantages of diagnostic tests using inflammatory mediators

Advantages

The main advantages are listed below:

- Only one mediator, GCF PGE$_2$, has been shown to be predictive of disease activity in longitudinal studies
- ELISA techniques can be used to detect cytokines and PGE$_2$, which could be developed into chairside kits that are simple to use
- ELISAs can be read after a short time
- They can be shown to the patient and related to the tooth site.

GCF PGE$_2$ is the best candidate for a marker in this group.

Disadvantages

The main disadvantages are listed and discussed below:

- The choice of the most appropriate biomarker may still be difficult with the present state of knowledge
- There is difficulty in determining the sites to sample and when to sample them
- If a moiety is associated with inflammation, this may mask its association with destructive disease
- Cost.

The choice of the most appropriate biomarker
Only GCF PGE$_2$ has been shown to be predictive, and IL-2 and IL-6 and possibly IL-1β show promise in this regard. However, in all cases further research is need to confirm this.

Determining the sites to sample and when to sample them
It is obviously not possible to sample all the sites in the mouth with any diagnostic test system, and for this reason the site(s) to be tested have to be preselected. This usually means testing sites that already show clinical signs of previous attachment loss, since these sites are slightly more likely to progress than other sites. However, the pattern of progression of periodontitis is very irregular and unpredictable, and this may make the choice of sites difficult.

Association of the marker with inflammation
All the inflammatory mediators are associated with gingival inflammation, and this association could produce false association with disease activity. It is therefore very important to show that a potential marker has a true association with periodontal disease activity that is independent of and stronger than any association it may have with gingival inflammation.

Cost
All diagnostic test systems are relatively expensive and for this reason cannot be used in NHS practice without incurring financial loss. The cost of the kit and time involved in obtaining, reacting and reading the sample(s) would need to be added to the patient's bill.

Hydrolytic enzymes of tissue origin

Inflammation leads to the accumulation of polymorphonuclear neutrophil leucocytes (PMNs), macrophages, lymphocytes and mast cells, which are very important in protecting the body against infection. The inflammatory cells contain destructive enzymes within their lysosomes, which are normally used to degrade phagocytosed material. These enzymes are, however, capable of degrading gingival tissue components if released. Such enzymes may be released by inflammatory cells during their function, or when they degenerate or die (see Chapter 5). The main enzymes released by these cells are listed below:

Proteolytic enzymes	Collagenase
	Elastase
	Cathepsin G
	Cathepsin B
	Cathepsin D
	Dipeptidylpeptidases
	Tryptase
Hydrolytic enzymes	Aryl sulphatase
	β-glucuronidase
	Alkaline phosphatase
	Acid phosphatase
	Myeloperoxidase
	Lysozyme
	Lactoferrin

Collagen degradation is a multistage process (*Figure 5.3*, Chapter 5), and the triple helical region can only be attacked by specific collagenases (MMP-1 and -8). The terminal peptides, which contain the sites of intra- and intermolecular cross-links can be attacked by a number of other metallo-serine and cysteine proteinases acting in concert (see Chapters 1 and 5)

The degradation of collagen is usually preceded by that of the proteoglycans. In proteoglycan degradation (*Figure 5.4*, Chapter 5) protein cleavage occurs first to release the GAGs from the protein core, and a number of metallo-, serine and cysteine proteinases can carry out this function. The released GAGs may remain intact, or be further degraded by other hydrolytic enzymes.

Thus, all these proteolyic and hydrolytic enzymes can play an important role in periodontal pathology.

Collagenase and related metalloproteinases

Collagenases are part of a family of matrix metalloproteinases (MMPs) that degrade collagen. They are synthesized by macrophages, neutrophils, fibroblasts and keratinocytes, and are secreted by these cells as latent enzymes when stimulated by some bacterial products and cytokines. There are two principal types of specific collagenase; MMP-8 is found in inflammatory cells such as PMNS and MMP-1 is found in fibroblasts and other cells (Birkedal-Hansen, 1993; Reynolds *et al.*, 1994; Reynolds, 1996). These cells also produce inhibitors known as tissue inhibitors of metalloproteinases (TIMP) (see Chapters 1 and 5).

Latent or pro-collagenases and related enzymes are activated by a number of proteolytic enzymes, including tissue plasmin produced from serum plasminogen by plasminogen activator, which is secreted by macrophages. They are inactivated by TIMPs and α_2-macroglobulin (Page, 1991).

Collagenase (MMP-8 and MMP-1) activity is present in gingival tissue, saliva and GCF, and can be assayed biochemically with collagen substrates (Sorsa *et al.*, 1990) or by using monoclonal antibodies with the ELISA technique (Ingman *et al.*, 1996; Matsuki *et al.*, 1996). MMP-1 (collagenase-1), MMP-8 (collagenase-2), MMP-2 (gelatinase-A) and MMP-9 (gelatinase-B) (see Chapter 1 and *Table 1.1*) are present in both GCF and saliva (Sorsa *et al.*, 1990; Ingman *et al.*, 1994; Makela *et al.*, 1994; Westerlund *et al.*, 1996), and in both situations MMP-8 and MMP-9 predominate. The main source of both these enzymes is PMNs. In addition, the MMP-8 present in both situations in untreated chronic periodontitis patients has been found to be predominantly in the active form, whilst that present in healthy or treated chronic periodontitis patients is mainly in the inactive or latent form (Uitto *et al.*, 1990; Hayakawa *et al.*, 1994).

Saliva
Salivary levels of MMP-8 and -9 are significantly higher in untreated chronic periodontitis patients than in healthy controls (Hayakawa *et al.*, 1994; Makela *et al.*, 1994; Ingman *et al.*, 1996; Matsuki *et al.*, 1996). Levels of MMP-8 also correlate with indices of disease severity (Sorsa *et al.*, 1994), and levels of MMP-8, -2 and -9 significantly decrease following periodontal treatment (Uitto *et al.*, 1990; Hayakawa *et al.*, 1994; Makela *et al.*, 1994). In addition, TIMP-1 is significantly lower in untreated chronic periodontitis patients than in healthy controls (Hayakawa *et al.*, 1994; Matsuki *et al.*, 1996).

By contrast, in localized juvenile periodontitis (LJP) salivary MMP-1 predominates, but the levels of collagenase present in this condition are significantly less than in either untreated or treated chronic periodontitis or healthy patients (Ingman *et al.*, 1993). In addition, the levels of TIMP-1 are significantly increased in LJP cases compared with those in either healthy or chronic periodontitis patients.

There are no longitudinal studies of salivary MMPs, because salivary samples relate to the whole oral cavity and are unable to give information on site-related periodontal disease progression.

GCF
The level of GCF collagenase in naturally occurring and experimental gingivitis correlated with the severity of inflammation (Kowashi *et al.*, 1979; Overall and Sodek, 1987). Collagenase levels also correlated with the amount of attachment loss in ligature-induced periodontitis in dogs, and latent enzyme predominated at healthy and gingivitis sites (Kryshalskyi *et al.*, 1986; Kryshalskyi and Sodek, 1987).

In human periodontitis, GCF collagenase activity has been shown to increase with increasing severity of gingival inflammation and increasing pocket depth and alveolar bone loss (Golub *et al.*, 1976; Larivee *et al.*, 1986; Overall and Sodek, 1987; Villela *et al.*, 1987; Häkkarainen *et al.*, 1988). Total enzyme and active enzyme levels are significantly higher and enzyme inhibitor levels are lower at diseased sites compared with healthy or treated sites (Larivee *et al.*, 1986).

More recently, it has been shown that the predominating collagenase in GCF is MMP-8, mainly from PMNs, and that GCF levels of MMP-8 and -9 are significantly higher in untreated chronic periodontitis patients than in healthy controls (Sorsa *et al.*, 1990; Makela *et al.*, 1994; Ingman *et al.*, 1996; Westerlund *et al.*, 1996). Furthermore, it has been shown that the relationship between MMPs and LJP is the same in GCF and saliva (Ingman *et al.*, 1993).

Also recently, it has been shown (Chen *et al.*, 1999) that total MMP-8 and MMP-8 concentration reduced significantly following periodontal treatment. It was also shown that this enzyme gave more significant correlations with clinical parameters and fell more after successful periodontal treatment than either elastase or cathepsin B. This might reflect more effective complexing of this enzyme with inhibitors as the periodontal condition improves, and this contention is supported by the finding in this study that the amount of the inhibitor α_2-macroglobulin also decreased significantly following treatment.

At the time of writing there has only been one longitudinal study of GCF collagenase levels and periodontal attachment loss (Lee *et al.*, 1995b). This study measured the relative amounts of active and latent collagenase relative to GCF by functional assays in a 12-month longitudinal cohort study. Comparisons were made between 14 subjects with inflammation and a previous history of progressive attachment loss (progressive periodontitis, Group 1), 27 subjects with inflammation and previous attachment loss but who were now clinically stable (stable periodontitis, Group 2), and 17 subjects with inflammation and no attachment loss (gingivitis, Group 3).

Subjects with progressive and stable periodontitis (Groups 1 and 2) were given basic periodontal treatment and monitored 3 months later. All subjects were then monitored monthly for attachment loss with a constant pressure probe, and a threshold of 2 mm was used for confirmed attachment loss. GCF samples were taken from six specific sample teeth in each subject, and from other teeth that lost attachment of 2 mm or more. Subjects in Group 1 were rejected from the study if they did not lose attachment after 1 year, and further subjects were recruited until 14 had lost attachment. The samples were all analysed at the end of the study so that all attachment loss sites were included. Inhibitors and blocking antibodies were used to determine the cellular source of GCF collagenase, and this was found to be PMNs.

There were 14 sites that lost attachment in excess of the tolerance level, one in each of the chosen patients in Group 1. Active collagenase activity was pooled from the six sites per subject for the group comparisons, and this was significantly higher in Group 1 subjects compared to Groups 2 and 3. In contrast, latent collagenase was twofold higher in Group 2 than in Group 1.

There was a wide variation in the site-specific active collagenase levels in sites with progressive attachment loss, and in these sites there was a significant increase with time. However, there were sharp elevations in active enzyme level at the time of attachment loss in only 8 out of the 14 sites that lost attachment. Furthermore, as seven sites that lost attachment did not show these elevations, the diagnostic sensitivity and specificity values for active collagenase as a predictor of attachment loss, although not calculated in this study, would have been low. In spite of the apparent poor predictive qualities of this enzyme, one commercial test kit has been developed (see below).

Most of the studies described above relating collagenases to periodontal disease severity or activity have used biochemical assays with collagen substrates. It was generally assumed that they were measuring neutrophil collagenases, but it is now known that this assay probably reflected the combined action of several collagenolytic enzymes, including collagenases 1, 2, 3 (MMP-1, -8, -13), gelatinases A and B (MMP-2, -9), membrane-type-1-MMP (MT-1-MMP, MMP-14) and bacterial collagenases in GCF. Now that ELISA assays have been developed for many individual MMPs, it is possible to assay for them individually. It has been shown, using these techniques, that the inflammatory cell MMP (MMP-8) relates positively to indices of periodontal severity and significantly reduces following treatment. It is therefore possible that MMP-8 might give better results in a longitudinal study than those from a mixture of enzymes in previous studies using biochemical assays.

Cysteine proteinases

Cathepsins B, L and H are a family of intracellular cysteine proteinases that can degrade extracellular components, including collagen. They act at acid pH and are primarily involved in intracellular degradation, but are also active extracellularly when released during inflammation. They are particularly active during bone resorption (see Chapter 5). They are produced principally by fibroblasts, macrophages (Kennett *et al.*, 1994a) and osteoclasts (Vaes, 1988). Ultrastructural studies have

also shown cathepsin B localized within lysosomes and associated with the surface membrane of macrophages (Kennett *et al.*, 1997b). In addition, cathepsin B was seen on the surface of collagen fibrils in the adjacent connective tissue to these cells, and this suggests that it could play a role in connective tissue degradation. Cysteine proteinases are inhibited by α_2-macroglobulin and the tissue inhibitors known as cystatins (Eley and Cox, 1991). Fibroblasts and some macrophages in human gingiva contain α_2-macroglobulin (Kennett *et al.*, 1994a), and the active cysteine proteinase activity in gingival tissue and GCF is a balance between enzyme and inhibitors.

Saliva

There are no studies on cysteine proteinase potential markers because there is a high level of cystatins (tissue inhibitors of cysteine proteinases) in saliva, which is sufficient to inhibit the activities of this group of enzymes in this situation.

GCF

Cathepsins B, L and H are present in gingival tissue and GCF (Cox and Eley, 1989a; Eley and Cox, 1991), as are the inhibitors (Eley and Cox, 1991). GCF levels of cathepsins B and L significantly correlate with increasing gingival inflammation, probing depth, probing attachment level and bone loss (Eley and Cox, 1992b, 1992c). In addition, levels of cathepsins B and L significantly reduce following periodontal treatment (Cox and Eley, 1992; Eley and Cox, 1992d). Zero or very low levels are present at healthy sites, low levels at gingivitis sites and high levels at periodontitis sites (Eley and Cox, 1993).

To date there has been only one longitudinal study of GCF cathepsin B activity and periodontal attachment loss (Eley and Cox, 1996b). This was a 2-year study of 75 patients using site, patient and population thresholds for probing attachment loss, measured with a Florida electronic probe and radiological measurements to determine confirmed progressive attachment loss. All clinical parameters and enzyme levels significantly reduced following basic periodontal treatment prior to baseline.

Over the 2 years there were 121 sites in 49 patients with confirmed attachment loss, giving an annual rate of 5.04% of sites. Ninety of these sites in 37 patients were rapid episodic attachment loss (RAL), and 31 sites in 21 patients showed gradual progressive attachment loss over a longer time period (GAL). Levels above critical values chosen for total cathepsin B activity and enzyme concentration were present at all RAL sites, both at the time of attachment loss and 3 months previously (predictive time). They were all significantly higher than control sites in the same patients.

These levels were also shown to be predictive of attachment loss in diagnostic testing. There were values of 100% (sensitivity) and 99.83% (specificity) for total enzyme activity, and 100% (sensitivity) and 99.75% (specificity) for enzyme concentration. In addition, there were values of 86.53% (positive prediction) and 100%

(negative prediction) for total enzyme activity and 81.08% (positive prediction) and 100% (negative prediction) for enzyme concentration.

The mean levels over the 2 years and the highest recorded values at GAL sites were also both above their respective critical values, and were statistically significantly higher than those values at control sites in the same patients. In addition, all comparisons of mean patient values in patients with or without attachment loss were statistically significant.

Thus, GCF cathepsin B appears to be a good predictor of future progressive attachment loss. A test system suitable for chairside use has been developed (Cox *et al.*, 1990), and has been shown to produce similar results to the laboratory system (see below).

Aspartate proteinases

Cathepsin D is found in gingival tissue, and GCF and GCF levels have been shown to correlate significantly with increasing gingival inflammation, probing depth, probing attachment level and bone loss (Ishikawa *et al.*, 1972). No longitudinal studies have been carried out relating this proteinase to periodontal attachment loss.

Serine proteinases

Elastase

Elastase in gingival tissue is produced by neutrophil polymorphonuclear leucocytes (PMNs), and is held in the cell in an inactive form probably bound with an inhibitor (Kennett *et al.*, 1995). It is inhibited in the tissues by α_1-proteinase inhibitor (α_1-PI) and α_2-macroglobulin (α_2-M). α_2-M is found in many fibroblasts and also some macrophages, which may also contain α_1-PI (Kennett *et al.*, 1995a).

Active elastase can only occasionally be detected in gingival tissue biochemically (Eley and Cox, 1990) or histochemically (Kennett *et al.*, 1995), and is probably only detectable in an active state where there is an enzyme–inhibitor imbalance. This is usually seen either adjacent to junctional epithelium where PMNs are migrating into the crevice or in granulation tissue at the advancing front of the lesion (Kennett *et al.*, 1995).

Elastase is able to degrade proteoglycans and can also activate latent collagenase (Eley and Cox, 1990). Collagenases are unable to degrade collagen until the terminal peptide region of the molecule, which contains intermolecular cross-links, is first cleaved. This can also be carried out by elastase. It may thus have an important role in periodontal pathology.

Elastase is present in both saliva and GCF, and can be biochemically assayed from these sources.

Saliva

Salivary elastase levels are very low in periodontally healthy patients and zero in edentulous patients (Pederson *et al.*, 1995). The mean elastase level rose significantly in successive patient groups from gingivitis to early periodontitis, to moderate periodontitis to advanced periodontitis. Its levels also correlated with indices of disease severity and with the number of deep pockets present (Uitto *et al.*, 1996). Eighty-five% of patients with one deep ($\geqslant 6$ mm) periodontal pocket had elevated levels of salivary elastase. Levels also decreased significantly following periodontal treatment (Nieminen *et al.*, 1993a). Importantly, salivary elastase levels are not a good indicator for gingivitis as only 45% of these patients had detectable elastase in their saliva (Uitto *et al.*, 1996). In addition, its levels did not significantly rise during the progression of experimental gingivitis. Finally, salivary elastase levels are much lower in untreated localized juvenile periodontitis than in untreated chronic periodontitis, and in fact are little different from control levels in healthy patients (Ingram *et al.*, 1993).

GCF

The GCF elastase level significantly correlates with increasing gingival inflammation, probing depth, probing attachment level and bone loss (Eley and Cox, 1992b, 1992c), and its level also significantly reduces following periodontal treatment (Cox and Eley, 1992; Eley and Cox, 1992d). Zero or very low levels are present at healthy sites, low to moderate levels at gingivitis sites, and very high levels at periodontitis sites (Eley and Cox, 1993).

A 6-month longitudinal study using a test kit system for elastase measurements has been reported (Palcanis *et al.*, 1992). This study used small thresholds of probing attachment loss of 0.4, 0.6 and 1 mm measured with a Florida probe (see Chapter 12) and bone loss detected by subtraction radiology (see Chapter 12) to determine when attachment loss occurred. It showed significant differences of total elastase activity at baseline in progressive and non-progressive sites assessed 2–6 months later.

Results from a 2-year longitudinal study of 75 patients using both a higher threshold and radiological examination to determine confirmed progressive attachment loss (Eley and Cox, 1996b) showed similar and better results. All clinical parameters and enzyme levels significantly reduced following basic periodontal treatment prior to baseline. Over the 2 years there were 119 sites in 48 patients with confirmed attachment loss, giving an annual rate of 4.96% of sites. Eighty-nine of these sites in 36 patients were rapid episodic attachment loss (RAL), and 30 sites in 21 patients showed gradual progressive attachment loss (GAL) over a long time period.

Levels above critical values chosen for total elastase activity and enzyme concentration were present at all RAL sites, both at the time of attachment loss and 3 months previously (predictive time). They were all significantly higher than values at control sites in the same patients.

These levels were also shown to be predictive of attachment loss in diagnostic testing. There were values of 100% (sensitivity) and 99.95% (specificity) for total enzyme activity, and 100% (sensitivity) and 99.91% (specificity) for enzyme concentration. In addition, there were values of 95.70% (positive prediction) and 100% (negative prediction) for total enzyme activity, and 68.46% (positive prediction) and 100% (negative prediction) for enzyme concentration.

The mean levels over the 2 years and the highest recorded values at GAL sites were both above their respective critical values, and were statistically significantly higher than those values at control sites in the same patients. In addition, all comparisons of mean patient values in patients with or without attachment loss were highly statistically significant.

In addition, the levels of GCF elastase have also been compared at healthy, gingivitis and histologically confirmed attachment loss sites in beagle dogs with ligature-induced periodontitis (Renvert *et al.*, 1998). At the attachment loss sites, maximum histological attachment loss was found to coincide with the period of maximum GCF elastase activity and there was significant correlation between the two during the first 7 days of ligature placement. In contrast, the healthy and gingivitis sites had minimal levels of enzyme activity throughout the study period.

Thus, GCF elastase appears to be a good predictor of future progressive attachment loss. A test system suitable for chairside use has been developed (Cox *et al.*, 1990) and has been shown to produce similar results to the laboratory system. A commercial system based on the same biochemistry has also been developed (Palcanis *et al.*, 1992).

Tryptase

Tryptase activity is present in large amounts in gingival tissue and in small amounts in GCF when measured biochemically (Eley and Cox, 1990; Cox and Eley, 1989a, 1989b, 1989c), and it has been localized to gingival mast cells (Kennett *et al.*, 1993). In the mast cell granules it is stabilized as an active tetramer by association with heparin, and is released by these cells on degranulation.

Tryptase can cleave the third component of complement and can activate latent collagenase. It can stimulate the release of collagenase from gingival fibroblasts, and in inflamed gingival tissues mast cell degranulation occurs in areas of connective tissue breakdown.

In dogs, an inhibitor of mast cell degranulation has been shown significantly to reduce the rate of alveolar bone loss (Jeffcoat *et al.*, 1985). Thus, tryptase could be involved in the pathogenesis of periodontitis.

In humans, GCF tryptase activity correlates with clinical parameters of disease severity, including probing attachment and bone loss (Eley and Cox, 1992b, 1992c), and significantly reduces following periodontal treatment (Cox and Eley, 1992; Eley and Cox, 1992d). Zero to very low levels are present at healthy sites, low levels at gingivitis sites, and moderately high levels at periodontitis sites (Eley and Cox, 1993). There have been no longitudinal studies with this enzyme. The test system for chairside use (Cox *et al.*, 1990) described in the previous section could be used with this enzyme.

Dipeptidylpeptidase (DPPs)

DPP II, which is active at acid pH, and DPP IV, which is active at alkaline pH, are present in gingival tissue and GCF (Cox and Eley, 1989; Cox *et al.*, 1992b).

Within gingival tissue, DPP II is a lysosomal enzyme present in fibroblasts (Kennett *et al.*, 1994b, 1996). In GCF smears it is also present in macrophages (Cox *et al.*, 1995; Kennett *et al.*, 1997). This may suggest that this enzyme within macrophages is in an inactive form in gingival tissue, but in an active form in migrated cells in GCF.

DPP IV is a lysosomal enzyme present in macrophages, T-lymphocytes and fibroblasts (Kennett *et al.*, 1994b, 1996a). Using immunogold localization with electron microscopy, DPP IV was found to be present on the surface membrane of T-lymphocytes, macrophages and fibroblasts (Kennett *et al.*, unpublished data).

GCF DPP II and IV need to be distinguished from bacterial DPPs, and selective assays have been developed for this purpose (Cox *et al.*, 1989; Eley and Cox, 1995a). They are able to cleave glycylprolyl residues and may play a role in collagen degradation after the action of other enzymes.

Both tissue DPP II and IV correlate with clinical parameters of disease severity and significantly reduce following periodontal treatment (Eley and Cox, 1992a, 1992b, 1992c, 1992d; Cox and Eley, 1992). Zero or very low levels are present at healthy sites, low levels at gingivitis sites, and high levels at periodontitis sites (Eley and Cox, 1993).

A 2-year longitudinal study of both GCF DPP II and DPP IV in 75 patients has recently been completed (Eley and Cox, 1995b). It used site, patient and population thresholds for probing attachment loss measured with a Florida electronic probe and radiological measurement to determine confirmed progressive attachment loss. All clinical parameters and enzyme levels significantly reduced following basic periodontal treatment prior to baseline.

Over the 2 years there were 120 sites in 49 patients with confirmed attachment loss, giving an annual rate of 5.0% of sites. Eighty-eight of these sites in 35 patients were rapid episodic attachment loss (RAL) sites, and 32 sites in 20 patients showed gradual progressive attachment loss (GAL) over a longer time period.

Levels above critical values chosen for both DPP II and DPP IV (total enzyme activities and enzyme concentrations) were present at all RAL sites, both at the time of attachment loss and 3 months previously (predictive time). They were all significantly higher than control sites in the same patients.

These levels were also shown to be predictive of attachment loss in diagnostic testing. These values were 100% (sensitivity) and 99.58% (specificity) for total enzyme activities and 100% (sensitivity) and 99.34% (specificity) for enzyme concentrations in respect of DPP II, and 100% (sensitivity) and 99.48% (specificity) for total enzyme activities and 100% (sensitivity) and

99.17% (specificity) for enzyme concentration in respect of DPP IV. In addition, there were values of 70.96% (positive prediction) and 100% (negative prediction) for total enzyme activity and 60.68% (positive prediction) and 100% (negative prediction) for enzyme concentration in respect of DPP II, and of 66.17% (positive prediction) and 100% (negative prediction) for total enzyme activity and 55% (positive prediction) and 100% (negative prediction) for enzyme concentration in respect of DPP IV.

The mean levels over the 2 years and the highest recorded values at GAL sites for both proteases were also above their respective critical values, and were statistically significantly higher than those values at control sites in the same patients. In addition, all comparisons of mean patient values in patients with or without attachment loss were highly statistically significant.

Thus, both GCF DPP II and DPP IV appear to be good predictors of future progressive attachment loss. A test system suitable for chairside use has been developed (Cox *et al.*, 1990) and has been shown to produce similar results to the laboratory system.

Protease inhibitors

The two main endogenous protease inhibitors, α_1-proteinase inhibitor (α_1-PI) and α_2-macroglobulin (α_2-M), are present in serum, saliva and GCF (Sandholm, 1986; Roa *et al.*, 1995). The levels of α_1-PI in saliva and GCF do not significantly vary in healthy and periodontal diseased patients. On the other hand, the levels of α_2-M are significantly higher in chronic periodontitis patients compared with gingivitis patients, and the levels in gingivitis patients are significantly higher compared to healthy patients (Pederson *et al.*, 1995).

Cystatins are tissue-derived inhibitors of cysteine proteinases. Cystatin C is produced by many cells and tissues and has a general distribution, whilst cystatins S, SA, SN and D are produced by glandular acinar cells and are mainly found in glandular secretions, including saliva. Cystatin A is produced by inflammatory cells and is the main cystatin in GCF. Saliva contains cystatins S, SA, SN and D produced by the salivary glands, cystatin C from other cells and possibly cystatin A from GCF. GCF contains cystatin A from inflammatory cells, and sometimes lesser amounts of cystatin C from other cells.

Total salivary cystatins were found to be significantly higher in chronic periodontitis patients compared to gingivitis patients, and in gingivitis patients compared to periodontally healthy patients (Heskens *et al.*, 1993a). However, the levels of protein and albumin followed the same pattern, so it is possible that the changes were due to differences in the salivary flow rate. It has also been found that the levels of cystatin C were also higher in chronic periodontitis patients compared to healthy patients (Heskens *et al.*, 1993b), and that saliva from healthy patients contains mainly cystatin S whilst that from chronic periodontitis patients contains both S and C (Heskens *et al.*, 1994, 1996a). In addition, it has also been shown that salivary total cystatins and cystatin C in chronic periodontitis patients reduce significantly following periodontal treatment (Heskens *et al.*, 1996b).

The level of cystatins in GCF is significantly lower than in saliva (Blankenvoorde *et al.*, 1997). Also, cystatins S and SN and C could not be detected in GCF, but cystatin A was found in every GCF sample analysed and was also found in saliva. Cystatin A in saliva could either come from GCF or from migrating inflammatory cells.

β-Glucuronidase and arylsulphatase

Extensive studies have been carried out on β-glucuronidase and arylsulphatase, and this work is reviewed in Lamster (1992) and Page (1992). Both of these enzymes are lysosomal and are found in PMNs. β-glucuronidase is an acid hydrolase that is considered to be a marker for primary granule release by these cells.

In cross-sectional studies, both these enzymes in GCF have been shown to have statistically significant correlations with gingival inflammation, pocket depth and alveolar bone loss. The levels of these enzymes are also higher in diseased relative to healthy sites, and their levels drop following periodontal treatment.

During a 4-week period of experimental gingivitis, the level of these enzymes increased for the first 3 weeks and then levelled out or dropped off. The levels of both enzymes increased with increasing pocket depths, and β-glucuronidase was also positively associated with spirochaetes, *P. gingivalis*, *P. intermedia* and lactose-negative black-pigmenting bacteria in the subgingival flora and negatively associated with cocci.

A 6-month longitudinal study, where GCF β-glucuronidase activity was related to disease activity defined as loss of attachment of 2.0 mm or more over that period, has been reported (Lamster *et al.*, 1988). Those sites that showed the highest β-glucuronidase activity at baseline and again at 3 months had the highest association with loss of attachment. Critical values at these sites had a sensitivity and specificity of 89% in diagnostic testing.

In a further study (Lamster *et al.*, 1991) 59 patients were similarly followed for a year, and it was shown that persistently elevated β-glucuronidase levels were associated with disease activity that could be predicted from 3 to 6 months in advance. In this study, critical values of β-glucuronidase had a sensitivity of 92% and a selectivity of 86% respectively in diagnostic testing. All of these results were related to total β-glucuronidase activity per 30-second sample, and not to enzyme concentration.

The association with disease activity has been confirmed in a multicentre trial in which 140 patients were followed up for 6 months, and this showed a total predictive value as high as 90% (Lamster, 1992). This has so far only been reported in oral presentations published as abstracts and reported in the review paper quoted. However, the baseline data for this study has been reported in full (Lamster *et al.*, 1994). Thus, total β-glucuronidase activity per 30-second sample appears to be a good predictor of future attachment loss.

A diagnostic kit based on GCF β-glucuronidase is being commercially developed by Abbott Laboratories, North Chicago, USA.

Alkaline phosphatase

Alkaline phosphatase is thought to play a role in bone metabolism and is found in PMNs. A cross-sectional study of GCF alkaline phosphatase in periodontitis patients showed that it positively and significantly correlated with pocket depth but not with bone loss (Ishikawa and Cimasoni, 1970), and is found at higher levels at diseased than at healthy sites (Chapple *et al.*, 1994). A longitudinal study (Binder *et al.*, 1987) that related GCF levels to periodontal attachment loss of more than 2 mm showed that active sites yielded 20 times the activity in serum and were significantly associated with periodontal disease activity. However, when the data was calculated in terms of false positives and negatives using the most favourable cut-off point, 73% of active sites were identified although 36% of the inactive sites were included. This would seem to indicate that its predictive value is low.

Acid phosphatase

Acid phosphatase is present in inflammatory cells and has been detected in GCF (Binder *et al.*, 1987). Levels do not, however, correlate with measurements of either disease severity or activity.

Myeloperoxidase, lysozyme and lactoferrin

Myeloperoxidase, lysozyme and lactoferrin are found in PMNs and can be detected in saliva and GCF.

Myeloperoxidase

Myeloperoxidase (MPO) is a potent antibacterial enzyme produced by PMNs. Salivary MPO levels are significantly higher in untreated chronic periodontitis patients compared with healthy control subjects, and their levels significantly reduce following periodontal treatment (Over *et al.*, 1993; Guven *et al.*, 1996; Suomalainen *et al.*, 1996). GCF MPO levels are higher at periodontitis sites than at control sites, and the levels decrease significantly following periodontal treatment. However, MPO activity was not found to correlate with clinical indices of disease severity (Smith *et al.*, 1986; Cao and Smith, 1989).

Lysozyme

Lysozyme (muraminidase) is an antibacterial enzyme found in body secretions, notably tears and saliva. It is also found in GCF. Salivary lysozyme levels have been reported to be significantly lower in chronic periodontitis and insulin dependent diabetes mellitus patients than healthy control subjects (Markkanen *et al.*, 1986; Pinducci *et al.*, 1996; Suomalainen *et al.*, 1996). Salivary lysozyme levels have also been shown not to vary between untreated localized juvenile periodontitis (LJP) patients and healthy controls.

In GCF it has been reported that the levels of lysozyme in untreated LJP patients is significantly higher than in healthy control subjects. It has also been shown that these levels reduce to normal following treatment (Suomalainen *et al.*, 1996). An elevation of the levels of GCF lysozyme harvested from diseased sites in patients with LJP relative to samples from patients with gingivitis or adult periodontitis has also been reported (Friedman *et al.*, 1983). Thus it appears that salivary and GCF lysozyme levels are decreased in chronic periodontitis and increased in LJP patients.

Lactoferrin

Lactoferrin is an antibacterial agent produced by inflammatory cells. The levels of salivary and GCF lactoferrin are significantly increased in untreated LJP patients compared with healthy controls, and decreased to normal levels following periodontal treatment (Suomalainen *et al.*, 1996).

However, all these studies indicate that none of these enzymes appear to have diagnostic potential.

Pseudocholinesterase

Pseudocholinesterase (PCE) is an esterase enzyme with some similarities to acetylcholinesterase, and acts as a scavenging enzyme in the tissues. It is present in many tissues and in serum, saliva and GCF. The PCE level in GCF is higher than that in saliva but lower than that in serum, and GCF may be the main source of salivary activity. The mean salivary and GCF PCE activity has been shown to be significantly higher in rapidly progressive periodontitis patients compared to either localized juvenile periodontitis patients or healthy controls (Yamalik *et al.*, 1990). The same group has also shown that the salivary PCE activity in chronic periodontitis patients significantly reduces following subgingival scaling and root planing, and reduces still further following periodontal surgery (Yamalik *et al.*, 1991).

Commercial diagnostic test kits

The commercial test kits based on some of the GCF factors described above that are currently available are listed below.

Periocheck (ACTech)

This system detects the presence of neutral proteinases such as collagenase in GCF.

A paper strip is used to obtain a GCF sample. This strip is then placed in contact with a collagen gel to which a blue dye has been covalently bonded. This is then incubated at 43°C. If the neutral proteinases are present in the sample, they will attack the collagen gel and release the blue dye. The released blue dye produces colour in the strip, the intensity of which is proportional to the amount of enzyme present in the sample. The intensity and the area of the blue colour is then scored on a scale of 0 to 2 by comparing it with three standards on a colour card provided with the test kit.

Prognostik (Dentsply)

This system detects the presence of the serine proteinase, elastase, in GCF samples.

A GCF sample is collected on special paper strips that have been impregnated with the appropriate peptidyl derivative of 7-amino-trifluoromethylcoumarin (AFC). The substrate used is MeOSuc-Ala-Ala-Pro-Val-AFC, which detects elastase and is linked to a fluorescent leaving group, AFC. If elastase is present in the sample it reacts with the substrate in 4–8 minutes, releasing the fluorescent leaving group, AFC. This produces green fluorescence in the strip, which can be seen under ultraviolet (UV) light using a UV light box. The intensity of the fluorescence is proportional to the amount of GCF in the sample, and this is scored by comparing it with AFC standards. The biochemical technology for this test system was developed by Enzyme System Products/Prototek, Dublin, California, USA for Dentsply.

The commercial firms owning these tests are constantly changing because some of them sell the rights to their products to others. For this reason, names of the firms cited as owning these tests may not remain accurate.

Potential diagnostic tests worthy of development

β-glucuronidase

A diagnostic kit based on β-glucuronidase is being commercially developed by Abbott Laboratories, North Chicago, USA. It probably uses a histochemical substrate for the enzyme coupled to a colour detection system, which is released if the enzyme attacks the substrate. The system used is probably very similar to that described by the Lamster research group (Lamster *et al.*, 1988, 1991, 1994).

Cysteine and serine proteinases

A test system suitable for chairside use has been developed in the research laboratory of one of the authors in conjunction with researchers from Enzyme System Pro-ducts/Prototek, Dublin, California, USA (Cox *et al.*, 1990). This firm synthesizes the peptide substrates and the 7-amino-trifluoromethylcoumarin (AFC) leaving group, which is considerably more sensitive than other fluorogenic leaving groups.

This system uses the same leaving group and basic biochemical technique as that used in the Dentsply system for elastase described above, but was developed 4 years before this system and has a number of advantages over it. These are that:

1. It can be modified to detect a number of different proteinases, including the serine proteinases elastase, tryptase and DPP II and IV and the cysteine proteinases cathepsins B and L. It can also be modified to detect the bacterial proteases gingivain and DPP in GCF, so this system could also be used for these proteases (see section above).
2. The GCF sample is collected on a normal paper strip and therefore the peptide substrate and leaving group are not introduced into the gingival crevice, as in the Dentsply system.
3. Most importantly, the assay buffer can be made appropriate for the enzyme in question by being of the correct pH and by including any necessary activators of the enzyme in question in the buffer. It can also include any necessary inhibitors of other potentially interfering proteases that can cleave the same substrate as the desired enzyme.
4. The colour detection method developed for this system is much more convenient for use in dental practice, as it requires no special apparatus.

The details of the system are described below.

Chromatography paper discs impregnated with the appropriate peptidyl derivative of 7-amino-trifluoromethylcoumarin (AFC) are placed in a multiwell plate and covered with the appropriate assay buffer. The GCF sample is taken on a standard chromatography paper strip and is eluted into the buffer in the appropriate well. If the enzyme is present, it reacts with the peptide substrate and splits off the AFC fluorescent leaving group (*Figure 13.5*). The intensity of the fluorescence can be detected under UV light, and is proportional to the amount of enzyme in the sample (*Figure 13.6a*). Alternatively, a simpler colour detection system can be used by adding p-dimethylamino-cinnamaldehyde to the well (*Figures 13.5* and *13.6b*). This molecule couples to the AFC leaving group, forming a coloured Schiff reagent. Semi-quantitative assessment of disc fluorescence or colour is made by comparison with AFC/substrate standards.

This system has been shown to be accurate and reliable by comparison with full biochemical quantitative fluorometric assays (Cox *et al.*, 1990). The colour system was more sensitive than fluorescence, and requires no special apparatus in the clinical setting. This system awaits a commercial sponsor to develop and market it for dental practice.

Amino acid
sequence

Blocking
group

Enzymic
cleavage

UV light   + cinnamaldehyde

Green fluorescence   Schiff Base purple colour

Figure 13.5 Diagram to show the use of the appropriate peptidyl derivative of 7-amino-trifluoromethylcoumarin (AFC) to detect proteolytic enzyme activity. It shows how the appropriate enzyme activity splits the substrate and releases AFC. This produces typical green fluorescence, which can be detected by ultraviolet (UV) light. It can also be reacted with cinnamaldehyde to produce a Schiff purple colour base. The amount of enzyme present is proportional to the intensity of the fluorescence or colour

Figure 13.6 Chairside diagnostic test system based on the technology illustrated in Figure 13.5. Chromatography paper discs impregnated with the appropriate peptidyl derivative of 7-amino-trifluoromethylcoumarin (AFC) are placed in a multiwell plate and covered with the appropriate assay buffer. The GCF sample is taken on a standard chromatography paper strip and is eluted into the buffer in the appropriate well. If the enzyme is present, it reacts with the peptide substrate and splits off the AFC fluorescent leaving group.
(a) Fluorescence detection system. The intensity of the fluorescence can be detected under UV light, and is proportional to the amount of enzyme in the sample.
(b) Colour detection system. A simple colour detection system can be used by adding p-dimethylamino-cinnamaldehyde to the well. This molecule couples to the AFC leaving group, forming a purple coloured Schiff reagent.
Semiquantitative assessment of disc fluorescence or colour is made by comparison with AFC/substrate standards.

Advantages and disadvantages of diagnostic tests using hydrolytic enzymes

Advantages

The main advantages are listed and discussed below:

- Some markers, e.g. cathepsin B, elastase, DPP II and IV and β-glucuronidase, are predictive of disease activity in longitudinal studies
- They are simple to use, particularly the colour detection systems
- They can be read after a short time
- They can be shown to the patient and related to tooth site.

All of the markers used in the commercially available test systems and those under development have been shown to be capable of detecting disease activity. However, only a few of the enzymes described above appear to be predictive of disease activity. Of the potential markers described in this article, cathepsin B, elastase, DPP II and IV and β-glucuronidase have been shown in longitudinal studies to be predictive of periodontal disease progression. One of these, elastase, is available in a commercial diagnostic test, and a test for β-glucuronidase is being developed by Abbott Laboratories, North Chicago, USA. Also, a simple chairside test system has been designed in one of the author's laboratories in conjunction with Enzyme System Products/Prototek, Dublin, California, USA, which can be used with cathepsin B, elastase, DPP II and IV and tryptase.

All of the test systems are simple to use, and can be read after relatively short periods. The colour detection systems are particularly easy to read and score.

Disadvantages

The main disadvantages are listed and discussed below:

- The choice of the most appropriate biomarker may still be difficult with the present state of knowledge
- There is difficulty in determining the sites to sample and when to sample them
- If a moiety is associated with inflammation, this may mask its association with destructive disease
- No account of biological control mechanisms is taken in present tests
- Cost.

The choice of the most appropriate biomarker

Of the potential markers described in this account, cathepsin B, elastase, DPP II and IV and β-glucuronidase have been shown in longitudinal studies to be predictive of periodontal disease progression. Collagenase, tryptase, alkaline phosphatase, arylsulphatase and myeloperoxidase have been shown in cross-sectional studies, and in some cases longitudinal studies, to be associated with disease severity and activity. However, they are not predictive of disease activity, and this is the basic requirement of a diagnostic test. Acid phosphatase, lysozyme and lactoferrin at present do not appear to be associated with either disease activity or severity.

Only one of the two commercially available tests use a marker, elastase, which has been shown to be predictive of disease activity. However, tests involving β-glucuronidase, cathepsin B, DPP II and IV could appear in the future. Also, tests which do not incorporate the reaction substrate on the GCF collection strip are to be preferred because the incorporation of an appropriate buffer in the reaction well can make the test much more selective for the marker.

Determining the sites to sample and when to sample them
It is obviously not possible to sample all the sites in the mouth with any diagnostic test system, and for this reason the site(s) to be tested have to be preselected. This usually means testing sites that already show clinical signs of previous attachment loss, since these sites are slightly more likely to progress than other sites. However, the pattern of progression of periodontitis is very irregular and unpredictable, and this may make the choice of sites difficult.

Association of the marker with inflammation
All enzymes released from inflammatory cells are likely to be associated with gingival inflammation. Since gingival inflammation is often present in the absence of disease activity (i.e. progressive periodontal attachment loss), this association with inflammation could produce false association with disease activity. It is therefore very important to show that a potential marker has a true association with periodontal disease activity, which is independent of and stronger than any association it may have with gingival inflammation. This is most clearly shown in comparisons of true and false positive and negative sites in respect of confirmed attachment loss, which are used to compute the sensitivity, specificity, and positive and negative predictive values quoted in the sections on each marker.

Biological control mechanisms
All diagnostic tests should reflect an understanding of the role played by biological control mechanisms in determining the levels of the test substance. For instance, protease levels in gingival tissue are determined partly by a balance between the enzyme and its natural inhibitors. Serine proteinases like elastase are inhibited by the serum inhibitor α_1-proteinase inhibitor and α_2-macroglobulin and cysteine proteases by α_2-macroglobulin and the tissue inhibitors, cystatins. The level of enzyme in the tissues, and to some extent GCF, must therefore depend upon the enzyme inhibitor balance. In addition, the level of inflammatory cell proteinases in GCF also depends on release from inflammatory cells that have migrated into the crevice.

Cost
All diagnostic test systems are relatively expensive and for this reason cannot be used in NHS practice without incurring financial loss. The cost of the kit and time involved in obtaining, reacting and reading the sample(s) would need to be added to the patient's bill.

Enzymes released by dead cells (cytosolic enzymes)

Enzymes released from dead cells (cytosolic enzymes) include:

1. Aspartate amino transferase (AST)
2. Lactate dehydrogenase (LDH).

Aspartate amino transferase (AST) and lactate dehydrogenase (LDH) are soluble cytoplasmic enzymes that are confined to the cell cytoplasm but are released by dead or dying cells. Since cell death is an integral and essential component of periodontal tissue destruction, they should be released during this process and pass with the inflammatory exudate into GCF.

Aspartate amino transferase

Levels of AST in serum and cerebrospinal fluid have been used for a number of years in medicine as an indicator of tissue necrosis and cell death. In dogs, GCF AST levels have been shown to increase during the development of ligature-induced experimental periodontitis (Chambers *et al.*, 1984). In experimental gingivitis in humans, levels in GCF samples harvested during the development and resolution of the condition were significantly associated with gingival inflammation (Persson *et al.*, 1990b). In a cross-sectional study, GCF AST was shown to correlate with clinical indices of disease severity (Imrey *et al.*, 1991).

In longitudinal studies, GCF AST levels have been related to confirmed attachment loss (Persson *et al.*, 1990c; Chambers *et al.*, 1991). These workers found that elevated GCF AST levels were strongly associated with disease active sites in contrast to disease inactive sites. Active sites contained 725 units of AFC more than inactive sites. Sites with severe inflammation also yielded more AST than less inflamed sites.

There is as yet no evidence to indicate that GCF AST levels are predictive of disease activity, because the positive correlations were made at the time of attachment loss rather than before it.

A multicentre trial was performed using a dichotomous colorimetric test, which becomes positive when 800 units or more of GCF AST are present. Samples were taken before and after periodontal treatment and showed that levels were reduced below the detection limit following treatment (Page, 1992).

A commercial diagnostic test kit based on GCF AST levels has been developed, and is marketed at present by Colgate.

Lactate dehydrogenase

LDH has been correlated with probing depth and other clinical indices of disease severity in cross-sectional studies. It has also been related to periodontal disease activity in a longitudinal study. However, in both cases the level of correlation was less than for β-glucuronidase, which was included in the same studies (Lamster *et al.*, 1988).

Sampling GCF for these components

Samples of GCF for the detection of both LDH and AST can be collected on conventional paper strips left *in situ* for 30 seconds.

Degradation products of degenerating cells

Epithelial cells produce the protein keratin, and this forms the cornified layer on the surface of stratified squamous epithelia. This keratin may be released into the environment of these cells when they turnover rapidly, are damaged or degenerate. This discarded keratin has been detected in saliva and GCF (McLaughlin *et al.*, 1996). In chronic periodontitis patients, the keratin concentration in GCF was found to be significantly greater at sites exhibiting gingivitis or periodontitis than at healthy sites, but no differences were detected between gingivitis and periodontitis sites. In addition, no differences in the salivary levels of keratin were seen for these groupings. The presence of keratin in GCF may reflect damage to the pocket epithelium, which occurs in these conditions. However, since this product is unable to distinguish between gingivitis and periodontitis in a cross-sectional study, it has no potential as a marker for periodontal disease activity.

Commercial test kit

The only commercial test kit based on factors released from tissue degradation is that based on GCF AST, which is released from dead cells. This is briefly described below. More details can be found in the AST section above and in a recent publication (Persson *et al.*, 1995).

Periogard (Colgate) AST in GCF test kit

The test kit uses paper point GCF samples and colorimetric detection.

The test kit consists of a tray with two test wells for each tooth and appropriate reagents for conducting the test. The strip containing the GCF sample is placed into an appropriate test well, and two drops of one reagent (10 mM Tris HCl with 0.067% Triton X-100, pH 6.0) is added. At the same time, positive and negative control wells are prepared using strips provided. Two drops of a solution provided (260 mM L-aspartic acid, 33 mM 2-oxogluteric acid, 4.3 mM disodium EDTA, 1.6% polyvinylpyrolidone, 0.067% Triton X-100, 2.7 mM sorbic acid in 100 mM Tris HCl, pH 6.0) are added to the wells and allowed to incubate at room temperature. After 9 minutes' incubation, the substrate/detection solution (1 mg Fast red RC diazotized salt in 1% methanol, 0.067% Triton X-100, in 230 mM Tris HCl, pH 8.0) is mixed and two drops are added at 10 minutes. Five minutes later the test results can be read by eye by comparing the test well colour to the colour of the positive control. A colour of greater intensity than that of the negative control is scored as a positive and one of lesser or equal intensity as a negative result. The test is designed to be positive at $\geqslant 800$ mIU AST activity and negative at values below 800 mIU.

The commercial firms owning tests may change (as stated earlier) because some of them sell the rights to their products to others. For this reason, names of the firms cited as owning these tests may not remain accurate.

Advantages and disadvantages of diagnostic tests using cytosolic enzymes

Advantages

The possible advantages are listed and discussed below:

- Both of these potential markers associate with disease activity but do not predict it
- Tests can be devised that are simple to use
- They can be read after relatively short periods
- They can be shown to patients and related to tooth site affected.

The marker used in the only commercially available test system in this group, AST, and those under possible development have been shown to be capable of correlating disease activity. However, neither AST nor any of the other markers in this section have been shown to be predictive for disease activity in human chronic periodontitis. The AST test system is relatively simple to use, and can be read after relatively short periods. The colour detection system is easy to read and score.

Disadvantages

The main disadvantages are listed and discussed below:

- The choice of the most appropriate biomarker is difficult with the present state of knowledge
- There is difficulty in determining the sites to sample and when to sample them
- Cost.

The choice of the most appropriate biomarker
Both the potential markers described above have been shown in longitudinal studies of human chronic periodontitis to correlate with parameters of disease severity. In addition, AST has been shown on the basis of human longitudinal studies to correlate with disease activity (i.e. correlate at the time the attachment loss was recorded). However, neither of them appears to be capable of predicting disease activity.

Determining the sites to sample and when to sample them
It is obviously not possible to sample all the sites in the mouth with any diagnostic test system, and for this reason the site(s) to be tested have to be preselected. This has already been discussed in the section above.

Cost
This has already been discussed above.

Markers of connective tissue degradation

During its passage through the inflamed tissue, GCF could pick up normal components of the extracellular matrix or tissue degradation products released during the destructive process. The components that could be involved in this process are listed below:

Connective tissue	Collagens I, III, V
	Proteoglycans
	Hyaluronan
	Fibronectin
Basement membrane	Collagen IV
	Laminin

The detection of the breakdown products of these macromolecules could be indicative of tissue breakdown. These include the following:

Component	Breakdown product
Collagen	Hydroxyproline
	Collagen cross-links
	N-propeptide
Proteoglycan	Glycosaminoglycans (GAGs)
GAGs	Heparan sulphate
	Chondroitin-4-sulphate
	Chondroitin-6-sulphate

Fibronectin

Fibronectin, a normal component of serum and the connective tissue matrix, is present in GCF, and more intact molecules are present in samples from healthy and treated sites than from diseased sites (Lopatin *et al.*, 1989; Talonpoika *et al.*, 1989). In addition, the number of intact molecules increased following treatment of the diseased sites. To date, there have been no longitudinal studies of this molecule.

Hydroxyproline-containing peptides

Hydroxyproline-containing peptides are released during collagen degradation. They have been shown to be present in GCF harvested from dogs during the development of experimental periodontitis (Svanberg, 1987). However, the relation of this peptide to human destructive periodontitis has not been studied to date.

Glycosaminoglycans

The extracellular ground substance of connective tissues contains a series of hexauronate-containing heteropolysaccharides termed glycosaminoglycans (GAGs), which are linked to a specific core protein to form high molecular weight aggregates called proteoglycans. The connective tissue breakdown that occurs during periodontitis includes proteoglycan degradation, and this process involves proteolytic enzymes, which release GAGs from the protein core. The GAGs may then pass into GCF via the inflammatory exudate, where they have been detected (Embery *et al.*, 1982).

The GAGs in GCF from individual sites of defined clinical conditions have been investigated with cellulose-acetate electrophoresis (Embery *et al.*, 1982; Last *et al.*, 1985). The non-sulphated GAG hyaluronic acid was present in all samples, and was the only major GAG found in chronic gingivitis patients. An additional sulphated GAG, identified by enzyme digestion as chondroitin-4-sulphate, was detected in GCF from sites with untreated advanced periodontitis. Initial GCF samples from early periodontitis and juvenile periodontitis also contained this GAG. This GAG was, however, not detected after periodontal treatment of these sites with subgingival scaling, pocket reduction surgery or daily irrigation of the pockets with a chlorhexidine solution.

Sulphated GAGs were also detected in GCF samples from around teeth undergoing orthodontic movement, teeth subject to occlusal trauma and from samples from healing tooth-extraction wounds. Thus, the presence of sulphated GAGs in GCF appears to correlate on a cross-sectional basis with those clinical conditions in which degradation changes are occurring in the deeper periodontal tissues (Last *et al.*, 1985). For this reason, the electrophoretic profile or the presence of chondroitin-4-sulphate in GCF may be a sensitive method of indicating active phases of destructive periodontal disease.

So far, no longitudinal studies have been carried out to relate GCF GAGs to periodontal disease activity. Also, unfortunately, it may be difficult to design a diagnostic test based on these techniques. This is for two reasons: first, because a large sample of GCF is required to detect GAGs, necessitating collection with a micropipette for 15 minutes; and second, cellulose-acetate electrophoresis and enzyme digestion is used for their detection and identification.

Proteoglycan degradation products
The degradation products (unsaturated disaccharide isomers) of enzymic degradation of chondroitin sulphate have been shown to be present in whole saliva (Okazaki *et al.*, 1996). This group has shown that the salivary levels of these products are significantly higher in untreated chronic periodontitis patients than in healthy control subjects.

Antioxidant activity and capacity

Inflammatory cells produce reactive oxygen species (ROS) within their phagolysosomes, and these may spill over into the tissues during phagocytosis or when they degenerate. This may cause bystander tissue damage around these cells. ROS have a great capacity to damage cells and tissues, and are scavenged for within the tissues by antioxidants.

The antioxidant capacity of saliva has been investigated in healthy and chronic periodontitis patients (Moore *et al.*, 1994). The major aqueous antioxidant component of whole saliva was found to be uric acid, with lesser contributions from ascorbic acid and albumin. Using biochemical methods, the antioxidant capacity of the saliva was not found to be compromised in chronic periodontitis patients, and this was attributed to increased salivary flow and antioxidant flow from GCF.

An enhanced chemiluminescent assay can be used to measure the total antioxidant (AO) capacity of serum, saliva and GCF (Chapple *et al.*, 1997). In saliva and GCF an AO response was found that was not present in the serum of the same patients. This group investigated the peripheral (serum) and local (saliva) AO capacities of chronic periodontitis and healthy patients. There were no differences in the serum AO capacities, but the salivary total AO concentrations were significantly lower in the chronic periodontitis group compared with the healthy group. Thus the saliva of chronic periodontitis patients may have a reduced AO capacity, which could result from increased ROS production by inflammatory cells. The enhanced chemiluminescent assay provides a rapid and simple method of measuring the total antioxidant defence in small volumes of biological fluid, and hence could have diagnostic use. However, much more work on its relationship to the progression of periodontal disease needs to be done before this can be properly assessed.

Sampling GCF for these components

GCF for the detection of fibronectin and hydroxyproline-containing peptides can be collected on paper strips. However, the detection of GAGs in GCF requires a large volume of fluid produced over long collection times of around 15 minutes using micropipettes. This is impractical in the clinical situation, and can also significantly affect GCF composition compared to that produced by short collection times. The longer collection time will collect fluid that consists mostly of continuously stimulated inflammatory exudate rather than the residual fluid and which additionally contains components from the local environment.

Methods of isolation and detection

The biochemical techniques used to isolate and detect some of these components are difficult to modify for chairside use. This is the case for GAGs, which are isolated and detected by cellulose-acetate electrophoresis and staining, with further characterization by enzyme digestion. These methods are listed below:

Hydroxyproline	High pressure liquid chromatography (HPLC), ion exchange chromatography
Collagen cross-links	HPLC
GAGs	Cellulose acetate extraction and staining

Problems with the possible clinical use of tissue degradation products

- Most involve complex and expensive techniques to isolate and detect
- If present in GCF, they usually require long collection times using a micropipette to obtain sufficient quantities to analyse
- Long GCF collection times affect its composition
- The normal cycle of synthesis and degradation of connective tissue and bone needs to be considered
- Most are not suitable for chairside use because it is difficult to develop a simplified detection system.

Diagnostic tests

Not surprisingly, no diagnostic tests have yet been developed for any of the potential markers in this section, and thus possible advantages and disadvantages will not be discussed further.

Bone resorption

Bone-specific proteins

Several bone morphogenic proteins are involved in bone mineralization, and some connective tissue proteins also play an important role in this process (Bowers *et al.*, 1989). Some of these, which are considered below, have been considered for possible markers of bone resorption and hence periodontal disease activity.

These proteins are listed below:

Osteonectin
Bone phosphoprotein (N-propeptide)
Osteocalcin
Telopeptides of type I collagen
Collagen I
Proteoglycans.

Osteonectin and bone phosphoprotein (N-propeptide)

Osteonectin is a normal component of bone matrix which is thought to play an important role in the initial phase of mineralization (Termine *et al.*, 1981). Bone phosphoprotein, which is an amino propeptide extension (N-propeptide) of the alpha-1 chains of type I collagen, appears to be involved in the attachment of connective tissue cells to the substratum (Bowers *et al.*, 1989).

Both of these proteins have been detected in GCF from patients with periodontitis (Bowers *et al.*, 1989). In addition, the total amount of both GCF osteonectin and bone phosphoprotein have been shown to increase in line with the site probing depth (Bowers *et al.*, 1989). They may therefore be associated with periodontal disease severity. However, no further cross-sectional or any longitudinal studies of these proteins have been reported to date.

Osteocalcin

Osteocalcin is a 5.4 kD calcium-binding protein of bone and is the most abundant non-collagenous protein of the mineralized tissues (Lian and Gundberg, 1988). It contains three residues of a specialized calcium-binding amino acid known as gamma-carboxyglutamic acid, and this allows specific confirmatory changes that promote hydroxyapatite binding and subsequent accumulation of bone (Hauschka *et al.*, 1975). Osteocalcin also chemotactically attracts osteoclast progenitor cells and blood monocytes (Glowacki and Lian, 1987; Mundy and Poser, 1987). In addition, it is stimulated by vitamin D_3 (Price and Baukol, 1980), producing concentrations that inhibit collagen synthesis in osteoblasts, promote bone resorption (Calalis and Lian, 1988) and stimulate the differentiation of progenitor cells capable of bone resorption (Lian *et al.*, 1985). Furthermore, elevated levels of osteocalcin are found in the blood during periods of rapid bone turnover, such as osteoporosis and fracture repair (Slovik *et al.*, 1984; Yasuruma *et al.*, 1987). For all these reasons, osteocalcin has been suggested as a possible marker for bone resorption and hence periodontal disease progression.

Osteocalcin can be assayed using polyclonal or monoclonal antibodies by an enzyme-linked immunosorbent assay (ELISA) or a radioimmune assay. An ELISA technique could be simplified and developed for use in a diagnostic test suitable for dental practice.

There have recently been two cross-sectional studies of the relation of GCF osteocalcin levels to periodontal disease severity. The first of these studied 19 patients, 5 with chronic gingivitis and 14 with chronic periodontitis at their initial visits (Kunimatsu *et al.*, 1993). Probing depth (PD), probing attachment level (PAL) and the gingival index (GI) were recorded and compared with the GCF osteocalcin levels. No significant amounts of osteocalcin were found in gingivitis patients, whereas in periodontitis patients varying levels of osteocalcin were found and these significantly correlated with the clinical parameters. The levels were highest at the sites with marked inflammation (GI = 3), and the results suggested that GCF osteocalcin levels reflected the degree of inflammation at the sampled sites.

The second cross-sectional study (Nakashima *et al.*, 1994) investigated 17 patients and compared the GCF osteocalcin levels at healthy, gingivitis and periodontitis sites. They found that osteocalcin was present at both healthy and diseased sites, and the mean concentrations in GCF were more than 10 times greater than normal serum levels. They also found that the total amounts of GCF osteocalcin at diseased sites were significantly higher than those at healthy or gingivitis sites. In addition, the total amounts of GCF osteocalcin significantly correlated with clinical parameters. However, when the GCF osteocalcin concentrations were compared, they correlated with GI but not with PD.

There have been no longitudinal studies in humans relating GCF osteocalcin levels to periodontal disease activity, but there has recently been one study relating these levels to the progression of ligature-induced experimental periodontitis in beagle dogs (Giannobile *et al.*, 1995). Thirty-six experimental sites and 36 control sites were examined longitudinally at 2-week intervals over 6 months. The GCF osteocalcin was measured by radioimmunoassays. Standardized radiographs were taken at 2-weekly intervals to measure the linear loss of alveolar bone, and the percentage bone loss at each 2-week interval was calculated using a previously described method (Jeffcoat and Williams, 1984). In addition, active bone loss was monitored monthly by assessing the uptake of a bone-seeking radioactive technetium compound (^{99}Tc-MDP) using a previously described nuclear medicine technique (Jeffcoat *et al.*, 1987).

The GCF osteocalcin levels increased significantly 2 weeks after the initiation of the disease, and this increase preceded significant increases in the bone-seeking radiopharmaceutical uptake (BSRU) by 2 weeks and the radiographical evidence of bone loss by 4 weeks. The BSRU was significantly elevated at experimental as compared to control sites at 4 weeks and 8 weeks post-disease initiation. GCF osteocalcin levels peaked at 8 and 10 weeks following ligature placement, at levels nearly 10-fold greater than those at contralateral control sites. Following the removal of the ligatures, the GCF osteocalcin levels dropped precipitously to approach control levels.

The diagnostic ratios of GCF osteocalcin concentration in predicting active bone loss were calculated at all time periods and these were 56% (sensitivity), 78% (specificity), 87% (positive prediction) and 34% (negative prediction). This indicates that GCF osteocalcin may serve as a predictor of active bone loss in experimental periodontitis, but the low figure for negative prediction means that it would fail to predict a significant number of truly active sites. If this were translated to a clinical situation, it would mean that these sites would not be treated.

Cross-linked carboxyterminal telopeptide of type I collagen

The pyridinoline cross-linked carboxyterminal telopeptide of type I collagen (CTP) is a 12–20 kD fragment of bone type I collagen (*Figure 13.7*) released by digestion with trypsin or bacterial collagenase (Risteli *et al.*, 1993). Type I collagen makes up about 90% of the organic matrix of bone. During synthesis of bone collagen, pyridinoline cross-links are formed between the telopeptide regions of

Carboxyterminal
peptide (telopeptide)   Triple Helix   Aminoterminal
peptide (telopeptide)

Figure 13.7 A diagram showing the pyridinoline cross-linked carboxyterminal telopeptide of type I collagen (CTP). This is found at the carboxyterminal end of bone type I collagen

an α_1 collagen molecule and a helical region of another such molecule, and this increases the mechanical stability of the structure.

CTP has recently been shown to correlate with bone turnover in myxoedema, thyrotoxicosis, primary hyperparathyroidism and post-menopausal osteoporosis (Eriksen *et al.*, 1993). Elevated CTP has also been shown to coincide with the bone resorptive rate (Eriksen *et al.*, 1993; Hassager *et al.*, 1994).

CTP has been detected in GCF (Talonpoika and Hämäläinen, 1994; Giannobile *et al.*, 1995) in periodontitis patients (Talonpoika and Hämäläinen, 1994), and in experimental periodontitis in dogs (Giannobile *et al.*, 1995).

There has been one recent cross-sectional study of GCF CTP in humans (Talonpoika and Hämäläinen, 1994). This studied 20 patients, who were divided into a periodontitis-affected group (13 subjects) and a periodontitis-free group (7 subjects). GCF was collected from 126 sites in all these patients. Four subjects from the periodontitis-affected group received periodontal treatment, and GCF samples were additionally collected 2, 5, 10, 20 and 40 days after treatment. GCF CTP was determined by a radioimmunological method. Significantly higher GCF CTP concentrations were found in the periodontitis-affected group compared to the periodontitis-free group, and the GCF levels were 100 times higher than serum reference levels. Significant positive correlations were found between the total amount of GCF CTP per site and pocket depth, radiological bone loss, papillary bleeding index and plaque index.

Periodontal treatment reduced the GCF CTP concentrations to levels found in healthy subjects. However, there were large variations in the amounts of GCF CTP found in individual patients and at individual sites within each patient. In this regard, some CTP levels below the detection limit were found in deep pockets and some high levels were found in periodontitis-free individuals. Thus, it is possible that GCF CTP levels reflect local type I collagen degradation in the periodontal tissues, which may or may not be reflected in the clinical parameters found at the site sampled.

There have been no longitudinal studies in humans relating GCF CTP levels to periodontal disease activity, but recently there has been one relating these levels to the progression of ligature-induced experimental periodontitis in beagle dogs (Giannobile *et al.*, 1995). This is the same study as has been described above for osteocalcin, and the experimental details are the same. GCF CTP was detected by radioimmunoassays. The GCF CTP levels increased

significantly 2 weeks after the initiation of the disease. This increase preceded significant increases in the bone-seeking radiopharmaceutical uptake (BSRU) by 2 weeks and the radiographical evidence of bone loss by 4 weeks. The BSRU was significantly elevated at experimental as compared to control sites at 4 and 8 weeks post-disease initiation. GCF CTP levels remained elevated throughout the entire disease progression phase.

The GCF CTP levels dropped precipitously following the removal of the ligatures and approached control levels. The diagnostic ratios of GCF CTP in predicting active bone loss were calculated at all time periods, and these were 95% (sensitivity), 81% (specificity), 87% (positive prediction) and 91% (negative prediction). These values were all considerably better than those for GCF osteocalcin, and indicate that GCF CTP levels relate positively to indices of active alveolar bone loss in experimental periodontitis and may serve as markers for future alveolar bone loss. Its use clinically, however, will depend on the results of human longitudinal studies.

Sampling GCF for these components

The detection of osteonectin requires the use of nitrocellulose strips, as it cannot be recovered from conventional strips (Bowers *et al.*, 1989). In contrast, GCF samples for the detection of osteocalcin and CTP (Giannobile *et al.*, 1995) were collected on conventional paper strips left *in situ* for 30 seconds. However, in some studies of osteocalcin and CTP, multiple strip collection was carried out using two strips in succession for 1 minute at the same site (Nakashima *et al.*, 1994), or three strips together at the same site for very short periods of collection (Talonpoika and Hämäläinen, 1994). Clearly, some standardization of collection technique is required if the data from such studies is to be compared.

Development of diagnostic tests

Most of the potential markers in this group could easily be adapted into test kits, as their detection involves the use of specific polyclonal or monoclonal antibodies. In this regard, the techniques for osteocalcin utilize either ELISA (Kunimatsu *et al.*, 1993; Nakashima *et al.*, 1994) or radioimmunoassays (Giannobile *et al.*, 1995), those for CTP utilize radioimmunoassays (Talonpoika and Hämäläinen, 1994; Giannobile *et al.*, 1995), and those for osteonectin and N-propeptide utilize ELISA (Bowers *et al.*, 1989).

Advantages and disadvantages of diagnostic tests using markers of bone resorption

Advantages

- Some of these potential markers associate with disease activity
- They are simple to use
- They can be read after relatively short periods
- They can be shown to the patient and related to the tooth site affected.

GCF CTP levels appear to predict active bone loss in experimental periodontitis in dogs, but have yet to be tested in a longitudinal study in humans.

Disadvantages

- The choice of the most appropriate biomarker is difficult with the present state of knowledge
- There is difficulty in determining the sites to sample and when to sample them
- Cost.

The choice of the most appropriate biomarker
Of the potential markers described in this section, none of them has been shown in longitudinal studies of human chronic periodontitis to predict disease activity. Osteocalcin and CTP seem, on the basis of cross-sectional human studies and studies on experimental periodontitis in dogs, to relate to alveolar bone resorption, and may thus have potential as markers. Their further development will, however, have to await the results of human longitudinal studies.

Determining the sites to sample and when to sample them
It is obviously not possible to sample all the sites in the mouth with any diagnostic test system, and for this reason the site(s) to be tested have to be preselected. This has already been discussed in the section above.

Cost
This has already been discussed above.

Clinical uses of a predictive diagnostic test

If a reliable predictive test were developed, it could predict future periodontal activity and thus enable site-specific treatment to be given before irreversible damage had occurred. For this to be the case, the marker, as already stated above, must have been shown in human longitudinal studies to have highly statistically significant correlations with confirmed attachment loss, both at the predictive and the attachment loss times. It should also have very high positive and negative predictive values in

diagnostic testing using 2×2 contingency tables. Multi-centre studies are also desirable. Only markers with these credentials should be used in clinical practice, and could be used for the reasons listed below:

- To help to prevent destructive disease
- To help to prevent progression of disease
- To identify high-risk patients
- To target treatment to specific sites
- To help to monitor the effects of periodontal treatment.

A periodontal diagnostic test could only help to prevent destructive disease if such a test was predictive of impending attachment loss at healthy gingival sites. If this were the case, it would only be possible to achieve this goal if all the sites in the mouth were tested regularly. Even if this were possible, disease progression could occur at any time between each test appointment, and could therefore easily be missed.

It is also no use using a marker that correlates with gingival inflammation because, although this always precedes attachment loss, it can be present for long periods in most patients without resulting in attachment loss. In addition, in some sites and some patients' mouths it may never result in attachment loss. Furthermore, gingival inflammation is simple to detect clinically and can be easily reversed with good plaque control and scaling providing no plaque retentive factors such as poor restorations are present.

Finally, since no attachment loss has occurred in the healthy patient, one has no idea of their susceptibility to periodontal disease as the amount of attachment loss cannot be related to their age. It is therefore not possible to determine how frequently to test the patient or, indeed, which sites in the mouth to test. If a test were ever used for this purpose it would probably be best to test the most common tooth sites to show attachment loss, such as mesially and distally to the first molars.

A predictive periodontal diagnostic test could be used to prevent progression of periodontal disease if tooth sites with previous attachment loss were regularly tested. However, it would still be possible for progression to occur between test visits, although this is less likely if these patients are on effective 3-monthly maintenance visits.

Some diagnostic tests may be capable of identifying high-risk patients by using mean values of the marker for the mouth from several sites. For this to be the case, a long duration longitudinal study must have shown highly statistically greater mean values for the marker in attachment loss patients (i.e. those which showed progressive attachment loss during the study) compared with non-attachment loss patients (i.e. those patients which did not show attachment loss during the study).

If a predictive test correctly identified a site with impending attachment loss, it could target treatment to that site and thus should prevent the attachment loss from occurring.

A test could also help to monitor periodontal treatment, as its level should reduce if the treatment is successful.

However, as periodontal disease is site-specific and its progression may be episodic, it is difficult to determine which sites to test or when to test them. This will therefore always be a problem, demanding sound clinical judgment.

References

Asikainen, S., Alaluusua, S. and Saxen, L. (1991) Recovery of *Actinobacillus actinomycetemcomitans* from teeth, tongue and saliva. *Journal of Periodontology* **62**, 203–206

Barnett, M.L., Ciancio, S.G. and Mather, M.L. (1980) The modified papillary bleeding index: comparison with gingival index during the resolution of gingivitis. *Journal of Preventive Dentistry* **6**, 135–138

Birkedal-Hansen, H. (1993) Role of matrix metalloproteinases in human periodontal diseases. *Journal of Periodontology* **64**, 474–484

Binder, T.A., Goodson, J.M. and Socransky, S.S. (1987) Gingival fluid levels of acid and alkaline phosphatase levels. *Journal of Periodontal Research* **22**, 14–19

Blankenvoorde, M.F., Heskens, Y.M., Van der Weijden, G.A. *et al.* (1997) Cystatin A in gingival crevicular fluid of periodontal patients. *Journal of Periodontal Research* **32**, 533–538.

Bowers, M.R., Fisher, L.W., Termine, J.D. and Somerman, M.J. (1989) Connective tissue-associated proteins in crevicular fluid: Potential markers for periodontal diseases. *Journal of Periodontology* **60**, 448–451

Bragd, L., Dahlén, G., Wikström, M. and Slots, J. (1987) The capability of *Actinobacillus actinomycetemcomitans*, *Bacteroides gingivalis* and *Bacteroides intermedius* to indicate progressive periodontitis. *Journal of Clinical Periodontology* **14**, 95–99

Calalis, E. and Lian, J.B. (1988) 1,25 dihydroxyvitamin D_3 effects on collagen and DNA synthesis in periosteum and periosteum-free calvaria. *Bone* **6**, 457–460

Cao, C.F. and Smith, Q.T. (1989) Crevicular fluid myeloperoxidase at healthy, gingivitis and periodontitis sites. *Journal of Clinical Periodontology* **16**, 17–20

Chambers, D.A., Crawford, J.M., Mukherjee, S. and Cohen, R.L. (1984) Aspartate aminotransferase increases in crevicular fluid during experimental periodontitis in beagle dogs. *Journal of Periodontology* **55**, 526–530

Chambers, D.A., Imrey, P.B., Cohen, R.L. *et al.* (1991) A longitudinal study of aspartate aminotransferase in human gingival crevicular fluid. *Journal of Periodontal Research* **26**, 65–74

Chapple, I.L., Glenwright, H.D., Matthews, J.B. *et al.* (1994) Site-specific alkaline phosphatase levels in gingival crevicular fluid in health and gingivitis: cross sectional studies. *Journal of Clinical Periodontology* **24**, 146–152

Chapple, I.L., Mason, G.I., Garner, I. *et al.* (1997) Enhanced chemiluminescent assay for measuring the antioxidant capacity of serum, saliva and crevicular fluid. *Annals of Clinical Biochemistry* **34**, 412–421

Chen, C.K., Dunford, R.G., Reynolds, H.S. and Zambon, J.J. (1989) *Eikenella corrodens* in the human oral cavity. *Journal of Periodontology* **60**, 611–616

Chen, H.-Y., Cox, S.W., Eley, B.M. *et al.* (1999) A comparison of matrix metalloproteinase-8 and elastase levels in gingival crevicular fluid from chronic adult periodontitis patients. *Journal of Clinical Periodontology*, in press

Cox, S.W. and Eley, B.M. (1989a) The detection of cathepsin B- and L-, elastase-, tryptase-, trypsin- and dipeptidyl peptidase IV-like activities in gingival crevicular fluid from gingivitis and periodontitis patients using peptidyl derivatives of 7-amino-4-trifluoromethylcoumarin. *Journal of Periodontal Research* **24**, 353–361

Cox, S.W. and Eley, B.M. (1989b) Identification of a tryptase-like enzyme in extracts of inflamed human gingiva by effector and gel-filtration studies. *Archives of Oral Biology* **34**, 219–221

Cox, S.W. and Eley, B.M. (1989c) Tryptase-like activity in crevicular fluid from gingivitis and periodontitis patients. *Journal of Periodontal Research* **24**, 41–44

Cox, S.W. and Eley, B.M. (1992) Cathepsin B/L-, elastase-, tryptase-, trypsin- and dipeptidyl peptidase IV-like activities in gingival crevicular fluid: a comparison of levels before and after basic periodontal treatment of chronic periodontitis patients. *Journal of Clinical Periodontology* **19**, 333–339

Cox, S.W., Cho, K., Eley, B.M. and Smith, R.E. (1990) A simple, combined fluorogenic and chromogenic method for the assay of proteases in gingival crevicular fluid. *Journal of Periodontal Research* **25**, 164–171

Cox, S.W., Gazi, M.I. and Eley, B.M. (1992) Dipeptidyl peptidase II- and IV-like activities in gingival tissue and crevicular fluid from human periodontitis lesions. *Archives of Oral Biology* **37**, 167–173

Cox, S.W., Kennett, C.N. and Eley, B.M. (1995) Evaluation of the cellular contribution to protease activities in gingival crevicular fluid. *Journal of Dental Research* **75** Abstr. 193, 846

Curtis, M.A., Griffiths, G.S., Price, S.J. *et al.* (1988) The total protein concentration of gingival crevicular fluid; variation with sampling time and gingival inflammation. *Journal of Clinical Periodontology* **15**, 628–632

Ebersole, J.L., Frey, D.E., Taubman, M.A. *et al.* (1984) Serological identification on oral *Bacteroides* sp. by enzyme-linked immunosorbent assay. *Journal of Clinical Microbiology* **19**, 639–644

Dinsdale, C.R.J., Rawlinson, A. and Walsh, T.F. (1997) Subgingival temperature in smokers and non smokers. *Journal of Clinical Periodontology* **24**, 761–766

Dzink, J.L., Tanner, A.R.C., Haffajee, A.D. and Socransky, S.S. (1985) Gram negative species associated with active destructive periodontal lesions. *Journal of Clinical Periodontology* **12**, 648–659

Dzink, J.L., Haffajee, A.D. and Socransky, S.S. (1988) The predominant cultivable microbiota of active and inactive lesions of destructive periodontal diseases. *Journal of Clinical Periodontology* **15**, 316–323

Eley, B.M. and Cox, S.W. (1990) A biochemical study of serine proteinase activities at local gingivitis sites in human chronic periodontitis. *Archives of Oral Biology* **35**, 23–27

Eley, B.M. and Cox, S.W. (1991) Cathepsin B and L-like activities at local gingival sites of chronic periodontitis patients. *Journal of Clinical Periodontology* **18**, 499–504

Eley, B.M. and Cox, S.W. (1992a) Crevicular fluid dipeptidyl peptidase activities before and after periodontal treatment. *Journal of Dental Research* **71**, 622

Eley, B.M. and Cox, S.W. (1992b) Cathepsin B/L-, elastase-, tryptase-, trypsin- and dipeptidyl peptidase IV-like activities in gingival crevicular fluid: correlation with clinical parameters in untreated chronic periodontitis patients. *Journal of Periodontal Research* **27**, 62–69

Eley, B.M. and Cox, S.W. (1992c) Correlation of gingival crevicular fluid proteases with clinical and radiological parameters of periodontal attachment loss. *Journal of Dentistry* **20**, 90–99

Eley, B.M. and Cox, S.W. (1992d) Cathepsin B/L-, elastase-, tryptase-, trypsin- and dipeptidyl peptidase IV-like activities in gingival crevicular fluid: a comparison of levels before and after periodontal surgery in chronic periodontitis patients. *Journal of Periodontology* **63**, 412–417

Eley, B.M. and Cox, S.W. (1993) Gingival crevicular fluid inflammatory cell proteases at healthy, gingivitis and periodontitis sites. *Journal of Dental Research* **72**, 705

Eley, B.M. and Cox, S.W. (1994) Bacterial proteases before and after periodontal treatment. *Journal of Dental Research* **73**, 799 Abst.

Eley, B.M. and Cox, S.W. (1995a) Bacterial proteases in gingival crevicular fluid before and after periodontal treatment. *British Dental Journal* **178**, 133–139

Eley, B.M. and Cox, S.W. (1995b) Correlation between gingival crevicular fluid dipeptidyl peptidase II and IV activity and periodontal attachment loss. A 2-year longitudinal study in chronic periodontitis patients. *Oral Diseases* **1**, 201–213

Eley, B.M. and Cox, S.W. (1996a) Correlation between gingivain/gingipain and bacterial dipeptidyl peptidase in gingival crevicular fluid and periodontal attachment loss in chronic periodontitis patients. A 2-year longitudinal study. *Journal of Periodontology* **67**, 703–716

Eley, B.M. and Cox, S.W. (1996b) The relationship between gingival crevicular fluid cathepsin B activity and periodontal attachment loss in chronic periodontitis patients. A 2-year longitudinal study. *Journal of Periodontal Research* **31**, 381–392

Eley, B.M. and Cox, S.W. (1996c) A 2-year longitudinal study of elastase in gingival crevicular fluid and periodontal attachment loss. *Journal of Clinical Periodontology* **23**, 681–692

Embery, G., Oliver, W.M., Stanbury, J.B. and Purvis, J.A. (1982) The electrophoretic detection of acid glycosaminoglycans in human gingival sulcus fluid. *Archives of Oral Biology* **27**, 177–179

Eriksen, E.F., Charles, P., Melsen, F. *et al.* (1993) Serum markers of type I collagen formation and degradation in metabolic bone disease: correlation with bone histomorphometry. *Journal of Bone Mineral Research* **8**, 127–132

French, C.K., Savitt, E.D., Simon, S.L. *et al.* (1986) DNA probe detection of periodontal pathogens. *Oral Microbiology and Immunology* **1**, 58–62

Friedman, S.A., Mandel, I.D. and Herrera, M.S. (1983) Lysozyme and lactoferrin quantifications in the crevicular fluid. *Journal of Periodontology* **54**, 347–350

Frisken, K.W., Tagg, J.R. and Laws, A.J. (1987) Suspected periodontopathic microorganisms and their oral habitats in young children. *Oral Microbiology and Immunology* **2**, 60–64

Garito, M.L., Prihoda, T.J. and McManus, L.M. (1995) Salivary PAF levels correlate with the severity of periodontal inflammation. *Journal of Dental Research* **74**, 1048–1056

Gazi, M.I., Cox, S.W., Clark, D.T. and Eley, B.M. (1994) Cathepsin B, tryptase and *Porphyromonas gingivalis* trypsin-like protease in gingival crevicular fluid. *Journal of Dental Research* **73**, 799

Gazi, M.I., Cox, S.W., Clark, D.T. and Eley, B.M. (1995) Comparison of host tissue and bacterial dipeptidylpeptidases in human gingival crevicular fluid by analytical isoelectric focusing. *Archives of Oral Biology* **40**, 731–736

Gazi, M.I., Cox, S.W., Clark, D.T. and Eley, B.M. (1996) A comparison of cysteine and serine proteinases in human gingival crevicular fluid with host tissue, saliva and bacterial enzymes by analytical isoelectric focusing. *Archives of Oral Biology* **41**, 393–400

Genco, R.J. (1992) Host responses in periodontal diseases: current concepts. *Journal of Periodontology* **63**, 338–355

Genco, R.C., Zambon, J.J. and Christersson, L.A. (1986) Use and interpretation of microbiological assays in periodontal diseases. *Oral Microbiology and Immunology* **1**, 73–79

Genco, R.C., Zambon, J.J. and Christersson, L.A. (1988) The origin of periodontal infections. *Advances in Dental Research* **2**, 245–259

Giannobile, W.V., Lynch, S.E., Denmark, R.G. *et al.* (1995) Crevicular fluid osteocalcin and pyridinoline cross-linked carboxyterminal telopeptide of type I collagen (ICTP) as markers of rapid bone turnover in periodontitis. A pilot study in beagle dogs. *Journal of Clinical Periodontology* **22**, 903–910

Glowacki, J. and Lian, J.B. (1987) Impaired recruitment by osteoclast progenitors by osteocalcin deficient bone implants. *Cellular Differentiation* **21**, 247–254

Golub, L.M., Siegel, K., Ramamurthy, N.S. and Mandel, I.D. (1976) Some characteristics of collagenase activity in gingival crevicular fluid and its relationship to gingival disease in humans. *Journal of Dental Research* **55**, 1049–1057

Greenstein, G. (1988) Microbiological assessments to enhance periodontal disease diagnosis. *Journal of Periodontology* **59**, 508–515

Guven, Y., Satman, I., Dinccag, N. and Alptekin, S. (1996) Salivary peroxidase activity in whole saliva of patients with insulin dependent (type 1) diabetes mellitus. *Journal of Clinical Periodontology* **23**, 879–881

Haffajee, A.D. and Socransky S.S. (1986) Attachment level changes in destructive periodontal disease. *Journal of Clinical Periodontology* **13**, 461–472

Haffajee, A.D., Socransky S.S. and Goodson, J.M. (1992a) Subgingival temperature. I. Relation to baseline clinical parameters. *Journal of Clinical Periodontology* **19**, 401–408

Haffajee, A.D., Socransky S.S. and Goodson, J.M. (1992b) Subgingival temperature. II. Relation to future attachment loss. *Journal of Clinical Periodontology* **19**, 409–416

Haffajee, A.D., Socransky S.S. and Goodson, J.M. (1992b) Subgingival temperature. III. Relation to microbial counts. *Journal of Clinical Periodontology* **19**, 417–422

Häkkarainen, K., Uitto, V.-J. and Ainamo, J. (1988) Collagenase activity and protein content of sulcular fluid after scaling and occlusal adjustment of teeth with deep periodontal pockets. *Journal of Periodontal Research* **23**, 204–210

Hassager, C., Jensen, L.T., Pødenphant, J. *et al.* (1994) The carboxyterminal pyridinoline cross-linked telopeptide of type I collagen in serum as a marker of bone resorption: the effect of nandrolone decanoate and hormone replacement therapy. *Calcified Tissue International* **54**, 30–33

Hauschka, P.V., Lian, J.B. and Gallop P.M. (1975) Direct identification of the calcium-binding amino acid gamma-carboxyglutamic acid in mineralized tissue. *Proceedings of the Royal Academy of Science USA* **72**, 3925

Hayakawa, H., Yamashita, K., Ohwaki, K. *et al.* (1994) Collagenase activity and tissue inhibitor of metalloproteinases-1 (TIMP-1) content in human whole saliva from clinically healthy and periodontally diseased subjects. *Journal of Periodontal Research* **29**, 305–308

Heskens, Y.M., Van der Velden, U., Veerman, E.C. and Nieuw-Amerongen, A.V. (1993a) Protein, albumin and cystatin concentrations in saliva of healthy subjects and of patients with gingivitis or periodontitis. *Journal of Periodontal Research* **28**, 43–48

Heskens, Y.M., Van der Velden, U., Veerman, E.C. and Nieuw-Amerongen, A.V. (1993b) Cystatin C levels of whole saliva are increased in periodontal patients. *Annals of the New York Academy of Science* **694**, 280–282

Heskens, Y.M., Veerman, E.C., Mantel, M.S. *et al.* (1994) Cystatins S and C in human whole saliva in glandular salivas in periodontal health and disease. *Journal of Dental Research* **73**, 1606–1614

Heskens, Y.M., Van den Keijbus, P.A., Veerman, E.C. *et al.* (1996a) Protein composition of whole and parotid saliva in healthy and periodontitis subjects. *Journal of Periodontal Research* **31**, 57–65

Heskens, Y.M., Van der Weijden, G.A., Van den Keijbus, P.A. *et al.* (1996b) Effects of periodontal treatment on the protein composition of whole and parotid saliva. *Journal of Periodontology* **67**, 205–212

Highfield, P.E. and Dougan, G. (1985) DNA probes for microbial diagnosis. *Medical Laboratory Science* **42**, 352–360

Hönig, C., Rordorf-Adam, C., Siegmund, C. *et al.* (1989) Increased interleukin beta (IL-1β) concentration in gingival tissue from periodontitis patients. *Journal of Periodontal Research* **24**, 362–367

Horowitz, A. and Folke, E.A. (1972) Hydrogen sulphide and periodontal disease. *Periodontal Abstracts* **2**, 59–62

Imrey, P.B., Crawford, J.M., Cohen, R.L. *et al.* (1991) A cross-sectional analysis of aspartate aminotransferase in human gingival crevicular fluid. *Journal of Periodontal Research* **26**, 75–84

Ingman, T., Sorsa, T., Konttinen, Y.T. *et al.* (1993) Salivary collagenase, elastase- and trypsin-like proteases as biochemical markers of periodontal tissue destruction in adult and localized juvenile periodontitis. *Oral Microbiology and Immunology* **8**, 298–305

Ingman, T., Sorsa, T., Lindy, O. *et al.* (1994) Multiple forms of gelatinases/type IV collagenases in saliva and gingival crevicular fluid of periodontitis patients. *Journal of Clinical Periodontology* **21**, 26–31

Ingman, T., Tervahartiala, T., Ding, Y. *et al.* (1996) Matrix metalloproteinases and their inhibitors in gingival crevicular fluid and saliva of periodontitis patients. *Journal of Clinical Periodontology* **23**, 1127–1132

Ishiwaka, I. and Cimasoni, G. (1970) Alkaline phosphatase in human gingival fluid and its relationship to periodontitis. *Archives of Oral Biology* **15**, 1401–1404

Ishiwaka, I., Cimasoni, G. and Ahmad-Zadeh, C. (1972) Possible role of lysosomal enzymes in the pathogenesis of periodontitis. A study of cathepsin D in human gingival fluid. *Archives of Oral Biology* **17**, 111–117

Jeffcoat, M.K. and Reddy, M.S. (1991) Progression of probing attachment loss in adult periodontitis. *Journal of Periodontology* **62**, 185–189

Jeffcoat, M.K. and Williams, R.C. (1984) Relationships between linear and area measurements of bone levels utilizing a simple computerized technique. *Journal of Periodontal Research* **19**, 191–198

Jeffcoat, M.K., Williams, R.C., Johnson, H.G. *et al.* (1985) Treatment of periodontal disease in beagles with lodoxamide ethyl, an inhibitor of mast cell release. *Journal of Periodontal Research* **20**, 532–541

Jeffcoat, M.K., Williams, R.C., Caplan, M.L. and Goldhaber, P. (1987) Nuclear medicine techniques for the detection of active alveolar bone loss. *Advances in Dental Research* **1**, 80–84

Jolley, M.E. (1996) Fluorescence polarization assays for the detection of proteases and their inhibitors. *Journal of Biomedical Screening* **1**, 33–38

Kennett, C.N., Cox, S.W., Eley, B.M. and Osman, I.A.R.M. (1993) Comparative histochemical and biochemical studies of mast cell tryptase in human gingiva. *Journal of Periodontology* **64**, 870–877

Kennett, C.N., Cox, S.W. and Eley, B.M. (1994a) Comparative histochemical, biochemical and immunocytochemical studies of cathepsin B in human gingiva. *Journal of Periodontal Research* **29**, 203–213

Kennett, C.N., Cox, S.W. and Eley, B.M. (1994b) Histochemical, immunocytochemical and biochemical studies of dipeptidyl peptidases in human gingival tissue. *Journal of Dental Research* **74** Abstr. 192, 845

Kennett, C.N., Cox, S.W. and Eley, B.M. (1995) Localization of active and inactive elastase, alpha-1-proteinase inhibitor and alpha-2-macroglobulin in human gingiva. *Journal of Dental Research* **74**, 667–674

Kennett, C.N., Cox, S.W. and Eley, B.M. (1996) The histochemical and immunocytochemical localization of dipeptidylpeptidase II and IV in human gingiva. *Journal of Periodontology* **67**, 846–852

Kennett, C.N., Cox, S.W. and Eley, B.M. (1997a) Investigations into the cellular contribution of host tissue protease activity in gingival crevicular fluid. *Journal of Clinical Periodontology* **24**, 424–431

Kennett, C.N., Cox, S.W. and Eley, B.M. (1997b) Ultrastructural localization of cathepsin B in gingival tissue from chronic periodontitis patients. *Histochemical Journal* **29**, 727–734

Kowashi, Y., Jaccard, F. and Cimasoni, G. (1979) Increase of free collagenase and neutral protease activities in the gingival crevice during experimental gingivitis in Man. *Archives of Oral Biology* **34**, 645–650

Kryshalskyi, E. and Sodek, J. (1987) Nature of collagenolytic enzyme and inhibitor activity in gingival crevicular fluid from healthy and inflamed periodontal tissues of beagle dogs. *Journal of Periodontal Research* **22**, 264–269

Kryshalskyi, E., Sodek, J. and Ferrier, J.M. (1986) Correlation of collagenolytic enzymes and inhibitors in gingival crevicular fluid with clinical and microscopic changes in experimental periodontitis in the dog. *Archives of Oral Biology* **31**, 21–31

Kunimatsu, K., Mataki, S., Tanaka, H. *et al.* (1993) A cross-sectional study of osteocalcin levels in gingival crevicular fluid from periodontitis patients. *Journal of Periodontology* **64**, 865–869

Lamster, I.B. (1992) The host response in gingival crevicular fluid: potential applications in periodontitis clinical trials. *Journal of Periodontology* **63**, 1117–1123

Lamster, I.B., Holmes, L.G., Gross, K.B.W. *et al.* (1994) The relationship of β-glucuronidase activity in crevicular fluid to clinical parameters of periodontal disease. Findings from a multicenter study. *Journal of Clinical Periodontology* **21**, 118–127

Lamster, I.B., Oshrain, R.L., Harper, D.S. *et al.* (1988) Enzyme activity in crevicular fluid for detection and prediction of clinical attachment loss in patients with chronic adult periodontitis. *Journal of Periodontology* **59**, 516–523

Lamster, I.B., Oshrain, R.L., Celenti, R.S. *et al.* (1991) Indicators of the acute inflammatory and humoral immune responses in gingival crevicular fluid: Relationship to active periodontal disease. *Journal of Periodontal Research* **26**, 261–263

Larivee, L., Sodek, J. and Ferrier, J.M. (1986) Collagenase and collagenase inhibitor activity in crevicular fluid of patients receiving treatment for localized juvenile periodontitis. *Journal of Periodontal Research* **21**, 702–715

Last, K.S., Stanbury, J.B. and Embery, G. (1985) Glycosaminoglycans in human gingival crevicular fluid as indicators of active periodontal disease. *Archives of Oral Biology* **30**, 275–281

Lee, H.-J., Kang, I.-K., Chang, C.-P. and Choi, S.-M. (1995a) The subgingival microflora and gingival crevicular fluid cytokines in refractory periodontitis. *Journal of Clinical Periodontology* **22**, 885–890

Lee, W., Aitken, S., Sodek, J. and McCulloch, C.A.G. (1995b) Evidence of a direct relationship between neutrophil collagenase activity and periodontal tissue destruction *in vivo*: role of active enzyme in human periodontitis. *Journal of Periodontal Research* **30**, 23–33

Lian, J.B. and Gundberg, C.M. (1988) Osteocalcin: biochemical considerations and clinical applications. *Clinical Orthopaedics and Related Research* **226**, 267–291

Lian, J.B., Couttes, M.C. and Canalis, E. (1985) Studies of the hormone regulation of osteocalcin synthesis in cultured fetal rat calvaria. *Journal of Biological Chemistry* **260**, 8706

Lin, M., Sugden, E.A., Jolley, M.E. and Stilwell, K.C. (1996) Modification of the *Mycobacterium bovis* extracellular protein MPB70 with fluoroscein for rapid detection of specific serum anitbodies by fluorescence polarization. *Clinical and Diagnostic Laboratory Immunology* **3**, 438–443

Listgarten, M.A. (1986) Direct microscopy of periodontal pathogens. *Oral Microbiology and Immunology* **1**, 31–36

Listgarten, M.A. (1992) Microbial testing in the diagnosis of periodontal disease. *Journal of Periodontology* **63**, 332–337

Listgarten, M.A. and Levin, S. (1981) Positive correlation between proportions of subgingival spirochaetes and motile bacteria and susceptibility of human subjects to periodontal deterioration. *Journal of Clinical Periodontology* **8**, 122–138

Listgarten, M.A., Schifter, C.C., Sulivan, P. *et al.* (1986) Failure of a microbial assay to reliably predict disease recurrence in a treated periodontitis population receiving regularly scheduled prophylaxes. *Journal of Clinical Periodontology* **13**, 768–773

Listgarten, M.A., Slots, J., Nowotny, A.H. *et al.* (1991) Incidence of periodontitis recurrence in treated patients with and without cultivable *Actinobacillus actinomycetemcomitans*, *Porphyromonas gingivalis* and *Prevotella intermedia*: a prospective study. *Journal of Periodontology* **62**, 377–386

Löe, H. (1967) The gingival index, the plaque index and the retention index systems. *Journal of Periodontology* **38**, 610–616

Loesche, W.J. (1986) The identification of bacteria associated with periodontal disease and dental caries by enzymatic methods. *Oral Microbiology and Immunology* **1**, 65–70

Loesche, W.J. (1992) DNA probe and enzyme analysis in periodontal diagnosis. *Journal of Periodontology* **63**, 1102–1109

Loesche, W.J., Bretz, W., Lopatin, D. *et al.* (1990) Multi-center clinical evaluation of a chairside method for detecting certain periodontopathic bacteria in periodontal disease. *Journal of Periodontology* **61**, 189–196

Lopatin, D.E., Caffessee, E.R., Bye, F.L. and Caffessee, R.G. (1989) Concentrations of fibronectin in the sera and crevicular fluid in various stages of periodontal disease. *Journal of Clinical Periodontology* **16**, 359–364

Makela, M., Salo, T., Uitto, V.J. and Larjava, H. (1994) Matrix metalloproteinases (MMP-2 and MMP-9) of the oral cavity: cellular origin and relationship to periodontal status. *Journal of Dental Research* **73**, 1397–1406

Macotte, H. and Lavoie, M.C. (1998) Oral microbial ecology and the role of salivary immunoglobulin A. *Microbiology and Molecular Biology Review* **62**, 71–109

Mandell, R.L. and Socransky, S.S. (1981) Selective medium for *Actinobacillus actinomycetemcomitans* and the incidence of the organism in juvenile periodontitis. *Journal of Periodontology* **52**, 593–598

Markkanen, H., Syrjanen, S.M. and Alakuijala, P. (1986) Salivary IgA, lysozyme and beta-2-microglobulin in periodontal disease. *Scandinavian Journal of Dental Research* **94**, 115–120

Masada, M.P., Persson, R., Kenney, J.L. *et al.* (1990) Measurement of interleukin-1α and 1β in gingival crevicular fluid: implications for the pathogenesis of periodontal disease. *Journal of Periodontal Research* **25**, 156–163

Matsuki, H., Fujimoto, N., Iwata, K. *et al.* (1996) A one-step sandwich enzyme immunoassay (EIA) system for human matrix metalloproteinase-8 (neutrophil collagenase) using monoclonal antibodies. *Clinica Chimica Acta* **31**, 244, 129–143

Matto, J., Saarela, M., Von Triol-Linden, B. *et al.* (1996) Similarity of salivary and subgingival *Prevotella intermedia* and *Prevotella nigrescens* isolates by arbitrarily primed polymerase chain reaction. *Oral Microbiology and Immunology* **11**, 395–401

Matto, J., Saarela, M., Alaluusua, S. *et al.* (1998) Detection of *Porphyromonas gingivalis* from saliva by PCR using a simple sample processing method. *Journal of Clinical Microbiology* **36**, 157–160

McLaughlin, W.S., Kirkham, J., Kowalik, M.J. and Robinson, C. (1996) Human gingival crevicular fluid keratin at healthy, chronic gingivitis and chronic adult periodontitis sites. *Journal of Clinical Periodontology* **23**, 331–335

Moore, S., Calder, K.A., Miller, N.J. and Rice-Evans, C.A. (1994) Antioxidant activity of saliva and periodontal disease. *Free Radical Research* **21**, 417–425

Moore, W.E.C., Moore, L.H. and Ranney, R.R. (1991) The microflora of periodontal sites showing active destruction progression. *Journal of Clinical Periodontology* **18**, 729–739

Muller, H.P., Heinecke, A., Borneff, M. *et al.* (1997) Microbial ecology of *Actinobacillus actinomycetemcomitans*, *Eikenella corrodens* and *Capnocytophaga* spp. in adult periodontitis. *Journal of Periodontal Research* **32**, 530–542

Mundy, G.R. and Poser, J.W. (1987) Chemical activity of the γ-carboxyglutamic acid-containing protein in bone. *Calcified Tissue International* **40**, 57

Nakashima, K., Roehrich, N. and Cimasoni, G. (1994) Osteocalcin, prostaglandin E$_2$ and alkaline phosphate in gingival crevicular fluid: their relations to periodontal status. *Journal of Clinical Periodontology* **21**, 327–333

Nieminen, A., Nordlund, L. and Uitto, V.J. (1993a) The effect of treatment on the activity of salivary proteases and glycosidases in adults with advanced periodontitis. *Journal of Periodontology* **64**, 297–301

Nieminen, A., Kari, K. and Saxen, L. (1993b) Specific antibodies against *Actinobacillus actinomycetemcomitans* in serum and saliva of patients with advanced periodontitis. *Scandinavian Journal of Dental Research* **101**, 196–201

Nieminen, A., Asikainen, S., Tokko, H. *et al.* (1996) Value of some laboratory and clinical measurements in the treatment plan for advanced periodontitis. *Journal of Clinical Periodontology* **23**, 572–581

Offenbacher, S., Odle, B.M. and Van Dyke, T.E. (1986) The use of crevicular fluid prostaglandin E$_2$ levels as a predictor of periodontal attachment loss. *Journal of Periodontal Research* **21**, 101–112

Offenbacher, S., Heasman, P.A. and Collins, J.G. (1993) Modulation of host PGE$_2$ secretion as a determinant of periodontal disease expression. *Journal of Periodontology* **64**, 432–444

Okazaki, J., Kamada, A., Gonda, Y. *et al.* (1996) High-performance liquid chromatography analysis of chondroitin sulphate isomers in human whole saliva in a variety of clinical conditions. *Oral Diseases* **2**, 224–227

Over, C., Yamalik, N., Yavuzyilmaz, E. *et al.* (1993) Myeloperoxidase activity in peripheral blood neutrophils, crevicular fluid and whole saliva of patients with periodontal disease. *Journal of the Nihon University School of Dentistry* **35**, 235–240

Overall, C.M. and Sodek, J. (1987) Initial characterization of a neutral metalloproteinase, active on 3/4-collagen fragments, synthesized by ROS 17/2.8 osteoblastic cells, periodontal fibroblasts, and identified in gingival crevicular fluid. *Journal of Dental Research* **66**, 1271–1282

Page, R.C. (1991) The role of inflammatory mediators in the pathogenesis of periodontal disease. *Journal of Periodontal Research* **26**, 230–242

Page, R.C. (1992) Host response tests for diagnosing periodontal diseases. *Journal of Periodontology* **63**, 356–366

Palcanis, K.G., Larjava, I.K., Wells, B.R. *et al.* (1992) Elastase as an indicator of periodontal disease progression. *Journal of Periodontology* **63**, 237–274

Patters, M.R., Niekrash, C.E. and Lang, N.P. (1989) Assessment of complement cleavage in gingival fluid during experimental gingivitis. *Journal of Clinical Periodontology* **16**, 33–37

Pederson, E.D., Stanke, S.R., Whitener, S.J. *et al.* (1995) Salivary levels of alpha-2-macrogobulin, alpha-1-antitrypsin, C-reactive protein, cathepsin G and elastase in humans with and without destructive periodontal disease. *Archives of Oral Biology* **40**, 1151–1155

Persson, S. Claesson, R and Carlsson, J. (1989) The capacity of the subgingival microbiota to produce volatile sulphur compounds in human serum. *Oral Microbiology and Immunology* **4**, 169–172

Persson, S., Edlund, M.B., Claesson, R and Carlsson, J. (1990a) The formation of H$_2$S and CH$_3$SH by oral bacteria. *Oral Microbiology and Immunology* **5**, 195–201

Persson, G.R., De Rouen, T.A. and Page, R.C. (1990b) Relationship between levels of aspartate aminotransferase in gingival crevicular fluid and gingival inflammation. *Journal of Periodontal Research* **25**, 17–24

Persson, G.R., De Rouen, T.A. and Page, R.C. (1990c) Relationship between gingival crevicular fluid levels of aspartate aminotransferase and active tissue destruction in treated chronic periodontitis patients. *Journal of Periodontal Research* **25**, 81–87

Persson, G.R., Alves, M.E., Chambers, D.A. *et al.* (1995) A multicenter clinical trial of Periogard in distinguishing between diseased and healthy sites. I. Study design, methodology and therapeutic outcome. *Journal of Clinical Periodontology* **22**, 794–808

Pinducciu, G., Micheletti, L., Piras, V. *et al.* (1996) Periodontal disease, oral microbial flora and salivary antibacterial factors in diabetes mellitus type l patients. *European Journal of Epidemiology* **12**, 631–636

Polychronopoulou, T. (1998) A study of a probe to measure volatile sulphides and clinical parameters in periodontal health and disease. M. Dent. Sci. Thesis. University of Liverpool

Price, P.A. and Baukol, S.A. (1980) 1,25(OH)$_2$D$_3$ increases the synthesis of the vitamin K dependent protein by osteosarcoma cells. *Journal of Biological Chemistry* **255**, 1160–1163

Rasch, M.S., Mealey, B.L., Woodard, D.S. *et al.* (1995) The effect of initial therapy on salivary platelet activating factor levels in chronic adult periodontitis. *Journal of Periodontology* **66**, 613–623

Reiff, R.L. (1984) Serum and salivary IgG and IgA response to initial preparation therapy. *Journal of Periodontology* **55**, 299–305

Reinhardt, R.A., McDonald, T.L., Bolton, R.W. *et al.* (1989) IgG subclasses in gingival crevicular fluid from active versus stable periodontal sites. *Journal of Periodontology* **60**, 44–50

Reinhardt, R.A., Masada, M.P., Kaldahl, W.B. *et al.* (1993) Gingival fluid IL-1 and IL-6 levels in refractory periodontitis. *Journal of Clinical Periodontology* **20**, 225–231

Renvert, S., Wikström, M., Mugrabi, M. *et al.* (1998) Association of crevicular fluid elastase-like activity with histologically-confirmed attachment loss in ligature-induced periodontitis in beagle dogs. *Journal of Clinical Periodontology* **25**, 368–374

Reynolds, J.J. (1996) Collagenases and tissue inhibitors of metalloproteinases; a functional balance in tissue degradation. *Oral Diseases* **2**, 70–76

Reynolds, J.J., Hembry, R.M. and Meikle, M.C. (1994) Connective tissue degradation in health and periodontal disease and the role of matrix metalloproteinases and their natural inhibitors. *Advances in Dental Research* **8**, 312–319

Risteli, J., Elomaa, I., Neimi, S. *et al.* (1993) Radioimmunoassay for the pyridinoline cross-linked carboxyterminal peptide of type I collagen: a new serum marker of bone collagen degradation. *Clinical Chemistry* **39**, 635–640

Roa, R.N., Balamuralikrishnan, K., Vasantkumar, A. *et al.* (1995) A study of antitrypsin and macroglobulin levels in serum amd saliva of patients with gingivitis. *Indian Journal of Dental Research* **6**, 41–46

Rossomando, E.F., Kennedy, J.E. and Hadjimichael, J. (1990) Tumor necrosis factor alpha in gingival crevicular fluid as a possible indicator of periodontal disease in humans. *Archives of Oral Biology* **35**, 431–434

Sandholm, L. (1986) Proteases and their inhibitors in chronic inflammatory periodontal disease. *Journal of Clinical Periodontology* **13**, 19–26

Sandholm, L. and Gronblad, E. (1984) Salivary immunoglobulins in patients with juvenile periodontitis and their healthy siblings. *Journal of Periodontology* **55**, 9–12

Sandholm, L., Tolo, K. and Olsen, I. (1987) Salivary IgG, a parameter of periodontal disease activity? High responder to *Actinobacillus actinomycetemcomitans* Y4 in juvenile and adult periodontitis. *Journal of Clinical Periodontology* **14**, 289–294

Savitt, E.D., Strzemoko, M.N., Vaccaro K.K. *et al.* (1988) Comparison of cultural methods and DNA probe analysis for the detection of *A. actinomycetemcomitans*, *P. gingivalis* and *B. intermedius* in subgingival plaque samples. *Journal of Periodontology* **59**, 431–438

Schade, S.Z., Jolley, M.E., Sarauer, B.J. and Simonson, L.G. (1996) BODIPY-α-casein, a pH-independent protein substrate for protease assays using fluorescence polarization. *Analytical Biochemistry* **243**, 1–7

Schmidt, E.F., Bretz, W.A., Hutchinson, R.A. and Loesche, W.J. (1988) Correlation of the hydrolysis of benzoyl-arginine-naphthylamide (BANA) by plaque with clinical parameters and subgingival levels of spirochaetes in periodontal patients. *Journal of Dental Research* **67**, 1505–1509

Slots, J. and Listgarten, M.A. (1988) *Bacteroides gingivalis*, *Bacteroides intermedius* and *Actinobacillus actinomycetemcomitans* in human periodontal diseases. *Journal of Clinical Periodontology* **15**, 85–93

Slots, J., Emrich, L.J. and Genco, R. (1985) Relationship between some subgingival bacteria and periodontal pocket depth and gain or loss of attachment after treatment of adult periodontitis. *Journal of Clinical Periodontology* **12**, 540–552

Slots, J., Bragd, L., Wikström, M. and Dahlén, G. (1986) The occurrence of *Actinobacillus actinomycetemcomitans*, *Bacteroides gingivalis* and *Bacteroides intermedius* in destructive periodontal disease in adults. *Journal of Clinical Periodontology* **13**, 570–577

Slovik, M., Gundberg, C.M, Neer, R.M. and Lian, J.B. (1984) Clinical evaluation of bone turnover by serum osteocalcin measurements. *Journal of Clinical Endocrinology and Metabolism* **59**, 228–230

Smith, Q.T., Hinrichs, J.E. and Melnyk, R.S. (1986) Gingival crevicular fluid myeloperoxidase at periodontitis sites. *Journal of Periodontal Research* **21**, 45–55

Socransky, S.S. and Haffajee, A.D. (1992) The bacterial etiology of destructive periodontal disease: current concepts. *Journal of Periodontology* **63**, 322–337

Sorsa, T., Suomalainen, K. and Uitto, V.J. (1990) The role of gingival crevicular fluid and salivary interstitial collagenases in human periodontal disease. *Archives of Oral Biology* **35** Suppl., 193S–196S

Sorsa, T., Ding, Y., Salo, T. *et al.* (1994) Effects of tetracyclines on neutrophil, gingival and salivary collagenases. A functional and western-blot assessment with special reference to their cellular sources in periodontal diseases. *Annals of the New York Academy of Science* **732**, 112–131

Sterne, J.A.C., Curtis, M.A., Gillett, I.R. *et al.* (1990) Statistical models for data from periodontal research. *Journal of Clinical Periodontology* **17**, 129–137

Suomalainen, K., Saxen, L., Vilja, P. and Tenovuo, J. (1996) Peroxidases, lactoferrin and lysozyme in peripheral blood neutrophils, gingival crevicular fluid and whole saliva of patients with localized juvenile periodontitis. *Oral Diseases* **2**, 129–134

Svanberg, G.K. (1987) Hydroxyproline determination in serum and gingival crevicular fluid. *Journal of Periodontal Research* **22**, 133–138

Talonpoika, J.T. and Hämäläinen M.M. (1994) Type I collagen carboxyterminal telopeptide in human gingival crevicular fluid in different clinical conditions and after periodontal treatment. *Journal of Clinical Periodontology* **21**, 320–326

Talonpoika, J.T., Heino, J., Larjava, H. *et al.* (1989) Gingival crevicular fluid fibronectin degradation in periodontal health and disease. *Scandinavian Journal of Dental Research* **97**, 415–421

Tanner, A.R.C., Socransky, S.S., and Goodson, J.M. (1984) Microbiota of periodontal pockets losing alveolar crestal bone. *Journal of Periodontal Research* **19**, 279–291

Termine, J.D., Kleinmann, H.K., Whitson, S.W. *et al.* (1981) Osteonectin, a bone-specific protein linking mineral to collagen. *Cell* **26**, 99–105

Theilade, E. (1986) The non-specific theory in microbial etiology of inflammatory periodontal diseases. *Journal of Clinical Periodontology* **13**, 905–911

Timmerman, M.F., Van der Weijden, G.A., Armand, S. *et al.* (1998) Untreated periodontal disease in Indonesian adolescents: clinical and microbiological baseline data. *Journal of Clinical Periodontology* **25**, 215–224

Uitto, V.J., Suomalainen, K. and Sorsa, T. (1990) Salivary collagenase. Origin, characteristics and relationship to periodontal health. *Journal of Periodontal Research* **25**, 135–142

Uitto, V.J., Nieminen, A., Coil, J. *et al.* (1996) Oral fluid elastase as an indicator of periodontal health. *Journal of Clinical Periodontology* **23**, 30–60

Vaes, G. (1988) Cellular biology and biochemical mechanism of bone resorption. *Clinical Orthopaedics and Related Research* **231**, 239–271

Van Os, J.H., de Jong, M.H., and Van der Hoeven, H. (1986) Growth of supragingival plaque organisms in enrichment cultures in saliva. *Journal of Dental Research* **65**, 836

Villela, B., Cogan, R.B., Bartolucci, A.A. and Birkedal-Hansen, H. (1987) Collagenolytic activity in crevicular fluid from patients with chronic adult periodontitis, localized juvenile periodontitis and gingivitis, and from healthy control subjects. *Journal of Periodontal Research* **22**, 381–389

Von Triol-Linden, B., Torkko, H., Alaluusua, S. *et al.* (1995) Salivary levels of suspected periodontal pathogens in relation to periodontal status and treatment. *Journal of Dental Research* **74**, 1789–1795

Von Triol-Linden, B., Alaluusua, S., Wolf, J. *et al.* (1997) Periodontitis patient and the spouse: periodontal bacteria before and after treatment. *Journal of Clinical Periodontology* **24**, 893–899

Vrecko, K., Staedtler, P., Mischak, I. *et al.* (1997) Periodontitis and concentrations of the cellular immune activation marker neopterin in saliva and urine. *Clinica Chimica Acta* **268**, 31–40

Wennström, J.L., Dahlén, G., Swensson, J. and Nyman, S. (1987) *Actinobacillus actinomycetemcomitans*, *Bacteroides gingivalis* and *Bacteroides intermedius*: predictors of attachment loss? *Oral Microbiology and Immunology* **2**, 158–163

Westerlund, U., Ingman, T., Lukinmaa, P.L. *et al.* (1996) Human neutrophil gelatinase and associated lipocalin in adult and localized juvenile periodontitis. *Journal of Dental Research* **75**, 1553–1563

Wolff, L.F., Koller, N.J., Smith, Q.T. *et al.* (1997) Subgingival temperature relation to gingival crevicular fluid enzymes, cytokines and subgingival plaque organisms. *Journal of Clinical Periodontology* **24**, 900–906

Yaegaki, K. and Sanda, K. (1992a) Biochemical and clinical factors influencing oral malodour in periodontal patients. *Journal of Periodontology* **63**, 783–789

Yaegaki, K. and Sanda, K. (1992b) Volatile sulfur compounds in mouth air from clinically healthy subjects and patients with periodontal disease. *Journal of Periodontal Research* **27**, 233–238

Yamalik, N., Ozer, N., Caglayan, F. and Caglayan, G. (1990) Determination of pseudocholinesterase activity in gingival crevicular fluid, saliva and serum from patients with juvenile periodontitis and rapidly progressive periodontitis. *Journal of Dental Research* **69**, 87–89

Yamalik, N., Ozer, N., Caglayan, F. *et al.* (1991) The effect of periodontal therapy on salivary pseudocholinesterase activity. *Journal of Dental Research* **70**, 988–990

Yasuruma, S., Aloia, J., Yeh, J. *et al.* (1987) Serum osteocalcin and total body calcium in normal, pre- and postmenopausal women and postmenopausal osteoporotic patients. *Journal of Clinical Endocrinology Metabolism* **64**, 681

Zambon, J.J., Nakamura, N. and Slots, J. (1985a) Effect of periodontal therapy on salivary enzyme activity. *Journal of Periodontal Research* **20**, 652–659

Zambon, J.J., Reynolds, H.S., Chen, P. and Genco, R.J. (1985b) Rapid detection of periodontal pathogens in subgingival plaque. Comparison of indirect immunofluorescence microscopy with bacterial cultures for detection of *Bacteroides gingivalis*. *Journal of Periodontology* **56**, 32–40

Zambon, J.J., Bochacki, V. and Genco, R.J. (1986) Immunological assays for putative periodontal pathogens. *Oral Microbiology and Immunology* **1**, 39–44

Further reading

Eley, B.M. and Cox, S.W. (1998) Advances in periodontal diagnosis. 3. Assessing potential markers of periodontal disease activity. *British Dental Journal* **184**, 109–113

Eley, B.M. and Cox, S.W. (1998) Advances in periodontal diagnosis. 4. Potential microbial markers. *British Dental Journal* **184**, 161–166

Eley, B.M. and Cox, S.W. (1998) Advances in periodontal diagnosis. 5. Potential inflammatory and immune markers. *British Dental Journal* **184**, 220–223

Eley, B.M. and Cox, S.W. (1998) Advances in periodontal diagnosis. 6. Proteolytic and hydrolytic enzymes of inflammatory cell origin. *British Dental Journal* **184**, 268–271

Eley, B.M. and Cox, S.W. (1998) Advances in periodontal diagnosis. 7. Proteolytic and hydrolytic enzymes link with periodontitis. *British Dental Journal* **184**, 323–328

Eley, B.M. and Cox, S.W. (1998) Advances in periodontal diagnosis. 8. Commercial diagnostic test kits based on GCF proteolytic and hydrolytic enzyme levels. *British Dental Journal* **184**, 373–376

Eley, B.M. and Cox, S.W. (1998) Advances in periodontal diagnosis. 9. Markers of cell death and tissue degradation. *British Dental Journal* **184**, 427–430

Eley, B.M. and Cox, S.W. (1998) Advances in periodontal diagnosis. 10. Markers of bone resorption. *British Dental Journal* **184**, 489–492

14

Basic treatment of chronic gingivitis and periodontitis

The basic treatment of periodontal disease is best divided into the treatment of chronic gingivitis and chronic periodontitis. The treatment of gingivitis mainly centres around plaque control, and is relatively simple. The treatment of periodontitis involves the meticulous debridement of the root surface within the periodontal pocket, and requires much skill and considerable time.

Chronic gingivitis

Treatment has three components, which are carried out concurrently:

1. Instruction in home care
2. Removal of plaque and calculus by scaling
3. Correction of plaque-retention factors.

These three exercises are interdependent. The removal of plaque and calculus cannot be completed without the correction of plaque-retention factors, and rendering the mouth plaque-free provides no benefit if no effort is made to prevent the recurrence of plaque deposition or ensure its swift removal after deposition.

In some patients, especially the young, calcified deposits may be negligible, and the treatment of gingival inflammation is largely a matter of plaque control (see Chapter 10). Where calcified deposits are present, scaling is needed. When deposits of calculus are heavy, it is rarely possible to remove them completely in one appointment; furthermore, resolution of gingival inflammation, especially when long-standing, may take a number of weeks. These facts must be explained to the patient. It is essential to establish a partnership of effort to restore gingival health (*Figure 14.1*).

Instruction in home care

Patients bear the major responsibility for their own dental health, and where disease is present the patients have a

(a)

(b)

Figure 14.1 *(a)* Gingival inflammation associated with poor oral hygiene prior to treatment. *(b)* The gingival condition after scaling and instruction in home care over the course of 8 weeks

special duty to themselves. The presence of disease indicates both past neglect and vulnerability to disease. The truth of the situation must be explained to the patient.

The organization of treatment needs to be very carefully planned, but it is impossible to prescribe a general timetable that could apply to every patient; each individual requires a personal schedule, but it is as well to make clear at the outset that gingival health will not be achieved overnight and that treatment is likely to take several months. Depending on the severity of the gingival inflammation, the state of oral hygiene, the presence of aggravating factors and the patient's perceived concern, a series of appointments can be made. Some instruction in home care must be given on the first visit, when scaling is started.

Where oral hygiene is poor, subsequent appointments may need to be made at weekly intervals, especially where there is a great deal of subgingival calculus. The proportion of time spent on scaling and on oral hygiene instruction must vary with individual needs, but in most cases the earlier appointments are largely given over to scaling and, as the patient feels and sees the improvement in gingival health that this brings, home care efforts can be stimulated. The patient is always advised to bring a toothbrush, and visits can be started by using a disclosing agent and enjoining the patient to 'get the stain off'. At this time, difficult areas are defined and modifications to the patient's technique devised. Encouragement is always helpful, criticism rarely; a positive approach is essential to patient co-operation.

Treatment should continue until both the oral hygiene and gingival condition are satisfactory. Recall appointments are then made at suitable intervals dictated by the patient's condition.

Scaling

This is the removal of all tooth deposits, supragingival calculus, subgingival calculus, plaque and stains. It must be carried out thoroughly; inflammation persists if all tooth deposits are not removed.

Scaling technique can be learned only by constant practice, but a number of conditions are essential to an effective technique:

1. The operation must be undertaken methodically, working around the mouth and around each tooth in an orderly manner.
2. The correct instrument should be used, i.e. one that fits well against the tooth surface to be cleaned. A fairly large-bladed instrument can be used to remove supragingival calculus; a much smaller one is necessary for the removal of subgingival calculus.
3. Each stroke of the instrument should be deliberate and effective. It is very easy to scratch around ineffectively or to use the instrument so that it actually damages the tooth surface (*Figure 14.2*). A firm finger rest on the teeth is essential for controlled use of the instrument. The movement of the instrument can be divided into two phases:
    (a) The exploratory stroke, in which the apical limit of deposits is defined. In the removal of sub-

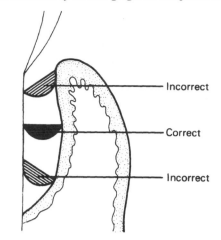

Figure 14.2 Diagram to show the angulation of a curette blade against the tooth surface. Incorrect positioning may make use of the instrument either ineffective or damaging

gingival calculus this is a blind procedure, and one carried out entirely by tactile sensation. The exploratory stroke must be gentle but deliberate so that the tissue, hard or soft, is not damaged.
    (b) The working stroke, which removes the deposits. In this action the instrument blade is pressed against the tooth surface and brought deliberately and slowly in a coronal direction, bringing the deposits with it.
4. The tooth surface should be rendered clean and smooth. The surface can be examined with a suitable instrument, e.g. the Cross calculus probe, to detect any residual deposits. Sometimes the gingival margin can be retracted and the subgingival tooth surface visualized by blowing warm air gently into the gingival crevice.

Scaling instruments

Hand instruments

A large number of instruments are available, and each operator will choose those that he or she finds most effective. The names of the instruments describe the design of the instrument and their mode of action: curettes, hoes, files, sickles and chisels. The instruments have three parts; a handle, a shank and blade. The handle needs to fit into the hand so that it is stable and cannot slip under pressure. The 'balanced grip' handle meets these requirements. The shank of the instrument varies in length and angulation so that all tooth surfaces are accessible to the blade, thus a short shank may be used in shallow pockets and a long shank in deep pockets and for interproximal sites at the back of the mouth. The blade has one or more edges designed to remove deposits from the tooth surface or soft tissue from the crevicular face of the gingiva. The edges of the blade must be kept sharp if the instrument is to be effective. Several instruments are now available with tungsten carbide blades, which do not need to be sharpened but do need to be replaced when blunt.

Curettes (*Figure 14.3a*) have a double-edged, spoon-shaped blade, which is curved to conform to the tooth surface. Most surfaces can be reached with a pair (left and right) of curettes. Because of the small size and shape of the blade it can be inserted under the gingival margin and, if necessary, can be used to clean the tooth surface and curette the gingival soft tissue simultaneously. The four most common types of curette are the McCall, Younger-Goode, Universal and Gracey. These instruments are mostly used for subgingival scaling and are described in more detail in the section on the treatment of chronic periodontitis.

Jacquette scalers (*Figure 14.3b*) have a blade that is triangular in cross-section and has two cutting edges. It is available in different sizes; the large blade is used for superficial scaling, the smaller blade for subgingival scaling. It comes in a set of three, with differently angulated shanks for use in different parts of the mouth.

Sickle scalers (*Figure 14.3c*) have a sickle-shaped blade, which is triangular in cross-section so that there are two cutting edges. The blade may also be curved in a lateral plane so that it fits against the tooth surface. Sickles are available in several sizes, the larger ones being used for superficial scaling.

Hoes (*Figure 14.3d*) are, as the name implies, hoe-shaped instruments that are available as a set of four, each shank angulated differently so that all tooth surfaces may be reached. In use, the blade is inserted lightly under the gingival margin, keeping the shank parallel to the axis of the tooth; the blade is then pressed against the tooth surface apical to the deposits of calculus and pulled in a coronal direction, detaching the calculus. These are mainly used for subgingival scaling (see below).

Files (*Figure 14.3e*) have very small dimensions so

they can be inserted extremely easily into the gingival crevice or pocket. They are used like hoes.

Chisels (*Figure14.3f*) *(watch-spring, push or Zerfing scalers)* are designed for the removal of interproximal deposits, and are especially useful in the front of the mouth.

The ultrasonic scaler

Ultrasonic vibrations, i.e. those above the range of normal hearing (above 20 000 Hz), can be used to remove tooth deposits. The ultrasonic scaler unit comprises an ultrasonic generator and a water supply. The instrument tip is vibrated between 25 000 and 42 000 Hz, and this action fragments deposits on the tooth surfaces against which it is placed. Special tips are used under a cooling water spray as the vibration creates heat. The water spray also has a detergent effect, which helps cleaning.

Several tips are available, and these include a chisel-shaped tip, a beaver-tail tip, a universal tip (shaped midway between a sickle and a curette) and a periodontal probe-shaped tip. The chisel-shaped tip is used to remove supramarginal ledges of calculus on anterior teeth, and is placed against the proximal tooth surface and used with a horizontal push stroke. The beaver-tail tip is used to remove very heavy supragingival calculus deposits, and a horizontal stroke is used on proximal surfaces and vertical strokes on buccal and lingual surfaces. The universal tip is the most commonly used to remove heavy submarginal deposits, and can be used supra- and subgingivally. It is used with vertical strokes on proximal surfaces and oblique strokes on buccal and lingual surfaces. The periodontal probe-shaped tip is used for subgingival scaling, and is particularly useful in furcation areas. An oblique stroke is used in all situations.

The instrument is applied to the tooth or root surface with soft stroking movements. Unlike a hand instrument, in using the ultrasonic scaler there is no tactile sensation in the operator's fingers, therefore it is essential to avoid excessive pressure.

The ultrasonic scaler can also be used to remove tooth stains and cement. It must be used with great care against ceramics. It can discolour composite restorations, as the metal tip can be abraded by the composite so that metal particles become incorporated in its surface. Some patients find that ultrasonic scaling is very painful, and in these cases it should not be used.

Its main advantages are that it removes heavy calculus and stain with less operator fatigue and less soft tissue trauma. In addition, fragments of calculus and other debris are flushed out by the water spray. However, it is more difficult to carry out definitive subgingival calculus removal with this instrument because of the lack of tactile sensation. It is also possible to produce surface irregularities of root cementum and dentine, or even enamel, if the tip is used incorrectly. Also, continuous contact with a surface or insufficient water coolant may result in heat build up giving rise to pulpal sensitivity.

It is best to use the ultrasonic instrument to remove

Figure 14.3 Diagram to show the blades of various scaling instruments: *(a)* curette, *(b)* Jacquette scaler, *(c)* sickle, *(d)* hoe, *(e)* file (much enlarged), *(f)* chisel

supragingival and the more superficial subgingival deposits, and then to complete the scaling with hand instruments. It can also be used effectively for repeat scaling of periodontal pockets at maintenance visits, provided that all subgingival calculus deposits have been removed previously by hand instruments at the first treatment visits. Special tips are available for subgingival scaling.

It can also be used to remove stains such as those from tobacco, tea, coffee or chlorhexidine, to remove cement and orthodontic bonding materials and even, with heavy inserts, to reduce or remove amalgam overhangs.

A chlorhexidine mouthwash given for 2 minutes before ultrasonic scaling reduces the number of salivary bacteria that are sprayed onto the operator from the aerosol produced during its use. It is essential to wear a mask and protective glasses to reduce operator exposure through this aerosol.

The ultrasonic scaler should *not* be used in:

- Patients with a pacemaker, since electromagnetic sound waves from the ultrasonic unit interfere with the electronic function of the pacemaker
- Patients suffering from contagious diseases, such as hepatitis, HIV infection, tuberculosis, throat and respiratory infections, since the micro-organisms are spread in the aerosol from the instrument
- Patients with uncontrolled diabetes
- Those with debilitating diseases or chronic nutritional deficiencies
- Patients with desquamative gingivitis or deep, pus-producing pockets
- Patients undergoing prolonged antibiotic or steroid therapy.

The ultrasonic scaler should also not be used adjacent to:

- Composite resin fillings, since the vibrations may cause marginal leakage and loss of retention
- Porcelain inlays or crowns, since the vibrations can cause porcelain margins to fracture.

In addition, ultrasonic scalers are not well tolerated by children. They are also poorly tolerated by patients with exposed, sensitive root surfaces, since acute pain may be produced by the vibrations and water spray. Finally, ultrasonic scalers may detect leaky fillings by stimulating pain, and painful sites should investigated for this possibility.

Tooth polishing

Rough surfaces become sites of plaque and calculus deposition; therefore, the tooth surface must be made smooth as well as free of calculus, plaque and stain. After scaling, any residual plaque and stain should be removed using rotating cup-shaped brushes or rubber cups and a small amount of abrasive polishing paste. The brush should be rotated fairly slowly and applied intermittently to the tooth surface to avoid overheating. An advantage of the rubber cup is that it can be taken below the gingival margin. Linen polishing strips can be used to polish interproximal tooth surfaces.

Correction of plaque-retention factors

Faulty restorations

Restorations may be rough and badly contoured, but the most frequent and important fault is the overhanging cervical margin (see *Figure 27.3*, Chapter 27), which collects plaque and prevents its removal. Very small overhangs may be removed using polishing burrs or strips, but in most cases it is necessary to replace the restoration, with careful attention given to the placement of the matrix band and the use of interdental wedges.

Marginal ridges and contact points must be properly designed. Under-contoured restorations should be replaced. Any caries under the margin of the restoration must be identified and a new restoration placed. Where possible, the margins of restorations should be placed coronal to the gingival margin (see Chapter 27).

Subgingival margins and, particularly, overhanging margins on posterior or anterior crowns (see *Figure 27.2*, Chapter 27) produce the worst problems and necessitate replacement of the offending restoration.

Faulty appliances

Removable prosthetic or orthodontic appliances may irritate the tissues in several ways (see Chapter 4). They can compress or rub the gingiva directly, or act to retain plaque against the gingiva. A removable partial denture should be designed so that, as far as possible, it is tooth-borne and gingiva-free. Where contact with the gingiva is unavoidable, the fit should be good and pressure on the tissue should be avoided. The model should never be carved to produce lines of pressure, nor should relief areas be provided in an attempt to avoid pressure, as these provoke gingival hyperplasia, which fills the relief chamber. Appliances must be kept scrupulously clean and not worn at night.

Fixed appliances must be designed so that they do not promote plaque stagnation or impede plaque removal. Fixed orthodontic appliances can present a difficult problem for the young patient to keep clean, and the patient must be taught how to look after the appliance without at the same time damaging it. Fortunately, young tissues recover quickly when the appliance is removed and thorough oral hygiene measures instituted.

Crowns and bridges

The margins of crowns and bridge abutments should fit precisely, without marginal excess or deficiency. The margins should also be accessible for cleaning. Faulty crowns and bridges associated with periodontal problems usually need replacing. In constructing these restorations, certain rules should be followed (see Chapter 27):

1. Restoration margins should be supragingival except on the labial face of upper incisors, where cosmetic considerations dictate that the crown margin should be just hidden.
2. The provision of adequate embrasure spaces is imperative; when crowns or pontics are being waxed up, a woodstick should be used to create a cleanable embrasure space. The design of pontics is particularly important; the ridge-lap pontics should be avoided where possible, and bullet-shape pontics or sanitary pontics should be used for posterior bridges. The pontics of anterior bridges usually need to slightly overlap the ridge labially for aesthetic reasons. These pontics can be made cleanable by sloping the ridge surface of the pontic so that it lies above the ridge palatally or lingually, and by keeping a sufficient embrasure space to allow the passage of floss via a threader or the use of superfloss.
3. Overcontouring crowns should be avoided and it is safer to err on the side of undercontouring, as this makes them easier to clean.

Lack of lip-seal

Although not a plaque-retention factor, lack of lip-seal does seem to render the exposed gingiva more vulnerable to plaque irritation. Once upon a time, the oral screen was prescribed to wear during sleep, the theory being that it would seal the mouth and prevent evaporation of saliva and dehydration of the tissues. Smearing the gingiva with petroleum jelly was a popular practice, and even taping the lips together was recommended! None of these measures were aimed at the cause of the problem, the plaque. Patients with lack of lip-seal need to have their particular vulnerability carefully explained so that they can co-operate intelligently. With a clean mouth, the patient can breathe through any respiratory orifice without jeopardizing gingival health.

Tooth malalignment

Frequently orthodontic treatment is carried out to correct tooth malalignment, which appears to be associated with gingival inflammation. A large proportion of this effort is wasted because the patient's home care is inadequate to clean even well-aligned teeth. On the other hand, some patients' efforts are effective enough to clean malaligned teeth and therefore do not need orthodontic treatment. Such treatment is justified where the patient is obviously trying to control plaque deposition and fails only in areas of malalignment.

Gingivoplasty

Gingival swelling creates gingival or 'false' pockets. When hyperplastic gingivitis has been present for a relatively short time the main component of the swelling is inflammation and, given adequate scaling, the inflam-

mation resolves and the swelling reduces. In the case of longstanding irritation, most frequently but not exclusively seen in the adult patient, there is a great deal of fibrous tissue formation, which does not resolve on scaling. The pocket persists and plaque redeposits so that inflammation is maintained. If pocketing and gingival swelling persist after repeated scaling and assiduous patient effort over a period of several months, surgical reshaping of the gingiva, i.e. gingivoplasty, is indicated. It may also be needed after recurrent episodes of acute ulcerative gingivitis where tissue destruction has resulted in the saucer-shaped gingival defects characteristic of this disease.

Gingivoplasty is a gingivectomy with the limited aim of improving gingival contour, i.e. producing a stream-lined contour with a knife-edged and scalloped margin and interdental sluice-ways *(Figure 14.4)*.

Details of the technique are given in Chapter 16.

(a)

(b)

Figure 14.4 *(a)* Hyperplastic gingivitis which did not resolve following a prolonged period of scaling and home care. *(b)* Gingival condition following surgical reshaping, i.e. gingivoplasty

Chronic periodontitis

Although chronic gingivitis may remain contained for many years, in many people failure to control the inflammation will eventually lead to periodontitis. The susceptibility to periodontitis is variable, and its rate of progression varies from one person to another and from one tooth to another. Traditionally, chronic periodontitis has been thought to advance slowly and progressively but, as described earlier, a number of longitudinal clinical studies of untreated chronic periodontitis have produced results that are inconsistent with this view (Goodson *et al.*, 1982; Socransky *et al.*, 1984). They suggest that the disease progresses by short and recurrent bursts of activity, probably of acute inflammation at specific sites, which are followed by long but variable periods of remission. Many tooth sites within an affected individual may remain free of destructive periodontal activity, and indeed some patients remain free from destructive periodontal disease throughout their lives. It is also suggested that destructive periodontal disease activity may occur more frequently during certain periods of an individual's life.

At the time of an examination many periodontal pockets may be inactive, so that periodontal examination will reveal evidence of past disease rather than present activity. Since there are currently no certain means either to diagnose current activity or to predict when disease activity will occur, the only way to be sure that periodontal disease is actually progressing is to keep it under careful longitudinal observation. This method, however, has the obvious disadvantage that further periods of destruction will have to occur before they can be detected and treated. Therefore, it is important to treat all periodontal pockets when they are first detected, to aim at the removal of all soft and hard deposits from the root surface, to create conditions that allow the patient to perform efficient plaque control and to eliminate all factors that would prevent the patient from maintaining that plaque control. Controlling dental plaque and supra- and subgingival scaling and root planing are often referred to as cause-related therapy, since these measures are directly aimed at controlling the factors causing the condition. The principal stages of this treatment are:

1. Treatment of any acute condition
2. Patient motivation (see Chapter 10)
3. Demonstration of oral hygiene techniques (See Chapter 10)
4. Anti-smoking advice
5. Supragingival scaling (see above)
6. Removal of any plaque-retention factors (see above)
7. Subgingival scaling and root planing (root surface debridement)
8. Occlusal adjustment if appropriate (see Chapter 24)
9. Monitoring response to therapy.

The objectives of this treatment are:

• To resolve the disease process

• To create conditions that will mitigate against recurrence of disease.

The methods of treatment are described in detail below.

Treatment of acute conditions

Acute conditions associated with chronic periodontitis should be treated without delay. The treatment of an acute lateral periodontal abscess and acute ulcerative gingivitis is described in Chapters 18 and 24.

In addition, a careful watch should be kept for sites of active disease, which should be treated immediately. Patients may complain of local symptoms at these sites, such as discomfort, itching or gingival bleeding, and they will usually show signs of acute inflammation with redness, swelling and bleeding on probing. These sites should be treated by immediate, careful subgingival scaling and root planing under local anaesthesia. The pocket can be washed out by subgingival irrigation with a 0.2% chlorhexidine solution, using a blunt needle and a 5 ml syringe. Local deposit antiseptics or antibiotics in slow release devices may also be used in these situations, and this is fully discussed in Chapter 15.

Treatment of chronic conditions

Subgingival scaling and root planing

All patients other than those with acute problems should first receive thorough supragingival scaling, as this will reduce gingivitis and bleeding. It is also important to have a full pocket chart before starting subgingival scaling.

Subgingival scaling is the most conservative method of pocket reduction and, where pocketing is shallow, it is the only treatment required. However, when pockets deepen to 5 mm or more, additional measures are required. The commonest of these is root planing, which seeks to remove embedded calculus and necrotic cementum and to smooth the root surface. This is an integral part of the subgingival scaling procedure in these situations.

Subgingival calculus is hard and tenaciously adherent to the root surface and CEJ, and is difficult to remove. It is firmly attached to the root because the calcification process involves filamentous bacteria, which may themselves penetrate into the surface cementum. Surface irregularities, such as the small pits previously occupied by Sharpey's fibres, are penetrated by apatite crystals, firmly locking the calculus to the root surface. It can be particularly adherent in areas with difficult access, such as furcations between multirooted teeth, and in grooves and concavities on the root surface.

The object of root planing is to remove necrotic cementum and embedded calculus and to smooth the root surface. It is also concerned with the removal of cementum infiltrated with toxic material of bacterial origin, such as endotoxin (LPS). However, recently it has been found that this material is only loosely associated with the root surface (Moore *et al.*, 1986) and can be removed by hand or ultrasonic scaling without the need for cementum removal. This indicates that the aim of scaling and root planing should be to produce a smooth, deposit-free root surface with the minimal removal of cementum.

Effects of subgingival scaling and root planing

Subgingival scaling and root planing significantly alter the bacterial composition of the pocket. Using dark ground microscopy techniques, it has been shown that this treatment results in a marked decrease in the number of motile rods and spirochaetes and a corresponding increase in cocci (Listgarten *et al.*, 1978). The time taken for bacterial repopulation to occur is variable and ranges from 1–6 months (Listgarten *et al.*, 1978; Mousques *et al.*, 1980). Cultural studies have also shown significant reductions in the numbers of obligate anaerobes and black-pigmented *Bacteroides* species (Walsh *et al.*, 1986). These significant and prolonged reductions in the numbers of Gram negative anaerobic bacteria and spirochaetes probably result from changes in the pocket environment, brought about by subgingival scaling, which makes it less favourable for the growth of these fastidious bacteria. It may reduce the nutritive sources for the proteolytic subgingival bacteria by reducing inflammation and thus GCF flow, and by removing subgingival calculus, which probably soaks up inflammatory exudate and slowly releases it to the adjacent bacteria. The rate of recolonization is affected by the standard of oral hygiene, since a regrowth of supragingival plaque will favour selective recolonization of the pocket (Magnusson *et al.*, 1984).

Recently, some studies using light microscopy, scanning electron microscopy and bacterial culture have shown that some bacteria may invade cementum and radicular dentine within the periodontal pockets of patients with chronic periodontitis (Adriaens *et al.*, 1984, 1987, 1988a, 1988b; Giuliana *et al.*, 1997). These studies have even suggested that the dentinal tubules may act as reservoirs of putative periodontal pathogens (see Chapter 5).

These findings suggest that radicular dentin could act as a bacterial reservoir from which periodontal pathogens can recolonize treated periodontal pockets, and could thus contribute to the recurrence of disease. Thus, root planing could reduce this potential source of recolonization (see below). However, some of these studies indicate that these bacteria may penetrate into the dentine tubules (Giuliana *et al.*, 1997), which is well beyond the reach of root planing.

Scaling and root planing are effective at reducing gingival inflammation and reducing pocket depth. When combined with good oral hygiene and regular maintenance, these effects can be prolonged over several years (Pihlstrom *et al.*, 1983; Ramfjord *et al.*, 1987; Badersten *et al.*, 1987). These studies indicate that these measures alone can be effective in treating and maintaining patients with moderate and even advanced chronic periodontitis, but it must be remembered that treatment is very time-consuming and demanding, particularly in patients with deep pocketing, and requires frequent maintenance visits. In the studies quoted above, the time taken for scaling and root planing ranged from 5–8 hours, and the patients were recalled for maintenance treatment every 2–4 months. Relapses did occur in some patients despite these measures. Obviously the patient's susceptibility to periodontal disease is a factor, but it is also becoming clear that it is very difficult to remove all calculus deposits from deep pockets by 'blind' subgingival scaling. Several studies have shown that some calculus frequently remains after careful subgingival scaling, and the incidence increases with increasing pocket depths (Rabbani *et al.*, 1981; Eaton *et al.*, 1985). This is less common following surgical exposure by flap procedures (Caffesse *et al.*, 1986).

Subgingival scaling and root planing are indicated for periodontal pockets of 4 mm or more, and if necessary should be carried out under local anaesthesia. Although ultrasonic scalers are equally as effective as hand scaling in removing calculus and root associated products, they have more limited access to deep pockets and fail to give the operator tactile information. They are therefore less capable of definitive subgingival calculus removal.

The techniques of subgingival scaling and root planing

The main hand instruments used for scaling and root planing are hoes and curettes, and it is essential that these instruments are sharp. The cutting edges of these instruments become blunted after use during a single treatment session, and therefore they need to be sharpened before they are next used (see below).

Hoes are used to remove resistant deposits of calculus, but care should be taken to avoid excessive pressure or incorrect positioning of the instrument, as this may groove the root surface (*Figure 14.5a*). The hoe should be gently manipulated to the base of the pocket and then carefully manoeuvred to engage the deep edge of the calculus deposit. It is then positively planed in a coronal direction, with its cutting edge being maintained in contact with the root surface, to remove the deposit. A firm finger rest and a finger pull movement are necessary to accomplish this movement (see below for details of use).

Curettes are used to remove residual fine deposits of calculus and to plane and smooth the root surface (*Figure 14.5b*). Again they are carefully manipulated to the base of the pocket to engage the deepest edge of the deposit, and are then planed upwards in contact with the root surface using a finger movement. In many situations it is easier to use curettes for the whole process of scaling and root planing (see below for details of use).

If the intention is to avoid trauma to the soft tissue, single-sided curettes such as the Gracey curette can be used. These are particularly good instruments for finishing and smoothing the root surface and for repeat subgingival scaling procedures at maintenance visits (see below for details of use).

Subgingival scaling and root planing may be painful,

Figure 14.5 Diagram to show the use of instruments and their correct placement in subgingival scaling and root planing: *(a)* a hoe is used to remove resistant deposits; *(b)* a curette is used to remove fine deposits and to root plane

Figure 14.6 Operator positions for scaling procedures related to the face of a 12-hour clock. This system is used in the text to describe these positions

due either to sensitivity of the soft tissues or the root surface, and these procedures are best carried out under local analgesia.

The patient may also experience some discomfort following root planing, and it may be wise to prescribe a mild analgesic following this procedure. Healing will take place over several days, and will be aided by meticulous oral hygiene.

Subgingival scaling

The first requirement is to decide on the instruments and technique, using a detailed knowledge of the root anatomy of individual teeth and the precise probing depths at all sites to be scaled. This is of particular importance when furcation involvement is present on molar or premolar teeth. The details of the essential factors in subgingival scaling technique are described below.

Operator and patient positions

The patient and operator positions are of great importance. With low seated dentistry, the patient's head is placed in the lap of the operator with the light directed into the mouth from a position vertically above it so that it is not impeded by the operator in any position round the patient. The operator can then rotate around the patient to gain access to particular tooth surfaces, and these positions can be related to the face of a clock projected over the face of the subject, with 12 o'clock above the midpoint of the top of the head and 6 o'clock below the midpoint of the chin (*Figure 14.6*). This is very clearly described in Shiffer Nield and Houseman (1982) for both right- and left-handed operators.

Using this system, the following positions are adopted, assuming a right-handed operator.

Mandibular teeth
- To access the buccal surfaces of the right mandibular molars and premolars and lingual surfaces of the left mandibular molars and premolars (*Figure 14.7a*):
  The operator is in the 9 o'clock position to the right side of the patient, looking down into mouth.
  The patient's head is positioned looking straight ahead with the chin inclined down. The patient's head is turned slightly away from the operator when required.
- To access the buccal surfaces of the left mandibular molars and premolars and lingual surfaces of left mandibular molars and premolars (*Figure 14.7b*).
  The operator is in either the 9 o'clock or the 11 o'clock position to the right side of the patient, looking down into mouth.
  The patient's head is turned towards the operator with the chin inclined down.
- To access the mandibular incisors, facial aspects:
  For tooth surfaces towards the operator (*Figure 14.7c*), the operator is in the 8 o'clock position on the right side of the patient, with the patient's head facing straight ahead and the chin inclined down.
- For tooth surfaces away from the operator (*Figure 14.7d*), the operator is in the 12 o'clock position behind the patient, with the patient's head facing straight ahead and the chin inclined down.
- To access the mandibular incisors, lingual aspects:
  For tooth surfaces towards the operator (*Figure 14.7e*), the operator is in the 8 o'clock position on the right side of the patient, with the patient's head facing straight ahead and the chin inclined down.
- For tooth surfaces away from the operator

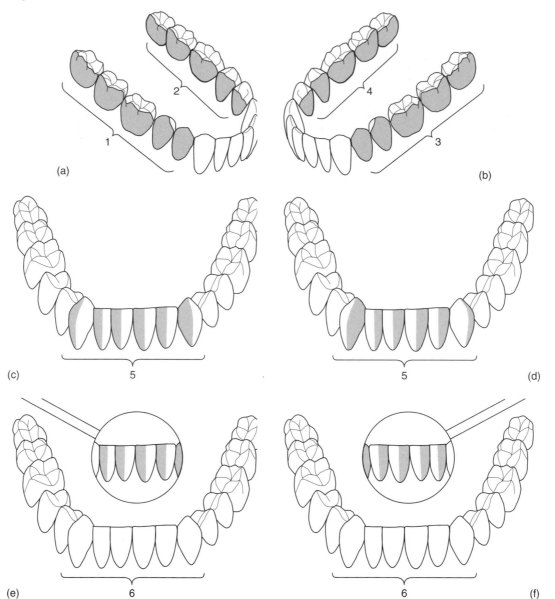

Figure 14.7 *(a)* Head position for buccal surface of right mandibular molars and premolars and lingual surfaces of the left mandibular molars and premolars; *(b)* head position for buccal surface of left mandibular molars and premolars and lingual surfaces of the right mandibular molars and premolars; *(c)* head position for facial aspects of mandibular incisors right aspects; *(d)* head position for facial aspects of mandibular incisors left aspects; *(e)* head position for lingual aspects of mandibular incisors right aspects using a mirror; *(f)* head position for lingual aspects of mandibular incisors left aspects using a mirror

(*Figure14.7f*), the operator is in the 12 o'clock position behind the patient, with the patient's head facing straight ahead and the chin inclined down.

Maxillary teeth
- To access the buccal surfaces of the right maxillary molars and premolars and the lingual aspects of the left maxillary molars and premolars (*Figure 14.8a*):
  The operator is in the 9 o'clock position to the right side of the patient.
  The patient's head is straight or slightly turned away from operator for the buccal surfaces and is always

turned away for the lingual surfaces. The patient's chin is inclined up.
- To access the buccal surfaces of the left maxillary molars and premolars and the lingual aspects of the right maxillary molars and premolars (*Figure 14.8b*):
  The operator is in either the 9 o'clock or the 11 o'clock position to the right side of the patient.
  The patient's head is turned towards the operator for both buccal and lingual aspects, with the chin inclined up.
- To access the mandibular incisors, facial aspects:
  For tooth surfaces towards the operator (*Figure*

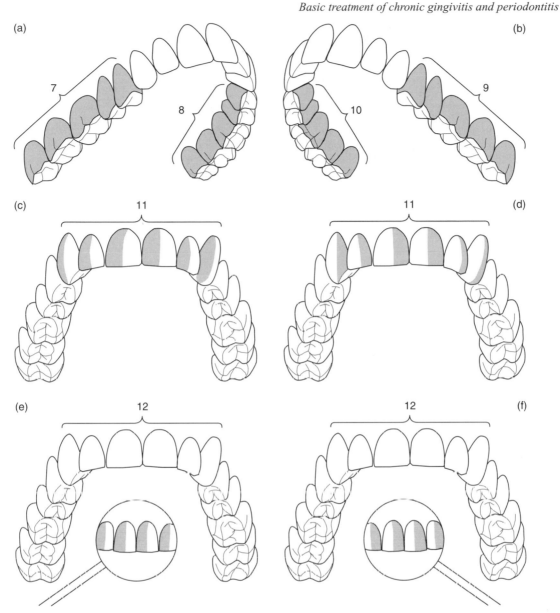

Figure 14.8 *(a)* Head position for buccal surface of right maxillary molars and premolars and palatal surfaces of the left maxillary molars and premolars; *(b)* head position for buccal surface of left maxillary molars and premolars and palatal surfaces of the right maxillary molars and premolars; *(c)* head position for facial aspects of maxillary incisors right aspects; *(d)* head position for facial aspects of maxillary incisors left aspects; *(e)* head position for palatal aspects of maxillary incisors right aspects using a mirror; *(f)* head position for palatal aspects of maxillary incisors left aspects using a mirror

14.8*c*), the operator should be in the 8 o'clock position to the right of the patient, with the patient's head facing straight ahead and the chin inclined up.

- For tooth surfaces away from operator (*Figure 14.8d*), the operator should be in the 12 o'clock position behind the patient, with the patient's head facing straight ahead and the chin inclined up.
- To access the mandibular incisors, lingual aspects:
  For tooth surfaces towards the operator (*Figure 14.8e*), the operator should be in the 8 o'clock position

to the right of the patient, with the patient's head facing straight ahead and the chin inclined up.
- For tooth surfaces away from operator (*Figure 14.8f*), the operator should be in the 12 o'clock position behind the patient, with the patient's head facing straight ahead and the chin inclined up.

These positions relate to right-handed operators, and would need to be reversed for left-handed operators. Full details can be found in Shiffer Nield and Houseman (1982), pages 17–59.

The parts of a subgingival scaler

A subgingival scaling instrument consists of a handle, with a variety of designs to aid gripping, a shank, extending from the handle to the working end, and the working end itself (*Figure 14.9*). These scalers are mostly double-ended, with a pair of complementary shanks and working ends per handle. These may be permanently attached to the handle or may screw into it and thus be replaceable. The shank may be straight, as in most anterior scalers, or angled or curved, as in posterior scalers to aid access to these teeth. They may be flexible, as in Gracey curettes, to increase tactile sense, or rigid or semi-rigid in most other scalers, to increase strength. The working end consists of a smooth, rounded back, which joins two lateral surfaces, which meet the face at the cutting edges (*Figure 14.10a*). The tip end of the face is known as the toe, the middle as the middle and the back end as the heel sections (*Figure 14.10b*). The tip may be pointed, as in the sickle scaler, or rounded in curettes. The working end usually has two functional cutting edges, as in universal curettes, but may only have one, as in hoes, or one functional one, as in Gracey curettes. The cutting edge(s)

Figure 14.9 The parts of a subgingival scaler (curette): A, handle; B, shank; C, working end

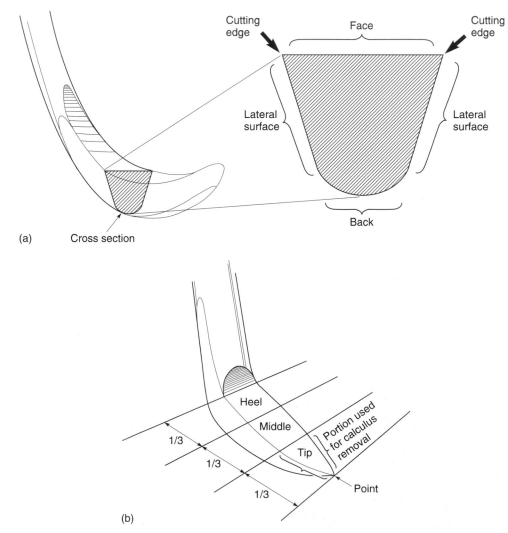

Figure 14.10 The parts of the working end of a scaler: *(a)* showing the cutting edges, face back and lateral surfaces; *(b)* showing the heel, middle, tip and point

must be kept sharp by regular sharpening, i.e. either after or before each use. Full details can be found in Shiffer Nield and Houseman (1982), pages 179–196.

Instrument grasp

Scalers are invariably held by a modified pen grasp (*Figure 14.11*). The tips of the thumb and index finger hold the scaler, and these fingers should be opposite one another near the junction of the handle and shank toward the working end of the instrument in double-ended scalers. The handle should rest against the hand somewhere between the thumb and the area behind the second knuckle of the index finger. When working on mandibular teeth, the handle usually rests against the index finger; when working on maxillary teeth, the handle usually rests closer to the thumb.

The middle finger rests lightly on the shank, and is used to feel the shank's vibration when the instrument's working surface is moving over the root surface. The pad of this finger contacts the instrument and helps to guide it. Another portion of its pad rests against the ring finger.

The ring finger contacts the patient's tooth to stabilize the hand in the patient's mouth. The hand and the instrument are balanced on this finger. The little finger has no function in scaling, and is held comfortably out of the way.

The index and middle fingers are bent and the thumb held straight or slightly curved, whilst the ring finger is held straight with the knuckles locked so that it balances the hand. A dental mirror may be held in the other hand when appropriate. The fingers of the other hand, or the mirror, may be used to deflect the lips, cheek or tongue when necessary.

Full details can be found in Shiffer Nield and Houseman (1982), pages 67–164.

Instrument insertion

The face of the scaler is placed flat against the tooth surface, with the toe third of the instrument in contact with the tooth (*Figure 14.14a*). The working end is then slid under the gingival margin and moved to the base of the pocket (*Figures 14.12, 14.14b*). In this position, the soft tissue wall of the pocket will only come in contact with the rounded back of the scaler and thus will not be traumatized. It must be ensured that the working end has passed over the calculus deposit so that the cutting edge can be subsequently positioned below its apical margin. When this position is reached, the instrument must be turned to bring the cutting edge in contact with the root surface at the correct working angulation. This is usually at an angle of 70–80 degrees to the root surface (*Figures 14.13, 14.14c*).

Instrument activation

Using this grasp, the scaler may be rocked using a wrist rotation for lateral movement, rotated by an action similar to turning a doorknob for a rotating curved movement, or moved up (apico-coronally) by a digital pulling movement over the root surface. The latter is the commonest scaling movement for most subgingival scaling procedures. With this technique the instrument is inserted below the calculus deposit and its sharp cutting edge is applied to the root surface (see above). The working tip is then planed over

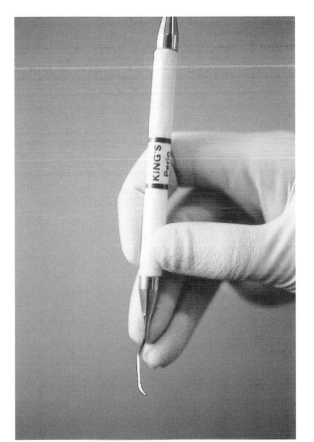

Figure 14.11 The modified pen grasp for scaling

Figure 14.12 Instrument insertion into the pocket

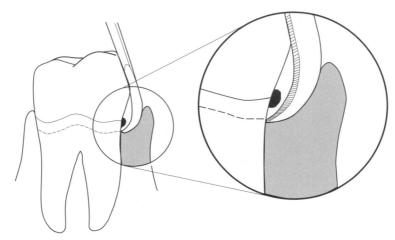

Figure 14.13 Scaler working end positioned for scaling stroke

Figure 14.14 The positioning of a subgingival scaling instrument (curette) ready for subgingival scaling: *(a)* scaler applied to tooth surface with steadying finger rest on adjacent teeth; *(b)* curette introduced into the pocket; *(c)* cutting edge positioned for scaling stroke

the root surface by an upward pull of the thumb and index finger, guided by the middle finger and stabilized against the teeth by the ring finger (*Figure 14.14*).

Working end design

The design of the main scalers has been already described, and this following description is confined to the working ends of the instruments and their uses.

Most working ends have a smooth back surface and a face. The face and the lateral surface in curettes, sickle scalers and jacquettes meet to form a cutting edge running along the full length of the face. There may be one or two cutting edges, depending on the design of the instrument. The cutting edge must be kept sharp for the instrument to function efficiently, and this is accomplished by grinding the lateral surface(s) and face with sharpening stones (see below). The rounded working end of a curette is known as a toe, and that of a sickle or jacquette as a tip. Both curettes and sickle scalers may have either straight or curved cutting edges.

Sickle or jacquette scalers have two cutting edges and are triangular in cross-section. They are strong instruments, mainly suited to supragingival scaling and the removal of heavy calculus deposits.

Curettes usually have two cutting edges and a spoon-shaped working end, and the cutting edges meet in a rounded toe. They have a rounded back and are semicircular in cross-section. Gracey curettes have one functional cutting edge, the lower, and are designed to avoid trauma to the gingival tissue adjacent to the root surface. Curettes are the main scalers for subgingival scaling.

Periodontal hoes have one cutting edge at a 99–100° angle to the shank. They can be used to remove heavy subgingival deposits, but must be used with care to avoid grooving the root surface. These scalers can only be used with a digital pull movement in an apico-coronal direction.

Push scalers or chisels have one straight cutting edge and a heavy, straight shank. They can only be used with a digital push movement to remove heavy interproximal supragingival deposits between the lower incisors.

Periodontal files have many cutting edges at 90–105° to the shank. They are mainly used to crush large calculus deposits or remove some overhanging margins.

Sharpening techniques

The cutting edge(s) of a scaler become easily blunted and need to be sharpened after each time it is used. A dull cutting edge will fail to remove subgingival calculus deposits, and could result in damage to the soft tissues. Scalers can be sharpened after use following cleaning and chemical disinfection. The sharpened scaler can then be autoclaved before it is next used. Alternatively, the sharpening stone may be sterilized to allow the instruments to be sharpened before use.

Frequent sharpening will minimize the amount of metal that is removed in the sharpening process. However, over time successive sharpenings will thin the working tip of the scaler to an extent that there is a danger of fracture during use. At this stage either the whole scaler, or working end or ends, must be replaced.

The design of the working end will dictate the sharpening technique. In this respect, cutting edges may be straight or curved, and this must be preserved in the sharpening process.

To sharpen a scaler one needs a properly prepared sharpening stone, a stable, flat working surface and a plastic testing stick. If the stone is of natural material, it should be lubricated on both sides with a few drops of oil. If it is synthetic, it should be lubricated on both sides with water.

Look carefully at the instrument to see whether it has straight or curved cutting edges, whether it ends in a rounded or pointed toe, and whether it has a rounded back. Divide the face into heel, middle and toe sections, since all three cannot be sharpened together because the entire edge may not be dull since the anterior two-thirds is most frequently used, and the instrument may have curved cutting edges. Sharpen each of these three sections in turn, starting at the heel. The extent of sharpening needed for any one of these sections depends on the state of their edges. The sharpening stone will be placed on the lateral surface so that it is in contact with the cutting edge of each section to be sharpened.

The grasp of the instrument is important in sharpening procedures because it maintains control of the instrument during the sharpening process and holds it at the correct angulation. First, grasp the instrument in a palm grip in the left hand if you are right-handed and in the right hand if you are left-handed. The instrument's handle should lie in the palm between the fingers and thumb, with the fingers and thumb wrapped around. Secondly, make a fulcrum on the edge of the stable working table with the inner edge of the hand so that the terminal shank of the scaler is perpendicular to the work surface, with the toe pointing direct towards you. The instrument should remain in this position throughout the sharpening procedure. Thirdly, grip the stone in between the tips of the fingers of the other hand, confining your grasp to the lower half of the stone. Fourthly, place the stone against the working end of the instrument, lying against the lateral surface to be sharpened, and establish a 90° angle between the face and the stone. Finally, close this angle to 70–80° by moving the stone closer to the lateral surface. The stone is now in the correct position to sharpen your instrument.

With the stone correctly positioned in contact with the heel section, sharpen this portion with rhythmic up and down strokes, always ending on a downward stroke. When the heel section is sharp, proceed to the middle section and then the toe section, up to the point or rounded end of the toe, using the same procedure. When this is complete, swing the stone around to contact the opposite cutting edge, using the surface of the stone closest to your hand. Then use the same procedure to sharpen the three sections of this surface. In this procedure the face should not be touched, because abrasion of this surface would quickly thin down the working tip and could result in its fracture during use.

Note that some instruments, such as Gracey curettes, have only one functional cutting edge, and in this situation only this edge should be sharpened. When sharpening a curette, use semicircular strokes around the back to bend in and smooth the junction with this surface.

Finally, using the plastic test stick, test the entire length of both cutting edges, remembering that the cutting edge should be at an 80° angle to the surface of the test stick.

The technique for sharpening periodontal hoes or files is obviously different. First, place the instrument horizontally on the table and hold it there firmly with the left hand (right hand if left-handed). Secondly, for a hoe, place the edge of the stone, held in your other hand, into the V-shaped groove adjacent to the single cutting edge so that its adjacent flat surface lies on the wall, ending at the cutting edge. Thirdly, sharpen this surface by moving the stone back and forth. For a file, repeat this process in each groove of the instrument.

Full details can be found in Shiffer Nield and Houseman (1982), pages 471–482.

Subgingival calculus removal

Any of the three strokes described, i.e. lateral, rotation and digital pull, may be used with curettes. Each separate stroke should progress around the tooth root in a systematic manner to cover the whole area of root within the pocket. One way of doing this is to divide the root surface into contiguous zones, which are instrumented sequentially. The curette must be sharp in order to function, and needs to be resharpened after each use.

A subgingival scaler can be used both as a scaler and as a calculus explorer. The working tip is first moved to the base of the pocket in the first zone and moved upward against the root until calculus is detected. It is then activated to remove the deposit. Following this, it is replaced to the base of the pocket in the same position and used as a calculus explorer to detect if any residual deposits are present. This is continued until this part of the root is smooth. The process then moves to the next zone of the root, and continues until the whole circumference of the root is smooth. It is then carried out on the next tooth until the planned area of subgingival scaling is completed.

Calculus removal in different areas of the mouth

Anterior teeth

Supragingival calculus can be removed by the use of sickle, jacquette 1 and push scalers (see above). The push scaler is used for heavy interdental calculus around the lower incisors, and the others for all other situations. The ultrasonic scaler can also be used.

Subgingival scaling is carried out with curettes and hoes. Hoes are used for heavy deposits in accessible areas. Anterior curettes can be of either the universal or the Gracey type (see below). The universal anterior curette has a straight shank and a working end with two parallel, straight cutting edges. The back is rounded and semicircular in cross-section. There are four Gracey curettes suitable for anterior teeth, Gracey 1, 2, 3 and 4, each with a straight shank and one functional straight cutting edge (see below).

Posterior teeth (molars and premolars)

Supragingival calculus can be removed by the use of sickles, jacquettes 2 and 3 and large spoon excavators (see above). The sickle and excavator are used for heavy deposits of calculus buccal to the molars and the jacquettes 2 and 3, with their angled shanks, for all other deposits, in particular those in interproximal areas.

Subgingival scaling is carried out with curettes and hoes. Hoes are used for heavy deposits, and curettes in all other situations. These instruments have angled and/or curved shanks to allow access to different areas. The curettes may be of the universal type with two cutting edges, or the Gracey type with only one functional cutting edge.

Gracey curettes

Gracey curettes were specifically designed to remove light calculus deposits on root surfaces within the periodontal pocket. They have special design features to carry out this function. First, since the working end must reach around the tooth into a deep periodontal pocket, these curettes have very long, curved functional shanks. Secondly, as these deposits are located within a periodontal pocket and cannot be seen, these curettes have flexible shanks to allow the operator to feel the calculus. Thirdly, they have a working end design that allows these curettes to be inserted to the base of the pocket without traumatizing the delicate periodontal tissues lining the pocket. The working ends are tilted so that one cutting edge will be at the correct angle to the root surface, whilst the opposite edge is angled away from the soft tissue wall of the pocket (*Figure 14.15*). Finally, the shanks and working ends of these curettes are designed to adapt to specific surfaces of individual teeth. Thus, Gracey 13 and 14 curettes will adapt to distal surfaces and 11 and 12 to mesial surfaces of posterior teeth.

The working end of a Gracey curette has two curved cutting edges that meet to form a rounded toe, and a rounded back, which is semicircular in cross-section. The working end is tilted in relation to the terminal shank, making one cutting edge lower than the other. This allows insertion into the pocket without trauma from the opposite edge. The lower functional edge then is placed at the correct angle to the root. Only the lower cutting edge is used for scaling, and *only* this edge should be sharpened. Each Gracey curette is area-specific, and this means that correct adaption to difficult areas can be achieved. However, several instruments are required to scale the whole mouth. These instruments have long functional shanks with multiple shank bends, and this design allows easy access to areas within deep pockets.

The flexibility of the shanks of Gracey curettes is ideal for the detection and removal of fine deposits, but makes the instruments unsuitable for the removal of heavy deposits, which is usually carried out with universal curettes. These have shorter rigid shanks. There are, however, situations with heavy subgingival deposits where access is impossible with universal curettes, and for these modified Gracey curettes with rigid shanks have been manufactured. These rigid shank Gracey curettes should not be used for definitive scaling and root planing because this design .results in limited transfer of tactile sensation to the operator, which in root planing could result in excessive removal of root surface.

Choosing the correct instrument

The area-specific curettes are combined in pairs to make double-ended instruments as follows:

Figure 14.15 The working end of a Gracey scaler showing the angled cutting edge

Gracey 1–2   Gracey 9–10   Gracey 13–14
Gracey 3–4   Gracey 11 12
Gracey 5–6   Gracey 11–14
Gracey 7–8   Gracey 12–13

A reasonable selection of these instruments suitable for most areas of the mouth would be one double-ended anterior and several double-ended posterior Gracey (G) curettes, e.g. G 1–2, G 11–14, G 12–13.

The correct Gracey curettes for different areas of the mouth are listed below:

Area of use	Gracey curette
Anteriors (incisors and canines)	Gracey 1
	Gracey 2
	Gracey 3
	Gracey 4
Anteriors and premolars	Gracey 5
	Gracey 6
Buccal and lingual surfaces of molars	Gracey 7
	Gracey 8
	Gracey 9
	Gracey 10
Buccal, lingual and mesial surfaces of molars	Gracey 11
	Gracey 12
Distal surfaces of molars	Gracey 13
	Gracey 14

In using these instruments, great care must be taken selecting the correct instrument, in determining the lower cutting edge of the instrument and placing this cutting edge at the correct angle to the tooth. If the correct curette is selected this criteria can be met by placing the shank nearest to the working end parallel to the tooth with the cutting edge against the tooth surface. This principle works for buccal, lingual, mesial and distal surfaces alike.

Insertion of a Gracey curette into the pocket

On proximal surfaces, a finger rest is established and the correct cutting edge is placed against the proximal surface. Next, the instrument handle is raised or lowered so that the whole working end face is in contact with the tooth surface, i.e. a zero face-to-tooth angulation. The working end is next slid along the tooth surface in an apical direction until the base of the pocket is reached. The finger rest is maintained whilst the instrument handle is adjusted so that the shank nearest to the working end is parallel to the proximal surface being instrumented. This places the lower cutting end at the correct angulation to the root surface.

On buccal or lingual surfaces a finger rest is established and the correct lower cutting edge is placed against the tooth surface. The handle is raised or lowered so that the toe of the working end is pointing directly into the pocket. The working end is then slid into the pocket until it reaches its base, and the handle is raised or lowered until the shank nearest to the working end is parallel to the tooth surface to be instrumented, which places the cutting edge at the correct angulation to start the working stroke.

Instrumentation

When instrumenting anterior teeth subgingivally using G 1–2, it is usual to start on the midline of the labial surface with the toe pointing towards the proximal surface and then to instrument across the root and onto the mesial surface. The working end of the double-ended instrument is then changed and positioned at the midline with the toe pointing distally so the rest of the labial surface and the distal aspect is instrumented. This is repeated for all the teeth, and again for the lingual surfaces. A combination of vertical and lateral working strokes can be used.

On posterior teeth it is usual to use vertical working strokes on proximal surfaces and mainly oblique working strokes on buccal and lingual surfaces. When instrumenting posterior teeth subgingivally using G 11–14 or G 12–13, it is usual to begin near the distobuccal or distolingual line angle and work across the root surface and onto the distal surface. The end is then changed and positioned with the toe at this line angle pointing mesially. The rest of the buccal (or lingual) surface is then instrumented, working onto the mesial surface. Overlapping strokes are used to avoid missing any area of the root. Each tooth is instrumented in order, completing one surface (buccal or lingual) before passing to the other.

Universal curettes

Universal curettes have paired, mirror image working ends, and two cutting edges per working end. Both cutting edges can be used for scaling, and both must be sharpened. The shank next to the working end is set perpendicular to the working end face. These instruments can be used to scale subgingivally in all areas of the mouth.

They have curved, semi-rigid shanks, and are therefore suitable for removal of moderately heavy or fine deposits of subgingival calculus. Each working end has two parallel, straight, cutting edges, which meet to form a rounded toe. They have rounded backs, which are semicircular in cross-section. Each universal curette has extensive applications throughout the mouth. The shanks of anterior universal curettes are straight, whilst those designed for posterior teeth are curved or angled.

Choosing the correct instrument

In order to determine the correct instrument to use, first choose either an anterior (straight shank) or posterior (curved or angled shank) instrument. The correct working tip for posterior teeth is then determined as follows. First hold the selected curette in the standard finger grip and establish a finger rest. Then place the working end on the buccal surface of the first lower right premolar, with the shank nearest to the working end approximately parallel to the tooth's long axis and resting on the tooth, with the tip of the toe pointing towards the front of the mouth. The handle should be directed out of the mouth and held as parallel as possible to the long axis of the tooth. If the shiny instrument face and both cutting edges are pointing inwards towards the tooth, then this is the right end to use. If they are pointing outwards, then the working end at the other end of the double-ended instrument is the correct one to use. The same working tip will be appropriate for the lingual surfaces of these teeth, and both cutting edges are used for one aspect of the sextant. The same system can be applied to the other upper or lower posterior sextants.

The correct working tip for anterior teeth is determined as follows. First, choose an anterior curette and hold the instrument in the standard finger grip to establish a finger rest. Place the working end of the instrument on the labial surface of a maxillary central incisor with the tip pointing in the direction in which you are working. The handle should be parallel to the long axis of the tooth. If the tip is directed distally and the face and cutting edges are turned inwards towards the tooth surface, then this is the correct end to use for surfaces facing away from you. If they turn away from the surface, then change to the other end of the instrument. Lingual areas can be tested in the same way. One working end of the anterior universal curette is used for surfaces turned away from you and the other for surfaces turned towards you in the same sextant.

Insertion of curette into the pocket

For proximal surfaces, first establish a finger rest and place the correct working end against the proximal surface with the face against the surface. Then align the handle so it is parallel to the occlusal surface of the posterior teeth or the incisor edge of the anterior teeth. The entire working end face should now be in contact with the tooth surface. Next, slide the working end along the side of the tooth and beneath the gingival margin and down to the base of the pocket. For buccal or lingual surfaces, place the appropriate working end on the buccal or lingual surface where you want to insert the instrument. Then, raise or lower the instrument handle until the toe of the working end is pointing towards the gingival margin with the face flush with the tooth surface. Finally, slide the working end under the gingival margin and down to the base of the periodontal pocket.

Instrumentation

When instrumenting anterior teeth subgingivally using the appropriate working end of an anterior universal curette, the same sequence is used as has been previously described for Gracey curettes. When the curette reaches the base of the pocket it is turned so that the appropriate cutting edge is at the correct angle with the root, and the active working stroke is commenced. A combination of vertical and lateral working strokes can be used. One working end will be used to scale the surfaces facing away from you and the other for surfaces facing towards you.

For posterior teeth, first choose one working end of the appropriate posterior universal curette. When the curette reaches the base of the pocket it is turned so that the appropriate cutting edge is at the correct angle with the root, and the active working stroke is commenced. On posterior teeth, it is usual to use vertical working strokes on proximal surfaces and mainly oblique working strokes on buccal and lingual surfaces. For lower teeth, start at the distal line angle of the lower right last molar and scale towards the distal proximal surface. Then scale from this point towards the mesial proximal surface and repeat this sequence on all the teeth in the sextant. One working end is used for all these surfaces, but one cutting edge is used on the distal sequence and the other cutting edge on the mesial sequence. This process is repeated on the lingual aspects of this sextant and then for the other mandibular and maxillary posterior sextants. In all cases, overlapping strokes are used to avoid missing any deposits. Full details can be found in Shiffer Nield and Houseman (1982), pages 201–304.

Root planing (root surface debridement)

This technique is used to remove surface irregularities encountered after subgingival calculus or necrotic cementum removal.

Roughness caused by instrumentation

Firm, scaling strokes used to remove subgingival calculus also remove a small amount of cementum, resulting in some notching of the root surface. Careful root planing needs to be carried out to smooth the root surface.

Necrotic cementum

Cementum exposed by the apical migration of the junctional epithelium is altered by exposure to subgingival plaque within the pocket. It may become hypermineralized, demineralized (root caries) or necrotic. Also, bacterial products may become superficially absorbed into its surface. For the tissues to heal following scaling, altered or necrotic cementum needs to be removed by root planing.

Embedded calculus

Some residual embedded calculus often remains following subgingival scaling and is removed by root planing.

Procedure

This procedure is required for all root surfaces exposed by periodontal disease within periodontal pockets. All subgingival scaling procedures should have been completed before this procedure is carried out.

Root planing is carried out with the appropriate Gracey curettes. These curettes must be freshly sharpened. A standard modified pen grip is used, with appropriate finger rest and light shaving pressures rather than a cutting action, and this can only be obtained with the flexible shanks of the Gracey curettes. The optimum angle to the root surface of 60–70° is necessary, and is obtained with the correct placement of the appropriate Gracey curette. The strokes should be long and made in various directions, e.g. vertical, oblique and circumferential, and numerous strokes, often 20–40, are needed to complete one surface. An efficient sequence similar to that for subgingival scaling needs to be carried out to cover all the teeth requiring this procedure. A good knowledge of root anatomy is necessary for this procedure.

Tissue response to scaling and root planing

The tissue response to even perfect scaling is variable. There are several possible consequences:

1. The pocket wall may shrink completely. This is most likely to happen when the pocket is fairly shallow and the inflammatory element in the pocket wall dominates over the fibrous tissue component. This is usually the case in young people, where the walls of pockets as deep as 6 mm may shrink completely (*Figure 14.16a*).
2. With resolution of inflammation the collagen bundles of the gingival fibre system are reformed so that the gingival cuff contracts against the tooth surface and the crevicular epithelium heals to form a long epithelial attachment, which may become connected to the tooth surface by hemidesmosomes. Thus a wide gingival cuff is formed, which is not supported by bone (*Figure 14.16b*). The integrity of this cuff depends on the length of the attachment, its strength of attachment to the tooth, the strength of the collagen bundles of the gingival fibres and the level of oral hygiene. If plaque-induced inflammation recurs, the cuff collapses readily.
3. Little shrinkage of the pocket wall may take place and the pocket may remain patent. This occurs most commonly when the pocket is deep and its wall is composed predominantly of fibrous tissue (*Figure 14.16c*).
4. Frequently, the gingival response represents a combination of the above possibilities.

Figure 14.16 Diagram to show some possible tissue changes that may follow scaling: *(a)* complete shrinkage of the pocket wall with resolution of inflammation; *(b)* reformation of gingival fibres plus some shrinkage of pocket wall to form wide gingival cuff with long epithelial attachment; *(c)* little shrinkage of the pocket wall and the pocket remains patent. The tissue change following scaling frequently represents a combination of these possibilities

5. There is a significant alteration in the bacterial composition of the pocket, with a marked decrease in the number of motile rods, Gram negative anaerobes and spirochaetes and a corresponding increase in cocci for periods of about 3 months. This brings about the resolution of inflammation, healing and formation of a long junctional epithelium, and maintains it for the duration of the bacterial changes, i.e. for approximately 3 months.

Effects of smoking on periodontal treatment

There is a strong relationship between smoking and periodontal disease severity and progression (see Chapter 4), and it would therefore be expected that smokers would respond poorly to periodontal therapy and require more treatment. This has been shown to be the case (Goultschin *et al.*, 1990). Smoking also appears to adversely alter the tissue response to various forms of periodontal treatment, and the clinical reductions in probing depth achieved by scaling and root planing have been shown to be significantly less in smokers than in non-smokers (Preber and Bergström, 1986; Ah *et al.*, 1994; Newman *et al.*, 1994). Thus, patients should be informed of this and should be actively discouraged from smoking.

Monitoring the response to therapy

Following subgingival instrumentation, a period of 6–8 weeks should elapse before any probing is performed. This is to allow resolution of inflammation and tissue healing to take place. Indeed, some studies show that final healing following these procedures may take longer than this period (Westfelt *et al.*, 1983). This monitoring should include an assessment of patient compliance, by assessing:

- Plaque and calculus deposits
- Gingival status
- Bleeding on probing
- Probing depths
- Gingival recession
- Tooth mobility.

Resolution of inflammation and healing should produce both a reduction in probing depth and some increase in gingival recession. This is brought about by a reduction in gingival swelling and hence false pocketing and a healing of junctional epithelium and gingival connective tissue, resulting in less probe penetration beyond the base of the true pocket. The extent of reduction in probing depths depends to some extent on the original depth and level of false pocketing recorded at the baseline examination. The reduction is usually between 1 and 3 mm. There should also be reductions in gingival inflammation and the values of any gingival and plaque indices taken at baseline. Complete resolution will produce an absence of bleeding on probing, and persistence of this sign is an indication of incomplete resolution and usually incomplete removal of root surface deposits during the treatment phase. Persistent bleeding on probing at a site is an indication for further subgingival scaling at that site. If bleeding still persists after two re-treatments, then adjuvant antimicrobial treatment may be indicated (see Chapter 15).

Patients demonstrating a good response to basic treatment with adequate oral hygiene and an absence of pocket activity, i.e. an absence of bleeding on probing and stable probing depths, will require a maintenance regimen to conserve the improvement achieved. The frequency of this will depend on the probing depths after treatment. If these are in excess of 4 mm, then further subgingival scaling will be necessary at these sites every 3 months. This is because the changes in the composition of the subgingival flora brought about by subgingival root debridement only last for this period.

Patients with good oral hygiene and persistent deep pockets or, more particularly, increasing pocket depth, radiographic evidence of further bone loss and persistent bleeding on probing may benefit from periodontal surgery (see Chapter 16).

Patients with poor compliance with oral hygiene techniques will not benefit from surgical intervention, but may benefit from regular maintenance care.

Summary

Subgingival scaling and root planing are difficult procedures, and ones that require considerable practice, skill and patience. The complete removal of soft and hard deposits from the root surface is difficult enough when the root is visible – as it is when surgically exposed – but when the procedures have to be undertaken 'blind', tactile sensibility has to be well developed to achieve anything approaching an immaculate, smooth root surface. Root proximity and rotation, concavities and ridges, grooves and pits, all compound cleaning problems. This is especially the case in the furcations of multirooted teeth.

These problems can only be overcome by careful instrumentation. Hill *et al.* (1981) spent 5–8 hours over the course of three to eight appointments, and Stambaugh *et al.* (1981) spent between 25 and 39 minutes on each posterior tooth to achieve root surfaces free of detectable roughness.

In a comparative study of open (surgical) versus closed scaling and root planing on multirooted teeth, Wylam *et al.* (1993) showed that, although the open approach was more effective on root surfaces, residual deposits often remained in furcation areas after both open and closed procedures. They concluded that hand instrumentation is inadequate for the debridement of furcations, and suggest that the use of ultrasonic instruments is necessary.

The deeper the pocket, the less the chance of complete debridement. It is possible to detect residual deposits with a special 'calculus probe', but using this presents the same problems as using a scaling instrument, and the persistence of gingival inflammation after scaling remains the best indicator of residual deposits, which can then be removed at successive scalings. Each scaling helps to reduce inflammatory swelling and allows a continually improving access to the root surface. It is essential to inform the patient at the outset that subgingival scaling and root planing require a commitment to multiple appointments.

The degree of pocket reduction following scaling and root planing must be carefully assessed before any decision about surgical treatment is made. Several months should elapse before reassessment of the patient, with a view to surgery, takes place.

Maintenance treatment

The changes in the subgingival flora brought about by subgingival scaling and root planing last about 3 months. Since these changes are responsible for the resolution that follows these procedures, the clinical situation will deteriorate after 3 months if periodontal pockets remain, since they cannot be reached by the patient's oral hygiene procedures. Therefore, if successful pocket elimination periodontal surgery is not carried out, maintenance subgingival scaling will be necessary every 3 months to produce a suitable bacterial flora to maintain periodontal stability. There is evidence that, even with good treatment of periodontal disease, the disease will return and progress unless an effective maintenance programme is established and carried out.

Maintenance involves:

- Regular monitoring of the periodontal status by regular periodontal charting.
- Further radiographs when indicated by clinical evidence of progression.
- Regular checks on oral hygiene.
- Simple scaling when necessary.
- Regular subgingival scaling of all residual periodontal pockets every 3 months. These are usually sites with probing depths of 4 mm or more. This is by far the most important procedure, since it is responsible for maintaining a 'healthy' subgingival bacterial flora.
- Treatment of recurrent periodontitis by appropriate means.

If effective subgingival scaling and root planing was carried out 3 months ago then no new subgingival calculus deposits are likely, but some residual fine deposits which remained even after these procedures could be present.

The residual pockets are best scaled with Gracey curettes, which are suited to the detection and removal of fine calculus deposits. If no residual deposits are detected, then fine, gently planing strokes with these instruments can be used. Alternatively, if suitable fine subgingival curette-shaped tip or probe-shaped tip inserts are available for an ultrasonic scaler, then this instrument can be used. It is also necessary to have the water spray outlet for the ultrasonic scaler incorporated into the tip so that the coolant water is carried down into the pocket. The tip should be passed to the base of each pocket and carried over all the root surfaces of the involved teeth.

Evidence for the beneficial effect of maintenance care

All the available evidence indicates that the maintenance of periodontal stability following a course of periodontal treatment depends on regular maintenance visits to monitor oral hygiene and carry out necessary supra- and subgingival scaling.

Lövdal *et al.* (1961) monitored 1428 subjects aged 20–40 years in an industrial company over 5 years following basic periodontal treatment. They were seen two to four times per year for maintenance treatment. There was a 60% improvement in their gingival condition, and tooth loss was reduced by 50%.

Suomi *et al.* (1971) monitored loss of attachment in young patients with gingivitis and early periodontitis. After periodontal treatment, one group received maintenance treatment every 3 months and the other (control group) received no further treatment. The plaque and gingivitis levels were significantly lower in the maintained group and the clinically measured loss of attachment per surface over the test period was 0.08 mm compared to 0.30 mm in the control group.

Ramfjord *et al.* (1973) carried out longitudinal clinical studies of the effect of maintenance on 104 patients of 13–64 years with advanced periodontitis. They were seen every 3 months for maintenance treatment over a 7-year period. This group recorded a low annual loss of attachment of 0.04 mm per tooth in these patients over this period. Better results were also found in those patients who maintained excellent plaque control compared with those with consistently poor oral hygiene (Knowles *et al.*, 1979; Ramfjord *et al.*, 1982).

Nyman *et al.* (1975) investigated 20 patients with advanced periodontitis who were treated with periodontal treatment, including periodontal surgery. They were divided into test and control groups, and the test group received professional cleaning and oral hygiene instruction every 2 weeks for 2 years, whilst the control group were recalled for scaling every 6 months but no efforts were made to maintain good oral hygiene. They found that the test group lost no further attachment over the 2 years, whilst the control group lost an average of 2 mm of attachment over the same time period.

Axelsson and Lindhe (1978, 1981a) investigated a test group of 375 patients aged 20–71 years and a similar control group over 3 years. The patients in the test group were given comprehensive maintenance treatment every 2 months for the first 2 years, and 3-monthly during the last year. Those in the control group were seen annually by their dentists for traditional dental care. The test group had probing depth reductions of about 0.5 mm and little or no attachment loss, whilst the control group had probing depth increases of about 0.5 mm and lost significant attachment, averaging between 0.17 and 0.3 mm per tooth surface.

Axelsson and Lindhe (1981b) also showed the value of maintenance treatment for patients treated for advanced periodontitis. They examined the patients before treatment, 2 months after the last surgical procedure, and after 3 and 6 years. Fifty-two patients were given maintenance treatment every 2 months for the first 2 years, and every 3 months for the last 4 years. The remaining 25 were sent back to their referring dentists with instructions for future care. The maintained group had low plaque scores and showed no loss of attachment over the whole time period. In contrast, the non-recalled group showed increasing plaque scores and gingivitis and signs of recurrent periodontitis. In the maintained group, 99% of teeth either improved or lost less than 1 mm of attachment, compared to 45% of the non-recall group, whilst the other 55% of teeth in this group had lost between 2 and 5 mm of attachment by the 6-year visit.

All the above studies were carried out in controlled conditions in dental schools, but their results are also supported by reviews of patients treated and maintained for up to 50 years in various dental practices (Oliver, 1969; Ross, 1971; Hirschfeld and Wasserman, 1978). The patients studied had all been referred to specialist periodontal practices, and the majority had advanced disease. In all three studies the average loss of teeth per year was dramatically reduced, so that fewer teeth were lost per patient than in the general population. One of the studies (Hirschfeld and Wasserman, 1978) reported the loss of teeth in 600 patients who had been maintained from 15–53 years. Over the entire observation period, the average loss was 1.8 per individual. Half the patients lost no teeth, 199 patients lost 1–3 teeth, whilst 25 patients (4.2% of total group) lost 13.3 teeth per individual. This last group was aptly described as the downhill group, and probably was comprised of the patients most highly susceptible to periodontal breakdown.

Thus, these studies clearly show the effectiveness of long-term maintenance treatment for periodontal patients, but also show a variation of response in some individuals.

Taken as a whole, all these studies show the great importance of regular and careful maintenance treatment for periodontal patients in maintaining periodontal stability. They also clearly show that failure to carry out effective maintenance treatment nearly always leads to periodontal breakdown and progression, irrespective of the type and quality of the original treatment.

Periodontal treatment in general dental practice

Since the vast majority of dental patients are treated in dental practices, and some stage of periodontal disease affects practically all patients, a minimum standard of basic periodontal treatment should be undertaken. Guidelines for this have been published by the British Society of Periodontology (1986) and the Royal College of Surgeons of England, Faculty of Dental Surgery (1997).

The appropriate basic periodontal treatment for general dental practice should include:

- Patient motivation
- Oral hygiene instruction
- Anti-smoking advice
- Supragingival scaling
- Removal of plaque-retention factors
- Subgingival scaling and root planing
- Monitoring response to therapy
- Possible use of adjunctive antimicrobial agents (only when clearly appropriate).

These procedures have all been described above. However, patients requiring more complex treatment are best referred for specialist care in either hospital periodontal departments or specialist periodontal practices.

The biggest drawback to effective periodontal treatment is the time it takes (see above). The restrictions of National Health Service (NHS) dentistry also make the provision of adequate treatment for periodontitis very difficult and, where appropriate treatment is allowed by the schedule, it is not rewarded with fees that adequately cover the time necessary to carry it out. Treatment of periodontitis is therefore much more suited to private dental practice. In spite of this, periodontal diagnosis and treatment has always had a recognized place in general dental practice since chronic periodontitis is one of the two major dental diseases treated by dentists (Smales, 1993).

However, recently the quality and appropriateness of the management of periodontal diseases in the general dental services have been questioned. The Green Paper on the future of NHS dentistry questioned whether the 14.6 million scale and polishes done in 1993/4 at a cost of £108 million were all essential on clinical grounds (Her Majesty's Stationery Office, 1994). The Scottish Dental Practice Board (1995) showed that in Scotland, while 1.3 million scales and polishes were carried out in the year 1994/5, only 2000 courses of multi-visit periodontal treatment were provided. This disparity between simple and complex treatment contrasts with the published data on the epidemiology of the severity of periodontal disease in this region, which shows that 15% of patients aged 35–44 years had advanced bone loss (Jenkins and Kinane, 1989).

The NHS fee structure has been cited as a major factor in limiting the provision of periodontal treatment in NHS general dental practice (Butterworth and Sheiham, 1991), and this in turn could diminish the diagnostic and treatment skills of many general dental practitioners. This view has been supported by a recent study to identify factors influencing the provision of periodontal care in dental practice (Chestnutt and Kinane, 1997). This survey analysed the returns to the Scottish Practice Board and data from 375 completed questionnaires from Scottish dental practitioners. It confirmed that the majority of periodontal treatment consisted of a simple scale and polish, with multi-visit periodontal treatment comprising less than 0.2% of all non-surgical periodontal treatment claimed from the Board. While the majority of survey respondents were confident in their ability to diagnose periodontal disease, only 40% were confident in treating it. Patient-related factors, such as difficulty in motivation and lack of compliance, were seen in this and in other studies (Nevins, 1996; Noaves *et al.*, 1996) as a major hindrance to disease management. Time factors and the low level of fees were also cited as major obstacles to NHS periodontal treatment by more than 50% of respondents.

Whilst about half of the respondents claimed that they would use the community periodontal index of treatment needs (CPITN) or its derivative, the basic periodontal examination (BPE), as a screening system on new patients, only 22% of respondents stated that they would probe all adults as part of their routine examination. As periodontal disease only gives rise to symptoms at an advanced stage, and earlier signs such as bleeding on brushing are so common as to be ignored by a majority of patients (Lang and Corbet, 1995), periodontal probing is essential to accurate periodontal diagnosis.

About half of the survey respondents (Chestnutt and Kinane, 1997) employed a hygienist in their practice. A similar percentage claimed to undertake complex periodontal treatment, and these were mostly dentists employing a hygienist and attending postgraduate courses. Only 89 of these dentists claimed to do this work themselves, and 107 referred these cases to their hygienist. In this regard, it has been clearly shown that practices employing hygienists provide a more periodontally-orientated mix of services (Brown, 1996). Furthermore, practitioners attending postgraduate courses most frequently request periodontal courses above all others (Davis and Pitts, 1994; Chestnutt and Kinane, 1997).

The discrepancy between the number of NHS claims for multi-visit subgingival scaling (0.2%) and the number of survey respondents claiming that they carried out this procedure (54%) suggests that most of these procedures were carried out under private rather than NHS contract. Private treatment for this procedure is encouraged by the low NHS fee, the need for prior approval and the fact that most NHS patients will be paying the full fee for the NHS procedure anyway.

Eighty-nine% of respondents (Chestnutt and Kinane, 1997) claimed to refer complex cases for specialist periodontal treatment, but only 4% of these did so once a month or more. It is now accepted that, whilst gingivitis is extremely prevalent, periodontitis has a more skewed distribution, with advanced disease affecting relatively few 'high-risk' individuals (Jenkins and Kinane, 1989). Such patients usually require specialist periodontal care.

However, many patients are becoming more informed about the nature of periodontal disease and, as they also become more litigation conscious, failure to provide adequate diagnosis and treatment of these conditions may render a practitioner liable to claims of malpractice (Killila, 1993). In addition, a recent report from a leading medical protection society (Dental Protection, 1996) has claimed that, over the last few years, it has recorded a steady increase in the number of complaints and claims that relate to the failure to identify, record and appropriately treat periodontal disease.

Whilst fiscal arrangements are no impediment to adequate periodontal care in private dental practice, either under a fee or insurance system, they are a major obstacle to its provision in NHS practice.

The results of the surveys quoted above indicate that there must be considerable doubt as to whether current arrangements for periodontal diagnosis and treatment are satisfactory in NHS general dental practice. Clearly there is an urgent need to develop evidence-based clinical guidelines and adequate fiscal arrangements to facilitate periodontal care under the NHS.

While all patients would benefit from oral hygiene instruction and simple scaling, greater emphasis needs to be placed on the appropriate treatment of early to moderate periodontitis. There is also a need to identify high-risk patients and refer them for specialist periodontal care.

Referral for specialist treatment

The following categories of patients should generally be referred for specialist care:

1. Patients with good compliance who have residual active periodontitis after basic treatment and might benefit from more complex treatment such as periodontal surgery. Patients with inadequate plaque control should not be referred until they can demonstrate motivation to improve this situation.
2. When a diagnosis of early onset periodontitis such as rapidly progressive periodontitis, juvenile periodontitis or prepubertal periodontitis is suspected.
3. Patients where complex treatment planning is required, e.g.
   Combined periodontal and endodontic lesions
   Combined periodontal and orthodontic treatment
   Planning of fixed prosthodontics and implants for periodontal cases.
4. Patients with medical conditions predisposing to gingival or periodontal disease or periodontal disease progression, e.g.
   Organ transplant patients
   Patients taking anti-convulsive drugs
   Diabetic patients
   Patients with immunosuppression
   Patients with renal disease.
5. Patients at special risk of complication from dental treatment, e.g.

Patients on anticoagulant therapy
Patients at risk for bacterial endocarditis.

Infection control in periodontal treatment

Good cross-infection control procedures are necessary for all dental procedures, and are particularly important in periodontal treatment. These procedures are well set out in a BDA advice sheet (BDA Advisory Service, 1996), and therefore will only be summarized here.

Most periodontal procedures such as subgingival scaling result in bleeding, and therefore blood contamination of instruments, the dental unit and the operator and staff is a major problem. For these reasons, cross-infection control measures are particularly important. Potentially infectious patients, such as those carrying viruses like hepatitis B/C or HIV, are a particular risk in these situations. However, these risks should be covered by universal cross-infection control measures, since an accurate history of these conditions is often not given or available.

Universal procedures

A thorough medical history should be obtained at the first visit and then regularly updated. Patients should not be refused treatment on medical grounds since it is unethical to do so, and also illogical, since many undiagnosed carriers of infectious disease pass undetected through practices or clinics every day. All information provided by the patient must be treated with complete confidentiality.

Equipment

The design of a surgery must allow easy cleaning of all surfaces and adequate ventilation. All equipment must be designed to allow cleaning and disinfection of all surfaces in the operative area, and all water lines should be appropriately treated. Foot rather than hand chair controls are to be preferred, as this cuts down on contamination. All surfaces likely to be contaminated during treatment must be cleaned and disinfected between patients and covered with a removable barrier, such as cling film, during the treatment session.

Instruments

All stainless steel instruments should first be cleaned to remove blood and debris and then autoclaved. The appropriate time and temperature for autoclaving must be adhered to, i.e. 134–138°C for at least 3 minutes, and longer times for lesser temperatures. If a hot air oven is used for any instruments, then a time of 120 minutes at 160°C must be used.

Presterilized disposable syringe needles and surgical blades should be used. Equipment that is difficult to clean, such as aspirator tips, saliva ejector tips and three-in-one air/water tips are also available as disposable items.

Operator

Single-use disposable gloves should be used for all clinical procedures, and these should be sterile for surgical procedures. Operators should wear appropriate clinical clothing, eye protection and masks. The latter two items are particularly important when using instruments that create an aerosol, as when carrying out ultrasonic scaling.

Staff

All staff must be fully trained in cross-infection control procedures.

Immunization

It is imperative that all staff are immunized against the common preventable infections, such as hepatitis B, poliomyelitis, rubella, pertussis, diphtheria, tetanus and tuberculosis. All clinical personnel must provide evidence of effective hepatitis B vaccination.

References

Adriaens, P.A., Claeys, G.W. and De Boever, J.A. (1984) Colonization of human dentin by a mixed flora of oral bacteria *in vitro*. *Caries Research* **18** Abstr. 21, 160

Adriaens, P.A., Loesche, W.J. and De Boever, J.A. (1987) Bacteriology of the flora present in the roots of periodontally diseased teeth. *Journal of Dental Research* **66** Abstr. 1855, 338

Adriaens, P.A., De Boever, J.A. and Loesche, W.J. (1988a) Bacterial invasion in root cementum and radicular dentin of periodontally diseased teeth in humans. *Journal of Periodontology* **59**, 222–230

Adriaens, P.A., Edwards, C.A., De Boever, J.A. and Loesche, W.J. (1988b) Ultrastructural observations on bacterial invasion in cementum and radicular dentin of periodontally diseased human teeth. *Journal of Periodontology* **59**, 493–503

Ah, M.K.B., Johnson, G.K., Kaldahl, W.B. *et al.* (1994) The effect of smoking on the response to periodontal therapy. *Journal of Clinical Periodontology* **21**, 91–97

Axelsson, P. and Lindhe, J. (1978) The effect of controlled oral hygiene procedures on caries and periodontal disease in adults. *Journal of Clinical Periodontology* **5**, 133–151

Axelsson, P. and Lindhe, J. (1981a) The effect of controlled oral hygiene procedures on caries and periodontal disease in adults. Results after 6 years. *Journal of Clinical Periodontology* **8**, 239–248

Axelsson, P. and Lindhe, J. (1981b) The significance of maintenance care in the treatment of periodontal disease. *Journal of Clinical Periodontology* **8**, 281–295

Badersten, A., Nilveus, R. and Egelberg, J. (1987) 4-year observations of basic periodontal therapy. *Journal of Clinical Periodontology* **14**, 438–444

British Dental Association Advisory Service (1996) *Infection Control in*

Dentistry. London: British Dental Association Advice Sheet 12

British Society of Periodontology (1986) *Periodontology in General Dental Practice in the United Kingdom. A First Policy Statement* (R.F. Mosedale, P.D. Floyd and F.C. Smales, eds). London: British Society of Periodontology

Brown, L.F. (1996) A comparison of patients attending practices employing or not employing dental hygienists. *Australian Dental Journal* **41**, 47–52

Butterworth, M. and Sheiham, A. (1991) Changes in the community periodontal index of treatment needs (CPITN) after periodontal treatment in general dental practice. *British Dental Journal* **171**, 363–366

Caffesse, R.G., Sweeney, P.L. and Smith, B.A. (1986) Scaling and root planing with and without periodontal flap surgery. *Journal of Clinical Periodontology* **13**, 205–211

Chestnutt, I.G., and Kinane, D.F. (1997) Factors influencing the diagnosis and management of periodontal disease by general dental practioners. *British Dental Journal* **183**, 319–324

Davis, M.N. and Pitts, N.B. (1994) Topics for general practitioner continuing education: survey of Scottish views. *European Journal of Prosthodontics* **1**, 23–25

Dental Protection (1996) Dentolegal aspects of periodontal disease. *Dental Protection – Dental News* **17**, 3–4

Eaton, K.A., Kieser, J.B. and Davies, R.M. (1985) The removal of root surface deposits. *Journal of Clinical Periodontology* **12**, 141–152

Giuliana, G., Ammatuna, P., Pizzo, G. *et al.* (1997) Occurrence of invading bacteria in radicular dentin of periodontally diseased teeth: microbiological findings. *Journal of Clinical Periodontology* **24**, 478–485

Goodson, J.R., Turner, A.C.R., Haffajee, A.D. *et al.* (1982) Patterns of progression and regression of advanced destructive periodontal disease. *Journal of Clinical Periodontology* **9**, 472–481

Goultschin, J., Sgan Cohen, H.D., Donchin, M. *et al.* (1990) Association of smoking with periodontal treatment needs. *Journal of Periodontology* **61**, 364–367

Her Majesty's Stationery Office (1994) *Improving NHS Dentistry*. London: HMSO

Hill, R.W., Ramfjord, S.P., Morrison, E.C. *et al.* (1981) Four types of periodontal treatment compared over 2 years. *Journal of Periodontology* **52**, 655–667

Hirschfeld, L and Wasserman, B. (1978) A long-term survey of tooth loss in 600 treated periodontal patients. *Journal of Periodontology* **49**, 225–237

Jenkins, W.M.M.J. and Kinane, D.F. (1989) The high-risk group in periodontitis. *British Dental Journal* **167**, 189–171

Killila, B.A. (1993) Dental profession liability issues. *Journal of Indiana Dental Association* **72**, 22–24

Knowles, J.W., Burgett, F.G., Nissle, R.R. *et al.* (1979) Results of periodontal treatment related to pocket depth and attachment level. Eight years. *Journal of Periodontology* **50**, 225–233

Lang, N.P. and Corbet, E.F. (1995) Periodontal diagnosis in daily practice. *International Dental Journal* **45**, 3–15

Listgarten, M.A., Lindhe, J. and Hellden, L. (1978) Effects of tetracycline and/or scaling on human periodontal disease. Clinical microbiological and histological observations. *Journal of Clinical Periodontology* **5**, 246–271

Lovdal, A., Arno, A., Schei, O. and Waerhaug, J. (1961) Combined effect of subgingival scaling and controlled oral hygiene on the incidence of gingivitis. *Acta Odontologica Scandinavica* **19**, 537–555

Magnusson, I., Lindhe, J., Yoneyama, T. and Liljenberg, B. (1984) Recolonization of the subgingival microbiota following scaling in deep pockets. *Journal of Clinical Periodontology* **11**, 193–207

Moore, J., Wilson, M. and Kieser, J.B. (1986) The distribution of bacterial lipopolysaccharide (endotoxin) in relation to periodontally involved root surfaces. *Journal of Clinical Periodontology* **13**, 748–751

Mousques, T., Listgarten, M.A. and Phillips, R.W. (1980) Effects of scaling and root planing on the composition of the human subgingival microbial flora. *Journal of Periodontal Research* **15**, 144–151

Nevins, M. (1996) Long-term periodontal maintenance in private practice. *Journal of Clinical Periodontology* **23**, 273–277

Newman, M.G., Kornman, K.S. and Holzman, S. (1994) Association of clinical risk factors with treatment outcomes. *Journal of Periodontology* **65**, 489–497

Noaves, A.B., Noaves, A.B. Jnr, Moares, N. *et al.* (1996) Compliance with supportive periodontal therapy. *Journal of Periodontology* **67**, 213–216

Nyman, S., Rosling, B. and Lindhe, J. (1975) Effect of professional tooth cleaning on healing after periodontal surgery. *Journal of Clinical Periodontology* **2**, 80–86

Oliver, R.C. (1969) Tooth loss with and without periodontal therapy. *Dental Abstracts* **17**, 8–9

Pihlstrom, B.L., McHugh, R.B., Oliphant, T.H. and Ortiz-Campos, C. (1983) Comparison of surgical and non-surgical treatment of periodontal disease. A review of current studies and additional results after 6.5 years. *Journal of Clinical Periodontology* **10**, 524–541

Preber, H. and Bergström, J. (1986) The effect of non-surgical treatment on periodontal pockets in smokers and non-smokers. *Journal of Clinical Periodontology* **13**, 319–323

Rabbani, G.M., Ash, M.M. and Caffesse, R.G. (1981) The effectiveness of subgingival root planing in calculus removal. *Journal of Periodontology* **52**, 119–123

Ramfjord, S.P., Knowles, J.W., Nissle, R.R. *et al.* (1973) Longitudinal study of periodontal therapy. *Journal of Periodontology* **44**, 66–77

Ramfjord, S.P., Caffesse, R.G., Morrison, E.C. *et al.* (1987) Four modalities of periodontal treatment compared over 5 years. *Journal of Clinical Periodontology* **14**, 445–452

Ramfjord, S.P., Morrison, E.C., Burgett, F.G. *et al.* (1992) Oral hygiene and maintenance of periodontal support. *Journal of Periodontology* **53**, 26–30

Ross, I.F. (1971) The results of treatment. A long-term study of 180 patients. *Parodontologie* **25**, 125–134

Royal College of Surgeons of England, Faculty of Dental Surgery (1997) *National Clinical Guidelines. Screening of Patients to Detect Periodontal Diseases*. London: Royal College of Surgeons

Scottish Dental Practice Board (1995) *Annual Report 1994/5*. Edinburgh: Scottish Dental Practice Board

Shiffer Nield, J. and Houseman, G.A. (1988) In *Fundamentals of Dental Hygiene Instrumentation*, pp. 17–482. Philadelphia: Lea and Febiger

Smales, F.C. (1993) Periodontology in general dental practice. *International Dental Journal* **43**, 193–199

Socransky, S.S., Haffajee, A.D., Goodson, J.M. *et al.* (1984) New concepts of destructive periodontal disease. *Journal of Clinical Periodontology* **11**, 21–32

Stambaugh, R.V., Dragoo, M., Smith, D.M. and Carasali, L. (1981) The limits of subgingival curettage. *Journal of Periodontal Restorative Dentistry* **1**, 31–41

Suomi, J.D., Greene, J.C., Vermillion, J.R. *et al.* (1971) The effect of controlled oral hygiene procedures on the progression of periodontal disease in adults: results after third and final year. *Journal of Periodontology* **42**, 152–160

Walsh, M.M., Buchanan, S.A., Hoover, C.I. *et al.* (1986) Clinical and microbiological effects of single dose metronidazole on scaling and root planing in treatment of adult periodontitis. *Journal of Clinical Periodontology* **13**, 151–157

Westfelt, E., Nyman, S., Socransky, S.S. and Lindhe, J. (1983) Significance of frequency of professional tooth cleaning for healing following periodontal surgery. *Journal of Clinical Periodontology* **10**, 148–156

Wylam, J.M., Mealey, B.L., Mills, M.P. *et al.* (1993) The clinical effectiveness of open versus closed scaling and root planing on multi-rooted teeth. *Journal of Periodontology* **64**, 243–253

Further reading

Shiffer Nield, J. and Houseman, G.A. (1988) In *Fundamentals of Dental Hygiene Instrumentation*. Philadelphia: Lea and Febiger

15

The chemotherapeutic approach to periodontal treatment

Antimicrobials used in periodontal treatment can be divided into two main groups:

1. Agents directed against supragingival plaque development.
2. Agents directed against subgingival bacteria.

Antimicrobial and anti-plaque agents used to inhibit bacterial plaque formation, and thus to prevent or resolve chronic gingivitis, can only affect supragingival plaque. They should be clearly distinguished from agents directed against subgingival plaque and therefore used to treat chronic periodontitis, which will be considered in the second section of this chapter.

Supragingival plaque control

A number of chemotherapeutic agents to control supragingival plaque have been studied. These agents can be divided into enzymes, bisdiguanide antiseptics, quaternary ammonium antiseptics, phenolic antiseptics, other antiseptics, metal ions, natural products and oxygenating agents (Addy, 1986), and are shown in *Table 15.1*.

These agents are discussed below.

Throughout this chapter, the terms plaque inhibitory, anti-plaque and anti-gingivitis have been used according to the clarification of terminology suggested by the European Federation of Periodontology at its second workshop. This defines a plaque inhibitory effect as one that reduces plaque to a level insufficient to prevent the development of gingivitis; an anti-plaque effect as one that produces a prolonged and profound reduction in plaque sufficient to prevent the development of gingivitis; and anti-gingivitis as an anti-inflammatory effect on the gingival health not necessarily mediated through an effect on plaque.

Enzymes

Two approaches to plaque control with enzymes have been tried:

Table 15.1 Chemical supragingival plaque control

Enzymes	Bisdiguanides	Quaternary ammonium compounds	Phenolic compounds
Protease	Chlorhexidine	Cetylpyridinium chloride	Thymol
Lipase	Alexidine	Benzalconium chloride	4-Hexylresorcinol
Nuclease	Octenidine		2-Phenylphenol
Dextranase			Eucalyptol
Mutanase			Listerine
Glucose oxidase			
Amyloglucosidase			

Fluorides	Metal ions	Oxygenating agents	Other antiseptics
Sodium fluoride	Copper	Peroxide	Iodine
Sodium monofluorophosphate	Tin		Povidone iodine
Stannous fluoride	Zinc		Chloramine-T
Amine fluoride			Sodium hypochlorite
			Hexetidine
			Triclosan
			Salifluor Delmopinol

(Reproduced from the *Journal of Clinical Periodontology* (1986) by kind permission of Dr. M. Addy and the Editor)

1. Studies of enzymes interfering with bacterial attachment, including dextranases and proteolytic enzymes. The results of these have been promising in animal studies, but inconclusive in humans (Addy, 1986).
2. Potentiation of host defences, which involves potentiation of salivary antibacterial activity using the enzymes amyloglucooxidase and glucose oxidase to produce hydrogen peroxide from dietary fermentable carbohydrates. This in turn converts thiocyanate to hypothiocyanite in the presence of salivary lactoperoxidase, which then acts as a bacterial inhibitor by interfering with cell metabolism. There is *in vitro* evidence for this process, but such activity in the mouth has not yet been demonstrated. Clinical studies of the use of this system as a mouthwash and a toothpaste (Zendium) have given conflicting results.

Bisdiguanide antiseptics

Several bisdiguanide antiseptics possess anti-plaque activity, including chlorhexidine, alexidine and octenidine (Addy, 1986). Chlorhexidine gluconate, however, is the most studied bisdiguanide and is the one on which there is most information on toxicology.

These antiseptics are able to kill a wide range of micro-organisms by damaging the cell wall. The anti-plaque properties of chlorhexidine are unsurpassed by other agents, and it has much greater effects than other antiseptics of similar or greater antibacterial activity. This appears to be due to the adsorption of the dicationic chlorhexidine molecule on to oral surfaces and its release at bacteriostatic levels for prolonged periods.

Chlorhexidine

The digluconate of chlorhexidine (1 : 6-Di-4′-chlorophenyl-diguanidohexane) is a synthetic antimicrobial drug that has been widely used as a broad spectrum antiseptic in clinical and veterinary medicine since 1953. It has been available in Europe for over 25 years, and has been successfully used in the dental field over that period. As an antimicrobrial agent, chlorhexidine is effective *in vitro* against both Gram positive and Gram negative bacteria (Davies *et al.*, 1954; Hennessy 1973; Emilson, 1977), yeasts and fungi (Budtz-Jorgensen and Löe, 1972) and facultative aerobes and anaerobes (Davies *et al.*, 1954). Its antibacterial action is due to an increase in cellular membrane permeability followed by coagulation of the cytoplasmic macromolecules (Hennesy, 1977). It has also been shown that chlorhexidine can reduce the adherence of *Porphyromonas gingivalis* to epithelial cells (Grenier, 1996). This effect is probably due to the binding of chlorhexidine to the bacterial outer membrane, and it could therefore have similar effects on the adherence of other plaque bacteria.

It has been shown that a 0.2% chlorhexidine gluconate mouthrinse will prevent the development of experimental gingivitis after the withdrawal of oral hygiene procedures (Hull, 1980; Addy, 1986). It has thus been shown to be an effective anti-plaque and anti-gingivitis agent. However, when used as an adjunct to normal oral hygiene measures, variable results are achieved, suggesting that chlorhexidine is more effective in preventing plaque accumulation on a clean tooth surface than in reducing pre-existing plaque deposits. It is thus able to inhibit plaque formation in a clean mouth, but will not significantly reduce plaque in an untreated mouth. For these reasons chlorhexidine mouthwash should never be given to patients before the necessary periodontal treatment has been carried out, and then should only be used for the specific reasons set out below.

Substantivity of chlorhexidine

The ability of drugs to adsorb onto and bind to soft and hard tissues is known as substantivity, and this property was first described for chlorhexidine in the 1970s (Rölla *et al.*, 1971; Bonesvoll *et al.*, 1974; Bonesvoll and Gjermo, 1978). Substantivity is influenced by the concentration of the medication, its pH and temperature, and by the length of time of contact of the solution with the oral structures (Bonesvoll *et al.*, 1974). This property of chlorhexidine was associated with its ability to maintain effective concentrations for prolonged periods of time (Gjermo *et al.*, 1974; Bonesvoll and Gjermo, 1978), and this prolongation of its action made it especially suitable for the inhibition of plaque formation.

Safety of chlorhexidine

The safety of an antimicrobial agent is tested in animal studies prior to its clinical use, and all side effects are then carefully investigated in human studies. The effects of antimicrobials and their metabolic products on the environment are now also frequently studied.

Animal experiments with radiolabelled chlorhexidine have shown that the primary route of excretion is through the faeces. There is minimal metabolic cleavage, and no evidence of formation of carcinogenic substances has been reported (Winrow, 1973). Chlorhexidine is poorly absorbed by the gastrointestinal tract and it therefore displays very low toxicity (oral LD_{50} is 1800 mg/kg and the intravenous LD_{50} is 22 mg/kg). No tetragenic alterations have been found following long-term use (Faulkes, 1973).

The most common side effect of chlorhexidine is the formation of extrinsic stain on the teeth and tongue following its use as a mouthwash (Addy, 1986).

Clinical usage

There are now quite a few commercially available chlorhexidine mouthwashes in the UK and the rest of Europe. Those in the UK, such as Corsodyl, contain 0.2% chlorhexidine, and recommend a 10 ml volume per rinse. The chlorhexidine mouthwash available in the USA, Peridex, contains 0.12% chlorhexidine and recommends a 15 ml volume per rinse. The factor governing the effectiveness of these mouthwashes is the dose of chlorhexidine delivered, and 10 ml of 0.2% solution delivers 20 mg and 15 ml of 0.12% solution delivers 18 mg (Binney *et al.*, 1995). Since both these amounts are similar and above the therapeutic dose, either of the formulations is equally effective.

Chlorhexidine and fluoride have valuable preventive roles in dental disease, and there is also evidence that in caries prevention they may act together to provide additional benefits. For this reason, combined chlorhexidine and fluoride have been investigated. One study (Jenkins *et al.*, 1993a) used a 0.12% chlorhexidine and 100 ppm F-mouthrinse in combination with toothbrushing in a randomized, double-blind parallel design involving 99 subjects over 6 weeks. At 6 weeks the plaque and gingivitis scores were significantly lower in the active mouthrinse group. As expected, some tooth staining also occurred. The anti-plaque effects were the same as with a conventional chlorhexidine mouthwash. Similar results were seen in a study using a 0.05% sodium fluoride and 0.05% chlorhexidine mouthwash (Joyston-Bechal and Hernaman, 1993).

It is more difficult to incorporate chlorhexidine into toothpastes and gels because of the binding of chlorhexidine to components in the toothpaste. This reduces its activity by decreasing the number of active cationic sites (Addy *et al.*, 1989). However, some formulations have been achieved that avoid this problem. In comparing the effect of potential plaque inhibitory ingredients in toothpastes, the plaque inhibitory effects of the other ingredients need to be taken into account. In this regard, it has been shown that commercial toothpastes containing various formulations of fluoride all reduced the rate of plaque regrowth compared to water in a 4-day study (Binney *et al.*, 1996).

More recently, toothpastes have been formulated to ensure a high availability of the contained antiseptic. A 1% chlorhexidine toothpaste of this type has been formulated, and has been investigated in a 19 day, randomized, double-blind, placebo-controlled, cross-over experimental gingivitis clinical trial (Jenkins *et al.*, 1993b). The toothpastes were used as slurries, which were rinsed around the mouth twice per day for 1 minute during the experimental period. Plaque and gingivitis scores were highly significantly reduced and stain scores were significantly increased in the active toothpaste period with respect to those in the placebo period. Thus, this particular formulation of chlorhexidine toothpaste does seem to provide a sufficient dose of chlorhexidine for a similar clinical effect to that seen with chlorhexidine mouthrinsing.

Chlorhexidine has also been incorporated into a sugar-free chewing gum (Fertin A/S, Vejle, Denmark), and in this form the chlorhexidine molecule remains unbound. The chewing gum contains 20 mg of chlorhexidine diacetate, and this has been compared to the effects of a 0.2% chlorhexidine mouthwash and a placebo gum in a clinical study (Smith *et al.*, 1996). One hundred and fifty-one subjects divided into three groups, one using the chlor-

hexidine gum, one using 0.2% chlorhexidine mouthwash and one a placebo gum, and were tested for their anti-plaque effects after 4 and 8 weeks. The subjects using the gum chewed two pieces twice per day for 10 minutes, and the mouthwash subjects rinsed twice per day for 1 minute. There were significant and similar anti-plaque effects with the chlorhexidine gum and mouthwash, and this was not seen with the placebo gum. Tooth staining was seen with both the chlorhexidine gum and the mouthwash, but the intensity and extent of stain was less with the gum.

In a similar study, the use of chlorhexidine gum has also been found to reduce plaque levels significantly more than the use of xylitol and sorbitol gums and also than the the subjects' regular plaque control routines (Tellefsen *et al.*, 1996). Therefore the use of chlorhexidine gum could be a good method of using chlorhexidine in longer-term users (see below).

Side effects of chlorhexidine usage

Although chlorhexidine is not toxic, it has an unpleasant taste, alters taste sensation and produces brown staining on the teeth, which is difficult to remove (*Figure 15.1*). This can also affect the mucous membranes and the tongue, and may be related to the precipitation of chromogenic dietary factors on to the teeth and mucous membranes. It is probable that one cationic group attaches chlorhexidine to the tooth or mucosal surface, whilst the other cationic group produces the bactericidal effect of damaging the bacterial cell wall. However, this cationic group can also attach dietary factors, such as gallic acid derivatives (polyphenols) found in food and many beverages including tea and coffee and tannins from wines, to the molecule and hence to the tooth surface. Chlorhexidine does also encourage supragingival calculus formation, and the resulting calcified and stained areas adhere strongly to the tooth (or restoration) surface and are difficult to remove.

Figure 15.1 Chlorhexidine tooth staining after 3 weeks of twice daily rinsing

The stained areas are resistant to polishing and can only be removed by scaling, and in this regard ultrasonic scaling is the most effective method. It also tends to stain the margins and surfaces of composite and glass ionomer restorations, and these stains are particularly resistant to removal by scaling. Scaling procedures are also liable to damage the surface of these restorations and therefore reduce their effective life.

For these reasons, it is important to advise patients using chlorhexidine mouthwash to avoid the intake of tea, coffee and red wine for the duration of its use. One should also severely restrict its use in patients with visible anterior composite and glass ionomer restorations.

It is also worth stating that chlorhexidine formulations that do not stain are ineffective in inhibiting plaque. This is because the second cationic group of the molecule has reacted with something in the formulation and thus is unavailable for either a beneficial bactericidal effect or the unwanted staining effect. This has been clearly shown in a comparison of a number of commercial chlorhexidine mouthwashes, which differed in their content of binding additives. Those that effectively bound up the chlorhexidine did not produce staining, but also lacked a significant anti-plaque effect (Addy and Wade, 1995; Harper *et al.*, 1995). Mouthwashes with this reduced effect include, at the time of writing, French Eludril. The formula of British Eludril has now been changed to prevent the binding of chlorhexidine, and as a result this product is now effective and causes tooth staining like the other effective products. However, at the time of writing, the formula of the French product has not been changed, and hence it remains ineffective and does not cause staining (Addy, personal communication).

In an effort to reduce staining, anti-adhesive molecules have also been combined with chlorhexidine in experimental mouthwashes. These combined mouthwashes have no effect on 4-day plaque regrowth and do not cause increased tea staining, almost certainly for the same reasons stated above (Moran *et al.*, 1995; Addy *et al.*, 1995).

Other much rarer side effects of chlorhexidine mouthwash are mucosal erosion and parotid swelling (Addy, 1986).

For these reasons, the prolonged use of chlorhexidine should be avoided in normal periodontal patients. It is useful for short periods (up to 2 weeks) when oral hygiene may be difficult or impossible, such as during acute oral infections or following periodontal surgery. It may occasionally be used as an adjunct to mechanical oral hygiene in initial periodontal treatment. In this regard, the gingivae may be sore after subgingival scaling and this may prevent normal toothbrushing.

After 2 weeks, normal brushing and flossing must be resumed and mouthwashing should stop. However, it is rarely necessary for more than 2–3 days, and normal brushing and flossing can be resumed at this stage.

Chlorhexidine mouthwash may also be used during periods of intermaxillary fixation following the treatment of fractures or skeletal surgery, when effective oral hygiene is not possible lingually and interdentally. During this period, the patient should also be seen regularly for professional cleaning by a dentist or hygienist to limit staining.

More prolonged use of chlorhexidine may be justified in physically and mentally handicapped patients, in medically compromised patients predisposed to oral infections and as an adjunct to oral hygiene in fixed orthodontic appliance wearers. All of these patients should also be seen for regular professional cleaning. In many of these special cases, the mouthwash or gel will be used over a prolonged period and severe staining will be a problem. This can be minimized by using concomitant toothbrushing and by avoiding the intake of certain foods and drinks, such as tea and coffee (see above).

With increasing pocket depth, subgingival plaque becomes inaccessible to both oral hygiene procedures and antibacterial mouthrinses, which are normally effective in preventing gingivitis. In this regard it has been shown that mouthwashes do not penetrate into the gingival crevice or periodontal pocket (Flotra *et al.*, 1972; Flotra, 1973). Therefore, antibacterial mouthrinses, toothpastes and gum have no place in the treatment or control of periodontitis.

It is also doubtful if antibacterial mouthrinses have any place in treating existing gingivitis, since in this situation there will be an established subgingival flora within the gingival (false) pocket and the mouthwash would not reach this vital area. Therefore, it is inappropriate to use any antiseptic mouthwash in the treatment of either gingivitis or periodontitis unless effective subgingival scaling has first been carried out. In this regard it is also worth noting that whilst chlorhexidine, because of its good substantivity, is effective in preventing plaque formation on a clean surface and thus the development of gingivitis, it is much less effective in penetrating a thick layer of established plaque in an untreated diseased situation.

Quaternary ammonium compounds

Quaternary ammonium compounds such as cetylpyridinium chloride (CPC) have moderate plaque inhibitory activity (Lobene *et al.*, 1977; Ciancio, 1986). Although they have greater initial oral retention and equivalent antibacterial activity to chlorhexidine, they are less effective in inhibiting plaque and preventing gingivitis. One reason for this may be that these compounds are rapidly desorbed from the oral mucosa (Holbeche *et al.*, 1975; Bonesvoll and Gjermo, 1978; Roberts and Addy, 1981). It has also been found that the antibacterial properties of these compounds are considerably reduced once adsorbed onto a surface, and this may be related to the monocationic nature of these compounds. The cationic groups of each molecule bind to receptors on the mucosa, producing the mucosal retention, but because of the monocationic nature of these molecules this process leaves few unattached sites available for its antibacterial function.

A CPC pre-brushing mouthrinse used as an adjunct to

mechanical oral hygiene has not been found to have a beneficial effect on plaque accumulation (Moran and Addy, 1991). With regard to conventional use, Jenkins *et al.* (1994) compared the plaque-inhibitory potential of 0.05% and 0.1% CPC, 0.05% chlorhexidine and control mouthrinses used twice daily during a 4-day period of non-brushing. The 0.1% CPC rinse had the lowest plaque scores, being approximately 26% lower than the control rinse and 7% lower than the 0.05% chlorhexidine rinse. The 0.05% CPC and chlorhexidine mouthwashes were very similar in their effects. The relatively poor effect of the 0.05% chlorhexidine and CPC mouthwashes is undoubtedly due to the low concentration in these formulations yielding too low a total dose for the expected effect. Also, the short duration of this study makes it impossible to detect an anti-plaque effect on gingivitis, which would be expected from a normal chlorhexidine mouthrinse. It does, however, show that the CPC 0.1% mouthwash produced a limited but statistically significant reduction in plaque growth.

A slow release system containing CPC has been tried to increase the retention time for CPC in the mouth (Vandekerchhove *et al.*, 1995). The plaque inhibitory effect of this device over 18 days was compared with those of a CPC mouthrinse, CPC lozenges (Cepacol®) and a chlorhexidine mouthrinse (Peridex®). As expected, the chlorhexidine mouthrinse (Peridex) had the most profound effects on plaque and gingivitis, and these were not approached by the other formulations. However, there were also no differences between any of the CPC formulations, which showed that the slow release system had no effect on the efficacy of CPC. All the CPC formulations and Peridex produced tooth staining, and this was worst with the CPC lozenges.

Phenolic antiseptics

Phenols, either alone or in combination, have been used in mouthrinses or lozenges for a considerable time. When used at high concentrations relative to other compounds, they have been shown to reduce plaque accumulation (Gomer *et al.*, 1972; Lusk *et al.*, 1974; Fornell *et al.*, 1975).

Listerine® is an essential oil/phenolic mouthwash that has been shown to have moderate plaque inhibitory effects and some anti-gingivitis effects. There have been a number of short- and long-term home use studies, which have shown these moderate plaque-inhibiting effects and some anti-inflammatory effects in reducing gingival inflammation (Lamster *et al.*, 1983; Gordon *et al.*, 1985; De Paula *et al.*, 1989). On the basis of these studies, it has been accepted by the American Dental Association to be an aid to home oral hygiene measures.

Its effect on 4-day plaque regrowth during abstinence from mechanical oral hygiene has been compared with those of chlorhexidine and anti-adhesive mouthwashes (Moran *et al.*, 1995). Chlorhexidine (0.2%) mouthrinse was significantly more effective

than Listerine, which was in turn more effective than the anti-adhesive mouthwashes alone or in combination with chlorhexidine, which it inactivates (see above). It was, however, found to be slightly more effective than triclosan mouthwash in plaque inhibition (Moran *et al.*, 1997). Its anti-inflammatory effects shown in the home use studies may be due to its antioxidative activity (Firatli *et al.*, 1994). Thus, Listerine has a moderate effect on plaque regrowth and some anti-inflammatory effect, which may reduce the severity of gingivitis. Its lack of profound plaque inhibitory effect is probably because, unlike chlorhexidine, it has poor oral retention.

Other antiseptics

Hexetidine

Hexetidine has some plaque inhibitory activity, but this is low in comparison with chlorhexidine (Bergenholz and Hanson, 1974; Roberts and Addy, 1981; Harper *et al.*, 1995; Addy and Wade, 1995). Its substantivity (oral retention) is between 1 and 3 hours (Harper *et al.*, 1995), which accounts for the reported plaque inhibitory effects of Oraldene®, the UK product (Roberts and Addy, 1981). However, one study that investigated its adjunctive effect on aphthous ulcer patients did not show any added benefit over mechanical oral hygiene (Chadwick *et al.*, 1991). It can cause oral ulceration at concentrations greater than 0.1% (Bergenholz and Hanson, 1974). It has also been shown that combining zinc with hexetidine improves its plaque-inhibiting activities, probably by acting synergistically with it (Giersten *et al.*, 1987).

Povidone iodine

Povidone iodine appears to have no significant anti-plaque activity when used as 1% mouthwash (Addy *et al.*, 1977), and the absorption of significant levels of iodine may make this compound unsatisfactory for prolonged use in the oral cavity (Fergerson *et al.*, 1978). Also, it could cause a problem of iodine sensitivity in sensitized individuals.

Triclosan

Triclosan, a trichlora-2'-hydroxydiphenyl ether, is a non-ionic antiseptic that lacks the staining effects of cationic agents. It has been used recently in a number of commercial toothpastes and mouthwashes, and produces moderate plaque inhibitory effects when used as a mouthwash in combination with zinc (Moran *et al.*, 1992; Schaeken *et al.*, 1994). In one study (Moran *et al.*, 1992) the combination mouthwash produced inhibition of plaque regrowth during a 4-day period with abstinence from mechanical oral hygiene, but this study raised doubts as to the individual contribution of triclosan to this effect. The use of a combination of zinc and triclosan arose from the concept that agents with different modes of action might have synergistic or additive effects, but the separate and combined effects of triclosan have been investigated and these are described below.

The effects of combination zinc and triclosan mouthwashes were investigated in a 3-week clinical trial (Schaeken *et al.*, 1994), where abstinence from brushing was produced by wearing an acrylic tooth shield over the test area of the mouth during brushing. Two experimental mouthwashes containing 0.4% zinc sulphate and 0.15% triclosan were compared with a 0.12% chlorhexidine mouthwash and a placebo (negative control) mouthwash. The two experimental mouthwashes differed only in their ethanol and humectant content. The mouthwashes were used twice daily for 3 weeks, after brushing. In the negative control subjects the plaque and gingival bleeding scores rose above their pre-study levels. In the subjects using the first zinc/triclosan mouthwash these levels were significantly lower than the control levels, but the change was not significant for the second zinc/triclosan mouthwash. The first zinc/triclosan mouthwash had higher concentrations of ethanol and humectant, which probably improved the effect by increasing the solubilization of triclosan, which has a low solubility in water. As expected, the plaque and gingivitis scores were the lowest in the subjects using chlorhexidine mouthwash.

The effects of these same two experimental zinc/triclosan mouthwashes were compared with a non-active control mouthwash over 28 weeks (Schaeken *et al.*, 1996). The subjects were divided into three groups and each was given one of the three mouthwashes, which they used twice per day after brushing. Assessments were made of the clinical status and levels of salivary *Streptococcus mutans*. At 4 weeks, plaque and calculus scores in all groups were low compared to baseline, but thereafter they progressively increased. Plaque and gingival bleeding scores were significantly lower in subjects using the experimental mouthwashes than in those using the control mouthwash. Calculus scores were also significantly lower at 28 weeks for the subjects using the second experimental mouthwash. No significant changes in salivary *Streptococcus mutans* numbers were seen. The only adverse effect seen was some tooth staining.

Another cross-over study (Ramberg *et al.*, 1996) compared the effect of 0.06% triclosan, 0.12% chlorhexidine and placebo mouthwashes on *de novo* plaque formation over 18 days at healthy and inflamed gingival sites of 10 volunteers. No significant differences in the gingivitis scores were found between the three mouthwashes, but both active mouthwashes produced significant reductions of plaque formation compared to the control mouthwash. These reductions were significantly greater for the chlorhexidine compared to the triclosan mouthwash. They also found that more plaque formed at inflamed sites than at healthy sites, regardless of which mouthwash was used.

Whilst triclosan itself has little or no substantivity, there is evidence that its oral retention can be increased by its combination with co-polymers of methoxyethylene and maleic acid (Gantrex®, ISP Corp.) (Deasy *et al.*,

1991; Lobene *et al.*, 1992). Furthermore, there is also evidence from two short-term (Deasy *et al.*, 1991; Lobene *et al.*, 1992) and two longer-term trials (Worthington *et al.*, 1993; Ayad and Berta, 1995) conforming to Council on Therapeutics, American Dental Association (1986) Guidelines that the combination of 0.03% triclosan with Gantrex® used as a pre-brushing rinse can produce significant adjunctive effects to mechanical oral hygiene in further reducing plaque levels and gingivitis.

Moreover, there is evidence that triclosan may also act as an anti-inflammatory agent in mouthrinses and toothpastes (Kjaerheim *et al.*, 1996). In this way it has been shown to reduce the inflammatory reaction to sodium lauryl sulphate on the gingiva (Waaler *et al.*, 1994a, 1994b) and skin (Barkvoll and Rölla, 1994), and the skin reaction to nickel hypersensitivity (Barkvoll and Rölla, 1995). In addition, it has been shown to reduce histamine-induced dermal inflammation and the severity and healing period of aphthous ulceration (Skaare *et al.*, 1996). The mechanism of this property has been investigated *in vitro* (Gaffar *et al.*, 1995), and it has been shown to inhibit both cyclo-oxygenase and lipoxygenase, thus reducing the synthesis of prostaglandins and leukotrienes.

This issue is further complicated by the fact that the anti-inflammatory and anti-bacterial properties of triclosan combinations are affected by the nature of the solvents in the formulation (Jenkins *et al.*, 1991; Kjaerheim *et al.*, 1994a, 1994b; Skaare *et al.*, 1997).

Thus, triclosan mouthwashes reduce plaque accumulation, but to a much lesser extent than chlorhexidine. However, the extent of their plaque inhibitory effects seems to be dependent both upon the presence of co-polymers in the formulation to increase the oral retention of triclosan and upon triclosan's anti-inflammatory and hence anti-gingivitis effect. The anti-inflammatory effect of triclosan depends upon its ability to penetrate into the gingival tissues, and this is in turn dependent upon the nature of the solvent(s) in the mouthwash formulation.

Triclosan has also been added to a number of experimental and commercial toothpastes with and without zinc, and it appears to produce moderate inhibition of plaque formation (Saxton, 1986; Jenkins *et al.*, 1989a). These and other studies have shown that zinc citrate and triclosan toothpastes (Saxton, 1986; Saxton *et al.*, 1987; Svaton *et al.*, 1987, 1989, 1990; Saxton and Van der Ouderaa, 1989; Jenkins *et al.*, 1989a; Stephen *et al.*, 1990) and triclosan/co-polymer toothpastes (Stephen *et al.*, 1990; Cubells *et al.*, 1991; Cummings, 1992; Deasy *et al.*, 1992) have produced greater reductions in plaque and gingivitis than brushing alone. However, one study has shown that it has plaque inhibitory effects that are little different from other detergent-based commercial toothpastes, regardless of whether it is present with or without zinc (Jenkins *et al.*, 1989b).

The effects of a triclosan dentifrice on the microbial composition of supragingival plaque over 6 months has also been studied (Walker *et al.*, 1994). One hundred and forty-four subjects were divided into two groups, and one was given 0.3% triclosan/0.2% co-polymer/0.243% sodium fluoride toothpaste and the other a placebo toothpaste. Both test and placebo dentifrice produced significant reductions in the total bacterial counts and a non-significant reduction in the anaerobic count. Neither dentifrice resulted in detrimental shifts in the microbial composition of the flora, nor to the emergence of periodontal or opportunistic pathogens. There was also no difference in the proportion of the flora resistant to triclosan, regardless of whether the triclosan or placebo toothpaste was used. Thus, the extended use of a 0.3% triclosan/0.2% co-polymer toothpaste appears to be safe to use and does not seem to disrupt the normal oral flora.

In another study (Renvert and Birkhed, 1995), the effects of three commercial triclosan toothpastes, Colgate Paradent (triclosan/co-polymer), Pepsodent Gum Health (triclosan/zinc citrate) and Dentosal Friskt Tandkött (triclosan/pyrophosphate), and a placebo toothpaste on plaque, gingivitis and the salivary microflora were compared over 6 months in 112 subjects. Over the 6-month study period, Colgate Paradent reduced plaque scores by 36% and Pepsodent Gum Health by 6%; there were increased scores of 5% for Dentosal Friskt Tandkött and 2% for the placebo. Gingival bleeding scores reduced in all groups, with no significant differences between them. There was an increase in the number of streptococci over time with Dentosal, Pepsodent and the placebo, but not the Colgate toothpaste. This would seem to indicate that only the triclosan/co-polymer formulation significantly reduced plaque levels with respect to the control during this period of normal usage.

Another study (Binney *et al.*, 1995) also compared the effects of a commercially available triclosan/co-polymer toothpaste, a sodium fluoride-containing toothpaste, a chlorhexidine rinse (positive control) and saline rinse (negative control) on 4-day plaque regrowth. The toothpastes were made into a slurry for rinsing around the mouth, so the compounding effect of mechanical brushing was avoided. Eighteen healthy volunteers took part in the study. On day 1 they suspended toothbrushing and rinsed twice daily with the allocated mouthrinse or toothpaste slurry. Chlorhexidine was significantly more effective than all the other agents tested, and both toothpastes were significantly better than the saline rinse. There was no significant difference between the two toothpaste rinses.

These studies show that triclosan toothpastes offer only moderate plaque inhibiting properties when compared with conventional toothpastes. However, they have also been shown to reduce gingival inflammation further than mechanical brushing alone when used as an adjuvent to normal brushing (Saxton, 1986; Saxton *et al.*, 1987; Svaton *et al.*, 1987, 1989, 1990; Jenkins *et al.*, 1989a; Saxton and Van der Ouderaa, 1989; Stephen *et al.*, 1990; Cubells *et al.*, 1991; Cummings, 1992; Deasy *et al.*, 1992), and this may be associated with triclosan's anti-inflammatory properties. However, these effects are much less profound when triclosan toothpastes are used as slurries to mitigate against the confounding effects of mechanical plaque removal, and in this form they are no more effective than a conventional toothpaste without triclosan or any other antimicrobial agent (Jenkins *et al.*, 1989; Binney *et al.*, 1995).

Delmopinol

Several substituted amine alcohols, such as octapinol hydrochloride, have been shown to inhibit plaque accumulation (Attström *et al.*, 1983; Brecx *et al.*, 1987). More recently, studies have been carried out on the related morpholino-ethanol derivative, delmopinol hydrochloride. Both *in vitro* (Simonsson *et al.*, 1991a) and *in vivo* (Collacrt *et al.*, 1992) studies show that it inhibits plaque growth and reduces gingivitis. One study has suggested that delmopinol has only limited substantivity in comparison to chlorhexidine, and in this regard inhibits salivary bacteria for only 30 minutes as compared to several hours for chlorhexidine (Moran *et al.*, 1992). However, the substantivity test used in this study was designed for antibacterial agents that act directly on bacteria and thus reduce their numbers. Since delmopinol is not a true antibacterial agent in this sense, and has virtually no inhibitory concentration, it is not correct to test its substantivity in this way.

A suggested mode of action for the plaque inhibiting effects of delmopinol is interference with plaque matrix formation and reduction of bacterial adherence (Simonsson *et al.*, 1991b). This would cause the plaque to be more loosely adherent to the tooth so that it would be more easily removed by mechanical cleaning procedures, and it would therefore be suitable for a pre-brush mouthrinse.

A trial of 0.1% and 0.2% delmopinol hydrochloride mouthrinses as adjuncts to normal oral hygiene has been carried out (Claydon *et al.*, 1996). This study was a 6-month home-use, placebo-controlled, double-blind, randomized parallel design, and was structured to conform with the ADA Council of Dental Therapeutics guidelines. Four hundred and fifty healthy subjects with moderate levels of plaque and gingivitis were recruited and were either given one of the delmopinol mouthrinses or a placebo mouthrinse. They were instructed to use 10 ml for 1 minute twice a day after brushing. At baseline and at 3 and 6 months they were scored for plaque, gingivitis, tooth stain and supragingival calculus, and plaque was collected for microbiological analysis. The oral mucosa was also examined, and they were questioned about adverse reactions. At the start and end of the trial a full medical examination, including haematological and biochemical tests, was carried out. A few adverse signs and symptoms were reported, and these included transitory numbness of the tongue, tooth and tongue staining, taste disturbance and, rarely, mucosal soreness and erosion. All these local side effects were less commonly reported at 6 months compared to 3 months, and only six subjects withdrew from the study because of adverse events. No systemic effects attributable to the agent were observed, and no shifts in haematological and biochemical parameters occurred. Both test groups showed significant decreases in plaque, gingivitis and calculus scores, with few differences between them, but there were some significant differences in plaque scores in favour of 0.2% delmopinol. Tooth staining was increased in the delmopinol groups, but not calculus.

The reductions in gingivitis seen in this study (Claydon *et al.*, 1996) suggests that delmopinol may have an anti-inflammatory and hence an anti-gingivitis effect. In addition, the reductions in both plaque and gingivitis also suggest that it may be a true anti-plaque agent.

The microbiological effects of the above study were investigated on plaque collected at 12, 24 and 36 weeks (Elworthy *et al.*, 1995). There were no consistent effects on the microscopic or total counts. However, there was a significant reduction in the proportion of dextran-producing streptococci in the active compared to the control group throughout treatment. There was no colonization by *Candida* or major shift in bacterial composition in the active group, nor was there any decrease in susceptibility to delmopinol. Thus, delmopinol seems to mediate its anti-plaque effect without causing a major shift in bacterial populations, apart from the reduction in dextran-producing streptococci.

The effectiveness of 0.2% delmopinol and 0.2% chlorhexidine mouthwashes has also been compared in a 4-week, double-blind, randomized, placebo-controlled clinical study of 57 patients with gingivitis (Halse *et al.*, 1995). The patients all received professional cleaning before baseline. They were given either delmopinol, chlorhexidine or placebo mouthwashes, and told to use 10 ml twice per day after brushing. The plaque index and plaque wet weight were used to score plaque and gingival fluid flow, and the bleeding on probing index to score gingivitis. With respect to plaque, both chlorhexidine and delmopinol significantly reduced scores relative to the placebo, and there were no significant differences between the effects of chlorhexidine and delmopinol. However, in respect of gingivitis, there were no significant differences between the effects of delmopinol or placebo mouthrinses. The same adverse effects as were described above were reported for both active mouthwashes. A transient anaesthetic effect on the oral mucosa was more commonly reported in the delmopinol group, whilst chlorhexidine produced more tooth and tongue staining than delmopinol.

This same group (Halse *et al.*, 1998a) compared the use of 0.2% delmopinol, 0.2% chlorhexidine and placebo mouthwashes over 6 months in 149 patients. It showed that both active mouthwashes significantly reduced the levels of plaque and gingivitis over this period. In respect of plaque, the chlorhexidine mouthwash produced somewhat greater reductions, but in terms of gingivitis there was no difference in the effects of the active mouthwashes. This study shows a much better effect of delmopinol on gingivitis over this longer period than its effect in the short term (Halse *et al.*, 1995), and this study also supports the previous findings of another group (Claydon *et al.*, 1996).

A further study by the same group (Halse *et al.*, 1998b) on 68 of these patients showed that neither mouthwash produced an undesirable shift in the bacterial flora in saliva or dental plaque. There were slight reductions in the total cultivated counts with both of them, but no changes in bacterial proportions and no increase in the growth of staphylococci, enteric bacteria or yeasts. Furthermore, there was no change in the MIC values for individual bacteria species in subjects using the 0.2% delmopinol mouthwash over this time period, which indicates that no adaption to this agent had taken place. Finally, neither delmopinol nor chlorhexidine showed any residual effects on the studied bacterial species after the end of treatment. Thus, the use of delmopinol seemed to be accompanied by a composition of the plaque and salivary flora associated with healthy conditions in the oral cavity.

A recent study has compared the plaque inhibitory effects of 0.1%, 0.2% delmopinol mouthwashes and a placebo mouthwash in 'slow' and 'rapid' plaque formers (Zee *et al.*, 1997). It confirmed the beneficial effects of both delmopinol mouthwashes versus the placebo, but found no differences in its effect on slow or rapid plaque formers.

Therefore, it would seem that delmopinol is well tolerated and may produce a true anti-plaque effect. It thus holds promise as a useful agent for mouthwashes and, possibly, toothpastes.

Salifluor

Salifluor is a salicylanide (5n-octanoyl-3'-trifluoro-methylsalicylanide) which has both antibacterial and anti-inflammatory properties (Genco, 1994). The possibility that 5-alkyl-salicylanides like salifluor may have a plaque inhibitory effect was suggested by Coburn *et al.* (1981) from *in vitro* studies. Recently, a combination of salifluor and polyvinylmethylether/malic acid (OVM/MA) have been investigated *in vitro* (Nabi *et al.*, 1996), and the combination was shown to enhance the uptake of salifluor on saliva-coated hydroxyapatite discs and to reduce plaque growth in an artificial mouth.

Also recently, three related double-blind, randomized, cross-over clinical trials into the effect of mouthrinses containing salifluor on plaque and gingivitis have been carried out (Furuichi *et al.*, 1996). In each study 10 medically and dentally healthy dental students were used, and the effects of 0.08%, 0.12% and 0.2% salifluor, 0.12% chlorhexidine and control mouthwashes were compared, with a washout period between each. In the first study they found that the salifluor mouthrinses were significantly more effective than control rinses and equally effective to 0.12% chlorhexidine in retarding 4-day plaque growth.

In the second study, oral hygiene was stopped for 2 weeks to induce gingivitis and the teeth were then professionally cleaned. Plaque was again allowed to form again for a further 4 days, during which time either the control, the 0.12% salifluor or the 0.12% chlorhexidine mouthwash was used. The results showed that mouthwashes containing 0.12% salifluor and 0.12% chlorhexidine inhibited plaque formation to the same extent at both inflamed and non-inflamed sites, but the effects of both mouthrinses were less at inflamed compared with non-inflamed sites.

In the third study, oral hygiene was stopped for 2 weeks and during this time one of the three mouthrinses was used. Clinical measurements and plaque samples for dark ground microscopy were taken at baseline and days 4, 7 and 14. The sequence was repeated for each mouthwash, with a washout period between each. There was no difference between 0.12% salifluor and 0.12% chlorhexidine mouthwashes in their ability to retard *de novo* plaque formation and the development of gingivitis during the 14-day period. The microbial examination showed that in the control group the percentage of cocci decreased and the percentage of filaments, fusiforms and spirochaetes increased, whilst in the salifluor and chlorhexidine groups no distinct changes occurred in the composition of the supragingival plaque.

Thus, the results of these three studies demonstrate the potential of salifluor as an effective anti-plaque agent. However, the mechanisms behind the anti-microbial and anti-inflammatory properties of salifluor are not yet properly understood. Therefore, the clinical use of salifluor should be further studied in the longer term to include a detailed evaluation of possible side effects before it can be released for routine clinical use.

Metal ions

A number of metal ions have been studied for their effects on plaque, and zinc, copper and tin have been shown to possess plaque inhibitory activity. Both copper and tin suffer from the local side effect of staining. Some fluoride compounds, such as stannous fluoride and amine fluorides, also have plaque inhibitory effects, but not as a result of the fluoride ion itself but rather due to the effect of the stannous ion or surface-active amine portion of the molecule.

Studies on the effect of metal ions on plaque accumulation have been contradictory (Addy, 1986), and factors like concentration and frequency of use may explain the differences. Of further interest is the apparent additive or synergistic effect of the combination of zinc and other metal ions with other antiseptics (Waaler and Rölla, 1980). This effect has been noted with zinc combined with hexetidine (Giertsen *et al.*, 1987), triclosan (Schaeken *et al.*, 1996) and sanguinarine (Southard *et al.*, 1987).

Little is known of the mechanisms by which metal ions exert their effects. It has been suggested that zinc may assist the inhibition of glycolysis by sanguinarine (Southard *et al.*, 1987), which could in turn limit plaque formation. It has also been reported to improve the bactericidal activities of sanguinarine against certain oral organisms and to enhance the efficiency of other antiseptics such as triclosan and hexetidine in inhibiting plaque. It has also been noted (Ingram *et al.*, 1992) that zinc is retained by dental plaque and inhibits its regrowth without disrupting the oral ecology.

Natural products

Studies on the plant extract *sanguinarine chloride* have shown that it produces moderate reductions in plaque and gingivitis. The zinc present in the formulations could be partly responsible for the effect.

Sanguinarine

Chemically, sanguinarine is a benzophenanthridine alkaloid derived from the alcoholic extraction of powdered rhizomes of the bloodroot plant *Sanguinaria canadensis*, which grows in Central and South America and Canada (Grenby, 1995). After precipitation and purification of the alcohol extract, an orange powder containing 30–35% sanguinarine is obtained. Sanguinarine contains the chemically reactive iminium ion, which is probably responsible for its activity. It appears to be retained in plaque for several hours after use and is poorly absorbed from the gastrointestinal tract (Grenby, 1995). Several clinical studies have been carried out into its effects.

A sanguinarine mouthrinse and toothpaste regimen given for 6 months during orthodontic treatment reduced plaque by 57%, gingival inflammation by 60% and bleeding on probing by 45%, compared to figures of 27%, 21% and 30% for the placebo control group (Hannah *et al.*, 1989).

A later study of sanguinarine mouthrinse and toothpaste (Kopczyk *et al.*, 1991) carried out under the ADA guidelines (see above) in 120 subjects showed 13–17% lower plaque scores and 16–18% less gingival inflammation, compared with a placebo group, after a 6-month treatment period.

Reviews on antimicrobial mouthrinses including sanguinarine (Mandel, 1988; Overholser, 1988) conclude that short-term studies on sanguinarine have shown variable but significant plaque inhibitory effects, but no effect on gingivitis. On the other hand, two reviews of sanguinarine toothpastes, used alone without the mouthwash, have shown no detectable plaque inhibitory or anti-inflammatory effects (Schonfeld *et al.*, 1986; Mallatt *et al.*, 1989).

In respect of its possible modes of action, it has also been shown that sanguinarine at a concentration of 16 μg/ml completely inhibited 98% of microbial isolates from human dental plaque (Dzink and Socransky (1985), and that sanguinarine and zinc act synergistically in suppressing the growth of various oral strains of streptococci and actinomyces (Eisenberg *et al.*, 1991).

Some studies have compared the activity of sanguinarine with other antimicrobial antiseptics. A small group of 14 healthy volunteers was involved in an experimental gingivitis study and subjects used either a sanguinarine-zinc (Veadent) or a chlorhexidine mouthwash (Moran *et al.*, 1988). This showed that the chlorhexidine mouthwash was significantly more effective than sanguinarine-zinc in inhibiting plaque formation and the development of gingivitis. The effects of various mouthwashes on 21 patients with gingivitis were examined by Wennström and Lindhe (1986), and this study showed that both chlorhexidine and sanguinarine mouthwashes produced significant plaque inhibition compared with a non-active placebo, but only chlorhexidine reduced gingivitis. Sigrist *et al.* (1986) compared the effectiveness of sanguinarine-zinc (Veadent®), chlorhexidine and essential oil/phenolic (Listerine®) mouthwashes with a placebo mouthwash in an experimental gingivitis study over 21 days. All these active mouthwashes significantly inhibited plaque accumulation with respect to the placebo, but only chlorhexidine was effective in preventing the development of gingivitis. In a further placebo-controlled study in the USA, the effectiveness of sanguinarine-zinc (Veadent), chlorhexidine and essential oil/phenolic (Listerine) mouthwashes were again compared with a placebo mouthwash, this time in a 6-month study (Grossman *et al.*, 1989). Again, all the active mouthwashes significantly reduced plaque scores compared to the placebo, but only chlorhexidine was able to significantly reduce gingival index and gingival bleeding scores.

It is doubtful to what extent zinc contributes to the plaque inhibitory properties of sanguinarine-zinc mouthwashes. The interaction of zinc and sanguinarine has been investigated in some detail by Southard *et al.* (1987), and they concluded that the effect on plaque was more determined by sanguinarine concentration than by the presence or absence of zinc. However, the addition of zinc did produce a slight enhancement of its effects.

In conclusion, sanguinarine appears to be an effective plaque inhibitory agent, but is less effective in this regard than chlorhexidine. Also, unlike chlorhexidine, it is not able to prevent the development of gingivitis. Furthermore, the mouthwash is a much more effective plaque inhibitory agent than the toothpaste, which may be devoid of activity. This may be due to the binding of other components in the toothpaste to the chemically reactive site of the sanguinarine molecule.

Propolis

Propolis (Murray *et al.*, 1997) is a naturally occurring bee product used by bees to seal openings in their hives. It mainly consists of of wax and plant extracts, and contains flavones, flavanones and flavanols. It has been used in homeopathic remedies as an antiseptic, anti-inflammatory, antimycotic and bacteriostatic agent and, because of these properties, it has been suggested as a constituent of a plaque inhibitory mouthwash.

A double-blind, parallel clinical study of the effectiveness of a propolis mouthwash has been carried out with negative and positive controls (Murray *et al.*, 1997). This showed that it had a very low level of clinical effectiveness and was not significantly better in inhibiting *de novo* plaque growth than the negative control. It does not therefore appear to have any use as a mouthwash.

Oxygenating agents

Oxygenating agents (such as hydrogen peroxide and buffered sodium peroxyborate and peroxycarbonate) in mouthrinses have a beneficial effect on acute ulcerative gingivitis, probably by inhibiting anaerobic bacteria (Wade *et al.*, 1966). As obligate anaerobes are important in the development of gingivitis and periodontitis, these effects could be useful. The information relating to the value of these agents in suppressing supragingival plaque formation is limited, although some retardation of plaque growth has been noted with the use of oxygenating mouthwashes (Wennström and Lindhe, 1979). In view of the importance of obligate anaerobic bacteria in the development of gingivitis and periodontitis, these compounds deserve further investigation (Addy, 1986).

The possible uses of antiseptic mouthwashes

The main uses of antibacterial mouthwashes are as follows:

1. To replace mechanical toothbrushing when this is not possible in the following situations:
    *   After oral or periodontal surgery and during the healing period.
    *   After intermaxillary fixation used to treat jaw fractures or following cosmetic jaw surgery.
    *   With acute oral mucosal or gingival infections, when pain and soreness prevents mechanical oral hygiene.
    *   For mentally or physically handicapped patients who are unable to brush their teeth themselves. However, these patients may also not be able to use a mouthwash so that swabbing of the gingival margins by a care worker may be the only option. This may not necessarily be easier for the care worker to carry out than brushing. The long-term use of effective agents has the major disadvantage of causing tooth staining.

2. As an adjunct to normal mechanical oral hygiene in situations where this may be compromised by discomfort or inadequacies:
    *   Following subgingival scaling and root planing, when the gingiva may be sore for a few days. The use of a mouthwash is usually only necessary for about 3 days in this situation.
    *   Following scaling, when there is cervical hypersensitivity due to exposed root surface. Its use needs to be combined with measures to treat the hypersensitivity, since the duration for the use of the mouthwash should not usually exceed 2 weeks in order to avoid tooth staining. However, patients vary considerably in the amount of staining they experience; some may have staining within a few days, and others show little after 1 month's use.
    *   Following scaling in situations where the patient's

oral hygiene remains inadequate. The inadequacy needs to be remedied quickly, since the duration of the mouthwash use should not exceed 2 weeks in order to avoid staining. It would be better to use a suitable antibacterial agent that does not cause significant staining in a toothpaste or pre-brush rinse, such as triclosan, for this purpose, in view of the above restriction.

Anti-plaque mouthwashes have no place in the treatment of existing periodontal disease – either gingivitis or periodontitis – since they cannot either reach the subgingival environment or penetrate thick layers of established plaque (see the section on chlorhexidine above).

All effective anti-plaque mouthwashes (bisguanides) cause staining (*Figure 15.1*), and this severely limits their use. They should therefore only be used for short periods (up to 2 weeks), in professionally cleaned mouths, to prevent the development of gingivitis when oral hygiene may be difficult or impossible (see above).

All patients using antibacterial mouthwashes for short periods should be told to avoid drinking tea, coffee and red wine in order to minimize the tooth staining. Such mouthwashes should not generally be used for smokers, since they would cause major tooth staining in this situation.

Whilst many of the agents discussed above have significant plaque inhibitory activity when compared with an inactive placebo, the extent of this varies amongst different agents and different formulations, e.g. mouthwash and toothpaste. Many of the more effective agents share the side effect of producing tooth staining, which may limit their longer-term use. Only one group of agents that are in general use, the bisguanides (of which chlorhexidine is the most effective), produce true anti-plaque activity and thus are able to prevent the development of an experimental gingivitis. This is because they combine substantivity (oral retentiveness) with antibacterial activity, and thus remain active in the mouth for long periods after their use.

Effective anti-plaque agents must have these combined properties to work. The bisguanides are therefore the only group of mouthwashes with therapeutic efficiency, and all the others are normally compared against this yardstick. All other agents have only plaque inhibitory effects, and thus are not therapeutically effective and can at best be used as adjuvants to mechanical cleaning measures such as toothbrushing.

Two other experimental agents, delmopinol and salifluor, also hold promise in this regard, and both of these have anti-inflammatory and hence anti-gingivitis effects in addition to plaque inhibitory effects.

Assessing manufacturers' claims about mouthwashes

The degree of effectiveness of a commercial mouthwash is very variable, and depends on the composition of both the active and various additional agents within the mouthwash. Their characteristics are best assessed under the following headings:

* Substantivity to the oral surface
* Range of antibacterial activity against the various plaque bacteria
* Possible anti-inflammatory effect
* Acceptable taste
* Ability to promote fresh mouth sensation.

They can be grouped into three categories on the basis of these properties: Groups A, B and C.

Group A

These are mouthwashes with good substantivity and a wide antibacterial spectrum, and they thus have true anti-plaque effects. The only agents with these properties are the bisguanides, the best of which is chlorhexidine. These can be used to replace mechanical cleaning methods for short periods when this is not possible. The main drawback of the bisguanides is staining, which is strongly linked to their substantivity. It precludes their prolonged use. Commercial chlorhexidine mouthwashes that do not produce staining are inactive, usually because the active chlorhexidine molecules have been bound to another constituent of the mouthwash.

Two other agents, salifluor and delmopinol, either achieve or come close to achieving these properties, but probably by rather different mechanisms to chlorhexidine.

Group B

These are agents with little or no substantivity but a good antibacterial spectrum. Therefore, they have plaque inhibitory effects but lack true anti-plaque effects. They cannot therefore be used to replace toothbrushing, but can be used as adjuvants to mechanical cleaning. They include cetyl pyridinium chloride, the essential oil/phenolic mouthwash, Listerine® and triclosan. In the case of triclosan, additional constituents such as zinc citrate or a co-polymer can enhance its plaque-inhibitory effects possibly, in the case of the latter, by increasing its retention time in the mouth when used as a constituent in mouthwashes or toothpastes.

Group C

These are antiseptic mouthwashes that have been shown to have antibacterial effects *in vitro*, but in clinical studies have been shown to have either plaque inhibitory effects varying from moderate to low, or to show no statistical difference from the negative control. These include hexetidine (Oraldene®), povidone iodine, oxygenating agents and the natural product sanguinarine (Veadent®), which is a benzophenanthridine alkaloid. These would have limited or no adjuvant effects when combined with mechanical cleaning, and therefore cannot be recommended for this purpose.

Subgingival plaque control

As periodontal disease is caused by bacteria, the use of antibacterial agents would appear to be reasonable in its treatment. However, for their use to be effective certain conditions need to be fulfilled:

1. They should be effective against the bacteria involved in the lesion
2. They should reach the site of infection in sufficient concentration for an adequate length of time
3. Their efficiency should outweigh all contraindications, e.g. side effects
4. They should not be used in situations where other conventional means of treatment are equally effective.

These agents can be taken systemically or applied locally into the periodontal pocket. Agents taken systemically must reach the periodontal pocket in a sufficient concentration to be inhibitory to the subgingival bacteria, whilst agents applied locally must also remain in a sufficient concentration for an adequate length of time.

Agents used systemically are always antibiotics, whilst those applied locally into the periodontal pocket can be either antibiotics or antiseptics.

Antiseptic agents

The association of bacteria with periodontal disease has given rise to considerable interest in the development and use of non-antibiotic antimicrobial agents for its management. These have to be applied locally into the periodontal pocket in slow release agents. Interest has centred mainly on their use as adjuvants to scaling and root planing.

The gingival crevice or periodontal pocket is not reached by chemical agents in mouthwashes or toothpastes, which have their effect purely on supragingival plaque. This is the main reason that such mouthwashes have no place in the treatment of established gingivitis or periodontitis. More recently local drug delivery systems have been developed to carry antibiotics into the pocket area, and some of these have been used to deliver antiseptics.

Chlorhexidine

Chlorhexidine is the most common antiseptic to be used in this way. It can be irrigated into the pocket using a 5 ml syringe and blunt needle, in either a liquid or gel form. It can also be incorporated into acrylic strips (Addy, 1986) and other slow releasing devices. Using an acrylic strip delivery system, chlorhexidine was shown to change markedly the subgingival bacterial composition as measured by dark ground microscopy. Comparative studies of the effect of subgingival delivery of either chlorhexidine or antibiotics have shown that it is less effective than tetracycline or metronidazole in changing the bacterial

flora and reducing gingivitis (Addy, 1986). It does not, however, suffer from the potential drawbacks of inducing bacterial resistance, and may therefore be more suitable for repeated use. In particular, chlorhexidine pocket irrigation is a useful and practical adjuvant to scaling and root planing deep pockets, particularly when marked inflammation is present.

Slow release devices

Slow release devices of various types have been used to deliver antibiotics into the periodontal pocket (see below), and these have also been used with antiseptic agents such as chlorhexidine. These systems allow the therapeutic agent to be delivered to the diseased periodontal site with increased therapeutic effect and minimal side effects.

The first slow release systems used to deliver chlorhexidine subgingivally were acrylic strips and dialysis tubing (Addy *et al.*, 1982), and these were effective in inhibiting the pocket flora but had to be placed for about a week and then removed. More recently, biodegradable slow release systems have been developed and used with chlorhexidine. The first of these were ethyl cellulose-based systems (Friedman and Golomb, 1982; Soskolne *et al.*, 1983). Soskolne *et al.* (1983) used such a system in a human study, producing a 3-day exposure to chlorhexidine, which released 80% of its dose in 72 hours. This produced drastic alterations in the pocket flora compared to the use of a placebo, reducing spirochaetes and motile rods in the pocket to negligible amounts. However, it was unable to maintain this effect for an extended period of time, and the bacterial numbers returned to their pretreatment levels after 14 days. Repeated placement of this system every 3 days for 9 days produced an extended delivery time in an attempt to prolong the suppression of the flora to clinically significant periods of time (Stabholz *et al.*, 1986). The devices were placed in 13 pockets of 5–8 mm depth in eight patients. There was a marked decrease in the relative proportions of spirochaetes and motile rods, and the total anaerobic count post-treatment and the probing depths were also reduced in all 13 pockets. These effects were maintained for 11 weeks post-treatment. This shows that a more prolonged exposure to chlorhexidine can suppress the pocket flora for more prolonged periods, along with accompanying clinical improvement. However, the changes are still no better than those obtained by subgingival scaling and root planing, which can produce such changes for up to 25 weeks.

Recently a new product known as the Blend-a-Med Perio Chip® has been developed, based upon this work, with the aim of prolonging the exposure from a single application. This product has now been marketed by Proctor and Gamble. It is a small chip suitable for placing in the periodontal pocket made of biodegradable polymer containing chlorhexidine (Heasman *et al.*, 1995). The polymer is made from 3.4 mg of cross-linked hydrolysed gelatin, 0.5 mg of gelatin and 0.96 mg of purified water, and contains 2.5 mg chlorhexidine. It is very simple to place into a periodontal pocket, and the swelling of the chip on contact with moisture retains it in place (*Figure 15.2*).

Release characteristics

A recent *in vitro* study (Lerner *et al.*, 1996) has demonstrated two phases of chlorhexidine release from the cross-linked protein matrix. The first phase was an initial burst effect in the first 24 hours, when 40% of the chlorhexidine was released, followed by a constant slower release over about 7 days, occurring partially in parallel with chip enzymatic degradation. An *in vivo* study on 12 patients confirmed this biphasic profile demonstrated in the *in vitro* model. Chlorhexidine concentrations of 800–1000 ppm were measured in the gingival crevicular fluid in the first 48 hours after the Perio Chip was placed. Lower concentrations of 100–500 ppm were found in GCF over the next 6 days. Concentrations well above the minimum inhibition concentration (MIC) for most pathogens (Å150 ppm) were seen for at least 7 days. This confirms that the amount of chlorhexidine in the periodontal pocket over a period of 7 days appears to be sufficient to eliminate pathogenic bacteria.

Clinical efficiency

A European multicentre study (Soskolne *et al.*, 1998) has been carried out into the prolonged delivery of chlorhexidine using this system as an adjunct to scaling and root planing. This was a blind, randomized, controlled, split mouth clinical study using 118 patients at three centres; Jerusalem (Israel), RAF Halton (UK) and Newcastle (UK). Two quadrants of the upper jaw with pockets of 5–6 mm were randomized to the two treatments, scaling and root planing alone or scaling and root planing plus Perio Chip. Probing depth, probing attachment level, bleeding on probing, gingivitis, plaque and tooth staining were measured before and at intervals after treatment for 6 months. The results found a statistically significant difference in these measurements in favour of the adjunctive

Figure 15.2 A Blend-a-Med Perio Chip® placed into a periodontal pocket

use of the chlorhexidine-containing chip. No differences in reported adverse effects were noted between the two treatments, and no tooth staining was noted throughout the trial.

Taken together, all the studies on prolonged subgingival delivery of chlorhexidine, which have recently been reviewed by Killoy (1998), show the following points. First, the Perio Chip can deliver the agent at effective levels over 7 days and disintegrates after this due to enzymatic degradation. Secondly, it can markedly reduce the numbers of bacteria in the pocket over this period, and can maintain these changes for up to 100 days. This is, however, no better than can be achieved by scaling and root planing. Thirdly, it appears to produce slightly better changes in clinical parameters than scaling alone. Fourthly, it appears safe and does not produce the tooth staining seen with the supragingival use of chlorhexidine. Finally, although similar results can be achieved with antibiotics, it does not suffer from the potential drawbacks of inducing bacterial resistance and hypersensitivity, and therefore may be more suitable for repeated use.

Sanguinarine

A biodegradable drug delivery system incorporating 5% sanguinarine has been produced under the trade mark ATRIGEL®. The delivery system consists of poly (DL-lactide) in a biocompatible carrier N-methyl-2-pyrrolidone, and this has flowable features, allowing it to be delivered into the pocket with a syringe. A two-centre trial of this system has been carried out (Polson *et al.*, 1996), and 201 chronic periodontitis patients with at least three pockets of 5–9 mm were studied over 3 months at the two centres using a four-quadrant split mouth design. Active gel was compared to placebo gel, scaling and root planing and supragingival plaque control, and probing pocket depth (PPD), probing attachment level (PAL), bleeding on probing (BOP) and plaque index (PI) were recorded at baseline, 14, 30, 60 and 90 days. Scaling and root planing was superior to all other treatments at all time points. The active gel failed to demonstrate consistent superiority to the placebo gel on a consistent basis. Thus, subgingival sanguinarine application is considerably less effective than conventional treatment and appears to have no place in periodontal therapy.

The Keyes technique

The Keyes technique consists of packing a mixture of NaCl, NaHCO$_3$ and H$_2$O$_2$ (3%) subgingivally, and then irrigating the pockets with an antiseptic solution such as an iodine solution (e.g. 0.5% povidone iodine (Betadine)). Used in combination with scaling, this has been reported to improve marginally the clinical effects of scaling and root planing alone (Rosling *et al.*, 1983). The mixture can also be used by patients during brushing, but this does not seem to produce any benefit over brushing alone. The use of the Keyes technique on its own is much less effective than scaling and root planing; therefore, the technique does not seem to offer any significant advantage in periodontal treatment.

Use of agents to raise redox potential

The growth of anaerobic bacteria in an ecosystem such as the periodontal pocket is dependent in part of the redox potential (Eh) (Finegold, 1989). It has been shown that redox potentials as low as -300 mV may exist in some parts of deep periodontal pockets, and this may enable strictly anaerobic bacteria to survive in this environment (Kenney and Ash, 1969). These researchers have also shown that the redox potential of the healthy gingival crevice (Eh $+70$ mV), with its very low proportion of anaerobes, is significantly higher than the average potential of the periodontal pocket (Eh -48 mV). By raising the redox potential it may be possible to create an environment that is incompatible with the growth of anaerobic periodontal pathogens.

A variety of substances, including redox dyes and transitional metal ions, can raise the redox potential in an ecosystem without producing molecular oxygen. One of the most promising of these is the redox dye methylene blue, which was partly chosen because of its low toxicity for humans (Gibson *et al.*, 1994).

This was first studied in a pilot study using chronic periodontitis patients (Wilson *et al.*, 1992). Methylene blue was applied by subgingival irrigation, and was shown after 28 days to have reduced gingival crevicular fluid flow and to have produced a shift in the bacterial flora towards one more compatible with health.

A recent study (Gibson *et al.*, 1994) compared subgingival methylene blue application with a negative control and scaling and root planing using a split mouth design; 24 chronic periodontitis patients were chosen because they had matched periodontal pockets in all four quadrants of 5 mm or more. One quadrant received subgingival irrigation of 0.1% methylene blue irrigation at baseline, 1 and 4 weeks; the second received sterile water irrigation (negative control); the third received scaling and root planing; and the fourth received a single subgingival application of methylene blue in a slow release device consisting of a biodegradable collagen alginate vicryl composite.

After 4 weeks there were no significant differences in the clinical measurements, although the gingival index and pocket depth reduced for all groups. Darkground microscopy showed an increase in cocci and a decrease in motile organisms for all groups. There were also reductions in the numbers of spirochaetes, and these were statistically significant both for methylene blue by slow release and for scaling and root planing. Bacterial cultures showed an increase in the aerobic/anaerobic ratio for all groups, with significant changes in both the methylene blue and the scaling and root planing groups. Methylene blue, irrigation and slow release also showed significant reductions in the numbers of black-pigmented anaerobics, and this change was not produced by either water irriga-

tion (negative control) or scaling and root planing. Furthermore, in contrast with scaling and root planing, very few patients complained of discomfort with methylene blue applications.

These results indicate that methylene blue, by raising the redox potential, is able to alter the microflora in the periodontal pocket to one more compatible with periodontal health. In most respects these changes are comparable to those achieved with scaling and root planing, but in some respects are better. It has none of the disadvantages associated with the use of antibiotics given either locally or systemically, such as the emergence of resistant bacterial strains and the development of hypersensitivity. Methylene blue may therefore have potential as a therapeutic agent in the treatment of chronic periodontitis.

It is not known precisely what dose of methylene blue is necessary in the periodontal pocket for the optimal effect of redox potential. However, *in vitro* studies have shown that *Porphyromonas gingivalis* is killed by the change in redox potential produced by methylene blue at 1.0 mg/ml (Fletcher and Wilson, 1993).

Antibiotics and periodontal treatment

Until recently, there has been a justifiable reserve in the dental profession regarding the use of antibiotics to treat periodontal disease. However, in the past few years, interest in the use of antibiotics for this purpose has increased, and many clinical trials of their use have been published.

Several criteria must be met before the use of antibiotics can be justified. These are that:

1. The nature of the bacterial flora associated with periodontal disease must be amenable to control by antibiotics
2. Antibiotics must be shown either to be superior to traditional clinical treatment in controlling the disease, or to act as useful adjuvants to it
3. Antibiotics used must be free from adverse side effects and from the induction of hypersensitivity or bacterial resistance
4. Antibiotics must achieve effective concentrations in the periodontal pockets where the causative bacteria reside.

The antibiotics most commonly used in the treatment of periodontal patients are:

* Penicillins
* Tetracyclines
* Metronidazole
* Erythromycin
* Clindamycin
* Vancomycin
* Gentamicin.

The antimicrobials most commonly used as adjuvants in

the treatment of chronic periodontitis are tetracyclines and metronidazole. Both of these antibiotics are broad-spectrum agents, aimed at many different bacteria within the periodontal pocket rather than a single pathogen. For this reason, the rationale for their use has to be questioned (see below).

Tetracyclines and an amoxycillin/metronidazole combination have been suggested to treat juvenile periodontitis, with the aim of eliminating *Actinobacillus actinomycetemcomitans* from the periodontal pocket (see Chapter 20).

Acute periodontal abscess should ideally be treated with the appropriate antibiotic determined by an antibiotic sensitivity test on a pus sample from the lesion (see Chapter 19). In this situation antibiotics should only be considered if the abscess fails to respond to drainage alone.

Metronidazole is the agent of choice in treating acute necrotizing ulcerative gingivitis (see Chapter 22).

Amoxycillin, erythromycin, clindamycin, vancomycin and gentamicin all have a place in the prophylaxis of transient bacteraemia in susceptible patients (see below). The factors involved in the possible use of antibiotics are considered in detail below.

Classification of antibiotics

Antibiotics of interest to dentists are classified according to their structures (Mandel and Petri, 1996a, 1996b; Chambers and Sande, 1996a, 1996b; Sande *et al.*, 1996; Tracy and Webster, 1996) into:

Beta-lactams	These contain a β-lactam ring nucleus, and include the penicillins, cephalosporins and cephalomycins
Aminoglycosides	These are either derived from various species of the *Streptomyces* fungi, and end in mycin (e.g. streptomycin and tobramycin), or from *Micromonospora purpura*, which is not a fungus, and hence end in micin (e.g. gentamicin and semi-synthetic drugs such as amikacin)
Sulphonamides	The names of this group contain sulpha or sulfa
Tetracyclines	These all have a four-ringed structure, and their names end in cycline
Azoles	These all contain an azole ring, and their names end in azole (e.g. metronidazole)
Quinolones	These are all structurally related to nalidixic acid and most end in oxacin, e.g. ciprofloxacin
Macrolides	e.g. erythromycin
Others	These are structurally unrelated to any of the above groups. They include chloramphenicol, clindamycin and vancomycin

Natural production of antibiotics by bacteria or fungi

Antibiotics are medically useful not only because of their effects on bacteria, but also because they do not have similar effects on human cells, which are sufficiently different from bacterial cells to escape destruction (Chambers and Sande, 1996a; Laurence *et al.*, 1997).

People tend to think of antibiotics as a human invention, but this is far from the truth. Ever since the British biologist Alexander Fleming discovered in 1928 the antimicrobial activity of a substance released from the *Penicillium* fungus, which was aptly called penicillin, people have realized that bacteria and fungi can manufacture powerful antibiotics. Thus, antibiotics are manufactured by the very classes of organisms they aim to destroy.

Scientists are still not clear why these organisms manufacture antibiotics. One theory is that they are designed to inhibit other competing species of the bacteria trying to inhabit a new environment, but this seems inconsistent with certain features of antibiotics. In this regard, one would expect an organism in search of a new environment to lack the resources to make complex antibiotics and therefore to be simple compounds (Amábile-Cuevas *et al.*, 1995). This is not the case, as antibiotics are complex molecules that require a good deal of energy for their manufacture. Furthermore, they are produced by organisms in a stationary stage of their life cycle, which seems incompatible with competition in a new environment.

On the other hand, workers such as Davies (1990) have proposed that antibiotics are vestiges of ancient metabolic systems, dating back to some of the very first organisms on earth. Many antibiotics bind to cellular structures, and could have facilitated the synthesis of biological molecules such as peptides or stimulated other metabolic pathways. As biochemistry evolved, it is likely that these ancient binding molecules were replaced by enzymes, which proved much more efficient. However, the ancient binding molecules may have persisted in bacteria and fungi, and now function as antibiotics.

The structure and origins of antibiotics

A variety of techniques have been used to determine the chemical structure of naturally produced antibiotics, and the detailed structure of most of these is now known.

Penicillin (Mandel and Petri, 1996b; Laurence *et al.*, 1997) originates from the *Penicillium* fungus, but since the structure of its nucleus was determined many new penicillins have been synthesized. This has vastly increased the antibacterial range of these antibiotics and increased their adsorptions from a variety of routes. This has been achieved by adding appropriate side chains to the β-lactam nucleus (*Figure 15.3*). Cephalosporins also contain the β-lactam nucleus, and individual cephalosporins are based on changes in two side chains (*Figure 15.4*).

Tetracycline (Chambers and Sande, 1996b; Laurence *et*

β-lactam nucleus

Side chains

benzyl penicillin

phenoxymethyl penicillin

ampillin $R_1 = H$

amoxycillin $R_2 = OH$

Figure 15.3 The chemical structure of the β-lactam nucleus and the side chains of penicillins in common use

Cephem nucleus

Cephalothin

Cephalexin

There are now 2nd, 3rd and 4th generation cephalosporins based on changes in R_1 and R_2

Figure 15.4 The chemical structure of cephalosporins: the cephem nucleus and two common side chains

al., 1997) is produced by species of *Streptomyces*. It has a four-ringed parent structure (*Figure 15.5*), and a family of tetracyclines has been produced by altering side chains.

Metronidazole (Tracy and Webster, 1996; Laurence *et al.*, 1997) is a benzimidazole (*Figure 15.6*), which was synthesized for use as an antihelminthic agent. Its action against anaerobic bacteria was discovered as a result of its administration to a patient with a trichomonal vaginitis who was also suffering from oral acute necrotizing ulcera-

tetracycline

Figure 15.5 The chemical structure of tetracyclines

Figure 15.6 The chemical structure of metronidazole

tive gingivitis (ANUG) (Shinn, 1962; Shinn *et al.*, 1965). It was found to bring about a swift resolution of the ANUG. It has been shown to be active against most strictly anaerobic bacteria.

Erythromycin (Sande *et al.*, 1996; Laurence *et al.*, 1997) is a macrolide antibiotic with a complex structure (*Figure 15.7*) produced by species of *Streptomyces*.

Clindamycin (Sande *et al.*, 1996; Laurence *et al.*, 1997) is produced by the soil bacterium *Bacillus fragilis*. Its structure is shown in *Figure 15.8*.

Gentamicin (Sande *et al.*, 1996; Laurence *et al.*, 1997) is an aminoglycoside antibiotic (*Figure 15.9*) produced by *Micromonospora purpura*.

Vancomycin (Sande *et al.*, 1996; Laurence *et al.*, 1997) is a complex tricyclic glycopeptide (*Figure 15.10*), and its structure has only recently been chemically determined. It is produced by a species of *Streptomyces*.

Mode of action of antibiotics

The precise chemical mode of action varies from one antibiotic to another. Antibiotics are either bactericidal, i.e. they kill sensitive bacteria, or bacteriostatic, i.e. they inhibit multiplication of sensitive bacteria. Bactericidal antibiotics are usually the first choice in treating infections but in general, provided that an adequate concentration of the antibiotic is achieved at the site of infection and the host defences are normal, there is little difference in the effectiveness of both types. Penicillin and metronidazole are examples of bactericidal antibiotics, and tetracycline and erythromycin examples of bacteriostatic ones.

The antibiotics used in periodontal therapy act by one of the following mechanisms (Amábile-Cuevas *et al.*, 1995):

- Inhibition of cell wall synthesis
- Reversible inhibition of protein synthesis
- Inhibition of DNA synthesis or DNA function by interfering with DNA coiling or gene expression
- Inhibition of folic acid synthesis.

These are illustrated in *Figure 15.11*.

Erythromycin

Figure 15.7 The chemical structure of erythromycin

Figure 15.8 The chemical structure of clindamycin

Gentamicin

Figure 15.9 The chemical structure of gentamicin

The penicillin family and the cephalosporins (β-lactams) disrupt the construction of the bacterial cell wall. Tetracyclines, macrolides (e.g. erythromycin), aminoglycosides (e.g. gentamicin, streptomycin) and chloram-

phenicol all inhibit bacterial protein synthesis, and sulphonamides and trimethoprin inhibit bacterial folic acid synthesis. Finally, other newer antibiotics inhibit DNA synthesis or function, and in this regard rifampicin inhibits bacterial gene expression and nalidixic acid and ciprofloxacin disrupt the proper coiling patterns of bacterial DNA.

The spectrum of action of antibiotics varies considerably. It is obviously necessary for the antibiotic of choice to be strongly active against the causative bacteria of the disease. An example of this affecting the choice of an antibiotic for periodontal purposes is in the use of metronidazole, which is strongly active against strictly anaerobic bacteria but is only weakly active against facultative, capnophilic aerobes such as *Eikenella corrodens*, *Capnocytophaga* species (spp.) and *Actinobacillus actinomycetemcomitans*. Generally, antibiotics with a lower potential for sensitization and bacterial resistance (see below) should be preferred for treating periodontal diseases.

Antibiotics are primarily used for treating specific bacterial infections, where the infection can be treated with a narrow spectrum antibiotic specifically directed against the foreign pathogen. During treatment the susceptible pathogens and any indigenous bacteria sensitive to the antibiotic will either be killed (bactericidal antibiotic) or stopped from multiplying (bacteriostatic antibiotic). Bacteriostatic antibiotics depend upon the host defence mechanisms to rid the body of the suppressed pathogens. The success of the treatment depends on which bacteria regrow after the treatment is stopped. If the indigenous bacteria regrow rapidly after treatment, they will prevent the re-establishment of the pathogens (Van Palenstein Heldermann, 1986).

The nature of periodontal infections

Although the primary cause of inflammatory periodontal disease is bacterial, no single causative pathogen has been found (Chapter 4). Thus, chronic periodontitis seems best regarded as a non-specific bacterial disease caused by a local imbalance in the local indigenous

Vancomycin

Figure 15.10 The chemical structure of vancomycin

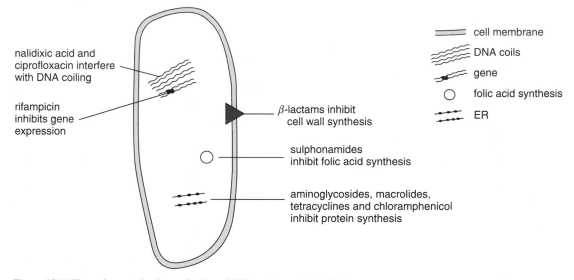

nalidixic acid and ciprofloxacin interfere with DNA coiling

rifampicin inhibits gene expression

β-lactams inhibit cell wall synthesis

sulphonamides inhibit folic acid synthesis

aminoglycosides, macrolides, tetracyclines and chloramphenicol inhibit protein synthesis

cell membrane
DNA coils
gene
folic acid synthesis
ER

Figure 15.11 The various mechanisms of action of different classes of antibiotics

bacterial population (Theilade, 1986). However, the bacteria in the subgingival plaque are the primary aetiological agents in periodontitis (Tonetti, 1994), which also results from the sequelae of quantitative and qualitative changes in both the composites of the subgingival microflora and the inflammatory response which results from its presence (Loesche, 1976). Certain indigenous bacteria may play a more important role in the disease process because they possess virulence factors that may enable them to damage host defences or degrade host tissues. However, there is no evidence that eradication of suspected pathogens of chronic periodontitis without the suppression of other members of the flora is effective in treating chronic periodontitis. If, as seems to be the case, all the suspected pathogens are members of the normal oral flora, their permanent eradication by antibiotics will

not be possible because they will re-establish themselves after treatment.

However, it is known that transient shifts in the subgingival bacterial flora can be produced both by scaling and root planing (see Chapter 14) and by the systemic administration or local application of some antibiotics. A number of studies have been carried out into the most promising antibiotics, tetracycline and metronidazole, and these will be described below.

There is a much stronger case for using certain antibiotics to treat acute necrotizing ulcerative gingivitis (Chapter 22) and juvenile periodontitis (Chapter 20), as they appear to be associated with selective growth of a much narrower range of bacteria.

However, because of the possibility of inducing bacterial resistance and antibiotic hypersensitivity by over-prescription of antibiotics, these drugs should *never* be prescribed if other means of treatment are possible.

The site of action of antibiotics for periodontal treatment

The site of action for an antibiotic treating periodontal disease is the periodontal pocket, and it is essential that the antibiotic should achieve a high concentration at this site (Van Palenstein Heldermann, 1986).

Antibiotics for treating periodontal disease can be administered either systemically or locally. The local method seems better for achieving high local concentrations of the drug and for minimizing the risks of developing bacterial resistance. This method should not be used with antibiotics, such as penicillin, that carry a high risk of sensitization. The inaccessibility of the pocket is a problem in this regard, as it cannot be reached by antibiotics in mouthrinses, ointments, toothpastes or chewing gum. This problem can be overcome by subgingival irrigation, but daily irrigation is not practical since it is patient-dependent. To avoid this problem, slow release devices have been developed that can be inserted by the dentist into the pocket, extending down to its base. These currently include hollow and monolithic fibres (Goodson *et al.*, 1979, 1983) and acrylic strips (Addy, 1986), and slow release gels (Norling *et al.*, 1992).

Systemically administered antibiotics can also reach the pocket via gingival crevicular fluid, which is an exudate. This has been shown to occur with tetracyclines (Gordon *et al.*, 1981), clindamycin (Walker *et al.*, 1981a), metronidazole (Notten *et al.*, 1982) and amoxycillin and an amoxycillin/clavulanic acid combination (Augmentin®) (Tenenbaum *et al.*, 1997). Tetracycline and its derivatives achieve higher concentrations in crevicular fluid than in serum, possibly by binding to calcium-containing substances (Baker *et al.*, 1983). The antibiotic concentrations in crevicular fluid, achieved using either the systemic route or local delivery systems, are higher than those necessary to inhibit the sensitive bacteria *in vitro* (Van Palenstein Heldermann, 1986).

Drawbacks to the use of antibiotics in periodontal treatment

The over-use and frequent misuse of antibiotics in medicine, dentistry, veterinary practice, farming and food production has severely reduced the clinical effectiveness of commonly used antibiotics in one of two ways:

1. By producing hypersensitivity reactions against specific antibiotics in many human subjects
2. By producing bacterial resistance, involving many species of important human pathogens, to antibiotics.

Hypersensitivity reactions against specific antibiotics

Some antibiotics can act as haptens and stimulate immune reactions against themselves, resulting in type 1 hypersensitivity reactions. This can occur with a number of antibiotics, including penicillins, tetracyclines and macrolide antibiotics such as erythromycin. These reactions occur more frequently in subjects genetically predisposed to hypersensitivity, such as sufferers of hay fever, eczema and asthma, and both the numbers of these subjects and the number of patients hypersensitive to antibiotics is increasing.

Hypersensitivity can result from both systemic and topical delivery of antibiotics, and its development is encouraged by frequent exposure.

All types of hypersensitivity can occur to antibiotics, ie types I, II, III and IV. The following clinical signs and symptoms have been described: angioneurotic oedema, urticaria and anaphylactic shock, red man syndrome, maculo-papular rashes, serum sickness-like syndromes, drug fever, erythema multiforme and adverse skin reactions in patients with lymphoid diseases (Riott, 1997).

When hypersensitivity to an antibiotic develops, it precludes the future use of that antibiotic (or family of antibiotics, in the case of penicillin) and therefore stops their use in potentially serious infections in the future.

Bacterial resistance to antibiotics

Frequent exposure to antibiotic produces the development of bacterial resistance in two main ways:

1. The antibiotic either kills or suppresses the bacteria sensitive to it, but does not affect those strains that are naturally resistant to it. This favours the growth of these resistant strains, which then increase in number. Further exposure to the same antibiotic, particularly a short time after it was last prescribed, progressively increases the number of resistant strains.
2. Bacteria resistant to a particular antibiotic possess gene(s) coding for factor(s) producing this resistance. Bacteria may pass genes to other bacteria in structures known as plasmids. The recipient bacteria could be of the same or closely related species, or in some cases different species. This process of gene transfer in plasmids may represent a primitive form of sexual reproduction. In this way, the genes concerned with antibiotic resistance can be passed from the resistant bacteria to other bacteria in the subject. The resistant bacteria can then spread to many other subjects by common means of transmission, either producing antibiotic resistant infections in the recipient subjects or passive carriage of the resistant strains in the commensal flora of their skin, nose or throat.

By the late 1950s and during the 1960s, an explosive search for new natural and synthetic antibiotics was under way, eventually yielding about 100 new drugs (Amábile-Cuevas *et al.*, 1995). As the costs of production of antibiotics dropped, they became overused in both appropriate and inappropriate ways. In addition to their medical and

veterinary uses, antibiotics became used, for purely commercial reasons, in supplements to animal feed, where they
were supposed to act as growth promoters. As a result of
this totally unnecessary use, thousands of pounds of antibiotics were and are being released into the environment
each year, killing off only the sensitive bacteria and leaving the resistant ones to grow and flourish. The combination of this totally illegitimate use and medical over-
prescription produced the obvious result, which was anticipated by Fleming himself, of a dramatic increase in the
number of bacteria resistant to the effects of antibiotics.

Antibiotics are so potentially destructive to micro-
organisms that they kill or suppress the very same organisms that make them. As a result of this undesirable effect
on the bacteria, many microbes develop mechanisms to
protect themselves from their own antibiotics. It is this
self-protective process that makes micro-organisms resistant to antibiotics. Furthermore, research has shown that
once a bacteria becomes resistant to an antibiotic, it can
potentially pass on this resistance to other members of its
own species and even to other species.

Mechanisms of resistance

The mechanisms of bacterial resistance are as varied as
the mechanisms of antibiotic activity. The main mechanisms used against particular antibiotics are:

- The release of enzymes that can dismantle the antibiotic, either outside or inside the cell
- Development of cellular pumps, which pump the
  antibiotic out of the cell
- Alteration of the shape of the molecule to which the
  antibiotic binds
- Synthesis of enzymes resistant to the effect of the
  antibiotic.

These are shown in *Table 15.2* and illustrated in *Figure 15.12*.

Dismantling enzymes
Enzymes are produced by the host bacteria that dismantle
the antibiotic. An example of this is the production and

Table 15.2 The mechanisms of action of antibiotics

Antibiotic	Resistance mechanism
β-lactams Aminoglycosides Chloramphenicol Erythromycin Tetracycline	Chemically modified by enzymes
Erythromycin Tetracycline	Actively removed from cell
Erythromycin	Enzymatic modification of target
β-lactams Fusidic acid	Proteins bind to and sequester antibiotics within target cell
Sulphonamides Trimethoprim	Synthesis of enzymes insensitive to the action of the drug

secretion of β-lactamases, which degrade the β-lactam
group of antibiotics (penicillins and cephalosporins) by
bacteria resistant to these antibiotics. This mechanism can
be circumvented by the use of a β-lactamase inhibitor
such as clavulanic acid, and this is used in the combination of amoxycillin with clavulanic acid in Augmentin®
(Farmer and Reading, 1982; Todd and Benfield, 1990).
Enzymes are also produced by other groups of resistant
bacteria, which chemically modify aminoglycosides such
as streptomycin and gentamicin and tetracyclines and
chloramphenicol.

Cellular antibiotic pumps
Some antibiotics, such as tetracycline or the macrolides
(erythromycin), enter the bacterial cell, but resistant bacteria have developed molecular pumps, which pump the
drug out again.

Change in antibiotic-binding molecules
Bacteria resistant to erythromycin and tetracyclines alter
the shape of the molecule to which the antibiotic binds.
The antibiotic is then unable to bind to this molecule and
is thus prevented from damaging the bacterial cell.

Synthesis of resistant enzymes
Bacteria resistant to sulphonamides and trimethoprim can
alter the target enzyme affected by the drug. In this way,
the enzyme can continue to function in spite of the
presence of the drug.

Genetic spread of resistance

Antibiotic resistance in bacteria is especially dangerous
because the genes encoding the resistance can be transferred between bacteria of the same species or between
bacteria of different and distantly related species (*Figure 15.13*). Genetic information (Holmes and Joblin, 1991)
can be passed between bacteria by 4 different mechanisms:
tranformation, transduction, conjunction and transposition
and the last two are particularly important. Transposons
are segments of DNA that can move from one site in a
DNA molecule to another in the same or a different DNA
molecule and this process is known as transposition. It can
move genes from the main chromosome to plasmids and
vice versa. Many of the genes that code for resistance
factors are found on small circular pieces of DNA known
as *plasmids*, which are independent of the main chromosome. A single bacterium can contain many different
plasmids, each with a different set of resistance genes on it
(*Figure 15.13a*). These resistance genes can be transferred
from one plasmid to another in the same bacterial cell, and
in this way a single plasmid can collect a number of
different resistance genes (*Figure 15.13b, c*). These multiple resistance gene plasmids also can be transferred from a
resistant to a susceptible bacteria along a conjunctive
bridge that forms between the two bacteria (conjugation)
(*Figure 15.13d, f*). An incredible number of genes encoding for inactivating enzymes and other resistance factors
are encoded on these structures. They include all the

Figure 15.12 The mechanisms by which bacteria gain resistance to antibiotics. Bacteria develop a variety of mechanisms to combat the effects of antibiotics. Some bacteria produce enzymes that can dismantle antibiotic molecules, and this is responsible for resistance to the β-lactams, aminoglycosides and chloramphenicol. These enzymes may be secreted and thus attack the antibiotics outside the cell before they enter it, or may attack antibiotics within the cell if they have already passed through the surface membrane. Other bacteria produce cellular pumps, which remove the antibiotics from the cell as soon as they enter it. This mechanism may produce resistance to tetracyclines and erythromycin. Another mechanism is the modification of the bacterial metabolic enzyme affected by the antibiotic so that the antibiotic may longer bind to it. Thus the enzyme may continue to function normally. This mechanism may produce resistance to sulphonamides and trimethoprim. In a similar way, other bacteria alter the target molecule affected by the antibiotic so that it can no longer key into its receptor site on the molecule. This mechanism may produce resistance to tetracyclines and erythromycin

resistance factors for β-lactams, aminoglycosides and many other antibiotics. Furthermore, new resistance genes are constantly forming in bacteria because of their high rate of mutation.

Other resistance factors are encoded on genes in the main DNA coil rather than on plasmids. However, it has recently been shown that genes can move from one DNA molecule to another (transposition). This allows genes on the main DNA cassettes to transfer to plasmids, or genes on one plasmid to spread to another. In this way most of the resistance genes can spread from one bacteria to another in plasmids. Thus, these processes greatly increase the genetic mobility of the resistance genes.

Some other separate resistance factors only encode on genes found on the main cassette, and these include the *mar* genes. These genes are turned on by the presence of an antibiotic, and at least two antibiotics, tetracycline and chloramphenicol, have been shown to stimulate this gene. When activated, these genes produce factors that inhibit pore formation on the bacterial cell wall. When this happens, the cell wall becomes totally impermeable to the antibiotic molecule. Another gene affected by antibiotics in a similar way is the bacterial *soxRS* gene which, when activated, makes the bacteria totally resistant to the effects

of superoxide produced by immune stimulated inflammatory cells. These last two systems are switched on in resistant bacteria by antibiotics, but as the genes remain on the main DNA cassette, these effects cannot be spread to other bacteria by plasmid exchange.

Significance of bacterial plaques

Interactions between bacteria allow them to associate together in close proximity in colonies and plaques, and in these relationships they are not affected by antibiotics as readily. Bacteria can in this way produce a biofilm on a variety of surfaces where they become protected from the effects of heat, ultraviolet light, viruses and antibiotics. These films can form on catheters, implants, dental units and tubing, endotracheal tubes, contact lenses and silicone surfaces. Bacteria living in multi-species biofilm or plaques, including dental plaque, live in a special microniche where nutrients are provided by neighbouring cells and diffusion. It has been shown that resistance to antibiotics can increase rapidly in these films, and the production of resistance disabling enzymes such as β-lactamase increase in these situations. Probably, close contact in the biofilm

Figure 15.13 The process of transfer of antibiotic resistance genes between bacteria (conjunction): *(a)* two plasmids with different resistance genes; *(b)* transfer of a resistance gene from one plasmid to another in the same bacterial cell by transposition or integration; *(c)* a bacterial cell containing a multiple resistance gene plasmid; *(d)* transfer of the genes on one multiple resistance gene plasmid to another bacteria across a conjunctive bridge; *(e)* donor and recipient bacterial cell after this process

greatly increases the chances of plasmid exchange. These factors are very pertinent to the practice of dentistry.

The large numbers of different bacteria within the periodontal pocket exist as interdependent microcolonies on the root surface, pocket epithelial lining and the pocket space itself. These represent highly organized microfilms, which operate in the ways described above. Concerning these, it should be realized that the minimum bactericidal concentrations (MBC) or minimum inhibitory concentrations (MIC) for antibiotics relate to their independent growth (planktonic conditions), and not to their growth in microfilms. As the target for the *in vivo* concentration of an antibiotic is often taken as its *in vitro* concentration, inhibiting or killing 90% of tested isolates (MBC$_{90}$ or MIC$_{90}$), the decreased susceptibility of bacteria in a biofilm needs to be taken into account. In this respect, there is no direct evidence on which to base an estimate of the MICs or MBCs of periodontal pathogens growing in organized biofilms. However, estimates from other

biofilm infections indicate that the necessary MICs and MBCs are at least 50 times higher than those for bacteria grown under planktonic conditions (Anwar *et al.*, 1992; Brown and Gilbert, 1993; Vorachit *et al.*, 1993). A recent study (Wright *et al.*, 1997) compared the MIC values for the effect of metronidazole on *Porphyromonas gingivalis* grown under planktonic conditions and as a biofilm on the surface of hydroxyapatite. Growth on the biofilm was still active after exposure to 20 μg/ml of metronidazole, which is 160 times the MIC for the planktonic growth of this bacteria. This bacteria within a biofilm would therefore be resistant to the concentrations of metronidazole found in tissues following systemic administration.

Antibiotic-resistant infections

The overuse of antibiotics and the spread of resistance genes by plasmid transfer has resulted in the development of bacterial infections resistant to one or more commonly prescribed antibiotics. Such infections are becoming increasingly common in humans and other animals. Unfortunately, some common bacterial infections are emerging which are resistant to most or, in a few cases, all known antibiotics. Such cases have been reported in increasing numbers across the world since 1963 (Amábile-Cuevas *et al.*, 1995). They have included *Neisseria gonorrhoeae* causing gonorrhoea infections resistant to penicillin, *Salmonella typhi* causing typhoid fever resistant to multiple drugs including chloramphenicol, streptomycin, tetracycline, ampicillin, cephaloridine, kanamycin, nalidixic acid and sulphonamides, *Shigella sonnei* causing dysentery resistant to ampicillin, tetracycline and sulphamethoxazole/trimethoprim, *Klebsiella pneumonia* infections resistant to multiple drugs, *Enterococcus faecium* and *faecalis* causing diarrhoea resistant to ampicillin, gentamicin, streptomycin and vancomycin, and *Mycobacterium tuberculosis* causing tuberculosis infections resistant to multiple anti-tuberculous drugs. The most dramatic increase in resistant infections recently has been in hospital-acquired wound infections (nosocomial infections). These include streptococcal infections resistant to penicillins and sulphonamides, *Staphylococcus aureus* infections resistant to penicillins, including the new penicillins, which are resistant to the effects of penicillinase, e.g. methicillin and flucoxacillin, and to cephalosporins and *Serratia marcescens* infections resistant to multiple drugs. Other common bacteria that show multiple resistance to antibiotics are *Pseudomonas* spp., *Proteus* spp. and *Escherichia coli*. It has also been demonstrated that the genes involved in multiple resistance can be spread between different species, and this has been shown to occur between a Central American *Shigella* strain and a Mexican *Salmonella* strain (Amábile-Cuevas *et al.*, 1995).

The infections that have wrought most damage to patients in British hospitals are the methicillin-resistant *Staphylococcus aureus* (MRSA) hospital wound infections. The bacteria causing these infections would probably more appropriately be called multiple antibiotic-resistant *Staphylococcus aureus*, since they are resistant to many of the most commonly used antibiotics. Many MRSA infections are currently resistant to all antibiotics except vancomycin, and a few (vancomycin-resistant MRSA) are also resistant to this antibiotic. These infections, including vancomycin-resistant MRSA, are becoming increasingly common in our hospitals, and when they occur they may result in closure of the ward, unit or hospital affected. Affected units must stay closed until the infection is eliminated. Passive carriage of multiple resistant *Staphylococcus aureus* in the nasopharynx and on the skin of contacts of the patients and hospital staff is also becoming increasingly common. Furthermore, carriage of MRSA by hospital staff may lead to them being laid off work if they are in contact with surgical patients.

Tuberculosis also is making a comeback in this country, mostly in the poor and deprived groups and in immigrants from affected countries. It may also be seen more commonly in HIV patients succumbing to AIDS. Many of these new cases of tuberculosis are resistant to commonly used anti-tubercular antibiotics, and in a few cases are resistant to all known anti-tubercular antimicrobial agents.

Control of the use of antibiotics

If inappropriate and excessive use of antibiotics on the scale of today continues, then it is likely that the majority of serious bacterial infections will become resistant to all the antibiotics currently available. It is also extremely unlikely that new antibiotics would appear at a fast enough rate to solve these problems, and even if they did, it would be very likely that bacteria would develop insensitivity to these new antibiotics in turn by the same mechanisms.

It is therefore extremely important that antibiotics are only prescribed when correctly indicated for infections known to be sensitive to the antibiotic in question. They should never be prescribed as blanket cover for the imprecise diagnosis of an infection, or for conditions that can be equally or better treated by other means. It is also vitally important that all other unnecessary uses of antibiotics, such as additives to farm animal feed, are totally eliminated.

In respect of periodontal disease, it is pertinent that no single pathogen is involved in its aetiology, so no precise antibiotic treatment to eliminate a single pathogen can be used. At the best, therefore, antibiotics used in periodontal treatment will suppress some of the bacteria in the subgingival flora for a variable period, after which they will grow back, since they are all members of the indigenous flora. This change in the subgingival flora can be equally or better achieved by subgingival scaling (see Chapter 14 and below), which has been shown to be effective for longer periods. Therefore, antibiotics can never be primary agents in treating periodontal diseases, and should only be used for the few situations where, for one reason or another, conventional treatment fails to be effective, even when it is efficiently carried out and repeated. These situations will be described below.

In addition, the prophylactic use of antibiotics should be reduced to the minimum by sensible management. Patients who give a history of rheumatic fever should be sent to a cardiologist for cardiac investigations to see whether the patient has actually suffered from rheumatic heart disease. When such patients are investigated in this way, many are found to have no cardiac disease and thus do not need prophylactic antibiotic cover. An examination by a cardiologist should also be arranged for apparently healthy patients reporting cardiac murmurs, if the exact status is not already known and available from their general medical practitioner.

If antibiotic prophylaxis is required for patients at risk from a transient bacteraemia, then treatment producing a bacteraemia should be organized in the minimum number of visits, and at least 6 weeks should elapse before antibiotic administration is repeated. Other prophylactic uses of antibiotics, such as following surgery, should be kept to the absolute minimum and only given if there is a high risk of infection.

Clinical trials of antibiotics in the treatment of chronic periodontitis

A number of clinical trials of the use of antibiotics for the treatment of chronic periodontitis have been carried out. They have used antibiotics either as the sole treatment, or in combination with scaling and root planing, and in both cases have compared the results obtained with those from scaling and root planing alone. All of these have involved the use of either a tetracycline or metronidazole.

Local application of antibiotics into the periodontal pocket would seem to have some advantages over systemic administration. Local application can produce a much higher concentration in the pocket, with a much lower total dose and very low systemic levels. This reduces the risk of resistant bacteria emerging and of the development of hypersensitivity. However, local application does not affect the reservoirs of bacteria at other sites in the mouth and only maintains bactericidal levels for about 24 hours. It is also much more expensive.

The effects of antibiotics as the sole agent

Short-term use of systemic or local tetracycline and metronidazole produces a marked reduction in Gram negative anaerobes and spirochaetes and improvements in the clinical condition, i.e. reduction in probing pocket depth (PPD) and bleeding on probing (BOP). Similar results have been shown with the local delivery of tetracycline in hollow or solid fibres (Goodson *et al.*, 1979, 1983; Lindhe *et al.*, 1979), or metronidazole in acrylic strips (Addy, 1986). Re-establishment of the pocket flora after antibiotic treatments occurs between 8 and 12 weeks (Lindhe *et al.*, 1979).

These studies show that, whilst marked reductions in the number of subgingival bacteria can be achieved with these antibiotics, these are often less than can be achieved by scaling and root planing, and tend to persist for shorter periods.

The effects of antibiotics as adjuvants to scaling and root planing

Since it is impossible to remove the whole pocket flora by scaling and root planing, the use of antibiotics as adjuvants to these procedures might enhance their effects. To test this possibility, a number of studies have been carried out to compare the combined effects of antibiotics and scaling and root planing with the effects of scaling and root planing alone (Lindhe *et al.*, 1979, 1983). In both groups, the changes in the flora were maintained for up to 25 weeks.

Long- and short-term systemic treatment with tetracyclines in combination with scaling and root planing have not shown any more benefit over scaling and root planing

alone. The effect of local tetracycline and metronidazole with local administration or slow release devices as an adjuvant to scaling and root planing has also been studied. Similar changes were seen with and without the adjuvants, and thus no additional benefit appeared to accrue (Lindhe *et al.*, 1979, 1983; Addy, 1986).

The results of some studies using systemic metronidazole in combination with scaling and root planing were similar to those from scaling and root planing alone (Lindhe *et al.*, 1983). However, there are other studies that show more marked and prolonged improvements in the clinical condition using systemic metronidazole as an adjuvant to scaling and root planing (Joyston-Bechal *et al.*, 1984, 1986; Loesche *et al.*, 1985, 1991; Söder *et al.*, 1990). In one study, these improvements had disappeared 3 years after treatment (Joyston-Bechal *et al.*, 1986).

Loesche and his co-workers have carried out three double-blind clinical trials of systemic metronidazole in the treatment of periodontal disease, and have observed each time a significant clinical improvement in the group receiving metronidazole (Loesche *et al.*, 1985, 1991, 1992). In these patients there was a significant rapid decline or disappearance of spirochaetes. Systemic metronidazole as an adjuvant to scaling was also found significantly to reduce the need for periodontal surgery (Loesche *et al.*, 1992). However, a few patients in the metronidazole groups appeared to be non-responsive to the drug. In another study (Loesche *et al.*, 1993), the compliance in taking the drug was investigated by measuring the reduction in spirochaetes, and it was found that only 10 patients out of 18 in the study were compliant in regularly taking the drug. These 10 patients experienced a significantly greater clinical benefit than the eight non-compliant patients.

Factors affecting local delivery of antimicrobial agents into the periodontal pocket

A pharmacological agent must reach its site of action and be maintained there at a sufficient concentration for a sufficient time for an effect to occur, and these three criteria affect the local delivery of agents to the periodontal pocket.

Site of action

The targets for locally delivered pharmacological agents include bacteria residing in the periodontal pocket, and bacteria possibly invading the junctional epithelium and adjacent connective tissue or the exposed root cementum or dentine (Saglie *et al.*, 1982, 1988; Adriaens *et al.*, 1988). Most methods of local delivery, including irrigating solutions, place the agent down at the base of the pocket (Pitcher *et al.*, 1980). However, it should be recognized that gaining access to the pocket does not necessarily mean gaining access to target bacteria. Extracellular components of the bacterial biofilm may impair diffusion or inactivate a significant proportion of the applied active agent, and thus may protect biofilm bacteria from the action of an antimicrobial agent. In addition, the biofilm may prevent the agent from diffusing into the the soft tissue wall or exposed root surface.

Concentration

To be effective against target bacteria, the antimicrobial agent should reach the site of action at a concentration higher than its minimal efficacious concentration. Definition of the desired concentration range is a key aspect in maximizing therapeutic efficiency of an agent and minimizing its expected side effects.

The first approximation of the desired concentration of antimicrobials comes from *in vitro* experiments looking at the susceptibility of the target bacteria to different concentrations of the drug in terms of its effects on growth inhibition (MIC) and bacterial killing (MBC). The *in vivo* concentration of an antimicrobial is usually based on the *in vitro* concentration of that agent that inhibits or kills 90% of the target bacteria in culture (MIC_{90} and MBC_{90}). It must, however, be realized that these *in vitro* concentrations are determined with the bacteria growing in culture under planktonic conditions, whereas the bacteria in the subgingival flora are residing in an organized biofilm. In these situations, the real therapeutic concentration is likely to be at least 50 times higher than the *in vitro* MIC_{90} or MBC_{90} (Anwar *et al.*, 1992; Brown and Gilbert, 1993; Vorachit *et al.*, 1993). However, it is also true that sub-MIC concentrations of antibiotics can also modulate bacterial metabolism and impair production of virulence and colonization factors, and may thus make bacteria more susceptible to the effects of the immune system (Hansberger, 1992).

It is necessary to adjust the therapeutic dose to take account of side effects of the drug, which are also associated with the local concentration. The pharmacological effect of any drug, including antibiotics, is characterized by a certain therapeutic range, which is the range of concentration above the minimal effective concentration but below the concentration that produces substantial toxicity or side effects. The most important concentration-dependent side effect of local delivery of antimicrobials is the overgrowth of non-susceptible micro-organisms, and this effect occurs at both ends of the concentration spectrum. After exposure to marginally effective concentrations, resistant bacteria may repopulate the whole ecological niche, while after exposure to highly effective concentrations, overgrowth of intrinsically non-susceptible micro-organisms (such as yeasts) is more likely to occur. Moreover, little attention has been paid to to the concentration-dependent side effects of local antibiotic therapy for periodontitis.

Time

Once a drug reaches the site of action in an effective concentration, it must remain at the site for long enough for its pharmacological effect to occur. Different classes of antibiotics inhibit or kill infecting bacteria by different mechanisms, e.g. interference with cell wall growth, inhibition of protein synthesis or inhibition of DNA synthesis. Antibiotics using these different specific mechanisms have been shown to require different durations of exposure to effective concentrations. Therefore, the duration of antimicrobial levels of the drug may be of critical importance in the case of some antibiotics.

Moreover, these assumptions are based on *in vitro* experiments and should be considered further when the target bacteria are not living in planktonic conditions such as in the periodontal pocket. In this respect, metronidazole requires rapidly proliferating bacteria to work effectively. However, in organized biofilms, most of the bacteria display a very slow growth rate, and this may seriously limit the effectiveness of many antibiotics (Evans *et al.*, 1990; Ashby *et al.*, 1994).

An inflammatory infiltrate, gingival crevicular fluid (GCF), constantly flows into the periodontal pocket. It has been estimated that the fluid present in a 5 mm periodontal pocket is replaced about 40 times per hour (Goodson, 1989), and such a high clearance is the result of a low volume and high flow rate (Binder *et al.*, 1987). Therefore it is apparent that, following subgingival placement of a drug, it will rapidly be removed from the pocket according to an exponential decay equation (Benet *et al.*, 1996).

The expected half-time of elimination of a subgingivally placed pharmacological agent (i.e. the time necessary to reduce its concentration by half) is about 1 minute. This is in good agreement with experimental observations of about 1.5 minutes obtained following subgingival irrigation with 1% ofloxacin solution (Higashi *et al.*, 1990) or the subgingival placement of fluorescein gel (Oosterwaal *et al.*, 1990).

This high rate of clearance of a drug placed into the periodontal pocket represents the major obstacle in attempting to maintain antimicrobial action following subgingival irrigation or placement of non-blinding substances. Therefore, longer antimicrobial action requires systems to establish drug reservoirs, which are able to release active medication in sufficient quantities to counteract the expected continuous loss over time effected by the flow of GCF.

Further studies on local delivery

Slow release gels

Further studies (Norling *et al.*, 1992) on local delivery of tetracycline and metronidazole have been carried out more recently, following the incorporation of these antibiotics into biodegradable slow release gels (*Figure 15.14a, b*). Studies of the release characteristics from these gels have shown that both the 2% minocycline (Dentomycin®) gel (Satomi *et al.*, 1987) and the 25% metronidazole (Elyzol®) gel (Stoltze, 1992) produce levels above the MIC for suspected pathogens for 12–24

(a)

(b)

Figure 15.14 Local delivery systems for antibiotic slow-release gels: *(a)* the delivery system for 2% minocycline (Dentomycin®); *(b)* the delivery system for 25% metronidazole (Elyzol®)

hours after treatment. It has also been shown that the systemic absorption, including that from swallowed excess gel, was less than that absorbed from one 200 mg metronidazole tablet taken orally (Stoltze and Stellfeld, 1992).

A single application of 5% metronidazole in a collagen slow release device used as an adjunctive to subgingival scaling has been compared to the effects of subgingival scaling alone (Hitzig *et al.*, 1997). Both treatments produced a marked decrease in the number of total anaerobes, black-pigmented anaerobes, spirochaetes and fusiform bacteria. Surprisingly, however, there was a greater reduction in the number of *Actinobacillus actinomycetemcomitans* in the metronidazole group. The reduction in clinical parameters was the same for both groups. Thus there seemed to be little advantage in using adjuvant metronidazole in this situation.

Further studies in human patients with these agents, using 2% minocycline gel (Van Steenberge *et al.*, 1993; Vandekerchhove, 1998), locally-delivered 10% doxycycline hyclate (Drisko, 1998) and 25% metronidazole gel

(Klinge *et al.*, 1992a; Ainamo *et al.*, 1992; Pedrazzoli *et al.*, 1992; Magnusson, 1998), produced similar findings to those reported for other local delivery agents in the previous section. It has also been shown that 25% metronidazole gel improved the clinical features of experimental periodontitis in dogs, and eliminated some of the bacteria associated with the condition (Klinge *et al.*, 1992b). Good results have also been achieved with topical irrigation with tetracycline-HCl solution (100 mg/ml), and this might in part be due to absorption of the compound onto root dentine and its subsequent release (Christersson *et al.*, 1993). Irrigation for long periods (5 minutes) is, however, necessary to achieve release of therapeutic concentrations of active antibiotic.

Recently, an 18-month, randomized, double-blind, parallel, comparative study (Timmerman *et al.*, 1996) has been carried out in 20 healthy patients with moderate to severe periodontitis, into the long-term efficacy and safety of locally applied minocycline. The adjuvant effect of either active or placebo gel and scaling and root planing was compared with regard to clinical and microbiological effects. The patients received oral hygiene instruction and supra- and subgingival scaling and root planing at baseline. The active or placebo gel was applied at baseline, 2 weeks, and 1, 3, 6, 9 and 12 months. Over the 18-month period, no differences were observed between test and control sites with regard to probing depth or probing attachment level. Over a 15-month period, there were significant reductions in the numbers of putative periodontal pathogens in all the treated sites, but there were no significant differences between test and placebo sites. *Candida albicans* and *Enterobacteriaceae* were only detected in small numbers at each time interval in a limited number of patients, and no changes in their proportions or prevalence were seen in any of these patients during the study. No adverse effects were observed in the trial period.

Thus, this group of patients responded favourably to scaling and root planing but did not benefit from the adjuvant use of minocycline gel. This study clearly shows that locally applied antibiotics do not have a place in the routine treatment of periodontitis patients.

Slow release fibres (Actisite®)

Two types of fibre system have been investigated for carriage of tetracycline for local delivery into the periodontal pocket. These are:

1. Drug filled hollow fibres (Goodson *et al.*, 1979)
2. Ethylene vinyl acetate co-polymer (EVA) fibres (Goodson *et al.*, 1985).

Monolithic fibres of EVA with a diameter of 0.5 mm containing 25% tetracycline have been used in a number of clinical trials, and are now been marketed by Stafford-Miller Ltd under the trade name of Actisite®.

It has been found that these fibres placed into the periodontal pocket maintained an average of 1590 μg/ml

(0.16%) of tetracycline over 10 days (Tonetti *et al.*, 1990), and this concentration is well above that necessary to inhibit growth of all the susceptible bacterial species, including those suspected as being periodontal pathogens (Walker *et al.*, 1981b).

Actisite® fibres are used to fill the periodontal pocket under treatment. The end of the fibre is first applied with a flat plastic instrument into the deepest part of the pocket, and then successive layers are then packed in, wrapping the fibre around the tooth so that all the subgingival areas are filled. A floss threader can be used to pass the fibre between the teeth. When the packing process is complete, excess fibre is cut off with scissors and the fibre is retained by applying a thin layer of cyanoacrylate adhesive to the tooth and top layers of the fibre at the gingival margin. The time taken to apply the fibre varies from 5 to 15 minutes per tooth, depending on the pocket depth and the position of the tooth. The fibre is left in the pocket for about 10 days, after which it is removed with a scaler or forceps. When the fibre is removed the pocket is dilated, and the root surface within the pocket can be clearly seen. This may reveal any residual calculus, which may have been left on the tooth following the preceding subgingival scaling procedures. This can be more easily seen and removed at this stage. The tissues then readapt to this clean root surface during the subsequent healing period.

Solid EVA fibres containing 25% tetracycline (EVA-TC fibres) have been subject to a number of laboratory and clinical studies.

Tonetti *et al.* (1990) investigated the delivery characteristics of these fibres in the periodontal pocket and compared them with subgingival irrigation. They found that following subgingival irrigation of 1% and 10% tetracycline solutions into the periodontal pocket, the gingival crevicular fluid (GCF) concentration decayed exponentially, with half-times of 4.2 and 12.2 hours respectively. In contrast, EVA-TC fibres packed into the pocket and left *in situ* for 10 days maintained a constant GCF concentration of 1590 μg/ml over the 10 days. These findings were in agreement with those expected from a steady-state model based on the release characteristics of the fibres and GCF flow rate. After removal of the fibres, the tetracycline concentration decreased exponentially with a half-time of 4.5 hours.

The serum concentration resulting from EVA-TC fibre placement has been studied by Rapley *et al.* (1992). They placed the fibres in eight deep pockets of four adult chronic periodontitis patients for 10 days, and took plasma samples at baseline, 1 hour, 3 hours, 3 days and 10 days. The amount of fibre used per patient ranged from 160–222 cm, and the maximum tetracycline local dose averaged 105 mg, with a range of 91–126 mg. This produced no detectable serum level greater than 0.1 μg/ml. This level was found in three out of four subjects at 3 hours after placement, and in one subject 3 days after placement. Transient and insignificant plasma levels were found after placement of multiple fibres, and the local dose was tolerated well by all the patients, with

no adverse effects. Thus, local EVA-TC fibre placement appears to result in insignificant systemic uptake of tetracycline.

The tissue concentration of tetracycline following EVA-TC fibre placement into periodontal pockets was studied by Ciancio *et al.* (1992). They sought to evaluate the tetracycline concentration in the gingival tissue adjacent to the fibre-treated periodontal pockets. Ten chronic periodontitis patients with two or more pockets in excess of 5 mm in each maxillary quadrant and with bleeding on probing were selected as subjects. After initial scaling and root planing, either placebo fibres or EVA-TC fibres were randomly assigned to two non-adjacent pockets in each subject. The fibres were left *in situ* for 8 days, after which the fibres were removed and periodontal surgery was performed. The flap incision allowed a biopsy of one interdental papilla to be taken from each of the two test sites in each quadrant. One biopsy was analysed for tetracycline concentration by high performance liquid chromatography (HPLC). The second biopsy was examined by light and ultraviolet (UV) fluorescence microscopy to determine the localization of residual tetracycline and intensity of inflammatory cell infiltrates in the adjacent periodontal tissues. They found a mean tissue tetracycline concentration of 64.4 ng/mg, which corresponds to 43 μg of tetracycline. The levels at placebo sites were below the detection limit of the HPLC system. Also, tetracycline fluorescence was seen in the soft tissue wall at depths ranging from 1–20 μm. Therefore, some tetracycline from the EVA-TC fibre placed in the periodontal pocket does pass through the damaged pocket epithelium into the adjacent periodontal tissue.

Morrison *et al.* (1992) studied the effect on the root surface within the pocket from a 10-day exposure to EVA-TC fibre placement. Eight patients with four teeth with terminal periodontitis, which required extraction, were selected for treatment. The teeth of each patient were randomly assigned to one of four treatment groups: no treatment control; scaling and root planing only; EVA-TC fibre only; and EVA-TC fibre plus scaling and root planing. The root surfaces were examined by fluorescent light microscopy (FLM), scanning electron microscopy (SEM) and energy dispersive spectroscopy (EDS). SEM revealed a visible reduction in the subgingival plaque on the root surfaces in the EVA-TC fibre and fibre plus scaling groups in comparison to the control group. In contrast, the scaling and root planing group showed randomly distributed areas of residual subgingival plaque and calculus with newly developed plaque fronts, which appeared to have formed over the 10 days following treatment. EDS analysis of large crystals adhering to the root surfaces of EVA-TC fibre and fibre plus scaling teeth revealed high chloride peaks, which were suggestive of residual tetracycline. These crystals were not present in the other groups. FLM examination of EVA-TC fibre and fibre plus scaling teeth showed a superficial penetration of tetracycline into the root surface to a depth of about 10 μm.

Areas of demineralized root exhibited slight tetracycline penetration into dentinal tubules. Thus, EVA-TC fibre treatment appears to be effective over 10 days in clearing subgingival plaque from the root surface, and also appears to result in some absorption of tetracycline into the root surface.

One of the main drawbacks to local antibiotic therapy is the possible development of bacterial resistance. For this reason, antibiotic resistance of the subgingival microbiota following EVA-TC fibre treatment has been studied (Goodson and Tanner, 1992). This was studied by three approaches. First, they assessed the ability of the subgingival microbiota to grow on media containing tetracycline. High percentages of tetracycline-resistant bacteria appeared at EVA-TC fibre-treated sites and within the saliva 1 week after treatment as compared with pretreatment levels. By 1 month post-treatment, the number had returned to levels comparable to those pretreatment. In a second approach, they took subgingival isolates following treatment and grew them on media without antibiotics. They then took selected isolates and determined their Gram stain and cell morphology characteristics. It showed that the subgingival sites became colonized with Gram positive cocci during the same time period in which the increase in the number of tetracycline-resistant bacteria developed. Since most Gram positive cocci are intrinsically resistant to tetracycline, this may account for the transient increase in tetracycline-resistant bacteria seen following EVA-TC fibre treatment. In a third approach, the antibiotic resistance of subgingival Gram negative bacteria was determined before and after EVA-TC fibre treatment. The predominant cultivable microbiota of nine sites from three subjects were isolated immediately before and 6 months after EVA-TC fibre treatment. Gram negative rods were characterized and tested for sensitivity to tetracycline (minimum inhibitory concentration (MIC) 1–128 μg/ml), penicillin at 80 μg/ml and erythromycin at 8 μg/ml. None of the Gram negative rods were resistant to tetracycline, either before or after treatment. Before treatment 98% were susceptible to tetracycline at 1–2 μg/ml, and after treatment 88% were susceptible. The percentage of Gram negative rods showing intermediate sensitivity (MIC 4–8 μg/ml) changed from 2% before treatment to 5.2% after treatment. In no case was penicillin or erythromycin resistance associated with increased resistance to tetracycline.

This study appears to show that no significant bacterial resistance develops following EVA-TC fibre therapy. This could be for three reasons. First, there is a high concentration of tetracycline in the pocket throughout the 10-day application, which is vastly in excess of the MIC (Tonetti *et al.*, 1990). This would inhibit virtually all the susceptible bacteria at this site. It could also inhibit bacteria on the root surface, as tetracycline appears to absorb into this surface following EVA-TC fibre treatment (Morrison *et al.*, 1992). Secondly, tetracycline from EVA-TC fibre treatment does find its way into the adjacent gingival tissues, and may thus inhibit any sus-

ceptible bacteria at this site (Ciancio *et al.*, 1992). Thirdly, tetracycline does not appear to become systemically absorbed to any significant level from the local site (Rapley *et al.*, 1992), and would thus not stimulate resistance at other sites.

However, this study does not take account of three important factors. First, tetracycline is bacteriostatic rather than bactericidal, and its effects on the susceptible bacteria are less prolonged and may thus allow the long-term development of resistance. Secondly, some strains of bacteria from species normally susceptible to an antibiotic are naturally resistant. Thus, inhibition of susceptible strains will select for these resistant strains and allow them to multiply. Thirdly, and most importantly, antibiotic-resistant bacteria can transfer antibiotic-resistance genes to non-resistant bacteria in plasmids, and this can involve bacteria of the same or different species. Since there is a significant reservoir of natural or acquired tetracycline-resistant bacteria in all periodontal pockets and gingival crevices, and these bacteria are in very close relationship with each other in this environment, there is a very real possibility of tetracycline resistance developing as a result of local tetracycline treatment. This applies equally to all other antibiotics used locally or systemically in periodontal treatment. Therefore, one should always be very cautious in using antibiotics, and should only use them for periodontal treatment when repeated conventional treatment is not effective.

Heijl *et al.* (1991) studied the clinical and microbiological effects of periodontal treatment with EVA-TC fibres and scaling. Ten chronic periodontitis patients with pockets of 6 mm or more and bleeding on probing in all four quadrants took part in the study. Supragingival plaque control was maintained throughout the study by weekly professional cleaning and 0.2% chlorhexidine mouthrinses. One quadrant of the mouth remained untreated, one was treated with subgingival scaling and root planing alone, one by EVA-TC fibres alone and one by scaling and root planing plus EVA-TC fibres. They were assessed at 10 and 62 days after treatment. All the treatments resulted in favourable clinical changes, which were not seen at the untreated sites, with reduced pocket depths, reduced bleeding on probing and decreased gingival index scores. Parallel to the clinical changes, all treatments reduced the total number of bacteria and the percentage of black-pigmented anaerobic rods, motile bacteria, non-motile rods and spirochaetes, and produced a proportional increase in cocci. Fibre therapy with or without scaling reduced bacterial counts by two orders of magnitude when evaluated 62 days post-therapy, and these effects were particularly favourable for a combination of fibre and scaling. Although some of the bacterial changes were better for fibre and scaling and fibre alone than for scaling alone, e.g. total plate colony counts, some were better for scaling alone than for fibre, i.e. reductions in spirochaetes and motile rods. In addition, in some patients no differences were seen between scaling and fibre placement. Therefore, whilst this study does show that EVA-TC fibre treatment is effective in producing favourable clinical and bacteriological changes, these effects are improved when it is combined with subgingival scaling and root planing. Furthermore, these combined treatment changes are very similar to those produced by subgingival scaling and root planing alone.

Goodson *et al.* (1991a, 1991b, 1991c) carried out a multicentre study of EVA-TC fibre treatment for chronic periodontitis. One hundred and seven subjects at five centres were chosen, and four sites with 6–10 mm pocketing which bled on probing were selected in each subject. These sites were randomly placed into one of four groups: EVA-TC fibre therapy alone; subgingival scaling alone; control fibre (i.e. EVA fibre without tetracycline); and untreated. EVA-TC fibre and EVA fibre alone were placed to fill the pocket and were sealed in with cyanoacrylate adhesive and removed after 10–12 days. Subgingival scaling was performed for 5 minutes per site under local anaesthesia. Following initial tooth cleaning procedures, probing depth, probing attachment level and bleeding on probing were measured with a controlled-force probe. They were measured at baseline and at 30 and 60 days following therapy. All these clinical parameters were reduced by both EVC-TA fibre and subgingival scaling treatments, but not by control fibre treatment or no treatment. The extent of these changes appeared to be greater with the EVA-TC fibre treatment than with scaling. No serious side effects attributable to EVA-TC fibre treatment were seen, and there were no cases of superinfection.

Microbiological samples were taken before and after treatment, and their analysis revealed significant reductions of *Fusobacterium nucleatum*, *Porphyromonas gingivalis*, *Prevotella intermedia*, *Eikenella corrodens* and *Campylobacter recta* in the sites by both tetracycline and scaling, with no significant differences between treatments (Goodson *et al.*, 1991c). The number of *Actinobacillus actinomycetemcomitans* were also reduced, but this did not reach significance, as only a few patients were infected with this bacteria. Thus, favourable bacterial changes are produced both by EVA-TC fibre treatment and scaling and root planing, with no statistical differences between them.

Another 6-month multicentre study has been carried out by Newman *et al.* (1994), in which 113 chronic periodontitis patients were recruited from seven private periodontal practices throughout the United States. Two non-adjacent sites in separate quadrants were selected on the basis of having pockets of 5–8 mm and bleeding on probing, which had been refractory to previous periodontal treatment. They were assigned to one of two groups: subgingival scaling and root planing alone, or EVA-TC fibre plus subgingival scaling and root planing. Probing depth, probing attachment level and bleeding on probing were measured at baseline and 1, 3 and 6 months. At 1, 3 and 6 months, EVA-TC fibre plus subgingival scaling and root planing was significantly better at promoting clinical attachment gain than subgingival scaling and root planing alone. Overall, these results indicate that EVA-TC fibre therapy enhances the effectiveness of subgingival scaling and root planing in the management of localized recurrent periodontitis sites, in patients receiving regular supportive periodontal treatment.

The effect of EVA-TC fibre treatment on recurrent lesions was also studied in a long-term study of 31 patients on maintenance care in a private periodontal practice (Corsair, 1994). Scaling and root planing were carried out on all the subjects 3 weeks before the start of the study. Sixty-one sites with moderate 4–6 mm (21) or deep 7 mm or more (40) pockets and bleeding on probing were treated with EVA-TC fibres. The fibres were removed after 1 week. Patients were evaluated 1, 3, 6, 12 and 24 months after therapy. Treated sites showed mean probing depth reductions of 2.5 mm at 6 months and 2.2 mm at 24 months, and clinical attachment gains of 2.4 mm at 1 month, 3 mm at 3 months and 2.5 mm at 6 months. Bleeding on probing was markedly reduced. Although there were no controls in this study, it did show that a combination of EVA-TC fibre treatment and scaling was effective in sites previously refractory to conventional treatment in a private practice situation.

Although all of these clinical studies (which have been recently reviewed by Tonetti, 1998) show that EVA-TC fibre treatment is effective, they do not show that it is significantly better than subgingival scaling and root planing in most situations. Therefore, one should always be very cautious in using antibiotics and should only use them for periodontal treatment when repeated conventional treatment is not effective at a local site.

Development of bacterial resistance of periodontal bacteria to antibiotics used in periodontal therapy

The use of systemic antibiotics can easily produce bacterial resistance by the methods described above, and this is particularly the case if:

1. Doses of the same antibiotic are repeated within relatively short time periods
2. Inappropriate antibiotics are prescribed
3. Suboptimal doses of antibiotic are given
4. The prescribed regimen is not adhered to by the patient.

Furthermore, oral administration of antibiotics also opens the possibility of the development of resistance in members of the gastrointestinal bacterial flora. Finally, the appropriateness of the use of antibiotic therapy for chronic periodontitis could be questioned in view of the non-specific nature of the bacterial cause of that disease.

Compared to systemic administration of antibiotics, local application reduces the risk of systemic side effects, as the total dose given is minimized. Also, the chance of the development of resistance in the gastrointestinal flora is markedly reduced, as the drug hardly reaches this area.

In this respect the use of excessive amounts of antibiotic gel should be avoided, as any that spills over into the mouth will be swallowed.

In the oral cavity, however, local application of antibiotics may pose an increased risk of the development and selection of resistant bacterial strains within the pocket flora, possibly causing further deterioration or recurrence of periodontal disease (Larson and Fiehn, 1997). Resistance may also be produced as a result of sub-inhibitory antibiotic concentrations developing in the periodontal pocket due to rapid wash out of the antibiotic from this site. Growth of bacteria at sub-inhibitory concentrations of antibiotic facilitates the development of resistance. In this regard, the emergence of a high proportion of resistant bacteria in periodontal pockets after the long-term low-dose administration of tetracycline, and this has been described by Kornman and Karl (1982) and Williams *et al.* (1979).

Local delivery of antibiotics to periodontal pockets initially produces very high concentrations but, as antibiotic is constantly washed out from the pocket, this is quickly succeeded by sub-inhibitory concentrations, which may well facilitate the development of bacterial resistance. A recent study (Larson and Fiehn, 1997) investigated the possible development of resistance in suspected periodontal pathogens after exposure to sub-inhibitory concentrations of the two most commonly used antibiotics for local application in the treatment of periodontal disease, minocycline and metronidazole. The minimum inhibitory concentration (MIC) of 18 reference strains and 12 clinical isolates was determined. Subsequently, all strains with a MIC of > 8 μg/l were exposed to serial passage on plates containing sub-inhibitory and gradually increasing concentrations of these antibiotics, until growth was inhibited. Initially most strains were inhibited at $\leqslant 0.25$ μg/ml of minocycline and 0.5 μg/ml of metronidazole, although *Actinobacillus actinomycetemcomitans* was resistant to metronidazole. After growth at sub-inhibitory concentrations, eight strains survived 1–2 times and 11 strains survived 8–32 times their initial MIC of metronidazole. With respect to minocycline, *A. actinomycetemcomitans* survived 8–64 times its initial MIC while all other strains survived 1–8 times their MIC. Thus, significant resistance to these antibiotics was shown to develop in suspected periodontal pathogens, and this could easily occur following their local application. Furthermore, widespread appearance of tetracycline resistance in medically important bacteria has limited the use of this antibiotic in the treatment of medical infections (Speer *et al.*, 1992).

In the oral cavity tetracycline resistance has also been shown to correlate to prior administration of this antibiotic, and whilst resistance was only seen in 1–7% of isolates in patients not treated with antibiotics, it was seen in over 20% of isolates following tetracycline treatment (Walker *et al.*, 1983; Fiehn and Westergaard, 1990; Olsvik *et al.*, 1995). In some studies of systemic administration (Hawley *et al.*, 1980; Heimdahl and Nord, 1983; Fiehn

and Westergaard, 1990), the percentage of resistant organisms has been shown to return to baseline levels after 3 months.

Studies of local application of tetracyclines (O'Connor *et al.*, 1990; Larson, 1991; Goodson and Tanner, 1992; Preus *et al.* 1995) have shown a similar pattern, possibly because of the very high concentration of antibiotic for the first 48 hours. However, the possibility that resistance may increase further upon repeated exposure to sub-inhibitory concentrations by the frequent use of subgingival antibiotics in maintenance patients cannot be excluded, and this could lead to resistance levels in periodontopathic bacteria, with clinical implications.

Common to all these studies was the maintenance of high inhibitory concentrations in the periodontal pocket for 1–3 weeks. In the older studies (Williams *et al.*, 1979; Kornman and Karl, 1982) resistance was determined after systemic administration of low, sub-inhibitory doses of tetracyclines over long periods, and these recorded resistance in up to 77% of isolates. One (Kornman and Karl, 1982) showed that 26% of isolates were still resistant 6–24 months after discontinuation of this antibiotic.

These studies show the importance of:

- Limiting the use of this antibiotic to situations when it is absolutely necessary
- Avoiding the repeat use of the same antibiotic within 3 months of its previous administration
- Achieving high inhibitory concentrations at the treatment site (the periodontal pocket) for the whole duration of the treatment, whether using systemic or local administration.

Resistance to metronidazole is much less common, in spite of the fact that this antibiotic has been used extensively (Edwards, 1993; Garcia-Rodriguez *et al.*, 1995). The development of metronidazole resistance has not been studied immediately following its use in periodontal patients, but one study of its local application (Pedrazzoli *et al.*, 1992) reported no increase in resistance 6 months after therapy.

However, in other parts of the body resistance to metronidazole has been described in *Bacteroides* species, and in *Helicobacter pylori* causing active gastritis and peptic ulcers (Sprott *et al.*, 1983; Edwards, 1993; Banatavala *et al.*, 1994; Noache *et al.*, 1994). *H. pylori* resistance has been shown to develop during antibiotic treatment (Goodwin *et al.*, 1988; Hirschl *et al.*, 1988), and the prevalence of resistance is associated with previous intake of metronidazole (Bantatvana *et al.*, 1994). In *Bacteroides* species, resistance to metronidazole has been shown to be transferable by several mechanisms (Garcia-Rodriguez *et al.*, 1995). Furthermore, in a group of patients with *H. pylori* gastric infection, pretreatment metronidazole-susceptible isolates were shown to be genetically identical to post-treatment metronidazole-resistant isolates, and this suggests that resistance had developed in the existing flora (Rautelin *et al.*, 1994).

These *in vivo* studies complement *in vitro* studies on the development of metronidazole resistance in *H. pylori*. The studies exposed the bacteria to serial passage on plates containing sub-inhibitory concentrations of metronidazole, and found increased resistance in up to 75% of the strains (Haas *et al.*, 1990; Van Zwet *et al.*, 1994). Furthermore, in the majority of isolates the acquired resistance was stable (Van Zwet *et al.*, 1994). This is in agreement with the study of Larson and Fiehn (1997), which showed that metronidazole resistance of 32 times the initial MIC developed in suspected periodontal pathogens, including *Porphyromonas gingivalis*, *P. anaerobius*, *Prevotella intermedia* and *Fusobacterium nucleatum*. This was shown to remain stable at a lower level.

Thus, it has been shown that bacterial resistance to metronidazole can develop in previously susceptible bacteria, including putative periodontal pathogens. Therefore, the use of this antibiotic should be restricted to situations where it is absolutely necessary, and should be subject to the same restrictions suggested for tetracycline above.

The non-antibiotic properties of tetracyclines

Tetracyclines (TCs) have been found to inhibit host-derived collagenases and some other matrix metalloproteinases (MMPs) by a mechanism independent of the well-known antimicrobial activity of these drugs (Golub *et al.*, 1983, 1984, 1985, 1987, 1991, 1992; Rifkin *et al.*, 1993; Ryan *et al.*, 1996). The first discovery that tetracyclines can inhibit host-derived MMPs by a mechanism independent of their antimicrobial properties was made in germ-free rats with experimentally induced diabetes, a model of excess collagenase activity (Golub *et al.*, 1983).

Available antimicrobial TCs with these properties are minocycline, doxycycline and tetracycline itself. Recently, however, Golub and co-workers (Golub *et al.*, 1987, 1991, 1992; Rifkin *et al.*, 1993) have synthesized 10 different analogues of the tetracycline molecule, which are known as chemical modified tetracyclines (CMTs), and all of these totally lack antimicrobial properties. In spite of this, nine of them exhibited strong collagenase inhibiting properties. The CMT that lost its anticollagenase activity was CMT-5, and this was the pyrazole analogue, in which the carbon-11 carbonyl oxygen and carbon-12 hydroxy groups were replaced by nitrogen atoms. This eliminated the important Zn^{2+} and Ca^{2+} binding sites in the tetracycline molecule, which is active at physiological pH.

The mechanism proposed to explain these anticollagenase properties concerned the Zn^{2+} and Ca^{2+} binding properties of the TC molecule, and explained the ability of TCs to inhibit already active collagenase or gelatinase in the extracellular matrix. It is supported by several pieces of recent evidence. First, adding excess Zn^{2+} or Ca^{2+} ions eliminates this property (Golub *et al.*, 1983; Yu *et al.*, 1991). Secondly, collagenase appears to contain secondary Zn^{2+} and Ca^{2+} ions outside the catalytic domain of the enzyme in addition to those within this domain. These secondary ions help to maintain the conformity and catalytic activity of the enzyme (Lovejoy *et al.*, 1994). The proposed mechanism suggested that TCs interacted with these secondary metal ions, in particular Zn^{2+} (Golub *et al.*, 1991). Thirdly, the mechanism of this action is not associated with fragmentation of the MMP molecule, and the results of *in vitro* experiments suggest a non-competitive action of these drugs (Sorsa *et al.*, 1994). Thus, these findings suggest that TCs other than CMT-5 may bind secondary Zn^{2+}, and to a lesser extent Ca^{2+}, in collagenase, thus altering the conformity of the enzyme molecule and blocking its catalytic activity.

TCs have been found to inhibit collagenases from a number of cell and tissue sources, including PMNs, macrophages, osteoblasts, osteoclasts, chondrocytes and tumour cells, rat skin and gingiva and human gingiva (Golub *et al.*, 1991; Rifkin *et al.*, 1993). Recent studies show that different tissues and cells vary in their susceptibility to TC collagenase inhibition, and members of the TC family vary in regard to their collagenase inhibitory activity. In respect of the first point, collagenase and other MMPs from PMNs (MMP-8, -9) are highly sensitive to TC inhibition, whilst those from fibroblasts (MMP-1, -2) are relatively resistant (Ingman *et al.*, 1993). With regard to the second point, the semi-synthetic TCs, doxycycline and minocycline and the CMTs, are more potent for this action than tetracycline itself (Rifkin *et al.*, 1993; Ryan *et al.*, 1996).

TCs and CMTs have also been found to inhibit bone resorption at concentrations within the normal therapeutic dose range of these drugs (Rifkin *et al.*, 1993). They appear to reduce the degradation of osteoid by inhibition of osteoblast collagenase and to increase bone formation by increasing alkaline phosphatase and collagen synthesis by these cells. They appear to decrease bone resorption by elevating osteoclast intracellular calcium levels, decreasing the osteoclast ruffled border, osteoclast acid production and osteoclast secretion of cysteine proteinases (cathepsins B and L) and by inhibiting osteoclast MMPs.

In animal model studies, three different models have been studied (Rifkin *et al.*, 1993). First, the effect of TCs was studied on the excessive alveolar bone loss seen in surgically desalivated rats, and it was found to reduce the bone loss in these animals compared to untreated controls with TCs. Secondly, its effect on accelerated periodontal disease in diabetic rats was studied. Severe disease was produced by inducing accelerated plaque formation, and this was then exacerbated by making the animals diabetic by the administration of streptozotocin. Daily tetracycline or CMT-1 administration decreased the excessive collagenase activity in their gingival tissue and reduced the severity of the disease. Interestingly, whilst tetracycline induced the emergence of tetracycline resistant bacteria in their oral cavities, the use of CMT-1 did not have this unwanted effect. Thirdly, their effects on gnotobiotic rats mono-infected with *Porphyromonas gingivalis* were studied (Rifkin *et al.*, 1993; Golub *et al.*, 1994). The infected animals showed marked gingival inflammation and bone loss compared with non-infected controls. Daily administration of either CMT-1 (with no antimicrobial properties) or doxycycline (with antimicrobial properties) for 8 weeks at normal therapeutic dosage resulted in significant reductions in both gingival inflammation and alveolar bone loss, and also significantly reduced gingival tissue collagenase concentration.

Finally, it has been found that CMT-1 administration can normalize the collagen metabolism in diabetic rats that otherwise exhibit severe collagen depletion in the skin and gingiva (Yu *et al.*, 1993).

In human studies, TCs given in normal therapeutic doses have been shown to reduce collagenase (in particular MMP-8) activity in gingival tissue, gingival crevicular fluid (GCF) and saliva (Golub *et al.*, 1985, 1991; Rifkin *et al.*, 1993; Sorsa *et al.*, 1994). The majority of gingival tissue extracellular collagenase and GCF collagenase activity comes from inflammatory cells rather than fibroblasts, and it is that form of MMP activity that is most susceptible to TCs. In addition, it has been found that a 3-week course of regular dose doxycycline reduced periodontal attachment loss in refractory periodontitis patients 7 months after stopping the treatment (Lee *et al.*, 1991). It has also been found that doxycycline inhibited both PMN-produced MMPs in gingival tissue and bacterial collagenase produced by *P. gingivalis* (Golub *et al.*, 1995).

The type of periodontal disease being potentially treated is important, since the type of the predominating MMP in gingival tissue, GCF and saliva varies (Ingman *et al.*, 1993). In adult chronic periodontitis the PMN-derived MMPs (MMP-8, -9) predominate, and these are highly sensitive to inhibition with TCs and CMTs. In localized juvenile periodontitis, however, the fibroblast-derived MMP-1 predominates, albeit at low levels, and this is relatively resistant to these drugs. In this regard it has been shown that MMP-8 was inhibited *in vitro* by doses of TCs of 75 μM/l, whilst MMP-1 was relatively insensitive to 100 μM/l (Ingman *et al.*, 1993; Sorsa *et al.*, 1994). MMP-1 was, however, inhibited by doses of 600 μM/l. It would therefore appear that adult chronic periodontitis is more likely to be effectively treated by the anti-collagenase effects of TCs than localized juvenile periodontitis.

Thus, it would appear that CMTs lacking antimicrobial effects, and hence the unwanted effects of inducing bacterial resistance, might have a therapeutic role in the treatment of adult chronic periodontitis in the future. Their proven abilities to both inhibit inflammatory cell MMPs and favourably modify bone metabolism would seem to be of major significance in this regard.

Possible indications for antibiotic use in periodontal treatment

It seems from current available evidence that, although systemic administration and local application of tetracycline and metronidazole can produce similar clinical and bacteriological effects to scaling and root planing, they appear to offer no significant advantages, and used on their own are generally inferior to scaling and root planing. There are also compelling reasons for avoiding antibiotics in situations where other treatments are equally effective because of the risks of developing bacterial resistance. It should also be realized that the concentration of antibiotics needed to kill or inhibit the growth of bacteria within a biofilm such as dental or subgingival plaque is 50–200 times higher than that for bacteria growing planktonically (Anwar *et al.*, 1992; Brown and Gilbert, 1993; Vorachit *et al.*, 1993; Wright *et al.*, 1997). This almost certainly means that bacteria in this situation are probably going to be resistant to the concentrations of antibiotic likely to present in the periodontal pocket following systemic administration of an antibiotic. However, the use of adjuvant antibiotic gels or fibres may be advantageous in the following few situations (Goodson, 1994):

- Deep pockets with very difficult access for scaling and root planing
- Deep pockets that fail to respond to repeated scaling and root planing
- Deep pocket sites in refractory or rapidly progressive periodontitis
- Pockets exuding pus
- Sites with acute lateral periodontal abscess (instead of systemic antibiotics).

Strategy for the use of adjuvant local antimicrobials

1. Subgingival antimicrobials should never be used alone, since mechanical disruption of the biofilm is necessary to achieve their penetration to the active sites (Anwar *et al.*, 1992, Brown and Gilbert, 1993; Vorachit *et al.*, 1993). Furthermore, even the best delivery systems with the best pharmacokinetic profiles and effecting substantial depression of subgingival microbiota are unable to completely disinfect a periodontal pocket. They should therefore only be used as adjuvant to scaling and root planing.
2. Since the changes in the bacterial flora by antimicrobials are similar in amount and duration to those produced by scaling and root planing, antimicrobials should only be used on pockets refractory to repeated use of this procedure.
3. Studies of recolonization kinetics of periodontal pockets indicate that disinfected pockets in disinfected mouths (i.e. following successful full mouth periodontal treatment) do not display significant recolonization of treated pockets (Tonetti *et al.*, 1995).

However, disinfected pockets in infected mouths demonstrate rapid rates of recolonization. These results seem to indicate that the residual oral flora is the primary source of recolonization. This implies that local delivery antimicrobial systems are most suited to the treatment of localized refractory and persistent lesions in otherwise stable mouths (Mombelli *et al.*, 1997). It also implies that regular maintenance treatment is necessary both at such sites and throughout the mouth to maintain stability. Also, with any form of periodontal therapy, a good level of oral hygiene is necessary for successful treatment (Kornman, 1993).

4. The choice of an appropriate antimicrobial to treat such localized refractory pockets is difficult, but a delivery system must be used that will maintain therapeutic levels of the agent for at least 7 days.
5. In general, the use of appropriate broad-spectrum antiseptics such as chlorhexidine should be preferred to antibiotics because they do not carry the risks of encouraging the development of a resistant flora.

Other uses of antibiotics in periodontal treatment

In the light of the studies described above, the use of antibiotics in periodontal treatment should be restricted to those cases where it will give benefits over and above those of conventional treatment. At the present time its use cannot be justified in the routine treatment of chronic periodontitis. Antibiotics should be restricted in the treatment of non-specific infections, particularly where other treatments are effective, since their prolonged use could give rise in some cases to hypersensitivity reactions, toxic reactions, the development of bacterial resistance and of superinfections with resistant organisms such as *Candida*. In spite of these restric-

tions, antibiotics could be of use in the following situations:

1. To protect against the possible effects of a transient bacteraemia in susceptible patients
2. In the treatment of acute ulcerative gingivitis
3. In the treatment of acute abscesses of periodontal origin
4. In the treatment of juvenile periodontitis

Protection against the effects of transient bacteraemia

The cardiac lesions that are known to predispose to infective endocarditis and those that do not are shown in *Table 15.3*. The patients at risk can be summarized as those with congenital or acquired cardiac defects, or those with prosthetic heart valves. Patients with mitral prolapse are only considered to be at risk when it is known to be associated with a systolic murmur.

Antibiotic prophylaxis should be given in these cases for extractions, scaling and periodontal surgery (Eley, 1983a). Transient bacteraemia may also arise from normal functional activity and tooth cleaning when gingivitis is present, and is best prevented by the maintenance of dental health and the prevention and early treatment of periodontal diseases. A good preventive programme in these patients from an early age should help to prevent dental caries and chronic periodontitis and thus obviate the need for dental extractions, subgingival scaling and other surgery requiring prophylactic antibiotics (Eley, 1983b). Good oral hygiene should also prevent gingivitis, which can lead to transient bacteraemia.

As already stated, patients who give a history of rheumatic fever should be sent to a cardiologist for cardiac investigations to see whether they have actually suffered

Table 15.3 Cardiac conditions that require/do not require antibiotic cover

Cardiac conditions requiring antibiotic cover	*Cardiac conditions not requiring antibiotic cover*
Ventricular septal defect (VSD)	Angina
Primum atrial septal defect (ASD)	Myocardial infarction
ASD repaired with prosthetic patch	Ventricular aneurysm
Post valvotomy	Innocent systolic murmur
Prolapsing mitral valve	Permanent pacemaker
Pulmonary stenosis	Ligated ductus arteriosus
Patent ductus arteriosus	ASD – unrepaired or repaired without patch
Coarctation of aorta	Coronary artery bypass graft unless within 6 months
Tetralogy of Fallot	Rheumatic fever without history and evidence of
Arteriovenous (AV) shunt	valvular disease – needs cardiac examination to confirm
Bicuspid aortic valve	
Murmurs of doubtful origin	
Rheumatic valvular stenosis or incompetence	
AV malformation or fistula	
History of infective endocarditis*	
Prosthetic valve replacement*	
Recent coronary artery bypass	
Hip prosthesis	

*High risk

from rheumatic heart disease, since many patients, when thoroughly tested, are found not to have rheumatic heart disease and therefore do not need prophylactic antibiotic cover. Apparently healthy patients reporting cardiac murmurs should also be examined by a cardiologist if the exact status is not already known and available from their general medical practitioner.

The role of antibiotic prophylaxis in patients with prosthetic joints who require dental treatment is controversial (Sandhu *et al.*, 1997). A Working Party of the British Society of Antimicrobial Chemotherapy (1992) recently suggested that there was no evidence to support the use of antibiotic prophylaxis in these patients. However, it has also been suggested that not all patients with prosthetic joints present a similar risk, and that certain patients may require cover (Tyne and Ferguson, 1991; Field and Martin, 1991; Mason *et al.*, 1992). These patients include those with rheumatoid arthritis, diabetes mellitus and immunosuppression, those on steroids and those with re-operated hips. Furthermore, a study (Jaspers and Little, 1985) indicated that over 90% of orthopaedic surgeons in the USA recommended the use of antibiotic cover for patients with prosthetic joints undergoing dental treatment.

This poses the question of who is in the best position to assess the need in these cases. Another recent study examined how closely the recommendations of the British Society for Antimicrobial Chemotherapy (BSAC) were being followed by British maxillofacial and orthopaedic surgeons, and the differences between these groups in the management of these patients (Sandhu *et al.*, 1997). This showed that 77.7% of the orthopaedic surgeons recommended the use of antibiotic cover for dental treatment, whilst only 29% of maxillofacial surgeons did so. There were were also differences in the antibiotic of choice between these groups. Most of the maxillofacial surgeons recommended the regimens described below, whilst the majority of orthopaedic surgeons recommended the use of cephalosporin, in spite of the fact that this is not the most efficacious antibiotic against oral streptococci, which are the the most likely infecting bacteria in these cases.

Thus this matter is far from resolved. It would seem appropriate for dental surgeons to follow the guidelines of the BSAC in not giving cover in most cases. In the case of the special risk groups described above, they should consult with the patient's orthopaedic surgeon. However, they should make sure that, if cover is recommended, the appropriate regimen is given.

Antibiotic prophylaxis for routine treatment, i.e. extractions, scaling or periodontal surgery under local anaesthesia, is usually 3 g amoxycillin orally 60 minutes before the procedure. Patients who are allergic to penicillin are usually given erythromycin stearate 2 g orally 2 hours before the procedure, followed by 500 mg orally 6 hours later. These orally administered regimens are obviously more convenient for dental practice. High-risk cases, such as patients with a history of previous infective endocarditis or with prosthetic heart valves, should be treated in hospital and should be given either amoxycillin (1 g i.m.) plus gentamicin (120 mg i.m.) or vancomycin (1 g i.v.) followed by gentamicin (120 mg i.v.). In addition, a chlorhexidine mouthwash should be given 5 minutes prior to treatment in all cases. As much treatment as possible should be given under the same antibiotic cover, and at least 6 weeks should elapse before antibiotic administration is repeated. A full plan of possible regimens is shown in *Figure 15.15*.

There are alternative regimens for some categories of cover when the patient is unable to take a drug in the regimen because of allergy or intolerance, or because it has been prescribed for any reason during the preceding period. These alternatives are shown in *Figure 15.16*.

Prescribing for children

Doses for children are usually based on body weight in kilograms or in age ranges, e.g. first month (neonate), up to a year (infant), 1–5 years, 6–12 years. The percentage method of drug doses using *Table 15.4* may be conveniently used to calculate children's doses, with a wide margin between the therapeutic and toxic dose.

Treatment of acute abscesses of periodontal origin

The treatment of an acute lateral abscess may include the use of an antibiotic (Chapter 19). These infections are usually sensitive to penicillin, and can be controlled with oral penicillin V 250 mg four times daily for 5 days. If the patient is allergic to penicillin, oral erythromycin stearate can be used in the same dosage. If an anaerobic infection is suspected, then metronidazole 200 mg three times per day for 5 days could be prescribed. This is contraindicated in patients who cannot be relied upon to refrain from alcohol, and during pregnancy. Local treatment with a slow release gel could be considered instead of systemic administration if the infection is completely localized. Minocycline (2%), metronidazole gel (25%) or Actisite tetracycline fibre could be used.

Drainage of any pus present and local atraumatic subgingival scaling with an ultrasonic scaler should be carried out when the patient is first seen (see Chapter 19).

Treatment of acute ulcerative gingivitis

Acute ulcerative gingivitis (Chapter 22) is an endogenous fusospirochaetal infection, and may be treated with penicillin or metronidazole. Metronidazole 200 mg three times per day for 3–4 days is the preferred regimen. This is fully described in Chapter 22.

Treatment of juvenile periodontitis

Juvenile periodontitis (Chapter 20) is associated with capnophilic, facultatively aerobic subgingival flora, and is best treated with either metronidazole 250 mg and amoxycillin 375 mg three times daily for 7 days (Van Winkelhoff *et al.*, 1989), or tetracycline 250 mg four

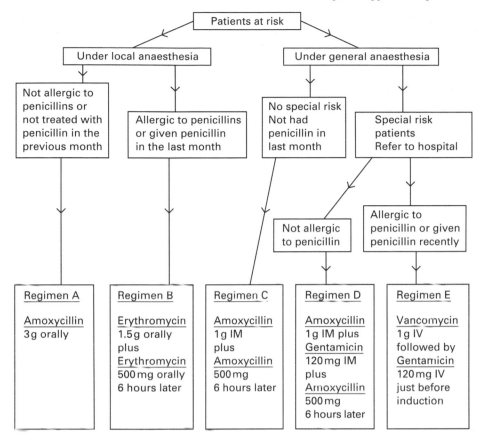

Special risk patients are those who:

a) need a general anaesthetic
b) have a prosthetic heart valve
c) have received penicillin more than once in the last month
d) are allergic to penicillin
e) have previously had endocarditis

Figure 15.15 Regimens for patients at risk from transient bacteraemia

1) For adults requiring regimen B

    Clindamycin orally 500 mg, 1 hour before procedure

2) For adults requiring regimen C

    either a) Amoxycillin 3g orally, 4 hours before anaesthesia plus a further 3g
          orally as soon as possible after the anaesthetic
    or b) Amoxycillin 3g plus probenecid orally, 4 hours before anaesthetic

Figure 15.16 Alternative regimens for patients at risk from transient bacteraemia

Table 15.4 The percentage of the adult dose used when prescribing for children

Age	Ideal body weight kg	lb	Height mm	in	Body surface area m^2	Percentage of adult dose
Newborn	3.4	7.5	500	20	0.23	12.5
1 month	4.2	9	550	22	0.26	14.5
3 months	5.6	12	590	23	0.32	18
6 months	7.7	17	670	26	0.40	22
1 year	10	22	760	30	0.47	25
3 years	14	31	940	37	0.62	33
5 years	18	40	1080	42	0.73	40
7 years	23	51	1200	47	0.88	50
12 years	37	81	1480	58	1.25	75
Adult						
Male	68	150	1727	68	1.80	100
Female	56	123	1626	64	1.60	100

times daily for 14 days (Slots and Rosling, 1983) before or during periodontal treatment. Ideally, antibiotic sensitivity of the bacteria, in particular *Actinobacillus actinomycetemcomitans*, should be determined in a microbiology laboratory.

The local application of 2% minocycline gel to the affected pockets could be considered. However, in this regard it should be noted that the results may not be as effective (Mandell *et al.*, 1986). This could possibly be related to the local invasive properties of *A. actinomycetemcomitans* resulting in local colonization of the periodontal tissues (Christersson *et al.*, 1987). Bacteria in the tissues may not be reached by local antibiotic in the pocket.

References

Addy, M. (1986) Chlorhexidine compared with other locally delivered antimicrobials. *Journal of Clinical Periodontology* 13, 957–964

Addy, M. and Wade W. (1995) An approach to efficacy screening of mouthrinses: studies on a group of French products. I. Staining and antimicrobial properties *in vitro. Journal of Clinical Periodontology* 22, 717–722

Addy, M., Griffiths, C., and Isaac, R. (1977) The effect of povidone iodine on plaque and salivary bacteria – a double-blind cross-over trial. *Journal of Periodontology* 48, 730–732

Addy, M., Rawle, L., Handley, R. *et al.* (1982) The development and *in vitro* evaluation of acrylic strips and dialysis tubing for local drug delivery. *Journal of Periodontology* 53, 693–699

Addy, M., Jenkins, S. and Newcombe, R. (1989) Studies of the effect of toothpaste rinses on plaque regrowth. (1) Influence of surfactants on chlorhexidine efficiency. *Journal of Clinical Periodontology* 16, 380–384

Addy, M., Moran, J., Newcombe, R .and Warren, P. (1995) The comparative tea staining of phenolic, chlorhexidine .and anti-adhesive mouthrinses. *Journal of Clinical Periodontology* 22, 923–928

Adriaens, P., De Boever, J. and Loesche, W. (1988) Bacterial invasion in root cementum and radicular dentin of periodontally diseased teeth in humans. *Journal of Periodontology* 59, 222–230

Ainamo, J., Lie, T., Ellingsen, B.H. *et al.* (1992) Clinical responses to subgingival application of metronidazole 25% gel compared to the effect of subgingival scaling in adult periodontitis. *Journal of Clinical Periodontology* 19, 723–729

Amábile-Cuevas, C.F., Cárdanas-Garcia, M. and Ludgar, M (1995). Antibiotic resistance. *American Scientist* 83, 320–329

Anwar, H., Strap, J. and Costerton, J. (1992) Establishment of ageing biofilms: possible mechanism of bacterial resistance to antimicrobial therapy. *Antimicrobial Agents and Chemotherapy* 36, 1347–1351

Ashby, M., Neale, J., Knott, S and Critchley, I. (1994) Effect of antibiotics on non-growing planktonic cells and biofilms of *Escherichia coli. Journal of Antimicrobial Chemotherapy* 33, 443–453

Attström, R., Matsson, L., Edwardsson, S. *et al.* (1983) The effect of octapinol on dentogingival plaque and development of gingivitis. III. Short-term studies in humans. *Journal of Periodontal Research* 14, 445–451

Ayad, F. and Berta, R. (1995) Effects on plaque and gingivitis of a triclosan/co-polymer pre-brush rinse: a 6-month study in Canada. *Journal of Canadian Dental Association* 61, 53–56

Baker, P.J., Evans, R.T., Coburn, R.A. and Genco, R.J. (1983) Tetracycline and its derivatives strongly bind to and are released from the tooth surface in an active form. *Journal of Periodontology* 54, 580–585

Banatavala, N., Davies, G.R., Abdi, Y. *et al.* (1994) High prevalence of *Helicobacter pylori* metronidazole resistance in migrants to east London: relation with previous nitroimidazole exposure and gastroduodenal disease. *Gut* 35, 1562–1566

Barkvoll, P and Rölla, G. (1994) Triclosan protects the skin against dermatitis caused by sodium lauryl sulphate exposure. *Journal of Clinical Periodontology* 21, 717–719

Barkvoll, P and Rölla, G. (1995) Triclosan reduces the clinical symptoms of the allergic patch reaction (APR) elicited with 1% nickel sulphate in sensitized patients. *Journal of Clinical Periodontology* 22, 485–487

Benet, L., Kroetz, D.L.J. and Sheiner, L. (1996) Pharmacokinetics: the dynamics of drug absorption, distribution and elimination. In *Goodman and Gilman's Pharmacological Basis of Therapy*, 9th Edn (A. Goodman-Gilman, J.G. Hardman, L.E. Limbird, *et al.*, eds), pp. 3–27. New York: McGraw-Hill

Bergenholz, A. and Hanstrom, L. (1974) The plaque inhibiting effect of hexidine (Oraldene®) mouthwash compared to that of chlorhexidine. *Community Dentistry and Oral Epidemiology* 2, 70–74

Binder, T., Goodson, J. and Socransky, S. (1987) Gingival fluid levels of acid and alkaline phosphatase. *Journal of Periodontal Research* 22, 14–19

Binney, A., Addy, M., McKeown, S. and Everatt, L. (1995) The effect of a commercially available triclosan-containing toothpaste compared to a sodium fluoride-containing toothpaste and a chlorhexidine rinse on 4-day plaque regrowth. *Journal of Clinical Periodontology* 22, 830–834

Binney, A., Addy, M., McKeown, S. and Everatt, L. (1996) The choice of controls in toothpaste studies. The effect of a number of commercially available toothpastes compared to water on 4-day plaque regrowth. *Journal of Clinical Periodontology* 23, 456–459

Bonesvoll, P., Lökken, P. and Rölla, G. (1974) Influence of concentration, time, temperature and pH on the retention of chlorhexidine in the human oral cavity after mouth rinses. *Archives of Oral Biology* 19, 1025–1029

Bonesvoll, P. and Gjermo, P. (1978) A comparison between chlorhexidine and some quaternary ammonium compounds with regard to retention, salivary concentration and plaque inhibitory effect in the human mouth after mouthrinses. *Archives of Oral Biology* 23, 289–294

Brecx, M., Theilade, J., Attström, R. and Glantz, P.-O. (1987) The effect of chlorhexidine and octapinol on early dental plaque formation. A light and electron microscopic study. *Journal of Periodontal Research* 22, 290–295

Brown, M. and Gilbert, P. (1993) Sensitivity of biofilms to antimicrobial agents. *Journal of Applied Bacteriology* 74 (Suppl.), 87–97

Budtz-Jorgensen, J. and Löe, H. (1972) Chlorhexidine as a denture disinfectant in the treatment of denture stomatitis. *Scandinavian Journal of Dental Research* 80, 457–464

Chadwick, B., Addy, M. and Walker, D.M. (1991) Hexidine mouthwash in the management of minor appthous ulceration and as an adjunct to oral hygiene. *British Dental Journal* 171, 83–87

Chambers, H.F. and Sande, M.A. (1996a) General considerations. In *Goodman and Gilman's The Pharmacological Basis of Therapeutics*, 9th Edn (A. Goodman-Gilman, J.G. Hardman, L.E. Limbird *et al.*, eds), pp. 1057–1072. New York: McGraw-Hill

Chambers, H.F. and Sande, M.A. (1996b) Antimicrobial agents – the aminoglycosides. In *Goodman and Gilman's The Pharmacological Basis of Therapeutics*, 9th Edn (A. Goodman-Gilman, J.G. Hardman, L.E. Limbird *et al.*, eds), pp. 1103–1123. New York: McGraw-Hill

Christersson, L.A., Albini, B., Zambon, J.J. *et al.* (1987) Tissue localization of *Actinobacillus actinomycetemcomitans* in human periodontitis. I. Light, immunofluorescence and electron microscopic studies. *Journal of Periodontology* 58, 529–539

Christersson, L.A., Norderyd, O.M. and Puchalasky, C.S. (1993) Topical application of tetracycline-HCl in human periodontitis. *Journal of Clinical Periodontology* **20**, 88–95

Ciancio, S.G. (1986) Chemotherapeutic agents and periodontal therapy. Their impact on clinical practice. *Journal of Periodontology* **57**, 108–111

Ciancio, S.G., Cobb, C.M and Leung, M. (1992) Tissue concentration and localization of tetracycline following site-specific therapy. *Journal of Periodontology* **63**, 849–853

Claydon, N., Hunter, L., Moran, J. *et al.* (1996) A 6-month home usage of 0.1% and 0.2% delmopinol mouthwashes. I. Effect on plaque, gingivitis, supragingival calculus and tooth staining. *Journal of Clinical Periodontology* **23**, 220–228

Coburn, R.A. Batista, A.J., Evans, R.T. and Genco, R.J. (1981) Potential salicylamide antiplaque agents. *In vitro* antibacterial activity against *Actinomyces viscosus. Journal of Medical Chemistry* **24**, 1245–1249

Collaert, B., Attström, R., DeBrune, N. and Movert, R. (1992) The effect of delmopinol rinsing on dental plaque formation and gingivitis healing. *Journal of Clinical Periodontology* **19**, 274–280

Corsair, A. (1994) Long-term effect of tetracycline fibres on recurrent lesions in periodontal maintenance patients. *Periodontal Clinical Investigations* (North Eastern Society of Periodontists) **16**, 8–13

Council on Therapeutics, American Dental Association (1986) Guidelines for acceptance of chemotherapeutic products for the control of plaque and gingivitis. *Journal of the American Dental Association* **112**, 529–532

Cubells, A.B., Dalmau, L.B., Petrone, M.E. *et al.* (1991) The effect of a triclosan/co-polymer/fluoride dentifrice on plaque formation and gingivitis: a 6-month clinical study. *Journal of Clinical Dentistry* **2**, 63–69

Cummins, D. (1992) Mechanisms of actions of clinically proven antiplaque agents. In *Clinical and Biological Aspects of Dentifrices* (G. Embery and G. Rölla, eds), pp. 205–228. Oxford: Oxford University Press

Davies, J. (1990) What are antibiotics? Archaic functions for modern activities. *Molecular Microbiology* **4**, 1227–1232

Davies, G., Francis, J. Martin, A. *et al.* (1954) 1 : 6Di-4′-chlorophenyl-diguanidohexane. Laboratory investigation into a new antibacterial agent of high potency. *British Journal of Pharmacology* **9**, 192–196

Deasy, M.J., Battista, G., Rustogi, K.N. and Volpe, A.R. (1991) Antiplaque efficacy of a triclosan/co-polymer prebrush rinse: a plaque prevention clinical study. *American Journal of Dentistry* **5**, 91–94

Deasy, M.J., Singh, S.M., Rustogi, K.N. *et al.* (1992) Effect of a dentifrice containing triclosan and a co-polymer on plaque formation and gingivitis. *Clinical Preventive Dentistry* **13**, 12–19

De Paula, L.G., Overholser, C.D., Meiller, T.F. *et al.* (1989) Chemotherapeutic inhibition of supragingival dental plaque and gingivitis development. *Journal of Clinical Periodontology* **16**, 311–315

Drisko, C.H. (1998) The use of locally delivered doxycycline in the treatment of periodontitis. Clinical results. *Journal of Clinical Periodontology* **25**, 947–952

Dzink, J.J. and Socransky, S.S. (1985) Comparative *in vitro* activity of sanguinarine against microbial isolates. *Antimicrobial Agents and Chemotherapy* **27**, 663–665

Edwards, D.I. (1993) Nitroimidazole drugs – action and resistance mechanisms. II. Mechanisms of resistance. *Journal of Antimicrobial Chemotherapy* **31**, 201–210

Eisenberg, A.D., Young, D.A., Fan-Hse, J. and Spitz, L.M. (1991) Interactions of sanguinarine and zinc on oral streptococci and *Actinomyces* species. *Caries Research* **25**, 185–190

Eley, B.M. (1983a) Infective endocarditis: a dentist's view. 1. Actiology and dental treatment. *Cardiology in Practice* **1(7)**, 35–38

Eley, B.M. (1983b) Infective endocarditis: a dentist's view. 2. Prevention. *Cardiology in Practice* **1(8)**, 16–19

Elworthy, A.J., Edgar, R., Moran, J. *et al.* (1995) A 6-month home usage of 0.1% and 0.2% delmopinol mouthwashes. II. Effects on plaque microflora. *Journal of Clinical Periodontology* **22**, 527–532

Emilson, C. (1977) Susceptibility of various micro-organisms to chlorhexidine. *Scandinavian Journal of Dental Research* **85**, 255–265

Evans, D., Allison, D., Brown, M. and Gilbert, P. (1990) Effect of growth rate on resistance of Gram negative biofilms to citrimide. *Journal of Antimicrobial Chemotherapy* **26**, 473–478

Farmer, T. and Reading, C. (1982) Beta-lactamases of *Brauhamella catarrhalis* and their inhibition by clavulanic acid. *Antimicrobial Agents and Chemotherapy* **21**, 506–508

Faulkes, E. (1993) Some toxicological observations of chlorhexidine. *Journal of Periodontal Research* **12** (Suppl.), 131–148

Fergerson, M.M., Geddes, D.A.M. and Wray, D. (1978) The effect of povidone iodine mouthwash on thyroid function and plaque accumulation. *British Dental Journal* **148**, 14–16

Fiehn, N.-E. and Westergaard, J. (1990) Doxycycline-resistant bacteria in periodontally diseased individuals after systemic doxycycline therapy and in healthy individuals. *Oral Microbiology and Immunology* **5**, 219–222

Field, E.A. and Martin, M.V. (1991) Prophylactic antibiotics for patients with artificial joints undergoing oral and dental surgery: necessary or not? *British Journal of Maxillofacial Surgery* **29**, 341–346

Finegold, S.M. (1989) Classification and taxonomy of anaerobes. In *Anaerobic Infections in Humans* (S.M. Finegold and W.L. George, eds), pp. 23–26. San Diego: Academic Press

Firatli, E., Unal, T., Onan, U. and Sandalli, P. (1994) Antioxidative activities of some chemotherapeutics: a possible mechanism of reducing inflammation. *Journal of Clinical Periodontology* **21**, 680–683

Fletcher, J.M. and Wilson, M. (1993) The effectiveness of a redox agent, methylene blue, on the survival of *Porphyromonas gingivalis in vitro*. *Current Microbiology* **26**, 85–90

Flotra, L. (1973) Different modes of chlorhexidine application and related side effects. *Journal of Periodontal Research* **12** (Suppl.), 41–44

Flotra, L., Gjermo, P., Rölla, G. and Waerhaug, J. (1972) A 4-month study of the effect of chlorhexidine mouthrinses on 50 soldiers. *Scandinavian Journal of Dental Research* **80**, 10–17

Fornell, J., Sundin, Y. and Lindhe, J. (1975) Effect of listerine on dental plaque and gingivitis. *Scandinavian Journal of Dental Research* **83**, 18–25

Friedman, M.A. and Golomb, G. (1982) New sustained dosage form of chlorhexidine for dental use. I. Development and kinetics of release. *Journal of Periodontal Research* **17**, 323–328

Furuichi, Y., Ramberg, P., Lindhe, J. *et al.* (1996) Some effects of mouthrinses containing salifluor on *de novo* plaque formation and developing gingivitis. *Journal of Clinical Periodontology* **23**, 795–802

Gaffar, A., Scherl, D., Affitto, J. and Colman, E.J. (1995) The effect of triclosan on the mediators of gingival inflammation. *Journal of Clinical Periodontology* **22**, 480–484

Garcia-Rodriguez, J.A., Garcia-Sanchez, J.E. and Munoz-Bellido, J.L. (1995) Antimicrobial resistance in anaerobic bacteria: current situation. *Anaerobe* **1**, 69–80

Genco, R.J. (1994) Pharmaceuticals and periodontal diseases. *Journal of the American Dental Association* **125**, 11S–19S

Gibson, M.T., Mangat, D., Gagliano, G. *et al.* (1994) Evaluation of the efficiency of a redox agent in the treatment of chronic periodontitis. *Journal of Clinical Periodontology* **21**, 690–700

Giersten, E., Svatun, B. and Saxton, A. (1987) Plaque inhibition by hexidine and zinc. *Scandinavian Journal of Dental Research* **95**, 49–54

Gjermo, P., Bonesvoll, P. and Rölla, G. (1974) Relationship between plaque inhibiting effect and the retention of chlorhexidine in the oral cavity. *Archives of Oral Biology* **19**, 1031–1034

Golub, L.M., Lee, H.M., Lehrer, G. *et al.* (1983) Minocycline reduces gingival collagenolytic activity during diabetes: preliminary observations and a proposed new mechanism. *Journal of Periodontal Research* **21**, 516–526

Golub, L.M., Ramamurthy, N.S., McNamara, T.F. *et al.* (1984) Tetracyclines inhibit tissue collagenase activity: a new mechanism in the treatment of periodontal disease. *Journal of Periodontal Research* **19**, 651–655

Golub, L.M., Wolff, M., Lee, H.M., *et al.* (1985) Further evidence that tetracyclines inhibit collagenase activity in human crevicular fluid and from other mammalian sources. *Journal of Periodontal Research* **20**, 12–23

Golub, L.M., McNamara, T.F., D'Angelo, G. *et al.* (1987) A non-antimicrobial chemically-modified tetracycline inhibits mammalian collagenase activity. *Journal of Dental Research* **66**, 1310–1314

Golub, L.M., Ramamurthy, N.S. and McNamara, T.F. (1991) Tetracyclines inhibit connective tissue breakdown: new therapeutic implications for an old family of drugs. *Critical Reviews in Oral Biology and Medicine* **2**, 297–322

Golub, L.M., Suomalainen, K and Sorsa, T. (1992) Host modulation with tetracyclines and their chemically modified analogues. Current science. *Current Opinions in Dentistry* **2**, 80–90

Golub, L.M., Evans, R.T., McNamara, T.F. *et al.* (1994) A non-antimicrobial tetracycline inhibits gingival matrix metalloproteinases and bone loss in *Porphyromonas gingivalis*-induced periodontitis in rats. *Annals of the New York Academy of Sciences* **732**, 96–111

Golub, L.M., Sorsa, T., Lee, H.-M. *et al.* (1995) Doxycycline inhibits neutrophil (PMN)-type matrix metalloproteinases in adult periodontitis gingiva. *Journal of Clinical Periodontology* **22**, 100–109

Gomer, R.M., Hobroyd, S.V., Fedi, P.F. and Ferrign, P.D. (1972) The effects of oral rinses on the accumulation of dental plaque. *Journal of American Society of Preventive Dentistry* **2**, 12–14

Goodson, J.M. (1989) Pharmacokinetics principles controlling efficacy of oral therapy. *Journal of Dental Research* **68**, 1625–1632

Goodson, J.M. (1994) Antimicrobial strategies or treatment of periodontal disease. *Periodontology 2000* **5**, 142–168

Goodson, J.M. and Tanner, A. (1992) Antibiotic resistance of the subgingival microflora following local tetracycline therapy. *Oral Microbiology and Immunology* **7**, 113–117

Goodson, J.M., Haffajee, A.D. and Socransky, S.S. (1979) Periodontal therapy by local delivery of tetracycline. *Journal of Clinical Periodontology* **6**, 83–92

Goodson, J.M., Holborow, D., Dunn, R. *et al.* (1983) Monolithic tetracycline containing fibres for control delivery to periodontal pockets. *Journal of Periodontology* **54**, 575–579

Goodson, J.M., Hogan, P.E. and Dunham, S.L. (1985) Clinical responses following periodontal treatment by local drug delivery. *Journal of Periodontology* **56**, 81–87

Goodson, J.M., Ugini, M.A., Kent, R.L. *et al.* (1991a) Multicenter evaluation of tetracycline fibre therapy. I. Experimental design, methods and baseline data. *Journal of Periodontal Research* **26**, 361–370

Goodson, J.M., Ugini, M.A., Kent, R.L. *et al.* (1991b) Multicenter evaluation of tetracycline fibre therapy. II. Clinical response. *Journal of Periodontal Research* **26**, 371–379

Goodson, J.M., Tanner, A., McArdle, S. *et al.* (1991c) Multicenter evaluation of tetracycline fibre therapy. III. Microbiological response. *Journal of Periodontal Research* **26**, 440–451

Goodwin, C.S., Marshall, B.J., Blincow, E.D., Wilson, D.H., Blackbourn, S. and Phillips, M. (1988) Prevention of nitroimidazole resistance in *Campylobacter pylori* by coadministration of colloidal bismuth subcitrate: clinical and *in vitro* studies. Journal of Clinical Pathology 41, 207–210.

Gordon, J.M., Walker, C.B., Murphy, J.C. *et al.* (1981) Tetracycline levels achievable in gingival crevice fluid and *in vitro* effect on subgingival organisms. Part 1. Concentrations in crevicular fluid after repeated doses. *Journal of Periodontology* **52**, 609–612

Gordon, J.M., Lamster, I.B. and Sieger, M.C. (1985) Efficacy of Listerine® antiseptic in inhibiting the development of plaque and gingivitis. *Journal of Clinical Periodontology* **12**, 697–704

Grenby, T.H. (1995) The use of sanguinarine mouthwashes and toothpastes compared with some other antimicrobial agents. *British Dental Journal* **178**, 254–258

Grenier, D. (1996) Effect of chlorhexidine on the adherence properties of *Porphyromonas gingivalis*. *Journal of Clinical Periodontology* **23**, 140–142

Grossman, E., Meckel, A.H., Issacs, R.L. *et al.* (1989) A clinical comparison of antimicrobial mouthrinses: effects of chlorhexidine, phenolics and sanguinarine on dental plaque and gingivitis. *Journal of Periodontology* **60**, 435–440

Haas, C.E., Nix, D.E. and Schentag, J.J. (1990) *In vitro* selection of resistant *Helicobacter pylori*. *Antimicrobial Agents and Chemotherapy* **34**, 1637–1641

Halse, J.C., Ainamo, J., Etemadzadeh, H. and Øttström, M. (1995) Plaque formation and gingivitis after mouthrinsing with 0.2% delmopinol hydrochloride, 0.2% chlorhexidine digluconate and placebo for 4 weeks following initial professional tooth cleaning. *Journal of Clinical Periodontology* **22**, 533–539

Halse, J.C., Øttström, R., Edwardsson, S. *et al.* (1998a) Six-month use of 0.2% delmopinol hydrochloride in comparison with 0.2% chlorhexidine digluconate and placebo. I. Effect on plaque formation and gingivitis. *Journal of Clinical Periodontology* **25**, 746–753

Halse, J.C., Edwardsson, S., Rundegren, J. *et al.* (1998b) Six-month use of 0.2% delmopinol hydrochloride in comparison with 0.2% chlorhexidine digluconate and placebo. II. Effect on plaque and salivary microflora. *Journal of Clinical Periodontology* **25**, 841–849

Hannah, J.J., Johnson, J.D. and Kuftinee, M.M. (1989) Long-term evaluation of toothpaste and oral rinse containing sanguinaria extract in controlling plaque and gingival inflammation and sulcular bleeding during orthodontic treatment. *American Journal of Orthodontics and Maxillofacial Orthopedics* **96**, 199–207

Hansberger, H. (1992) Pharmacodynamic effects of antibiotics. Studies on bacterial morphology, initial killing, post-antibiotic effect and effective regrowth time. *Scandinavian Journal of Infectious Disease* **81** (Suppl.), 1–52

Harper, P.R., Milsom, S., Wade, W. *et al.* (1995) An approach to efficacy screening of mouthrinses: studies on a group of French products. I. Inhibition of salivary bacteria and plaque *in vivo*. *Journal of Clinical Periodontology* **22**, 723–727

Hawley, R.J., Lee, L.N. and LeBlanc, D.J. (1980) Effects of tetracycline on the streptococcal flora of periodontal pockets. *Antimicrobial Agents and Chemotherapy* **17**, 372–378

Heasman, P.A., Soskolne, A., Smart, G. and Newman, H.N. (1995) Subgingival administration of Perio Chips® in patients with chronic periodontitis. *Journal of Dental Research* **74** Abstr. 644, 481

Heijl, L., Dahlen, G., Sundin, Y. *et al.* (1991) A four-quadrant comparative study of periodontal treatment using tetracycline-containing drug delivery fibres and scaling. *Journal of Clinical Periodontology* **18**, 111–116

Heimdahl, A. and Nord, C.E. (1983) Influence of doxycycline on the normal oral flora and colonization of the oral cavity and colon. *Scandinavian Journal of Infectious Diseases* **15**, 293–302

Hennessy, T. (1973) Some antibacterial properties of chlorhexidine. *Journal of Periodontal Research* **8** (Suppl.), 61–67

Hennessy, T. (1977) Antibacterial properties of Hibitane®. *Journal of Clinical Periodontology* **4**, 36–48

Higashi, K., Morisaki, K., Hayashi, S. *et al.* (1990) Local ofloxacin delivery using a controlled-release insert (PT-01) in the human periodontal pocket. *Journal of Periodontal Research* **25**, 1–5

Hirschl, A.M., Hentschel, E., Schütze, K. *et al.* (1988) The efficiency of antimicrobial treatment of *Campylobacter pylori*-associated gastritis and duodenal ulcers. *Scandinavian Journal of Gastroenterology* **23**, 76–81

Hitzig, C., Fosse, T., Charbit, Y. *et al.* (1997) Effects of combined topical metronidazole and mechanical treatment on the subgingival flora of deep periodontal pockets in cuspids and bicuspids. *Journal of Periodontology* **68**, 613–617

Holbeche, J.D., Ruljancich, M.K. and Reade, P. (1975) A clinical trial of cetylpyridinium chloride mouthwash. *Australian Dental Journal* **20**, 397–404

Holmes, R.K. and Joblin, M.C. (1991) Genetics In Medical Microbiology, 3rd Edn. (S. Baron ed.) Chap 5, pp 91–122. New York: Churchill Livingstone

Hull, P. (1980) Chemical inhibition of plaque. *Journal of Clinical Periodontology* **7**, 431–442

Ingman, T., Sorsa, T., Konttinen, Y.T. *et al.* (1993) Salivary collagenase, elastase- and trypsin-like proteases as biochemical markers of periodontal tissue destruction in adult and localized juvenile periodontitis. *Oral Microbiology and Immunology* **8**, 298–305

Ingram, G.S., Horay, C.P. and Stead, W.J. (1992) Interaction of zinc with dental mineral. *Caries Research* **26**, 248–253

Jaspers, M.T. and Little, J.W. (1985) Prophylactic antibiotic coverage in patients with total arthroplasty: current practice. *Journal of American Dental Association* **111**, 943–948

Jenkins, S., Addy, M. and Newcombe, R. (1989a) Toothpastes containing 0.3% and 0.5% triclosan. I. Effects on 4-day plaque regrowth. *American Journal of Dentistry* **2**, 211–214

Jenkins, S., Addy, M. and Newcombe, R. (1989b) Studies of the effect of toothpaste rinses on plaque regrowth. II. Triclosan with and without zinc citrate formulations. *Journal of Clinical Periodontology* **16**, 385–387

Jenkins, S., Addy, M. and Newcombe, R. (1991) Triclosan and sodium lauryl sulphate mouthrinses. II. Effects on 4-day plaque regrowth. *Journal of Clinical Periodontology* **18**, 145–148

Jenkins, S., Addy, M. and Newcombe, R. (1993a) Evaluation of a mouthrinse containing chlorhexidine and fluoride as an adjunct to oral hygiene. *Journal of Clinical Periodontology* **20**, 20–25

Jenkins, S., Addy, M. and Newcombe, R. (1993b) The effects of a chlorhexidine toothpaste on the development of plaque, gingivitis and tooth staining. *Journal of Clinical Periodontology* **20**, 59–62

Jenkins, S., Addy, M. and Newcombe, R. (1994) A comparison of cetylpyridinium chloride, triclosan and chlorhexidine mouthrinse formulations for the effect on plaque regrowth. *Journal of Clinical Periodontology* **21**, 441–444

Joyston-Bechal, S., Smales, F.C. and Duckworth, R. (1984) Effect of metronidazole on chronic periodontal disease in subjects using a topically applied chlorhexidine gel. *Journal of Clinical Periodontology* **11**, 53–62

Joyston-Bechal, S., Smales, F.C. and Duckworth, R. (1986) A follow-up study 3 years after metronidazole therapy for chronic periodontal disease. *Journal of Clinical Periodontology* **13**, 944–949

Joyston-Bechal, S. and Hernaman, N. (1993) The effect of a mouthrinse containing chlorhexidine and fluoride on plaque and gingival bleeding. *Journal of Clinical Periodontology* **20**, 49–53

Kenney, E.B. and Ash, M. (1969) Oxidation-reduction potential of developing plaque, periodontal pocketing and gingival sulci. *Journal of Periodontology* **40**, 630–633

Killoy, W.J. (1998) The use of locally-delivered chlorhexidine in the treatment of periodontitis. Clinical results. *Journal of Clinical Periodontology* **25**, 953–958

Kjaerheim, V., Waaler, S.M. and Rölla, G. (1994a) Organic solvents and oils as vehicles for triclosan mouthrinses: a clinical study. *Scandinavian Journal of Dental Research* **102**, 306–308

Kjaerheim, V., Waaler, S.M. and Rölla, G. (1994b) Significance of choice of solvents for the clinical effect of triclosan-containing mouthrinses. *Scandinavian Journal of Dental Research* **102**, 202–205

Kjaerheim, V., Skaare, A., Barkvoll, P., and Rölla, G. (1996) Anti-plaque, antibacterial and anti-inflammatory properties of triclosan mouthrinses in combination with zinc citrate or polyvinylmethylether maleic acid (PVA-MA) co-polymer. *European Journal of Oral Science* **104**, 529–534

Klinge, B., Kuvatanasuhati, J., Attström, R. *et al.* (1992a) The effect of topical metronidazole therapy on experimentally-induced periodontitis in the beagle dog. *Journal of Clinical Periodontology* **19**, 702–707

Klinge, B., Attström, R., Karring, T. *et al.* (1992b) Three regimes of topical metronidazole therapy compared with subgingival scaling on periodontal pathology in adults. *Journal of Clinical Periodontology* **19**, 708–714

Kopczyk, R.A., Abrams, H., Brown, A.T. *et al.* (1991) Clinical and microscopical effects of sanguinaria-containing mouthrinse and dentifrice with and without fluoride during 6 months of use. *Journal of Periodontology* **62**, 617–622

Kornman, K. S. (1993) Controlled-release local delivery antimicrobials in periodontics: prospects for the future. *Journal of Periodontology* **64**, 782–791

Kornman, K. S. and Karl, E.H. (1982) The effect of long-term, low-dose tetracycline therapy on the subgingival microflora in refractory adult periodontitis. *Journal of Periodontology* **53**, 604–610

Lamster, I.B., Alfano, M.C., Sieger, M.C. and Gordon, J.M. (1983) The effect of Listerine® antiseptic on reduction of existing plaque and gingivitis. *Clinical Preventive Dentistry* **5**, 12–15

Larson, T. (1991) Occurrence of doxycycline-resistant bacteria in the oral cavity after local administration of doxycycline in patients with periodontal disease. *Scandinavian Journal of Infectious Diseases* **23**, 89–95

Larson, T. and Fiehn, N.-E. (1997) Development of resistance to metronidazole and minocycline *in vitro*. *Journal of Clinical Periodontology* **24**, 254–259

Laurence, D.E., Bennett, D.N. and Brown, M.J. (1997) Infection and inflammation. In *Clinical Pharmacology*, 8th Edn, pp. 187–248

Lee, W., Aitken, S., Kulkarni, G. *et al.* (1991) Collagenase activity in recurrent periodontitis: relationship to disease progression and doxycycline therapy. *Journal of Periodontal Research* **26**, 479–485

Lerner, E., Barak, M., Landau, I. Palmer, K., Kolatch, B. and Soskolne A. (1996) Chlorhexidine release profile from a Perio Chip *in vitro* and *in vivo* studies. *Journal of Dental Research* **75**, 431 (Abst.3308)

Lindhe, J., Heijl, L., Goodson, J.M. and Socransky, S.S. (1979) Local tetracycline delivery using hollow fibre devices in periodontal therapy. *Journal of Clinical Periodontology* **6**, 141–149

Lindhe, J., Liljenberg, B., Adielson, B. and Börjesson, I. (1983) Use of metronidazole as a probe in the study of human periodontal disease. *Journal of Clinical Periodontology* **10**, 100–111

Lobene, R.R., Lobene, S. and Soparker, P.M. (1977) The effect of cetylpyridinium chloride mouthrinse on plaque and gingivitis. *Journal of Dental Research* **56**, 595

Lobene, R.R., Singh, S.S., Garcia, L. *et al.* (1992) Clinical efficacy of a triclosan/co-polymer pre-brush rinse: a plaque removal study. *Journal of Clinical Dentistry* **3**, 54–58

Loesche, W.J. (1976) Chemotherapy of dental plaque infections. *Oral Science Review* **9**, 65–107

Loesche, W.J., Syed, S.A., Morrison, E.C. *et al.* (1985) Metronidazole in periodontitis. I. Clinical and bacteriological results after 15 to 30 weeks. *Journal of Periodontology* **55**, 325–335

Loesche, W.J., Schmidt, E., Smith, B.A. *et al.* (1991) Effects of metronidazole on periodontal treatment needs. *Journal of Periodontology* **62**, 247–257

Loesche, W.J., Giordano, J.R., Hujoel, P.P. *et al.* (1992) Metronidazole in periodontitis: reduced needs for surgery. *Journal of Clinical Periodontology* **19**, 103–112

Loesche, W.J., Grossman, N. and Giordano, J.R. (1993) Metronidazole in periodontitis. IV. The effect of patient compliance on treatment parameters. *Journal of Clinical Periodontology* **20**, 96–104

Lovejoy, B., Cleaby, A., Hassell, A. *et al.* (1994) Structure of the catalytic domain of fibroblast collagenase complexed with an inhibitor. *Science* **263**, 375–377

Lusk, S.S., Bowers, G.M., Tow, H.D. *et al.* (1974) Effects of an oral rinse on experimental gingivitis, plaque formation and formed plaque. *Journal of the American Society of Preventive Dentistry* **4**, 31–37

Magnusson, I. (1998) The use of locally delivered metronidazole in the treatment of periodontitis. Clinical results. *Journal of Clinical Periodontology* **25**, 959–963

Mallatt, M.E., Beiswanger, B.B., Drook, C.A. *et al.* (1989) Clinical effect of a sanguinaria dentifrice on plaque and gingivitis in adults. *Journal of Periodontology* **60**, 91–95

Mandel, I.D. (1988) Chemotherapeutic agents for controlling plaque and gingivitis. *Journal of Clinical Periodontology* **15**, 488–498

Mandell, G.L. and Petri, W.A. (1996a) Antimicrobial agents – sulphonamides, trimethoprim-sulphamethoxazole, quinolones and agents for urinary infections. In *Goodman and Gilman's The Pharmacological Basis of Therapeutics*, 9th Edn (A. Goodman-Gilman, J.G. Hardman, L.E. Limbird *et al.*, eds), pp. 1057–1072. New York: McGraw-Hill

Mandell, G.L. and Petri, W.A. (1996b) Antimicrobial agents – penicillins, cephalosporins and other β-lactams. In *Goodman and Gilman's The Pharmacological Basis of Therapeutics*, 9th Edn (A. Goodman-Gilman, J.G. Hardman, L.E. Limbird *et al.*, eds), pp. 1073–1102. New York: McGraw-Hill

Mandell, R.C., Tripodi, L.S., Savitt, E. *et al.* (1986) The effect of treatment on *Actinobacillus actinomycetemcomitans* in localized juvenile periodontitis. *Journal of Periodontology* **57**, 94–99

Mason, J.C., Dollery, C.T., So, A. *et al.* (1992) An infected prosthetic hip – is there a role for antibiotic prophylaxis? *British Medical Journal* **205**, 300–302

Mombelli, A., Lehmann, B., Tonetti, M. and Lang, N.P. (1997) Clinical response to local delivery tetracycline in relation to overall and local periodontal conditions. *Journal of Clinical Periodontology* **24**, 470–477

Moran, J. and Addy, M. (1991) The effects of a cetylpyridinium chloride prebrushing rinse as an adjunct to oral hygiene and gingival health. *Journal of Periodontology* **62**, 562–564

Moran, J., Addy, M. and Newcombe, R. (1988) A clinical trial to assess the efficacy of sanguinarine-zinc mouthrinse (Veadent®) compared to a chlorhexidine mouthwash. *Journal of Clinical Periodontology* **15**, 612–616

Moran, J., Addy, M. and Roberts, S. (1992) The comparison of a natural product, triclosan and chlorhexidine mouthwashes on 4-day plaque regrowth. *Journal of Clinical Periodontology* **19**, 578–582

Moran, J., Addy, M., Wade, W.G. *et al.* (1992) A comparison of delmopinol and chlorhexidine on plaque regrowth over a 4-day period and salivary bacterial counts. *Journal of Clinical Periodontology* **19**, 749–753

Moran, J., Addy, M., Newcombe, R. and Warren, P. (1995) The comparative effects of phenolic, chlorhexidine and anti-adhesive mouthrinses. *Journal of Clinical Periodontology* **22**, 929–934

Moran, J., Addy, M., and Newcombe, R. (1997) A 4-day plaque regrowth study comparing an essential oil mouthrinse with a triclosan mouthrinse. *Journal of Clinical Periodontology* **24**, 636–639

Morrison, S.L., Cobb, C.M., Kazakos, G.M. and Killoy, W.J. (1992) Root surface characteristics associated with subgingival placement of monolithic tetracycline-impregnated fibres. *Journal of Periodontology* **63**, 137–143

Murray, M.C., Worthington, H.V. and Blinkhorn, H.S. (1997) A study to investigate the effect of a propolis-containing mouthrinse on the inhibition of de novo plaque formation. *Journal of Clinical Periodontology* **24**, 796–798

Nabi, N., Kashuba, B., Lucchesi, S. *et al.* (1996) *In vitro* and *in vivo* studies of salifluor/PVM/MA co-polymer/NaF combination as an antiplaque agent. *Journal of Clinical Periodontology* **23**, 1084–1092

Newman, M.G., Kornman, K.S. and Doherty, F.M. (1994) A 6-months multi-center evaluation of adjunctive tetracycline fibre therapy in conjunction with scaling and root planing in maintenance patients: clinical results. *Journal of Periodontology* **65**, 685–691

Noache, L.A., Langenberg, W.L., Bertola, M.A. *et al.* (1994) Impact of metronidazole resistance on the eradication of *Helicobacter pylori*. *Scandinavian Journal of Infectious Diseases* **26**, 321–327

Norling, T., Lading, P., Engström, S. *et al.* (1992) Formulation of a drug delivery system based on a mixture of monoglycerides and triglycerides for use in the treatment of periodontal disease. *Journal of Clinical Periodontology* **19**, 687–692

Notten, F., Koek-van Oosten, A. and Mikx, F. (1982) Capillary agar diffusion assay for measuring metronidazole in human gingival crevicular fluid. *Antimicrobial Agents and Chemotherapy* **21**, 836–837

O'Connor, B.C., Newman, H.N. and Wilson, M. (1990) Susceptibility and resistance of plaque bacteria to minocycline. *Journal of Periodontology* **61**, 228–233

Olsvik, B., Hansen, B.F., Tenover, F.C. and Olsen, I. (1995) Tetracycline resistant micro-organisms recovered from patients with refractory periodontal disease. *Journal of Clinical Periodontology* **22**, 391–396

Oosterwaal, P., Mikx, F. and Reggli, H. (1990) Clearance of a topical applied fluorescein gel from periodontal pockets. *Journal of Clinical Periodontology* **17**, 613–615

Overholser, C.D. (1988) Longitudinal clinical studies with antimicrobial mouthrinses. *Journal of Clinical Periodontology* **15**, 517–519

Pedrazzoli, V., Kilian, M. and Karring, T. (1992) Comparative clinical and microbiological effects of topical subgingival application of metronidazole 25% dental gel and scaling in the treatment of adult periodontitis. *Journal of Clinical Periodontology* **19**, 715–722

Pitcher G., Newman, H. and Strahan, J. (1980) Access to subgingival plaque by disclosing agents using mouthwashes and direct irrigation. *Journal of Clinical Periodontology* **7**, 300–302

Polson, A.M., Stoller, N.H., Hanes, P.J. *et al.* (1996) Two multi-centre trials assessing the clinical efficacy of 5% sanguinarine in a biodegradable drug delivery system. *Journal of Clinical Periodontology* **23**, 782–788

Preus, H.R., Lassen, J., Aass, A.M and Ciancio, S.G. (1995) Bacterial resistance following subgingival and systemic administration of minocycline. *Journal of Clinical Periodontology* **22**, 380–384

Ramberg, P., Furuichi, Y., Volpe, A.R. *et al.* (1996) The effects of antimicrobial mouthrinses on de novo plaque formation at sites with healthy and inflamed gingiva. *Journal of Clinical Periodontology* **23**, 7–11

Rapley, J.W., Cobb, C.M., Killoy, W.J. and Williams, D.R. (1992) Serum levels of tetracycline during treatment with tetracycline-containing fibres. *Journal of Periodontology* **62**, 817–820

Rautelin, H., Tee, W., Seppälä, K. and Kosunen, T.U. (1994) Ribotyping patterns and emergence of metronidazole resistance in paired clinical samples of *Helicobacter pylori*. *Journal of Antimicrobial Chemotherapy* **32**, 1079–1082

Renvert, S and Birkhed, D. (1995) Comparison between three triclosan dentifrices on plaque, gingivitis and salivary microflora. *Journal of Clinical Periodontology* **22**, 63–70

Rifkin, B.R., Vernillo, A.T. and Golub, L.M. (1993) Blocking periodontal disease progression by inhibiting tissue destructive enzymes: a potential role of tetracyclines and their chemically modified analogues. *Journal of Periodontology* **64**, 819–827

Riott, I.M. (1997) Hypersensitivity In *Riott's Essential Immunology 9th Edn*. Chap 16, pp 328–352. Oxford: Blackwell Science Ltd.

Roberts, W.R. and Addy, M. (1981) Comparison of the *in vivo* and *in vitro* antibacterial properties of antiseptic mouthrinses containing chlorhexidine, alexidine, cetylpyridinium chloride and hexidine. *Journal of Clinical Periodontology* 8, 295–310

Rölla, G., Löe, H. and Schiöt, C. (1971) Retention of chlorhexidine in the human oral cavity. *Archives of Oral Biology* 16, 1109–1116

Rosling, B.G., Slots, J., Webber, R.L. *et al.* (1983) Microbiological and clinical effects of topical subgingival antimicrobial treatment on human periodontal disease. *Journal of Clinical Periodontology* 10, 487–514

Ryan, M.E., Ramamurthy, S. and Golub, L.M. (1996) Matrix metalloproteinases and their inhibition in periodontal treatment. *Current Opinion in Periodontology* 3, 85–96

Saglie, R., Newman, M., Carranza, F. and Pattison, G. (1982) Bacterial invasion of gingiva in advanced periodontitis in humans. *Journal of Periodontology* 53, 217–222

Saglie, R., Pertuiset, J., Rezende, M. *et al.* (1988) *In situ* correlation immuno-identification of mononuclear cells and invasive bacteria in diseased gingiva. *Journal of Periodontology* 59, 688–696

Sande, M.A., Chambers, H.F. and Kupusnik-Uner, J.E. (1996) Antimicrobial agents – tetracyclines, chloramphenicol, erythromycin and other miscellaneous antibacterial agents. In *Goodman and Gilman's The Pharmacological Basis of Therapeutics*, 9th Edn (A. Goodman-Gilman, J.G. Hardman, L.E. Limbird *et al.*, eds), pp. 1123–1174. New York: McGraw-Hill

Sandhu, S.S., Lowry, J.C., Reuben, S.F. and Morton, M.E. (1997) Who decides on the need for antibiotic prophylaxis in patients with major arthroplasties requiring dental treatment: is it a joint responsibility? *Annals of the Royal College of Surgeons of England* 79, 143–147

Satomi, A., Vraguchi, R., Ishikawa, I. *et al.* (1987) Minocycline hydrochloride concentration in periodontal pockets after administration of LS-007. *Journal of Japanese Association of Periodontology* 29, 937–943

Saxton, C.A. (1986) the effects of a dentifrice containing zinc citrate and 2.2.4′-hydroxydiphenol. *Journal of Periodontology* 57, 555–562

Saxton, C.A. and Van der Ouderaa, F. (1989) The effect of a dentifrice containing zinc citrate and triclosan on the develop of gingivitis. *Journal of Periodontal Research* 24, 75–80

Saxton, C.A., Lane, R.M. and Van der Ouderaa, F. (1987) The effects of a toothpaste containing a zinc salt and a non-cationic antimicrobial agent on plaque and gingivitis. *Journal of Clinical Periodontology* 14, 144–148

Schaeken, M.J.M., Van der Hoeven, J.S., Saxton, C.A. and Cummins, D. (1994) The effect of mouthrinses containing zinc and triclosan on plaque accumulation and development of gingivitis in a 3-week clinical test. *Journal of Clinical Periodontology* 21, 360–364

Schaeken, M.J.M., Van der Hoeven, J.S., Saxton, C.A. and Cummins, D. (1996) The effect of mouthrinses containing zinc and triclosan on plaque accumulation, development of gingivitis and formation of calculus in a 28-week clinical test. *Journal of Clinical Periodontology* 23, 465–470

Schonfeld, S.E., Farnoush, A. and Wilson, S.G. (1986) *In vivo* antiplaque activity of a sanguinarine-containing dentifrice in comparison with conventional toothpastes. *Journal of Periodontal Research* 21, 298–303

Shinn, D.L. (1962) Metronidazole in acute ulcerative gingivitis. *Lancet* 1, 1191

Shinn, D.L., Squires, S. and McFadzean, J.A. (1965) The treatment of Vincent's disease with metronidazole. *Dental Practitioner* 15, 275–280

Sigrist, B.E., Gusberti, F.A., Brecz, M.C. *et al.* (1986) Efficacy of supervised rinsing with chlorhexidine gluconate in comparison to

phenolic and plant alkaloid compounds. *Journal of Periodontal Research* 21 (Suppl.), 60–73

Simonsson, T., Bondesson, H., Rundegren, J. and Edwardsson, S. (1991a) Effect of delmopinol on *in vitro* dental plaque formation, bacterial acid production and the number of micro-organisms in human saliva. *Oral Microbiology and Immunology* 6, 305–309

Simonsson, T., Arnebrant, T. and Peterson, L. (1991b) The delmopinol on the salivary pellicles, the wettable tooth surfaces *in vivo* and bacterial cell surfaces *in vitro*. *Biofouling* 3, 251–260

Skaare, A.B., Herlofson, B.B., and Barkvoll, P. (1996) Mouthrinses containing triclosan reduce the incidence of recurrent aphthous ulcers (RAU). *Journal of Periodontology* 23, 778–781

Skaare, A.B., Kjaerheim, V., Barkvoll, P. and Rölla, G. (1997) Does the nature of the solvent affect the anti-inflammatory capacity of triclosan? *Journal of Clinical Periodontology* 24, 124–128

Slots, J. and Rosling, B. (1983) Suppression of periodontopathic microflora in localized juvenile periodontitis by systemic tetracycline. *Journal of Clinical Periodontology* 10, 465–486

Smith, A.J., Moran, J., Dangler, L.V. *et al.* (1996) The efficacy of an antigingivitis chewing gum. *Journal of Clinical Periodontology* 23, 19–23

Söder, P., Frithiof, L., Wikner, S. *et al.* (1990) The effect of systemic metronidazole after non-surgical treatment in moderate and advanced periodontitis in young adults. *Journal of Periodontology* 61, 281–288

Sorsa, T., Ding, Y., Salo, T. *et al.* (1994) Effects of tetracyclines on neutrophil, gingival and salivary collagenases. A functional and Western-blot assessment with special reference to their cellular sources in periodontal diseases. *Annals of the New York Academy of Science* 732, 112–131

Soskolne, A., Golomb, G., Friedman, M. and Sela, M.N. (1983) New sustained release dosage form of chlorhexidine for dental use. II. Use in periodontal therapy. *Journal of Periodontal Research* 18, 330–336

Soskolne, A., Heasman, P.A., Smart, G. and Newman, H.N. (1998) European multi-centre study: sustained local delivery of chlorhexidine as an adjunct to scaling and root planing in the treatment of periodontal diseases. *Journal of Periodontology*, in press

Southard, G.L., Parsons, L.G., Thomas, L.G. *et al.* (1987) The relationship of sanguinaria extract concentration and zinc ion to plaque and gingivitis. *Journal of Clinical Periodontology* 14, 315–319

Speer, B.S., Shoemaker, N.B. and Salyers, A.A. (1992) Bacterial resistance to tetracycline: mechanisms, transfer and clinical significance. *Clinical Microbiology Reviews* 5, 387–399

Sprott, M.S., Ingham, H.R., Hickman, J.E. and Sisson, P.R. (1983) Metronidazole resistant anaerobes. *Lancet* 8335, 1230

Stabholz, A., Sela, M.N., Friedman, M. *et al.* (1986) Clinical and microbiological effects of sustained release chlorhexidine in periodontal pockets. *Journal of Clinical Periodontology* 13, 783–788

Stephen, K.W., Saxton, C.A., Jones, C.L. *et al.* (1990) Control of gingivitis and calculus by a dentifrice containing a zinc salt and triclosan. *Journal of Periodontology* 61, 674–679

Stoltze, K. (1992) Concentration of metronidazole in periodontal pockets after application of a 25% metronidazole dental gel. *Journal of Clinical Periodontology* 19, 698–701

Stoltze, K. and Stellfield, M. (1992) Systemic absorption of metronidazole after application of a 25% metronidazole dental gel. *Journal of Clinical Periodontology* 19, 693–697

Svaton, B., Saxton, C.A., Van der Ouderaa, F. and Rölla, G. (1987) The influence of a dentifrice containing a zinc salt and a non-cationic antimicrobial agent on the maintenance of gingival health. *Journal of Clinical Periodontology* 14, 457–461

Svaton, B., Saxton, C.A., Rölla, G. and Van der Ouderaa, F. (1989) One-year study of the efficacy of a dentifrice containing a zinc citrate and triclosan to maintain gingival health. *Scandinavian Journal of Dental Research* 97, 242–246

Svaton, B., Saxton, C.A. and Rölla, G. (1990) Six-month study of the effect of a dentifrice containing a zinc citrate and triclosan on plaque, gingival health and calculus. *Scandinavian Journal of Dental Research* **98**, 301–304

Tellefsen, G., Larsen, G., Kaligithi, K. *et al.* (1996) Use of chlorhexidine chewing gum significantly reduces dental plaque formation compared to similar xylitol and sorbitol products. *Journal of Periodontology* **67**, 181–183

Tenenbaum, H., Jehl, F., Gallion, C. and Dahan, M. (1997) Amoxycillin and clavulanic acid concentrations in gingival crevicular fluid. *Journal of Clinical Periodontology* **24**, 804–807

Theilade, E. (1986) The non-specific theory in microbial etiology of inflammatory periodontal diseases. *Journal of Clinical Periodontology* **13**, 905–911

Timmerman, M.F., van der Weijden, G.A., van Steenbergen, T.J.M. *et al.* (1996) Evaluation of the long-term efficacy and safety of locally-applied minocycline in adult periodontitis patients. *Journal of Clinical Periodontology* **23**, 707–716

Todd, P.A. and Benfield, P. (1990) Amoxycillin/clavulanic acid. An update of its antibacterial activity, pharmacokinetic properties and therapeutic use. *Drugs* **39**, 264–307

Tonetti, M.S. (1994) Etiology and pathogenesis. In *Proceedings of the 1st European Workshop on Periodontology* (N.P. Lang and T. Karring, eds), pp. 54–89. Berlin: Quintessence Publishing Co. Ltd

Tonetti, M.S. (1998) Local-delivery of tetracycline: from concept to clinical application. *Journal of Clinical Periodontology* **25**, 969–977

Tonetti, M.S., Cugini, M.A. and Goodson, J.M. (1990) Zero-order delivery with periodontal placement of tetracycline-loaded ethylene vinyl acetate fibres. *Journal of Periodontal Research* **25**, 243–249

Tonetti, M.S., Mombelli, A., Lehmann, B. and Lang, N. (1995) Impact of oral ecology on the recolonization of locally treated pockets. *Journal of Dental Research* **74** Abstr. 642, 481

Tracy, J.W. and Webster, L.T. (1996) Trypanomiasis, leishmaniasis, amebiasis, giardiasis, trichomoniasis and other protozoal infections. In *Goodman and Gilman's The Pharmacological Basis of Therapeutics*, 9th Edn (A. Goodman-Gilman, J.G. Hardman, L.E. Limbird *et al.*, eds), pp. 987–1008. New York: McGraw-Hill

Tyne, G.M. and Ferguson, J.W. (1991) Antibiotic prophylaxis in patients during dental treatment in patients with prosthetic joints. *Journal of Bone and Joint Surgery* **73B**, 191–194

Vandekerchhove, B.N.A., Van Steenberge, D., Tricio, J. *et al.* (1995) Efficacy on supragingival plaque control of cetylpyridinium chloride in a slow-release dosage form. *Journal of Clinical Periodontology* **22**, 824–829

Vandekerchhove, B.N.A., Quirynen, M. and Van Steenberge, D. (1998) The use of locally delivered minocycline in the treatment of chronic periodontitis. A review of the literature. *Journal of Clinical Periodontology* **25**, 964–968

Van Palenstein Heldermann, W.H. (1986) Is antibiotic therapy justified in the treatment of human chronic inflammatory periodontal disease? *Journal of Clinical Periodontology* **13**, 932–938

Van Steenberge, D., Bercy, P., Hohl, J. *et al.* (1993) Subgingival minocycline hydrochloride ointment in moderate to severe chronic adult periodontitis: randomized, double-blind, vehicle-controlled, multi-centre study. *Journal of Periodontology* **64**, 637–644

Van Winkelhoff, A.J., Rodenberg, A.J., Goené, R.J. *et al.* (1989) Metronidazole plus amoxycillin in the treatment of *Actinobacillus actinomycetemcomitans* associated periodontitis. *Journal of Clinical Periodontology* **16**, 128–131

Van Zwet, A.A., Thijs, J.C., Schievink-de Vries, W. *et al.* (1994) *In vitro* studies on stability and development of metronidazole resistance in

Helicobacter pylori. Antimicrobial Agents and Chemotherapy **38**, 360–362

Vorachit, M., Lam, K., Jayanetra, P. and Costerton, J. (1993) Resistance of *Pseudomonas pseudomallei* growing on a biofilm on silastic discs to ceftazidine and co-trimoxazole. *Antimicrobial Agents and Chemotherapy* **37**, 2000–2002

Waaler, S.M. and Rölla, G. (1980) Plaque inhibition effect of combinations of chlorhexidine with metal ions zinc and tin. *Acta Odontologica Scandinavica* **38**, 213–217

Waaler, S.M., Rölla, G., Skjörland, K.K. and Ögaard, B. (1994a) Effects of oral rinsing with triclosan and sodium lauryl sulfate on dental plaque formation: a pilot study. *Scandinavian Journal of Dental Research* **101**, 192–195

Waaler, S.M., Rölla, G., and Kjaerheim, V. (1994b) Triclosan containing mouthwashes: does the nature of the solvent influence their clinical effect? *Scandinavian Journal of Dental Research* **102**, 46–49

Wade, A.B., Blake, G.C. and Mirza, K.B. (1966) Effectiveness of metronidazole in treating the acute phase of ulcerative gingivitis. *The Dental Practitioner* **16**, 440–443

Walker, C.B., Gordon, J.M., Cornwall, H.A. *et al.* (1981a) Gingival crevicular fluid levels of clindamycin compared with its minimal inhibitory concentrations for periodontal bacteria. *Antimicrobial Agents and Chemotherapy* **19**, 867–871

Walker, C.B., Gordon, J.M., McQulkin, S.J. *et al.* (1981b) Tetracycline: levels achievable in gingival crevice fluid and *in vitro* effect on subgingival organisms. Part II. Susceptibilities of periodontal bacteria. *Journal of Periodontology* **52**, 613–616

Walker, C.B., Gordon, J.M. and Socransky S.S. (1983) Antibiotic sensitivity testing of subgingival plaque samples. *Journal of Clinical Periodontology* **10**, 422–432

Walker, C.B., Borden, L.C., Zambon, J.J. *et al.* (1994) The effects of a 0.3% triclosan-containing dentifrice on the microbial composition of supragingival plaque. *Journal of Clinical Periodontology* **21**, 334–341

Wennström, J. and Lindhe, J. (1979) The effect of hydrogen peroxide on developing plaque and gingivitis in Man. *Journal of Clinical Periodontology* **6**, 115–130

Wennström, J. and Lindhe, J. (1986) The effect of mouthrinses on parameters characterizing human periodontal disease. *Journal of Clinical Periodontology* **13**, 86–93

Williams, B.L., Østenberg, S.K.Å. and Jørgensen, J. (1979) Subgingival microflora of periodontal patients on tetracycline therapy. *Journal of Clinical Periodontology* **6**, 210–221

Wilson, M., Gibson, M., Strahan, J.D. and Harvey, M. (1992) A preliminary evaluation of the use of a redox agent in the treatment of periodontal disease. *Journal of Periodontal Research* **27**, 522–527

Winrow, M. (1973) Metabolic studies with radiolabelled chlorhexidine in animals and Man. *Journal of Periodontal Research* **12** (Suppl.), 45–48

Working Party of the British Society of Antimicrobial Chemotherapy (1992), reported in *Lancet* **339**, 301

Worthington, H.V., Davies, R.M., Blinkhorn, A.S. *et al.* (1993) A 6-month clinical study of the effect of a pre-brush rinse on plaque removal and gingivitis. *British Dental Journal* **75**, 322–326

Wright, T.L., Ellen, R.P., Lacroix, J.-M. *et al.* (1997) Effects of metronidazole on *Porphyromonas gingivalis* biofilms. *Journal of Periodontal Research* **32**, 473–477

Yu, L., Smith, G., Hasty, K. and Brandt, K. (1991) Doxycycline inhibits type XI collagenolytic activity of extracts from human osteoarthritic cartilage and of gelatinase. *Journal of Rheumatology* **18**, 1450–1452

Yu, Z., Ramamurthy, N.S., Leung, M. *et al.* (1993) Chemically-modified tetracycline normalizes collagen metabolism in diabetic rats: a dose response study. *Journal of Periodontal Research* **28**, 420–428

Zee, K.-Y., Rundegen, J. and Attström, R. (1997) Effect of delmopinol hydrochloride mouthrinse on plaque formation and gingivitis in 'rapid' and 'slow' plaque formers. *Journal of Clinical Periodontology* **24**, 486–491

16

Surgical periodontal treatment

Introduction

As described in Chapter 14, there are limitations to what can be achieved by subgingival scaling and root planing. Increased pocketing and the presence of defective restorations, especially overhanging margins, limit what can be accomplished by this 'blind' procedure. It has been claimed that a pocket depth of about 5 mm represents the limit for efficient debridement, but there is much debate about this. Many studies have compared the results of surgical (open) and non-surgical (closed) procedures (among them, Hill *et al.*, 1981; Brayer *et al.*, 1989; Wylam *et al.*, 1993). The Wylam study is especially interesting, as it compared the clinical effectiveness of the open and closed techniques on multi-rooted teeth and demonstrated heavy residual deposits in furcations after both procedures; better results were obtained on external root surfaces using the open procedures. These workers state that hand instrumentation alone is inadequate for debridement in furcations, and they suggest that ultrasonic instrumentation or rotating burrs are necessary. Kaldahl *et al.* (1993) have reviewed over 20 longitudinal studies that compared the results of surgical and non-surgical treatment, and they conclude that:

1. Both surgical and non-surgical procedures produce improvement in clinical parameters, i.e. gingival inflammation and bleeding, and reduction in pocket depth
2. Surgical procedures produced greater short-term reduction in probing depth, but long-term results were mixed
3. Comparison of those surgical procedures that did not include manipulation of alveolar bone with those that included bone resection showed mixed results.

One must conclude from the very mixed results of so many studies that much rests on:

- The appropriateness of the technique used to the pathological situation. This highlights the crucial nature of precise diagnosis and the identification of all the factors involved in the production of the lesion.
- The competence of the operator in executing different procedures.
- The production of a tissue anatomy that facilitates the patient's home care efforts which, whatever the operator may do, remain central to long-term success.

The type of surgical treatment necessary depends upon the form of the lesion, which can be described as:

1. Simple or suprabony, in which all the walls of the lesion are in soft tissue and are uncomplicated by mucogingival problems.
2. Intrabony, where the base of the pocket is apical to the bone margin and therefore one or more of the pocket walls are bounded by bone.
3. Those pockets complicated by mucogingival problems such as high muscle attachments or the absence of attached gingiva.

The most difficult lesions to treat are those intrabony defects associated with mucogingival problems and furcation involvement.

Contraindications to surgery

Contraindications to surgery may be oral or systemic, and include the following:

1. Patients of advanced age where teeth may last for life without resorting to radical treatment. Procedures indicated in someone of 60 may not be justified in someone of 70 years.
2. The presence of systemic disease, such as severe cardiovascular disease, malignancy, kidney and liver disease, blood diseases and bleeding disorders, uncontrolled diabetes, etc. Consultation with the patient's physician is essential.

3. Where thorough subgingival scaling and conscientious home care will remove or control the lesion.
4. Where patient motivation is obviously inadequate.
5. In the presence of acute infection.
6. Where the post-operative appearance would be so poor as to cause patient distress.
7. Where the prognosis is so poor that tooth loss is inevitable.

Some situations may require delay, or special pre-operative attention. An inadequately controlled diabetic patient will need to be stabilized. Surgery in the pregnant patient is best delayed until after parturition, except where acute lesions develop.

Patients with a history of valvular disease, open heart surgery and hip prostheses must have pre-operative antibiotic cover (see Chapter 15). Patients on various drugs, anticoagulants, steroids and antidepressants require special attention as directed by their physician. A thorough medical history is always essential.

Smoking and periodontal surgical treatment

Smoking is known to adversely affect all forms of periodontal treatment (see Chapters 4 and 14), and this is particularly important in surgical treatment. In longitudinal studies of groups of smokers and non-smokers who had undergone periodontal surgery (Preber and Bergström, 1990; Ah *et al.*, 1994), smokers exhibited greater post-treatment probing depths and less gain in clinical attachment levels than non-smokers. Smokers have also been shown to have poorer success rates in bone graft and implant procedures (Jones and Triplett, 1992), guided tissue regeneration procedures and soft tissue grafting procedures (Miller, 1987), which are described in Chapters 17, 18, 26. Thus, consideration should be given as to whether surgical treatment is ever justified in smokers and, if it is carried out, patients should be warned of the adverse effects of their smoking on the response achieved. All periodontal patients, and particularly potential surgery patients, should be actively discouraged from smoking.

Preparation for surgery

Patients should have completed basic treatment and reassessment and have good oral hygiene before being considered for surgery. They must be provided with information about what surgery can achieve in their case, about prognosis, limitations or complications, and the problems of the post-operative period.

Information also must be provided about the available anaesthesia and analgesia. The most common method of organization of the surgery is to carry it out in stages on sections of the mouth, either a segment or quadrant at one time, under local anaesthesia in the dental chair. Where full-mouth surgery is required, this will involve the patient in several procedures over many weeks. Alternatively, full-mouth surgery can be carried out under general anaesthesia in hospital. As full-mouth surgery can be an extremely lengthy procedure, involving an extended general anaesthetic, post-operative overnight stay in hospital is recommended. A third option, where several surgical stages are to be avoided, is to carry out surgery under local anaesthesia plus intravenous sedation. Which of the alternatives is used depends on patient preference, their emotional state, work and domestic commitments. Comprehensive information and discussion are essential to meet the patient's needs.

Periodontal surgical techniques

The aims of periodontal surgery are:

1. To arrest the progress of periodontal disease and prevent its recurrence.
2. To attempt to produce regeneration of tissue destroyed in the disease.

Thus, the various surgical techniques may also be divided into these same two groups. These are:

1. Those that are limited to eliminating disease and producing conditions that obviate against its recurrence. These can be further divided into two subgroups:
   - Procedures aimed at pocket elimination or reduction:
       Gingivectomy
       Inverse bevel gingivectomy
       Apical reposition flap.
   - Procedures to expose the root surface for open scaling and root planing:
       Replaced flap (modified Widman flap). This procedure will produce a long junctional epithelium.
2. Those that eliminate disease and also aim to produce regeneration of periodontal tissue that has been destroyed by disease, and thereby produce increased attachment level:
   - Guided tissue regeneration (GTR)
   - Bone grafting.

In this context it is important to distinguish two forms of healing:

1. The adherence of a long junctional epithelium to the root surface so that clinical probing depth may be reduced.
2. The formation of new connective tissue attachment consisting of periodontal ligament fibres embedded into bone and cementum.

These end-results are illustrated in *Figure 16.1*.

Simple suprabony pockets can be treated by any of these procedures, choosing whichever is most appropriate. Compound intrabony pockets require access by means of a flap procedure, and their treatment is discussed in Chapter 17. Mucogingival problems associated with

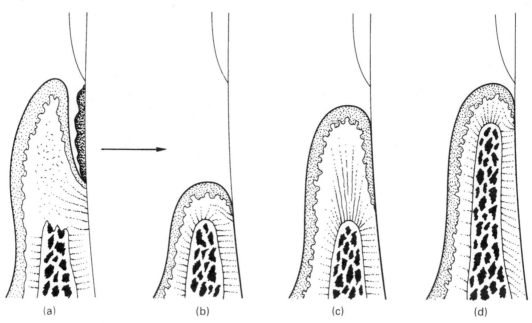

(a)   (b)   (c)   (d)

Figure 16.1 *(a)* Periodontal lesion; *(b)* the result of radical elimination of the lesion, e.g. by gingivectomy or apically repositioned flap; *(c)* the result of a replaced flap with long epithelial attachment; *(d)* regeneration of alveolar bone plus fibrous attachment

periodontal pockets that extend close to or beyond the mucogingival junction must be treated by an apically repositioned flap in order to increase the zone of attached gingiva.

Procedures for pocket elimination

Gingivectomy

Gingivectomy is the complete removal of the soft tissue wall of the pocket.

Indications for gingivectomy

1. The presence of suprabony pockets > 5 mm, which persist despite repeated subgingival scaling and root planing and conscientious home care, and where gingivectomy would leave an adequate zone of attached gingiva.
2. The presence of persistent gingival swelling where 'real' pocketing may be shallow but there is considerable gingival enlargement and deformity. If the gingival tissue is fibrous, gingivectomy may be the treatment most likely to produce a satisfactory result.
3. The presence of furcation involvement (without associated bone defects) where there is a wide zone of attached gingiva.
4. A gingival abscess, i.e. an abscess contained entirely by soft tissue.
5. A pericoronal flap.

Gingivectomy is a radical procedure that has been largely replaced by more conservative flap techniques. However, it remains the treatment of choice where recontouring of deformed tissue is needed, and where access and a precise and predictable anatomy are required to facilitate restorative treatment.

The procedure is given in detail, as it provides a model for other surgical procedures.

Procedure

1. *Pocket marking.* For complete removal of the pocket wall, the apical limit of the pocket must be identified and marked using either pocket marking forceps (*Figure 16.2*) or a periodontal probe. A series of such markings on both facial and lingual gingivae provides a guide for gingivectomy incision.
2. *The gingivectomy incision.* The incision can be made with several knives: e.g. Swann–Morton Nos 12 or 15 on a conventional scalpel handle; the Blake knife, which uses disposable blades; or special gingivectomy knives, such as the Kirkland, Orban or Goldman–Fox knives, which have to be sharpened. The choice of knife is entirely personal, but where possible the use of disposable blades is to be recommended. The incision must be made apical to the markings, i.e. apical to the base of the pocket, and at an angle of 45° so that the blade completely perforates the gingiva to the base of the pocket (*Figure 16.2*). A continuous incision (not an interrupted scalloped incision) that follows the base of the pockets is made. The correct incision will both remove the pocket wall and produce a streamlined tissue contour;

Figure 16.2 Pocket-marking forceps defining the approximate depth of the pocket. Note that the position of the gingivectomy incision is apical to the marking and that the angle of the incision is about 45°

Position of gingivectomy incision

if the incision is too flat, the post-operative contour will be unsatisfactory. The most common fault is to incise in a coronal position so that the base of the pocket wall is retained, with the possibility of disease recurrence. Following the bevelled incisions, horizontal incisions are made between each interdental space, with a No. 12 blade on a conventional scalpel handle, in order to separate the remaining interdental wedges of tissue.

3. *Tissue removal.* If the incision has completely separated the pocket wall from the underlying tissue, the pocket wall can be removed easily with a large curette or scaler, e.g. the Cumine scaler. Remnants of fibrous connective tissue and granulation tissue are removed thoroughly with sharp curettes to reveal the root surface. Efficient suction is essential, but once granulations have been removed bleeding reduces significantly.

4. *Root scaling and planing.* The root surfaces should be inspected for evidence of residual calculus deposits, and where necessary the root surfaces should be scaled and root planed. If necessary, further trimming and reshaping of the gingivae can be carried out using scalpel, fine scissors or diathermy. Sterile swabs are placed over the wound to control bleeding so that the periodontal dressing can be applied to a relatively dry wound area.

5. *The periodontal dressing.* A dressing to cover the wound serves a number of purposes:
   - It protects the wound from irritation.
   - It keeps the wound clean.
   - It controls bleeding
   - It controls exuberant granulation tissue production.

The dressing thereby promotes healing and provides post-operative comfort. The requirements of a satisfactory periodontal dressing are as follows:
- It should be non-irritant, and should not induce an allergic response.
- It should be adaptable to the teeth and tissues and flow between the teeth so that it is well retained; a slow setting-time allows manipulation.
- It should exclude food and saliva.
- It should have antibacterial properties to inhibit bacterial growth.
- It should set fairly hard so that it is not easily displaced.
- Its taste should be acceptable.

It is essential to apply the dressing carefully so that it covers the wound and fills the interdental spaces completely. It should be muscle trimmed by movement of the cheeks, lips and tongue, and all excess dressing on occlusal surfaces removed. A number of dressings based on zinc-oxide-eugenol are available, but many people find the taste of eugenol unacceptable and some reports of contact allergy to eugenol have been made. For these reasons eugenol-free dressings have been devised, e.g. Coe-Pack, Peripak, Septopak. These are easy to apply and well tolerated by the patients.

Post-operative care

It is very important to provide the patient with comprehensive information about post-operative care. The following advice should be given in writing:

1. Avoid eating or drinking for 1 hour.
2. Avoid hot drinks and alcohol for 24 hours. Do not rinse mouth for first day.
3. Avoid eating hard, sharp or sticky foods, and eat on the unoperated side.
4. Take an analgesic if there is pain when the anaesthetic wears off. Aspirin is contraindicated for 24 hours.
5. Use warm saline mouthwashes after the first day. A 0.2% chlorhexidine mouthwash is used morning and night, as mechanical plaque control is not possible. This can be used on the first day, provided it is not swished around the mouth. Tea, coffee and smoking should be avoided when using a chlorhexidine mouthwash to reduce staining.
6. If there is bleeding, exert pressure on the dressing for 15 minutes with a clean, boiled handkerchief; do not rinse; contact the surgery if the bleeding does not stop.
7. Use a toothbrush only on unoperated parts of the mouth.
8. If the immediate post-operative phase is uneventful but pain and swelling occur 2 or 3 days later, report immediately to the surgery.

A post-operative antibiotic is only prescribed in certain cases, e.g. possibly for a diabetic or any individual who may be debilitated. For routine purposes the dressing is usually removed after 1 week. All debris must be completely removed and the wound irrigated with warm water. If the wound is not sufficiently well epithelialized and is tender, a new dressing is applied for a further week.

After the dressing has been removed, further instruction in home care is needed. The chlorhexidine mouthwash can be used morning and night for a further week only, as prolonged use will cause staining, which is very difficult to remove. The patient is encouraged to start gentle toothbrushing with a soft toothbrush in warm water that evening. Either a gentle roll or Charter's technique is used at this stage. The Bass technique and interdental cleaning are avoided for a week. The patient is advised to avoid cold and hard food.

After 2 weeks, the wound is inspected and the teeth cleaned. The patient's oral hygiene must be reviewed until entirely satisfactory and until the healing is complete, after which a 3–6-monthly recall regimen, as appropriate, is established.

Healing after gingivectomy

The connective tissue wound is covered by a blood clot. The area beneath this undergoes a brief phase of acute inflammation, which is followed by demolition and organization. Epithelial cells migrate from the edge of the wound beneath the clot. They cover the wound in 7–14 days, and keratinize in 2–3 weeks. The formation of a new epithelial attachment may take as long as 4 weeks. Good oral hygiene is essential during the healing period.

The limitations and drawbacks of gingivectomy

1. The gingivectomy procedure creates an open wound, which heals by secondary intention.
2. Tissue that could be used to close the wound and obtain healing by primary intention is wasted.
3. Alveolar bone defects are not revealed and therefore cannot be treated adequately.
4. The zone of attached gingiva may be eliminated.
5. The clinical crown may be lengthened considerably, and in the front of the mouth this may be unsightly and unacceptable to the patient. It is important to explain before surgery that 'the teeth will look longer' (*Figure 16.3*).
6. Exposed root may be sensitive. Some sensitivity to cold and sweet immediately after gingivectomy is extremely common, but this symptom is usually transient. If it persists, it will require the use of desensitizing agents.

Despite the above limitations, the gingivectomy technique has a place in periodontal treatment. It is extremely easy to carry out, and gives an excellent result in the appropriate cases.

(a)

(b)

Figure 16.3 *(a)* Before gingivectomy; *(b)* after gingivectomy, showing the increase in clinical crown length

Flap techniques

The flap techniques have several obvious advantages over gingivectomy:

1. They allow access to the root and alveolar bone.
2. Tissue that can be used to close the wound is conserved.
3. The soft tissues can be manipulated if necessary to achieve an improved soft tissue morphology.

In raising a flap, certain basic requirements must be satisfied:

- The flap must be big enough to expose any underlying bone defects
- The base of the flap must be wide enough to maintain an adequate blood supply
- The incisions must allow movement of the flap without tension
- No important vessels or nerves should be damaged in raising the flap.

There are three basic flap shapes:

1. The full flap, made by a gingival incision and two releasing incisions
2. The triangular flap, with a gingival incision and one releasing incision
3. The modified flap, with only a gingival incision and no releasing incisions.

Flaps have also been divided into two types:

- A full-thickness flap, which consists of the complete mucoperiosteum and is raised by a periosteal elevator.
- The split-thickness flap, in which the gingiva is dissected from the underlying periosteum, which is left on the bone. This type of flap is more difficult to raise and its use is restricted to the special situations described below.

Flaps are further divided into those that are raised and replaced into their original position, and flaps that are moved into apical, coronal or lateral positions.

Flap procedures used to treat chronic periodontitis are described below.

The replaced flap (modified Widman technique)

The debate about 'open' and 'closed' approaches to subgingival scaling and root planing represents the most recent aspect of a historical conflict in periodontics between the conservative and radical approaches to treatment. In the early part of this century, as a reaction to gingivectomy, a mucoperiosteal flap approach to the periodontal lesion was described by Neuman (1912) and Widman (1918). This technique involved raising a full-thickness flap which, after scaling and root planing, was replaced in its original position to produce a closed wound, which was more comfortable and healed more rapidly than the open wound produced by gingivectomy.

Morris (1965) introduced the internal bevel incision, which separated the pocket wall from the rest of the mucoperiosteal flap and produced a healthy, thin and flexible margin to the flap. This was used by Ramfjord and Nissle (1974) in what they called the 'modified Widman flap' procedure, which allowed open access to the periodontal lesion and then much closer adaptation of the replaced flap to the tooth surface than had been possible with the unmodified full-thickness flap. The flap approach also allows access to alveolar bone defects (Chapter 17). A further advantage is that there is less post-operative root exposure than after gingivectomy, which is especially important in the front of the mouth.

When introduced, it was thought that the technique would produce a physiological dentogingival junction, and therefore lead to permanent pocket elimination, but this is not possible (Caton and Nyman, 1980, Caton *et al.,* 1980).

The long junctional epithelium produced by this procedure is inherently less stable than the physiological junctional epithelium, and demands much higher standards of plaque control and higher frequencies of recall for maintenance than pocket elimination procedures. However, it has been shown that this technique can successfully treat and stabilize cases with moderate and advanced chronic periodontitis. There have been many longitudinal studies over periods ranging from 2 to 6 years that have compared non-surgical and surgical treatment techniques, including both replaced and pocket elimination flap techniques (Pihlstrom *et al.*, 1983; Ramfjord *et al.*, 1987). These all show that both non-surgical scaling/root planing and surgical replaced flap/pocket elimination techniques can effectively control moderate to advanced chronic periodontitis, preventing further attachment loss. However, all of these workers used regular and often long maintenance visits at intervals of 3 months or less throughout the period of study; this factor could have been at least as important as the technique itself in preventing relapse. The effect of maintenance in preventing deterioration following treatment has been clearly shown in a number of studies (Nyman *et al.*, 1975). These studies also showed that cases with deep pockets needed retreatment more often when treated with scaling alone. This is consistent with reports that residual deposits of subgingival calculus are commonly left in deep pockets following subgingival scaling, and that this is significantly less common when surgical techniques are used (Chapter 14). Therefore this would seem to justify the use of periodontal flap techniques for open scaling and root planing, which is the main purpose of the replaced flap technique.

Procedure

1. *Incision.* An inverse bevel incision is made up to 1 mm from the gingival margin on both the facial and lingual sides of either the upper or lower arches. The aim of this incision, as with other flap techniques, is to separate the pocket epithelium and inflamed connective tissue (cervical wedge) from the flap (*Figure 16.4a*). No vertical relieving incisions are made unless necessary for reflection purposes. Two further incisions were described by Ramfjord and Nissle (1974). The first is an incision made from the base of the pocket to the bone crest. The second, which is made after flap reflection, is a horizontal incision made from the crest of the bone to the tooth surface. The purpose of these additional incisions is to allow the cervical wedge to be removed easily and to minimize damage to the underlying periodontal ligament. These incisions are not totally necessary and obviously serve no purpose if intrabony defects are present, which have to be curetted.

   Another suggested modification is to exaggerate the scalloping of the palatal inverse bevel incision in order to lengthen the interdental papillae so that they completely cover the interdental space on closure.

Figure 16.4 Diagram to show the replaced flap procedure: *(a)* inverse bevel incision; *(b)* the flap is reflected to reveal the alveolar margin; *(c)* the flap is replaced and sutured in its original position; *(d)* long junctional epithelium following healing

2. *Reflection of flap.* A full-thickness mucoperiosteal flap is reflected with a periodontal elevator in order to expose the roots of the teeth and the bone margin (*Figure 16.4b*).

3. *Curettage, scaling and root planing.* The cervical wedge is removed and the root surfaces are scaled and root planed. Great care should be taken with this process, as a totally clean and smooth root surface is necessary to ensure that the long junctional epithelium, which will form following healing, will adhere to it. Failure of this adherence will lead to the re-establishment of pocketing. Any bony craters and deeper defects should be totally cleared of granulation tissue to create the best conditions for bone regeneration (Chapter 17).

4. *Suturing.* The flaps are then replaced in their original position and secured by tight interdental suturing (*Figure 16.4c*). Every effort is made to ensure total interdental coverage and to avoid any root exposure. There is no need to place a periodontal dressing, as it has no supporting function in this procedure. However, it can be placed if required for patient comfort, and in this case it need cover only the gingival margin.

5. *Post-operative management.* Post-operative instructions are the same as those for the gingivectomy. Post-operative swelling with this procedure is usually slight because of the smaller amount of flap retraction involved. Sutures are removed after a week, and the chlorhexidine mouthwash is continued for a further week. Brushing is started with an extra soft brush. Flossing is usually started a week post-operatively, although some discretion needs to be exercised in this regard. It must be carried out with great care to avoid gingival trauma. The patient should be seen every 4 weeks until healing is complete and plaque control perfect. Maintenance visits will be necessary every 3 months thereafter, as the long junctional epithelium is more liable to break down and a very careful check must be kept for pockets reforming. This procedure is likely to be more stable around single-rooted anterior teeth, since they are more accessible for home care and for professional maintenance. Posterior teeth are likely to be complicated by furcation involvements, which are extremely difficult to maintain if situated subgingivally.

6. *Healing.* Following acute inflammation, healing will begin by the organization of the blood clot between the flap and the tooth into granulation tissue. This is then slowly replaced by collagenous connective tissue over the next 2–5 weeks. Epithelium proliferates over the connective tissue wound, to its pre-operative position. If the root surface is free of irritant, the long junctional epithelium can adhere to it. However, the longer the junctional epithelium, the more unstable this situation becomes and the greater the risk of the re-establishment of pocketing. A mature long epithelial attachment may take several weeks to form, and care should be taken not to disrupt it by probing during this period. Quite frequently gingival recession will occur following replaced flaps, and this has the effect of both producing some root exposure and reducing the length of the long junctional epithelium (*Figure 16.4d*).

Root conditioning with citric acid

A further approach to obtaining new connective tissue attachment has been attempted using citric acid conditioning of the root surface (Polson and Proye, 1982). Root cementum is first removed from the affected part of the root by planing with curettes. Citric acid at pH 1 is then applied to the dentine surface for 3 minutes. The superficial zone of the dentine becomes demineralized, leading to the exposure of collagen fibrils in the matrix. It has been claimed that a connective tissue attachment will reform by the interdigitation of new and existing collagen fibres on the root surface, but if this occurs at all the amount is limited. The usual result is the development of a long junctional epithelium, and this method does not therefore seem to offer any advantage over flap techniques alone (Moore *et al.*, 1997).

Apically repositioned flap

This procedure was first described by Friedman in 1962. It is indicated for the elimination of periodontal pocketing and increasing the zone of attached gingiva. Pocketing separates the attached gingiva from the tooth, and deep pockets may extend below the mucogingival junction, i.e. through the whole width of the attached gingiva. In these circumstances gingivectomy techniques would leave either a narrow zone of attached gingiva or none at all, and are therefore contraindicated. Replaced flap techniques (see above) cannot increase the zone of attached gingiva, and are thus not indicated for pockets extending to or beyond the mucogingival junction.

The apically repositioned flap achieves pocket elimination by moving the flap in an apical direction. Adequate mobility of the flap is necessary for this, and is obtained by extending the releasing incisions to the base of the vestibule and further dissection of the flap from the underlying tissues. Apical repositioning will leave the flap just covering the alveolar crest, thus eliminating the pocketing. During healing, the merging of the connective tissue on the inner surface of the flap with the bone will recreate a mucoperiosteal attached gingival zone.

Procedure

1. *Incisions.* Two vertical releasing incisions are made through to bone at either end of the operative area. They should be made mesial or distal to the last interdental periodontal pocket to be treated, and must not be positioned interdentally. They should be parallel to each other and should extend into the alveolar mucosa at the base of the vestibule.

   An inverse bevel incision is made along the gingival margin (*Figure 16.5*). It should start up to 1 mm

Figure 16.5 Position of blade for inverse bevel incision. The incision is discontinuous and scalloped, following the contour of each tooth

from the gingival margin and extend down to the crest of the alveolar bone (*Figure 16.6a*). It is discontinuous and scalloped around the neck of each tooth, and may be made in two stages, a superficial outlining incision and a deepening incision. This allows the interdental papilla to be deflected outwards when making the deepening incision, which allows the blade to be angled more acutely. The aim of these incisions is to separate the pocket lining and inflamed connective tissue from the inner wall of the flap. This tissue is left on the surface of the tooth when the flap is raised, and is referred to as the cervical wedge.

In the lower jaw, care should be taken lingually with the distal relieving incision to ensure that there is no risk to the lingual nerve. Care should also be taken not to damage or bruise the submandibular ducts in raising the flap. Palatal gingiva is treated by means of an inverse bevel gingivectomy incision, as obviously palatal tissue cannot be apically positioned. The angle of the incision can be varied according to

Figure 16.6 The apically repositioned flap procedure: *(a)* inverse bevel incision; *(b)* the flap is reflected and dissected from the alveolar process, so that *(c)* it can be moved in an apical direction; *(d)* the flap is sutured in an apical position, just covering the bone margin

the thickness of the tissue, and may be used to fillet out hyperplastic tissue.

2. *Raising the flap.* A periosteal elevator is used to separate attached gingiva from the alveolar process so that a full-thickness flap is lifted (*Figure 16.6b*). It should peel away easily from the tooth and bone and clearly separate from the cervical wedge. If it does not separate easily, the marginal inverse bevel incision should be deepened. The flap may be released in two stages, the first to expose the bone to allow curettage and the second to detach the flap further, just before apical positioning. In this way bone exposure is reduced to the minimum.

In the case of upper teeth, the palatal tissue is raised to expose the margin of the bone and to give sufficient access for the removal of the large wedge of tissue produced by the inverse bevel gingivectomy incision.

3. *Removing the cervical wedge and granulation tissue.* The separated cervical wedge is removed with curettes and scalers. All granulation tissue attached to the tooth surface, bone margin or within bone defects should be carefully and comprehensively curetted away to leave a clean tooth and bone surface. Efficient aspiration is necessary to ensure good visibility. Bleeding will reduce dramatically when this tissue has been removed. The treatment of intrabony pocketing and furcation involvement is discussed in Chapter 17.

4. *Root scaling and planing.* The exposed roots must be scaled to remove any residual calculus and planed.

5. *Apical repositioning.* The flap is reflected to the base of the vestibule. Once released the flap tends to contract and fold up, so that apical positioning often takes place spontaneously. One should ensure that the flap is displaced apically so that its edge just covers the alveolar crest (*Figure 16.6c*).

6. *Suturing.* It is important to be sure that the flap is not pulled coronally when suturing. Sutures should be placed first at the mesial and distal vertical incisions. The suture should be placed near to the margin of the free flap and sufficiently apically on the attached gingiva of the fixed tissue to ensure the degree of apical positioning required.

The margin of the flap can be secured with either loose separate interdental sutures or by means of a continuous suspensory suture (*Figure 16.7a, b*). Continuous suspensory suturing is useful in allowing manipulation of the flap margin where the bone margin is irregular and where the width of attached gingiva varies. Care should be taken not to pull the suture too tight, as this will drag the flap coronally. The tension on the suture can be adjusted at each loop, rather like loosening or tightening the lace of a shoe. The tension should be adjusted so that the flap margin just covers the bone margin (*Figure 16.6d*). It must be remembered that the continuous suture does not hold the flap in an apical position, but simply suspends it from the necks of the teeth. The degree of

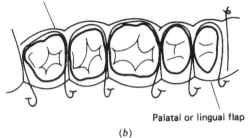

Figure 16.7 Diagram to show the continuous suspensory suturing technique: *(a)* a single tie is made at the anterior papilla and the buccal flap is suspended from the lingual root surfaces; *(b)* following adjustment of the apical position, the palatal or lingual flap is suspended against the buccal root surfaces. The suture is tied off at the end left on the single tie at the anterior papilla

apical positioning will be maintained by the correct placement of the periodontal pack.

7. *Placing the periodontal dressing.* It is usual to use Coe-Pack. Close adaptation of the flap to the underlying bone can be assured by pressing damp swabs over the flap while the periodontal dressing is being mixed. The dressing must be placed when it is freely mouldable. It should occupy the area between the flap margin and the crowns of the teeth so that it prevents any coronal displacement of the flap, and should also extend down to the base of the vestibular to maintain the vestibular depth. It should be carefully muscle trimmed.

8. *Healing.* The inner surface of the flap in contact with the bone and tooth undergoes inflammation, demolition, organization and healing. The blood clot, which should be thin, is replaced by granulation tissue in about a week. This matures into collagenous connective tissue in 2–5 weeks. The inner surface of the flap will unite with the bone to produce a mucoperiosteum, which increases the attached gingival zone.

About 2 days after surgery the epithelium will begin to proliferate from the flap margin over the connective tissue wound. It will migrate apically at the rate of 0.5 mm per day to produce a new junctional epithelium. As the margin of the flap just covers the bone, this will be of physiological length.

A mature epithelial attachment takes about 4 weeks to form. Some resorption of the alveolar bone margin will occur as the result of raising a flap, but with careful management this will be in the order of 0.5 mm. Connective tissue attachment will reform between the marginal tissues and the root cementum from the bone margin to the base of the junctional epithelium. It will prevent further apical migration of the junctional epithelium.

9. *Post-operative care*. The post-operative care is the same as for gingivectomy. The patient should however also be warned of facial swelling. This will develop over the first 3 post-operative days and then slowly reduce. The dressing and sutures are removed after 1 week, and the chlorhexidine mouthwash is usually discontinued a further week after this. The patient should be encouraged to return to normal brushing and flossing as soon as possible, and certainly no longer than 7 days after suture removal. An extra soft toothbrush should be used for 2–3 weeks. Particular care is necessary with plaque control during the first few weeks after surgery, since the tissues will be healing during this period and are particularly vulnerable to damage. Modification of these regimens must be made to take into account individual variation in healing.

Careful maintenance is necessary after this procedure. However, once immaculate plaque control is achieved, recall periods can be extended to 6 months as all pockets have been eliminated and a physiological length of junctional epithelium results.

Because apical repositioned flaps are often carried out in cases where bone loss is quite advanced, it is inevitable that the clinical crown will be lengthened. Patients must be warned of this beforehand.

This procedure can give excellent long-term results, providing that good oral hygiene is carried out by the patient and regular maintenance is carried out by the dentist and hygienist.

Comparison of apical repositioning and replaced flap techniques

It can be seen from the foregoing that the apically repositioned flap results in pocket elimination and the formation of a normal or physiological length of junctional epithelium, whereas the replaced flap results in the formation of a long junctional epithelium, which may adhere to the root surface (*Figure 16.4d*).

A long junctional epithelium must be regarded as inherently unstable because it lacks the mechanical support of gingival fibres passing into it from the crest of the bone and adjacent cementum. The stability of the delicate biological seal between the junctional epithelium and the root would seem to depend on a very high standard of oral hygiene and frequent regular maintenance visits. If any plaque is allowed to mature at the margin there is the risk

that subgingival plaque will become re-established and will proliferate apically to detach the epithelium and reform the pocket.

The result of an apically repositioned flap is much more stable, since pockets are eliminated and the dento-gingival junction is normal. This is particularly important for posterior teeth with furcation involvement.

Treatment of tuberosity involvement

The maxillary tuberosity may be large, flabby, unsupported by bone and related to a distal pocket on the last molar. It can be removed by making a radical gingivectomy incision, but this creates a large open wound that bleeds readily, can be painful and heals slowly. The retromolar pad in the lower jaw can present similar problems. Both situations can be dealt with by using the 'distal wedge' technique (*Figure 16.8*). Facial and lingual incisions are made through the tuberosity or retromolar pad to form a triangular wedge. The incisions must be deep enough to allow clean separation of the soft tissue wedge from the underlying bone. When the wedge is removed, any loose tags of tissue are trimmed and the distal root surface of the adjacent tooth cleaned. The edges of the wound are then sutured and the wound closed as completely as possible.

This procedure works well where the tissue is firm and fibrous, as it usually is with the maxillary tuberosity. However, it may be difficult or impossible to produce the desired result in the lower retromolar area when the tissue is soft and flabby.

Treatment of the edentulous ridge

If teeth involved in surgery are adjacent to an edentulous ridge that is covered by fibrous or flabby tissue, this can be removed by gingivectomy. However, the situation is

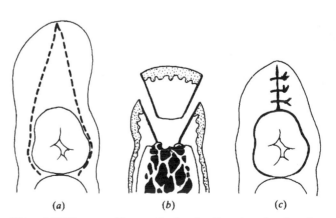

Figure 16.8 Diagram to illustrate distal wedge dissection of a tuberosity: *(a)* incision lines; *(b)* vertical section to show the wedge of tissue; *(c)* wound sutures

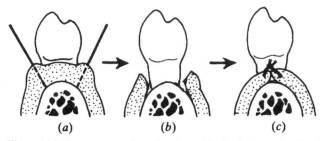

Figure 16.9 The treatment of an edentulous ridge is similar to the distal wedge. *(a)* Incisions mark out flabby ridge tissue, which is removed *(b)*. The wound is sutured *(c)*

better managed using a flap technique. Inverse bevel incisions are continued from around the teeth along the facial and lingual aspects of the edentulous ridge to dissect out a wedge of tissue with its base on the bone. This wedge of tissue is removed with curettes from the surface of the ridge. The edges of the flaps are then trimmed and sutured (*Figure 16.9*). The apical movement of the flaps will remove soft tissue pocketing mesial and distal to the two bordering teeth.

References

Ah, M.K.B., Johnson, G.K., Kaldahl, W.B. *et al.* (1994) The effect of smoking on the response to periodontal therapy. *Journal of Clinical Periodontology* **21**, 91–97

Brayer, W.K., Mellonig, J.T., Dunlap, R.M. *et al.* (1989) Scaling and root planing effectiveness: The effect of root surface access and operator experience. *Journal of Periodontology* **60**, 67–72

Caton, J. and Nyman, S. (1980) Histometric evaluation of periodontal surgery. 1. The modified Widman flap procedure. *Journal of Clinical Periodontology* **7**, 212–223

Caton, J., Nyman, S. and Zander, H. (1980) Histometric evaluation of periodontal surgery. II. Connective tissue attachment levels after four regenerative procedures. *Journal of Clinical Periodontology* **7**, 224–231

Friedman, N. (1962) Mucogingival surgery: the apically repositioned flap. *Journal of Periodontology* **33**, 328–340

Hill, R.W., Ramfjord, S.P., Morrison, E.C. *et al.* (1981) Four types of periodontal treatment compared over 2 years. *Journal of Periodontology* **52**, 655–662

Jones, J.K. and Triplett, R.G. (1992) The relationship of cigarette smoking to intra-oral wound healing: a review of evidence and implications for patient care. *Journal of Maxillofacial Surgery* **50**, 237–239

Kaldahl, W.B., Kalkwarf, K.L. and Patil, K.D. (1993) A review of longitudinal studies that compared periodontal therapies. *Journal of Periodontology* **64**, 243–253

Lindhe, J. and Nyman, S. (1984) Long-term maintenance of patients treated for advanced periodontal disease. *Journal of Clinical Periodontology* **11**, 504–514

Miller, P.D. Jnr (1987) Root coverage with free gingival graft. Factors associated with incomplete coverage. *Journal of Periodontology* **58**, 674–681

Moore, J.A., Ashley, F.P. and Waterman, C.A. (1984) The effect on healing of the application of citric acid during replaced flap surgery. *Journal of Clinical Periodontology* **14**, 130–135

Morris, M.L. (1965) The unrepositioned mucoperiosteal flap. *Periodontics* **3**, 141–151

Neumann, R. (1912) *Die Alveolar-Pyorrhea und ihre Behandlung.* Berlin: H. Meusser

Nyman, S., Rosling, B. and Lindhe, J. (1975) Effect of professional tooth cleaning after periodontal surgery. *Journal of Clinical Periodontology* **2**, 80–86

Pihlstrom, B.L., McHugh, R.B., Oliphant, T.H. and Ortiz-Campos, C. (1983) Comparison of surgical and non-surgical treatment of periodontal disease. A review of current studies and additional results after 6.5 years. *Journal of Clinical Periodontology* **10**, 524–541

Polson, A.M. and Proye, M.P. (1982) Effect of root surface alterations on periodontal healing. II. Citric acid treatment of the denuded root. *Journal of Clinical Periodontology* **9**, 441–454

Preber, H. and Bergström, J. (1990) Effect of cigarette smoking on periodontal healing following surgical therapy. *Journal of Clinical Periodontology* **17**, 324–328

Ramfjord, S.P. and Nissle, R.R. (1974) The modified Widman flap. *Journal of Periodontology* **45**, 601–607

Ramfjord, S.P., Caffesse, R.G., Morrison, E.C. *et al.* (1987) 4 modalities of periodontal treatment compared over 5 years. *Journal of Clinical Periodontology* **14**, 445–452

Widman, L. (1918) The operative treatment of pyorrhoea alveolaris. A new surgical method. *Svensk Tandlakare-Tidskrift* (special issue)

Wylam, J.M., Mealey, B.L., Mills, M.P. *et al.* (1993) The clinical effectiveness of open versus closed scaling and root planing on multi-rooted teeth. *Journal of Periodontology* **64**, 1023–1028

17

Management of bone defects and furcation involvement

As the periodontal lesion advances, the alveolar crest is resorbed and cancellous spaces are opened up. To compensate for resorption, some deposition may take place at sites more distant from the inflammation. The result of this remodelling process is the formation of bone defects, or 'intrabony' defects, of an infinite number of shapes. In Chapter 8 these have been classified as marginal defects, intra-alveolar defects, furcation defects and perforations, and can be further subdivided according to the number of bone walls bounding the defect.

The objectives of treatment of these defects are:

1. To eliminate the periodontal lesion
2. To achieve a tissue shape that will allow the patient to carry out efficient plaque control
3. If possible, to obtain some bone formation, increase in tooth attachment and improved tooth support.

Careful radiographic examination is essential to diagnosis, but even good radiographs may not reveal the presence of a bone defect or its precise morphology. This limitation can be overcome only by direct examination of the alveolar process, and all bone lesions are approached by lifting full-thickness mucoperiosteal flaps. In all cases granulations are curetted and root surfaces planed clean. When these procedures have been carried out it should be possible to examine the alveolar crest, define the morphology of any bone defect and decide on the mode of treatment.

Three basic options are available:

1. To shape the bone so that after healing and remodelling the resultant alveolar architecture will allow effective oral hygiene measures to be carried out (*Figure 17.1a*). This procedure, osteoplasty, must be undertaken with great care. Attempts to impose a stereotype of 'normal anatomy' are not justified. Cutting bone induces subsequent bone resorption, so that the final result could be loss of tooth support; therefore, osteoplasty should be resorted to only where gross bone deformity is present, e.g. buccal

ledges often associated with craters that extend into furcation areas.
2. To attempt to obtain some fill-in of the bone defect. This may be achieved with or without bone graft (*Figure 17.1b*).
3. To attempt to obtain new connective attachment. To date, this has been obtained only by guided tissue regeneration techniques and possibly some bone grafting techniques.

In practice the first two options are frequently used together, depending on the morphology of the bone defect. A three-walled intrabony defect offers a better chance of bony in-fill than a two-walled defect. A narrow, deep defect is more likely to be bridged by bone than a wide, shallow defect.

Bone reshaping

Osteoplasty is the term used for shaping bone that is not directly attached to the tooth. Ostectomy (osteo-ectomy) is the removal of bone that is directly involved in tooth support. Frequently these two procedures are carried out together. Bone may be removed by chisels or by rotating instruments, burs or diamond stones. If a rotating instrument is not adequately cooled, excessive bone loss may follow. If chisels are used to remove bone, the fragments may be used to fill in the bone defects. Small chisels, e.g. the Ochsenbein chisel, can be used with hand pressure. In attempting to obtain an acceptable bone shape, especially where there is a great deal of bone loss, a compromise must often be made to effect a balance between adequate tooth support and a cleanable tissue shape. No attempt should be made to reproduce some ideal bone architecture, as bone remodelling always follows surgery.

Bone reshaping is usefully applied to thickened and uneven alveolar margins, to marginal gutters (providing they are not very deep), interdental craters and two-walled

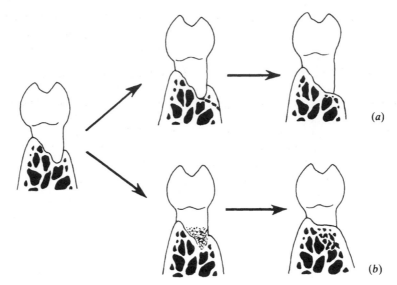

Figure 17.1 A bone defect may be treated by *(a)* bone reshaping to produce a cleanable tissue contour, or *(b)* an attempt to obtain fill-in (with or without graft) and reattachment

intrabony defects. When carrying out bone resection, the removed fragments may be used as an autograft in an attempt to obtain some fill-in of the defect.

Bone 'swaging' is the name given to a technique whereby a piece of bone is incompletely detached from its base (by a chisel) and swung into a neighbouring bone defect with some of its blood supply maintained. There is some clinical evidence of success following this procedure.

Periodontal tissue regeneration

The term 'reattachment' is used to describe the reunion of root and connective tissue separated by incision or injury, and the term 'new attachment' to describe the union of connective tissue with a previously pathogenically altered root surface. The cells with regenerative potential in the periodontal wound are junctional epithelial cells, gingival connective tissue cells, bone cells and periodontal ligament cells. The role of these tissues has been studied by clinical investigations and by the use of animal models, in particular the technique of producing experimental periodontitis in monkey teeth by placing orthodontic elastics into the gingival crevice (Caton and Zander, 1975).

Clinical investigations have shown that:

1. Alveolar bone has good regenerative capacity within two- and three-walled intrabony defects following inverse bevel flap surgery and curettage to remove all granulation tissue. Claims of success in obtaining bony in-fill of such defects vary greatly from 15–70%. These assessments are based, however, upon measurements of clinical attachment levels, radiographic measurements and clinical observation

following re-entry procedures, all of which are unreliable to varying degrees (Nyman *et al.*, 1990).

2. Bone regeneration may be encouraged or enhanced by the use of autograft cancellous bone or red bone marrow implants. With the latter material this may be complicated in some cases by root resorption and ankylosis unless it is frozen before use (Nyman *et al.*, 1990).

Melcher (1976) postulated that the cells that populate the root surface after surgery determine the nature of the healing process. These tissues will now be considered separately below.

Junctional epithelium

Junctional epithelium has a high regenerative capacity and will rapidly proliferate over the connective tissue wound surface. Using the monkey, Caton *et al.* (1980) studied the effect of four surgical procedures on the healing of experimental periodontal lesions:

1. Root planing and curettage
2. Replaced flap and curettage
3. Replaced flap followed by implantation of previously frozen autograft red marrow
4. Replaced flap followed by implantation of a bone substitute – beta tricalcium phosphate.

They found that all four procedures resulted in the formation of a long junctional epithelium to the presurgical level and extending to the base of the intrabony defects. Where bone regeneration occurred in intrabony defects, which was a frequent occurrence with all the open techniques, the epithelium always interposed itself between the new bone and the root surface. No new connective tissue attachment occurred.

Gingival connective tissue and bone

The effect of gingival connective tissue and bone on the healthy exposed root surface and the diseased root surface was studied in monkeys by Nyman *et al.* (1990). Extracted, partially periodontally diseased roots were buried below the surface of the edentulous ridge with one surface in contact with gingival connective tissue and one with bone. Reattachment occurred around the healthy portion of the root, but no reattachment occurred around the diseased portion. Both the bone and gingival connective tissue induced resorption of the diseased root surface. These experiments showed that granulation tissue derived from bone or gingival connective tissue does not have the capacity to form new connective tissue attachment to diseased root surfaces. It also shows that, in the clinical situation, the formation of a long junctional epithelium protects the root surface from resorption.

Periodontal ligament cells

The fact that new cementum with connective tissue attachment may occasionally form at the most apical portion of the periodontal wound suggests that coronal migration of periodontal ligament cells may be responsible for this (Melcher, 1976). This was confirmed by Nyman *et al.* (1990), using a monkey model that prevented junctional epithelial cells and gingival connective tissue cells from populating the wound. A portion of the buccal root surface of the canine tooth was exposed between the apex and the margin, then root planed to remove the cementum. The preservation of the marginal tissues prevented interference from apical migration of junctional epithelium, and the placement of a plastic filter barrier over the bony fenestration prevented ingress of gingival connective tissue cells when the wound was closed. After 3 months, new attachment had spread over the root surface from the margins of the fenestration and included new cementum, fibrous attachment and bone. This suggests that periodontal ligament cells have the capacity to develop new attachment if epithelium and gingival connective tissue are excluded from the wound during healing (Nyman *et al.*, 1990).

Methods aimed at the regeneration of periodontal tissues

Curettage for bony in-fill

The complete removal of inflammatory tissue from bony defects and careful root planing will often result in some bone in-fill produced by the activity of osteoblasts from the surrounding marrow spaces. No new cementum will form on the root surface, which will be covered by the junctional epithelium, and this will interpose itself between the new bone and the root, preventing resorption. A number of factors can prevent this from happening:

1. Choosing the wrong type of defect, i.e. one that is too wide and shallow, with too few bone walls. The ideal is the deep three-walled defect.
2. Failure to curette away all inflamed connective tissue and granulations.
3. Failure to clean the root surface completely.
4. Failure to close the flaps completely over the bone defect.
5. Infection and disintegration of the blood clot.
6. Excessive tooth mobility, which can disturb the healing tissues. Temporary immobilization of a very mobile tooth may help to protect the lesion from mechanical stress.

The surgical procedure to gain access may be an apically repositioned or replaced flap procedure, depending on the situation (Chapter 16). Particular attention is paid to closing the soft tissue wound over the bone lesion.

Eliminating the bone defect by reshaping is a more predictable procedure than curettage; therefore, in a situation where there is doubt about the treatment of the bone defect, the position of the lesion may well provide an answer to the dilemma. However, it must be borne in mind that in many cases bone resection will further reduce tooth attachment and is therefore contraindicated. In the posterior segment it may be better to treat the bone defect definitively by bone reshaping, whereas in anterior segments one needs to conserve bone to preserve the appearance.

Bone grafts

Attempting to obtain some fill-in of the bone defect and reattachment by simple curettage of the bone defect is an unpredictable procedure, and a number of different types of graft material have been tried. Graft materials are of four general types:

1. *The autograft*, which is bone from the same individual
2. *The allograft*, which is bone from an individual of the same species
3. *Xenografts*, which are bone from a different species, treated with ethylene diamine to remove the organic and antigenic fraction
4. *Grafts of bone substitutes and synthetic materials.* There are five types of alloplastic synthetic grafts available for clinical use, and these are:
   - *porous hydroxyapatite*
   - *non-porous hydroxyapatite*
   - *beta tricalcium phosphate*
   - *HTR polymer* (Mellonig, 1990)
   - *Bio-active glasses and ceramics* (Wilson and Low, 1992).

One of these, 'Periograft' or 'Durapatite', a non-porous hydroxyapatite, is illustrated in *Figure 17.2*.

The essential requirements of a graft material are that:

1. It should be immunologically acceptable
2. It should have osteogenic potential, i.e. it should contain viable bone cells which become active in the new site, or contain some chemical factor with osteogenic potential.

It would seem that graft materials that lack osteogenic potential act simply as a replacement for the blood clot, which usually breaks down, or as an inert scaffold on

Figure 17.2 Three radiographs showing a man of 50 years: *(a)* bone lesion between |45 caused by a lateral abscess; *(b)* post-operative radiograph showing graft (Periograft); *(c)* 1 year post-operative radiograph showing graft partly resorbed

which some bone formation takes place prior to the resorption of the graft. This is because cellular events of periodontal regeneration involve the controlled integration of a number of cell signalling systems for bone, cementum and periodontal ligament. Unless these are present in the graft material and/or the adjacent tissues in the right proportions, controlled regeneration cannot take place. However, regeneration of new cementum, periodontal ligament and alveolar bone can be achieved to some degree in intrabony defects with some grafting techniques, including autograft bone and marrow (Rosenberg, 1971; Hiatt and Schallhorn, 1973), human freeze-dried, demineralized bone allograft (Mellonig *et al.*, 1976; Rummelhart *et al.*, 1989), with bone substitutes such as bio-active glass (Wilson and Low, 1992) and possibly HTR polymer (Stahl *et al.*, 1990), and with guided tissue regeneration, GTR (see below).

Bone autograft

Bone autografts using iliac crest marrow (Hiatt and Schallhorn, 1973) or cancellous bone from oral sites (Rosenberg, 1971) have been used with some success. Cancellous bone and marrow can be obtained from a number of sites in the mouth, such as the tuberosity, extraction sockets or the edentulous ridge. The ideal autograft is obtained from the iliac crest, but it is doubtful whether tapping this site is justifiable. Also, fresh marrow tissue often produces root resorption and ankylosis; it must be frozen before use to prevent this. Shavings of cortical bone obtained from the neighbourhood of the bone defect, although not as useful or as effective as cancellous bone, may also be used. Unless bone formation is very rapid, as with fresh bone marrow tissue, junctional epithelium will usually migrate apically over the connective tissue wound to cover the root surface and protect it from root resorption.

Bone allograft

More recently, freeze-dried bone allograft has been used to treat periodontal osseous defects. Two types of bone allograft are in clinical usage. These are freeze-dried undemineralized bone allograft (FDBA) and freeze-dried demineralized bone allograft (FDDBA). Originally introduced as a periodontal material in 1976, it has been used successfully in clinical medicine for more than four decades (Mellonig, 1990). The freeze-drying permits storage within a vacuum for an indefinite shelf life, and also markedly reduces the antigenicity of the graft (Turner and Mellonig, 1981; Friedlaender, 1987; Quattlebaum *et al.*, 1988).

Clinical studies have shown that the use of the graft in intrabony defects following debridement produces more than 50% bony in-fill in 63% of the defects (Sanders *et al.*, 1983). Using a combination of FDBA and autograft bone to produce a composite graft produces this result in over 80% of defects (Sanders *et al.*, 1983). Although there is relatively little difference in the clinical results with

FDBA and FDDBA, the latter has largely superseded the former as a periodontal grafting material (Rummelhart *et al.*, 1989). FDDBA appears to have superior bone induction properties, and clinical studies indicate that sites grafted with this material produce more than 50% bony in-fill in 78% of sites, compared with only 38% of sites for debridement alone (Urist, 1965; Urist and Strates, 1971; Mellonig *et al.*, 1976; Mellonig, Bowers and Baily, 1981; Quintero *et al.*, 1982). In addition, human histological studies (Bowers *et al.*, 1989a, 1989b, 1989c) have provided evidence for regeneration of new bone, ligament and cementum using this material (see below). Furthermore, it has been shown that bone matrix contains bone inductive proteins (Sampath and Reddi, 1983), and several osteo-inductive signal molecules have been purified from FDDBA powder. These include bone morphogenic proteins (BMP) 2 and 7 (Sampath *et al.*, 1990) and six other distinct bone-derived growth factors (Hauschka *et al.*, 1986). It has also been suggested that the collagen matrix of the demineralized graft acts as a substrate for attachment, proliferation and differentiation of new osteoprogenitor cells (Sampath and Reddi, 1983).

The fate of FDDBA grafts in human intrabony defects has been studied in 12 patients with 32 grafted sites (Reynolds and Bowers, 1996). These lesions were removed *en bloc* after 6 months, and were examined histologically. This revealed that 72% of the grafted sites exhibited residual FDDBA particles, and these appeared amalgamated with new viable bone. Defects harbouring residual graft material showed significantly greater amounts of new attachment formation, including new bone, cementum and associated periodontal ligament, than sites without evidence of residual graft material.

However, some difficulties have been encountered in the placement and retention of particulate FDDBA grafts, especially in accessible and freely bleeding sites, when the material may be flushed out. In an effort to overcome these difficulties and improve the biological and physical handling properties, these bone grafts have been combined with microfibrillar collagen (Blumenthal *et al.*, 1986). The combined graft helped to bind and retain the particles, created a space between the particles and acted as a scaffold for cell and blood vessel ingrowth. In addition, it was claimed that the collagen material became bound to the root surface and prevented epithelial downgrowth. The material consists of a combination of human freeze-dried bone powder with human tendon collagen. Following rehydration it can be layered into a defect and expands to fill it. Clinical studies and experimental studies with dogs have been carried out with this material (Blumenthal *et al.*, 1986). Clinical re-entry was performed 5 months after the procedure, and found a mean 61% bone in-fill. Histological studies showed evidence of bone formation, periodontal regeneration and prevention of epithelial migration. The material has also been used successfully in humans (Blumenthal, 1994).

The possibility of disease transfer with bone allografts obtained from human cadaver material exists, but is nonetheless very unlikely if the material is procured and processed using established tissue banking protocols, which incorporate medical and social screening, antibody testing, direct antigen tests, serological tests, bacterial culturing and follow-up studies (American Association of Tissue Banks, 1984; Martin *et al.*, 1985; Quinnan *et al.*, 1986; Resnick *et al.*, 1986; Friedlaender, 1987; Buck *et al.*, 1989, 1990; Mellonig, 1990). The risk of disease transmission with FDDBA is 1 in 8 million. The HIV virus has been cultured from bone (Buck *et al.*, 1990), but is likely to be detected by the above tests and inactivated in the event of being missed in the screening process by the sterilization procedures used in the preparation of these materials.

It seems likely that most grafts act both as a replacement for the blood clot, which usually breaks down, and as a scaffold on which some bone formation takes place. There then follows a progressive resorption and replacement of the graft by new bone.

Bone xenograft

In contrast to FDDBA, bone mineral for implantation has also been produced which is free of organic component. This product, a xenograft, is known as bovine anorganic cancellous bone (BACB), or commercially as Bio-Oss®. It is produced from bovine bone by a special process, which removes its organic components but retains its inorganic structure. This product contains biological apatite crystals, and is either produced as cancellous blocks or granules. The same company also produces a porcine non-antigenic collagen (PNAC), known commercially as Bio-Oss® collagen. This is produced from healthy pigs and the collagen undergoes prolonged alkaline treatment, which produces a bilayer structure and eliminates any risk of bacterial or viral contamination. During further processing the terminal peptides (telopeptides) (see Chapter 5) are split off from the collagen molecules, and this process removes the areas most concerned with the antigenicity of the molecule. Also, specific purification processes remove any residual fat or protein from the processed collagen. PNAC is produced as a block, which can be cut or crushed to the desired size or consistency.

The antigenicity of grafts of BACB and composite BACB/PNAC have been compared with that of resorbable hydroxyapatite (see below) by implanting these materials subcutaneously into Wistar rats (Cohen *et al.*, 1994). The nature of the cellular infiltration around these materials in biopsies taken at 3 days and 1, 2, 4, 6 and 8 weeks was examined using immunocytochemistry. Biopsies of sites with all of the materials showed a transient infiltration of macrophages, which was maximal at 3 days, but this had resolved to normal levels by 6–8 weeks. Lymphocytic infiltration was not seen, and antibodies to bovine or porcine serum proteins or collagen were not detected. These data indicate that neither systemic nor local immune reactions developed in response to any of these materials.

The osteoconductive potential of BACB (Bio-Oss®), human FDDBA and resorbable hydroxyapatite (Osteogen®) have been compared in beagle dogs receiving dental implants (Wetzel *et al.*, 1995). Titanium dental implants (ITI®) (see Chapter 26) were placed into prepared edentulous sites, which were extended into the maxillary sinus by elevating the sinus floor. The area below the raised sinus floor contained the protruding implant tip, and was packed with one of these materials. The implanted material was placed so that it surrounded the implant tip and extended to the bone margin below. Sites implanted with human FDDBA showed no signs of new bone formation, whereas those implanted with BACB (Bio-Oss®) or resorbable hydroxyapatite (Osteogen®) did show significant new bone formation in this area. The use of bone markers (tetracycline or calcein green) revealed rapid bone formation and remodelling, especially around the BACB particles. Thus, both BACB and resorbable hydroxyapatite were shown to be osteoconductive in this situation.

The regenerative potential of composite grafts of BACB (Bio-Oss®) and PNAC (Bio-Oss®collagen) were studied by placing them into intrabony periodontal defects prepared in eight healthy beagle dogs (Clergeau *et al.*, 1996). The experimental lesions were either treated with a replaced flap plus curettage (control sites) or with additional composite BACB/PNAC grafts (test sites). After 6, 18 and 32 weeks post-operatively, non-decalcified block specimens were removed and examined by microscopy and contact microradiology. In the control sites, no significant bone regeneration was observed at any time period. In contrast, in the test sites bone trabeculae undergoing mineralization were seen at 6 weeks around the implanted particles above the reference notch. At 18 and 36 weeks, significant bone regeneration was seen. The periodontal ligament space adjacent to the new bone was always clear, and the only signs of ankylosis were seen within the reference notch at 18 weeks in one animal of the test group and at 36 weeks in one animal of the control group. Therefore, this combined graft material appears to have osteogenic potential in periodontal intrabony defects.

The main drawback with these materials is a very low risk of transmission of bovine or porcine viruses or other infective agents.

Synthetic bone substitutes

Synthetic bone substitutes are also available for clinical use. These materials avoid the problems of finding suitable autograft bone and the small risk of infective risks inherent in the use of human cadaver materials or other animal tissue. Five types of synthetic bone substitute are available, and all seem to produce better results than surgical debridement alone.

Porous and non-porous hydroxyapatite

Porous hydroxyapatite has a uniform pore size, which facilitates vascular ingrowth and subsequent new bone formation (Mellonig, 1990). Controlled studies in humans shows that it produces more bone in-fill in intrabony lesions than surgical debridement alone (Kenney *et al.*, 1985; Yukna *et al.*, 1986). Kenney *et al.* (1986) also showed histological evidence of new bone formation on the surface of and within the pores of porous hydroxyapatite. He placed this material into intrabony lesions of teeth with advanced periodontitis in human subjects, and removed the teeth and surrounding tissues for light and scanning electron-microscopical examination. Spreading osteoblasts and new bone were seen in contact with the particles.

In a 5-year follow-up study (Yukna *et al.*, 1989), non-porous hydroxyapatite has also been shown to be superior to surgical debridement in producing bony in-fill. It also showed that the condition remained stable for long periods following this treatment. Porous and non-porous hydroxyapatite and surgical debridement have been compared in the treatment of intrabony defects (Krejci *et al.*, 1987), and this study showed that non-porous hydroxyapatite produced the most consistent results. It is available commercially under the trade names of Periograf® and Alveolagraf®.

Tricalcium phosphate

Tricalcium phosphate has been shown to stimulate bone formation, and is comparable or in most cases superior in this regard to hydroxyapatite (Fetner *et al.*, 1994). It is produced commercially under the trade names of Synthagraft® and Augmen®. Its use in periodontal intrabony defects has been compared with hydroxyapatite (see above) and bio-active glass, Bioglass® (see below), in primates. It has been shown to stimulate bone formation to a greater extent than hydroxyapatite, but to a much lesser extent than Bioglass (Wilson and Low, 1992; Fetner *et al.*, 1994). However, it did not stimulate complete regeneration of the periodontium and did not retard epithelial downgrowth. In these regards it was similar to the effect of hydroxyapatite but unlike that of Bioglass (see below).

HTR polymer

HTR polymer is a non-resorbable, microporous biocompatible composite of poly-methylmethacrylate (PMMA) and polyhydroxyethylmethacrylate (PHEMA). This material has been used in the fabrication of contact lenses, lens transplants and prosthetic heart valves over many years. The polymer does not produce an inflammatory or immune response in contact with bone or soft tissue (Yukna, 1990). PMMA beads of 550–880 μm diameter with pores of 50–300 μm form the core of this material. These are coated with liquid PHEMA without the addition of any catalysts or inducers. The composite beads are then coated with calcium hydroxide/calcium carbonate. Thus, the actual surface interface with bone is the calcium surface layer, and both fibrous tissue and bone can form on and attach to this layer. The composite is provided in a fine granular form for use in periodontal intrabony defects.

Stahl *et al.* (1990) used this material in five volunteer patients with advanced periodontitis, and they provided 11 intrabony defects. These were surgically debrided and implanted with HTR polymer and the lesions were followed for 4–26 weeks. After this time, the teeth and blocks of tissue were removed for histological examination. The clinical observations showed a reduction in probing depth due to both gingival recession and a gain in clinical attachment level. The patients showed no untoward symptoms or signs during this period. Histological examination showed that the grafts became surrounded by connective tissue capsules, and some limited bone deposition was present on the surface of some implanted particles. The 11 lesions showed varied responses, and there were different responses between both patients and different sites in the same patient. In seven sites there was a long junctional epithelium between the root surface and the graft, whilst in four sites there was limited evidence of new attachment.

Yukna (1990) investigated the effectiveness of HTR polymer in treating intrabony lesions in 21 adult patients with moderate to advanced chronic periodontitis. Some sites were treated by surgical debridement alone, and some by debridement followed by implantation of HTR polymer. They were followed by clinical and radiographical measurements for 6 months, after which surgical re-entry procedures were carried out. The re-entry procedures showed that the sites implanted with HTR polymer showed significantly better mean bony in-fill (60.8%) than those treated by debridement alone (32.2%). Clinical and radiological measurements also showed significantly better results for the polymer group. These studies show that HTR polymer synthetic alloplast does show some promise for repair of periodontal osseous defects.

Bio-active glasses and ceramics

Certain types of glasses, glass–ceramics and ceramics composed primarily of SiO_2–CaO–Na_2O–P_2O_5 have been widely used in conjunction with medical and dental implants because they develop a layer of hydroxy-carbonate-apatite on their surface following exposure to body fluids. When used on the surface of metal implants, this layer incorporates collagen fibrils and in this way produces a mechanically strong bond between the implant and the adjacent bone surface (Hench and Wilson, 1984; Hench, 1986, 1994; Hench and West, 1996). Comparisons of SiO_2–CaO–Na_2O–P_2O_5 glasses with various other glass ceramics, SiO_2–CaO–P_2O_5 glasses, SiO_2 glasses, multi-component bio-active glasses and synthetic hydroxyapatites show that they all produce a strong interface bond with bone. However, most of these have a flexural strength, strain to fracture and fracture toughness less than bone. Also, the elastic modulus of the stronger and tougher bio-active glasses are greater than both cortical and cancellous bone. This would lead to excessive stress shielding of bone, and could eventually produce

fracture of bone distal and proximal to the implant. For these reasons their use with stress-bearing implants is limited, and is usually restricted to coating metal implants in non-load bearing areas or areas subject to compressive forces, such as vertebrae.

They have also been used for the treatment of periodontal intrabony defects (Wilson and Low, 1992), primarily because of their high bio-activity (see below).

Theory of bio-activity

The bio-activity of these materials is graded by their bio-active index, which depends on the rate of bone stimulation by these materials. The index is defined as the inverse of the time required for 50% of the implant surface to be bonded to bone.

Larger differences in the rate of bone bonding to bio-active implants indicates that different biochemical factors may occur at the implant tissue interface with different materials. The highly bio-active glass particulates show both osteoproduction and osteoconduction, whereas those with lower bio-activity show only osteoconduction (Hench, 1994; Hench and Wilson, 1995; Hench and West, 1996). Osteoproduction has been defined as the process in which the bio-active surface is colonized by osteogenic stem cells from the adjacent bone, whereas osteoconduction relates to the properties of the bio-active interface surface, which facilitate the migration of bone over it.

Wilson *et al.* (1994) have compared the effectiveness of a highly bio-active glass, 45S5 Bioglass®, with autogenous bone in the augmentation of canine ribs. They have shown that the 45S5 Bioglass® produced more bone formation than autogenous bone. They also showed that an equal mixture of Bioglass and autogenous bone was even more effective, and resulted after 6 weeks in the formation of twice the amount of new bone when compared with autogenous bone alone.

Oonishi *et al.* (1994), using the rabbit tibial model, have shown that 45S5 Bioglass® particulate enhanced new bone formation many times faster than hydroxyapatite particulate.

The same research group (Oonishi *et al.*, 1997) compared Bioglass® particulate and hydroxyapatite as a bone graft substitute. Holes 6 mm in diameter were drilled bilaterally in the femoral condyles of mature rabbits and, after haemostasis, these were filled with either particulate Bioglass or hydroxyapatite, with one material on each side providing its own control. The animals were sacrificed after 1, 2, 3, 6 and 12 weeks, and the areas were examined histologically. By 1 week, new bone was present on the surface of the Bioglass particles to the centre of the defect; by 2 weeks, all the particles were covered and those at the periphery were joined by trabecular bone. By 3 weeks all the particles were connected by thick bony bridges, and by 6 weeks they were all encased by new bone. By 12 weeks, the calcium and phosphate rich area extended throughout the remaining parts of the particles. The bone formation was much slower with the hydroxyapatite particulate, and whereas full restoration of bone was complete in 2 weeks with Bioglass, a comparable response took 12 weeks with hydroxyapatite. The Bioglass particulate was used up in this process, and therefore any problems associated with the production of a composite of bone and biological material are avoided in the fully restored bone.

In vivo studies have shown that there are probably two classes of bio-active materials, known as classes A and B. Class A bioactivity leads to osteoproduction, and class B to osteoconduction. Osteoproduction is thought to occur (Hench, 1994) when a material produces both intracellular and extracellular responses at its interface. Osteoconduction is thought to occur when a material produces only an extracellular response at its interface.

All class A bio-active materials release soluble silicon in the form of silicic acid due to surface ion exchange with H^+ and H_3O^+ on contact with body fluids, and this reaction occurs immediately on contact (Hench, 1994). The concentration of silicon in the solution rises until the solubility limit is reached, which is dependent on the pH and the relative concentrations of other chemical species, which can lead to the formation of complex silicate phases. Class A compounds release silicon by ion exchange and network dissolution, whereas class B materials have either low or zero ion exchange and release either very low or zero amounts of silicon.

It was first shown (Schwartz and Milne, 1972; Carlisle, 1986) that the released silicon is chemically combined with glycosaminoglycan–protein complexes, which surround collagen and elastic fibrils and cover the surface of cells.

Studies by Keeting *et al.* (1992) on human osteoblast-like cells have shown that soluble silicon is a potent mitogen for these cells. It was shown to increase the mitotic rate three-fold, and enhanced the release of alkaline phosphatase and osteocalcin from these cells. They found that the induction of genetically controlled intracellular autocrine factors appeared to be responsible for this response, and that the levels of mRNA for transforming growth factor beta (TGFβ), which is a potent mitogen for osteoblasts, were increased. Soluble silicon increased the release of latent TGFβ into the medium within 6 hours of stimulation.

Vrouwenvelder *et al.* (1993) grew human osteoblast-like cells on the surface of 45S5 Bioglass® and class B (hydroxyapatite) materials. They found that by 6 days there was enhanced alkaline phosphatase release from the cells on 45S5 Bioglass®, and by 8 days the amount released had doubled. The DNA content of the cells on this material was also increased. These changes were not seen with the cells grown on hydroxyapatite.

It has been proposed (Hench, 1994; Hench and West, 1996) that class A bio-active glasses provide both an intracellular effect by the release of silicon and an extracellular effect by the chemoabsorption of bone growth promoting factors such as TGFβ onto their surface. It has been shown that soluble silicon also accelerates the precipitation of an amorphous calcium phosphate phase from solution. This phase forms within the pores of the silica gel layer, where the porosity and silanols provide a heterogeneous nucleation mechanism for hydroxy-carbonite-apatite crystallization. Thus, the crystalline hydroxy-carbonite-apatite layer develops within a few hours on class A materials, whereas it may take many days or even weeks to develop on class B. The negatively charged silica gel and defect hydroxy-carbonite-apatite crystals provide sites for chemisorption of TGFβ and other growth factors released from proliferating osteoblasts. The absorbed growth factors are then thought to enhance differentiation and mitosis of stem cells, which migrate into the area from the adjacent bone marrow spaces. This then may create an autocatalytic growth of bone and other tissues.

The use of bio-active glasses in the treatment of periodontal intrabony defects

Wilson and Low (1992) compared the use of particulate 45S5 Bioglass® with commercially available hydroxyapatite (Periograf® and Alveolagraf®) and tricalcium phosphate (Synthagraft® and Augmen®) materials. Prepared periodontal intrabony defects were surgically created in the alveolar bone of six adult patus monkeys. In order to resemble pathological periodontal lesions, the root surface of the adjacent tooth was root planed. Eighteen such sites were prepared; 12 were filled with Bioglass particulate, two with hydroxyapatites, two with tricalcium phosphate materials, and the remaining two were left unfilled. The animals were killed after 4 weeks (1), 4 months (2), 6 months (2) and 9 months (1). The alveolar bone and attached soft tissues were removed and examined microscopically, with particular reference to the tooth/defect interface and the position and length of the junctional epithelium. They looked for particular histological evidence of regeneration of all the elements of the periodontium, i.e. bone, cementum and inserting periodontal ligament fibres.

Hydroxyapatite only resulted in partial restoration of bone by osteoconduction over the particles by 9 months, there was a long junctional epithelium, and no new attachment was seen. Tricalcium phosphate was very reactive throughout the study period and there was significant bone production and, in some sites, root resorption and ankylosis. Cementoid lined the defect quite quickly but failed to allow the regeneration of normal periodontium, and a long junctional epithelium formed. The use of Bioglass particulate did, however, allow the regeneration of a normal periodontium. Immediately after implantation, fibroblasts laid down collagen above the level of the particulate, and this collagen appeared to attach to the superficial particles, immobilizing them in the soft tissue and restoring the transeptal connections of the periodontium. This appeared to prevent epithelial downgrowth, which only occurs to the point at which it meets adherent collagen fibres overlying the restoring bone. Beneath this layer the particles induced a rapid production of bone and cementum, and by 9 months the particles were seen within the repairing bone and cementum. A normal periodontal ligament was seen between these tissues.

Fetner *et al.* (1994) compared the extent of periodontal regeneration in surgically created bony defects in six patus monkeys of 45S5 Bioglass® (PerioGlas® and Fluoride PerioGlas®) compared with tricalcium phosphate (Synthagraft® or Augmen®) or hydroxyapatite (Alveolagraf®). Each animal had a total of 18 sites in which 4 mm osseous defects were prepared; most of these were two-walled interproximal defects, but some were palatal and lingual three-walled defects. Adjacent root surfaces were planed and existing periodontal ligament and cementum was removed. Twelve sites were filled with Perioglas® particulates, two each with hydroxyapatite and tricalcium phosphate, and two remained as unfilled controls. Histological analyses were carried out at 1, 4 and 6 months. Histologically, Perioglas® sites showed superior bone and cementum regeneration to the other materials, with statistically higher percentages of both new cementum and bone. Perioglas® was also much more effective in retarding epithelial downgrowth than the other materials, and this could be one reason for its superiority.

The two properties of the Bioglass particulate that appeared to contribute to these favourable results seem to be first, the increased rate of reaction *in vivo* that it possesses in comparison to the other materials as a result of its release of silicon (see above), and secondly, that it appeared to bond with connective tissue collagen. Because of its high bio-activity, the reaction layers appear to form within minutes of its implantation and the osteogenic cells freed by the surgery can rapidly colonize the particles. This process supplements the bone, which grows by osteoconduction from the alveolus, and these two processes combined have been termed osteoproduction (Wilson *et al.*, 1987). This results in more rapid filling of the defects than occurs with other less active materials, such as hydroxyapatite. This may also result from a more rapid accumulation of bone morphogenic proteins and other growth factors on the surface of bioactive particles (Watanabe *et al.*, 1990). The prevention of epithelial downgrowth is probably the result of the rapid establishment of collagen over the coronal surface of the implanted particles, and could be explained by a direct inhibitory effect on epithelium or to the rapid deployment and attachment of collagen fibres beneath the advancing epithelium.

Bioglass particulate has also been used to stimulate bone formation in extraction sockets, and to thus maintain the alveolar ridge height (Hench *et al.*, 1991; Wilson *et al.*, 1993; Hench and Wilson, 1995).

Cementum formation stimulants

Enamel matrix derivative (Emdogain®)

The use of enamel matrix derivatives (EMD) for periodontal regeneration has been suggested because it is thought that this process might mimic the way these materials behave in normal tooth development. In this regard, studies during the last 20 years have indicated that enamel-related proteins appear to be involved in the formation of cementum.

The initial formation of cementum and root formation are intimately related. It was previously thought that Hertwig's epithelial root sheath (HERS) induced mesenchyme cells of the dentine papilla to form mantle predentine before it disintegrated to expose the mesenchymal cells of the dental follicle to the newly formed dentine. This event was then believed to induce cementogenesis (Bosshardt and Schroeder, 1996). However, it has now been shown that exposure of follicular cells to slices of root dentine does not provide a sufficient stimulus for cementoblast differentiation (Thomas and Kollar, 1988). The HERS is the apical extension of the dental organ and the inner layer of the sheath represents extension of the ameloblast layer in the dental organ, and this has led to the proposal that enamel-related proteins from the epithelial root sheath are involved in the formation of cellular cementum (Stavkin, 1976).

Enamel matrix proteins were first demonstrated on the root-analogue surfaces of rabbit incisors (Schonfield and Slavkin, 1977), and their role was further suggested by the finding that the HERS cells of the developing rat molars contained organelles suggestive of secretory activity (Owens, 1978, 1979).

Further support was gained from scanning electron microscope and autoradiographic studies on developing monkey incisors (Lindskog, 1982a, 1982b; Lindskog and Hammarström, 1982). This demonstrated that the inner layer of the epithelial root sheath had a secretory stage, and that an enamel-like material was formed in the root surface prior to cementum formation or as an initial step in this process. It was also shown that a cellular cementum contains proteins that are immunologically related to proteins present in enamel matrix (Slavkin *et al.*, 1989a, 1989b).

An association between enamel and cementum formation is also supported by the fact that coronal cementum is a normal structure on the enamel surface of a variety of rodents and herbivora such as elephants, sheep, cows, rabbits and guinea pigs (Ainamo, 1970). Coronal cementogenesis seems to be initiated by the exposure of the cells of the dental follicle to the developing enamel.

The major proteins of the enamel matrix are known as amelogenins, and they constitute about 90% of the matrix (Brookes *et al.*, 1995). The dormant protein known as amelogenin exists in several different sizes, which together form aggregates. These are markedly hydrophobic and play a major role in crystal formation. Other enamel matrix proteins have been identified recently by cloning and DNA sequencing, and these have been termed ameloblastin (Krebsbach *et al.*, 1996) and amelin (Cerny *et al.*, 1996).

Immunohistochemical (Thomas *et al.*, 1986) and *in situ* hybridization studies (Luo *et al.*, 1991) on developing rat molars have indicated that the enamel proteins expressed during root formation are not identical to amelogenin. It has also been shown by *in situ* hybridization that amelin is expressed by cells of HERS in rat molars during root formation (Fong *et al.*, 1996).

However, recently a number of further studies have been carried out on the role of enamel proteins in cementogenesis. The dominating constituent of enamel matrix, amelogenin, has been shown by immunohisto-chemistry to be expressed at the apical end of the forming root of human teeth, and also to be present in the Tomes granular layer of such teeth (Hammarström, 1997). This study, using a rat model, showed that, when the mesenchymal cells of the dental follicle were exposed to enamel matrix, a non-cellular hard tissue closely resembling cellular cementum was formed at the enamel surface. It was also shown that the application of porcine enamel matrix into prepared experimental cavities of the roots of monkey incisor teeth induced the formation of acellular cementum that was well attached to dentine. Control roots in these monkeys, which were sham operated and not treated with enamel matrix, formed a cellular, poorly attached hard tissue.

The ability of enamel matrix proteins to induce cementum formation and periodontal regeneration was first investigated in a buccal dehiscence monkey model (Hammarström *et al.*, 1977). Buccal mucoperiosteal flaps were raised from canine to first molar on each side of the maxilla, and the buccal alveolar bone plate, exposed periodontal ligament and cementum were removed. The exposed roots were then conditioned with citric acid and rinsed with saline. Various preparations of porcine enamel matrix with or without vehicles were applied before the flaps were reapplied and sutured.

After 8 weeks, the healing was evaluated by light microscopy and morphometric measurements. It was found that the application of homogenized enamel matrix or acidic extract of the matrix containing the hydrophobic, low molecular weight proteins, amelogenins, resulted in almost complete regeneration of acellular cementum firmly attached to the dentine and with collagenous fibres extending over to newly formed alveolar bone – i.e. complete regeneration of periodontium. In contrast, application of fractions obtained by neutral EDTA extraction containing the acidic, high molecular weight proteins of enamel matrix produced very little new cementum and hardly any new bone. This lack of regeneration was also seen in control animals in which no test substance was applied before the repositioning of the flaps. Three vehicles for enamel matrix proteins, propylene glycol alginate (PGA), hydroxyethyl cellulose and dextran, were tried, and it was shown that only PGA in combination with the amelogenin fraction resulted in significant regeneration of periodontium.

The effects of PGA formulations of enamel matrix proteins on cell kenetics and colonization were investigated using cell culture techniques and rat, pig and monkey models (Gestrelius *et al.*, 1997a). It was shown that enamel matrix derivatives (EMD) can be dissolved in PGA at an acid pH, resulting in a highly viscous solution. At neutral pH and body temperature the viscosity decreases and EMD precipitates, and it has been shown that it absorbs to hydroxyapatite, collagen and denuded dental roots. By using radiolabelled preparations in rats and pigs it was shown that it forms insoluble spherical complexes on the tooth surface and remains in detectable amounts at the site of application for 2 weeks. Using a monkey model, they also showed by scanning electron microscopy that EMD in PGA promoted a repopulation of the root surface by fibroblast-like cells during the first weeks after application.

Further cell culture studies on periodontal ligament cells and EMD were carried out (Gestrelius *et al.*, 1997b). These investigated the effects of EMD on migration, attachment, proliferation, biosynthetic activity and mineral nodule formation of these cells, and their ability to absorb a large range of polypeptide growth factors and cytokines. In culture, EDM formed protein aggregates that appeared to provide ideal conditions for cell–matrix interactions. Under these conditions, EMD enhanced the proliferation of periodontal ligament (PDL) cells but not epithelial cells, increased the protein and collagen production of PDL cells and promoted mineral nodule formation by these cells. However, it appeared to have no effect on the migration, attachment and spreading of these cells, nor did they absorb any of the growth factors or cytokines that were tested.

The ability of EDM to produce periodontal regeneration in the buccal dehiscence model was also tested in one human experimental defect (Heijl, 1997). This defect was produced in a volunteer on a lower incisor, which was to be removed for orthodontic treatment of incisor crowding. A defect was created on this tooth in a similar manner to that described in the monkey model above. The EMD was applied to the conditioned surface and the flaps were replaced and sutured. After 4 months, the experimental tooth together with the surrounding soft and hard tissues were removed surgically for histological evaluation. This revealed the formation of new acellular extrinsic fibre cementum, which was firmly attached to the underlying dentine. A new periodontal ligament with inserting and functionally orientated collagen fibres and associated alveolar bone was also present. The new cementum covered 73% of the original defect, and the new bone covered 65% of the presurgical bone height.

The clinical safety of the commercially developed PGA-EMD product (Emdogain[®]) was tested in an open controlled study design in 10 Swedish specialist clinics, and 107 patients were treated with the product (Zetterström *et al.*, 1997). Two surgical procedures were carried out on most patients, at local intrabony sites. In addition, a control group of 33 patients underwent flap surgery without the application of Emdogain[®] at one comparable site. Serum samples were taken from the test patients for the analysis of total and specific IgG and IgE antibody levels. None of the samples, even from allergy-prone patients, produced any deviations of antibody levels from baseline ranges, and this indicates that the immunogenic potential of Emdogain[®] is extremely low when used in this way. Comparisons of test and control patients indicated the same frequency of post-surgical experiences. About half the patients were evaluated again after 3 years. There was a significant difference between the test and control results at 8 months post-treatment, and this difference had increased further at the 3-year follow up. There was a 2.5–3 mm gain of clinical attachment and bone levels, assessed clinically and radiographically, in the test subjects.

The ability of Emdogain® to treat intrabony periodontal defects effectively has also been studied in a placebo-controlled, randomized multicentre trial involving 33 patients with 34 paired test and control sites (Heijl et al., 1997). It was designed to compare the long-term effects of this material as an adjunct to modified Widman flap (MWF) surgery with the effect of MWF plus placebo treatment. The design required two comparable interproximal intrabony lesions, appropriately separated in the same jaw, with probing pocket depths greater than 6 mm and intrabony defects at least 4 mm deep. Only predominantly one- and two-walled defects were included, to allow radiographical assessment. Clinical and radiographic assessments were made at baseline, 8, 16 and 36 months post-treatment. Mean values for probing attachment level gains in test and control sites at 8 months were 2.1 mm and 1.5 mm respectively; at 16 months, 2–3 mm and 1–7 mm respectively; and at 36 months, 2.2 mm and 1.7 mm respectively. The radiographic bone level continued to increase over the 36 months at the test sites, whilst it remained close to the baseline level at control sites. There was a statistically significant gain in radiographic bone level at 36 months of 2.6 mm at the test sites, which corresponded to a 66% fill of the original bony defect.

This study (Heijl et al., 1997) has indicated that the topical application of Emdogain® to the conditioned root surface of diseased teeth with intrabony defects will promote a gain in clinical attachment and bone following MWF surgery compared to control (placebo application) in the same patient.

Taken together, all of these studies show that EMD will stimulate the regeneration of firmly attached acellular cementum in experimentally prepared root surfaces and will also produce complete regeneration of periodontium in the buccal dehiscence models. Furthermore, it has been shown to produce good clinical and radiographical indications of attachment and bone gain when used to treat naturally occurring, diseased intrabony defects. In addition, the role of EMD in promoting acellular cementum formation in these situations appears to mimic its role in the normal development of teeth. However, it must be emphasized that not all research in this area supports these findings and two research group show findings that cast doubt on some of these concepts. (Thomas et al., 1986; Luo et al., 1991).

Possible formation of new attachment following bone grafting procedures or the use of cementum stimulating agents

The ability of new attachment to form between bone and the treated root surface during the healing of intrabony defects has been extensively studied in human subjects by Bowers et al. (1989a, 1989b, 1989c). This was investigated on human subjects with advanced periodontitis who had teeth destined for extraction. These teeth were subjected to the experimental procedures and then removed 6 months later with a block of surrounding bone for histological examination. The intrabony defects were exposed surgically and thoroughly debrided, and the root surfaces were then scaled and root planed. Some intrabony defects were grafted with freeze-dried demineralized bone allograft (FDDBA). Some teeth were left exposed in the mouth, and others had their root surfaces submerged. This was done by cutting off the crown level with the highest level of the alveolar bone and coronally advancing the buccal flap to completely cover the root face (Bowers et al., 1989a).

They found that, on the teeth with osseous defects receiving debridement only, no new attachment formed on the exposed teeth. All of these lesions healed by the formation of a long junctional epithelium, which extended down the treated root surface. However, new attachment apparatus, consisting of new bone, new cementum and new periodontal ligament, did form on the submerged root surfaces (Bowers et al., 1989a). They also found that grafting the intrabony defect with FDDBA did significantly increase the amount of new attachment apparatus that formed on submerged roots (Bowers et al., 1989b). However, the formation of some new attachment apparatus was also seen on exposed teeth with defects that were additionally grafted with FDDBA (Bowers et al., 1989c). New cellular cementum formed equally well on treated old cementum or dentine. No evidence of extensive root resorption, ankylosis or pulp death was seen on any of the exposed teeth or submerged roots. Thus, some new attachment apparatus may form in intrabony lesions grafted with FDDBA, and could possibly also occur with other graft materials.

Bioglass® particulate used in prepared intrabony defects (Wilson and Low, 1992) has been claimed to result in retardation of epithelial downgrowth and the restoration of alveolar bone, cementum and periodontal ligament (see above). This is by far the best result claimed for any bone or bone substitute graft.

The ability of enamel matrix derivative (Emdogain®) to stimulate the formation of firmly attached acellular cementum appears to then stimulate the regeneration of the other associated tissue of the periodontium, i.e. inserting periodontal ligament fibres and alveolar bone. In this regard it has been shown to be capable of producing full regeneration of the periodontal supporting apparatus in experimental buccal dehiscence defects in monkeys and humans (Hammarström et al., 1977, Heijl, 1997). It may therefore have the potential to bring about a similar regeneration when used to treat diseased sites such as intrabony and furcation defects, and there is good clinical and radiographic evidence that it may do so (Zetterström et al., 1997; Heijl et al., 1997).

Summary of treatments of intrabony defects

In summary, it can be said that new bone formation can regularly occur in surgically treated intrabony defects. The studies reported above indicate that surgical debridement of the lesion alone can result in up to 30% bony infill, whilst the additional use of autogenous bone grafts, freeze-dried bone allografts, demineralized freeze-dried bone allografts, grafts of bovine anorganic cancellous bone and porcine non-antigenic collagen, alone or together, and synthetic bone substitutes produce varying responses, but usually result in greater levels of bony infill up to a maximum of 60–70%. The extent of gain in new attachment is very variable with bone grafts but can sometimes occur, presumably by the material acting as a barrier to epithelial downgrowth (see below). It is possible that some of the grafting materials, e.g. FDDBA, may also contain growth factors, which may promote connective tissue, bone and cementum regeneration (see above). It is also possible that, in the future, synthetic bone allografts such as HTR-polymer may act as vehicles for selective growth promoting factors as the precise functions of these become known. Bio-active materials like Bioglass® appear to result in regeneration of periodontium by their active stimulation of bone and cementum growth and attachment of collagen fibres (see above).

The use of bone substitutes, bovine anorganic cancellous bone or porcine non-antigenic collagen (PNAC) avoid the tiny risk of human disease transfer with carefully prepared allografts of human cadaver bone such as FDDBA. The use of bovine or porcine xenografts also carries a tiny risk of transfer of animal disease to humans, but whether this is possible is unsure. However, human, bovine and porcine materials are all very carefully prepared and tested to avoid this problem (see above).

Guided tissue regeneration (GTR)

The capacity of the various periodontal tissues to regenerate has been discussed previously. Alveolar bone and cementum have good powers of regeneration, provided that the necessary cell types and cell signals are present. The same is true for periodontal ligament, but for this to form a functional attachment, the collagen fibres must become enclosed by newly formed bone on one surface and cementum on the other. This requires the regeneration of the three tissues to be finely integrated. Also, for any new attachment to form, junctional epithelium, which proliferates over exposed connective tissues, must be excluded from the wound. Gingival connective tissue must also be excluded and prevented from providing any cells to the healing area, and at the same time a space needs to be created between the membrane and the root surface of the tooth to allow the periodontal ligament and/ or the alveolar marrow space cells to migrate, differentiate, proliferate and eventually repopulate the previously exposed root surface (Nyman *et al.*, 1982a, 1982b; Wikesjo *et al.*, 1992; Gottlow, 1993).

Early studies

Early experimental animal studies involved the use of barrier membranes to facilitate the proliferation of the various periodontal tissue components and thereby alter the healing response following periodontal surgery (Nyman *et al.*, 1982a; Gottlow *et al.*, 1984; Aukhil *et al.*, 1987; Caffesse *et al.*, 1988).

It was shown first in monkeys that periodontal ligament cells can proliferate over planed root surfaces if epithelial cells, bone cells and gingival connective tissue cells are excluded from the healing wound by the placement of a membrane (Nyman *et al.*, 1982b; Gottlow *et al.*, 1984). Similar results were reported in clinical studies on human teeth with advanced periodontitis and intrabony defects (Nyman, 1982a, 1983; Gottlow *et al.*, 1986). Some new attachment in the form of cementum with embedded collagen fibres and bone or bone-like tissue was formed using this technique, and this has been demonstrated histologically both on monkey teeth (Nyman *et al.*, 1982b; Gottlow *et al.*, 1984) and on extracted human teeth (Nyman, 1982a, 1983). It has also been observed by longitudinal clinical observation on retained human teeth (Gottlow *et al.*, 1986). The basis of the technique is the exclusion of epithelium and gingival connective tissue from the wound by the membrane to allow time for periodontal ligament cells to migrate coronally and differentiate into functional cells for the three periodontal tissues – bone, cementum and periodontal ligament.

Barrier membranes

There are five criteria considered to be important in the design of barrier membranes used for GTR (Greenstein and Caton, 1993; Scantlebury, 1993; Hardwick *et al.*, 1995). These include:

1. Biocompatibility
2. Cell-occlusiveness
3. Spacemaking
4. Tissue integration
5. Clinical manageability.

In order to achieve the mechanical tissue separation and support, various types of materials have been developed, which can be grouped together as either non-resorbable or resorbable membranes.

Non-resorbable membranes

The first membranes used experimentally by Nyman's group in their initial work were constructed from Millipore® (cellulose acetate) filters, since these were easily available in the laboratory and were packed and stored in sterile conditions.

However, as the potential of this technique was realized, commercial membranes were developed for clinical use. The first of these were made from Teflon® (expanded polytetrafluoroethylene, ePTFE). This material was chosen because it had been found to be biocompatible in the human body, and has been used for some time in reconstructive vascular surgery for replacement arteries.

This membrane consisted of two parts: a collar portion, having open pores to allow ingrowth of connective tissue and to prevent epithelial migration; and an occlusive portion, preventing the flap tissues from coming into contact with the root surface (Scantlebury, 1993). Because the space defined and protected by the membrane determined the volume of tissue that could be regenerated, the material was redesigned with a stiff central portion to treat osseous defects (Scantlebury, 1993; Hardwick *et al.*, 1995) and reinforced with titanium for both osseous and periodontal defects (Hardwick *et al.*, 1995; Cortellini *et al.*, 1995a; Sigurdsson *et al.*, 1995b).

Since these membranes are made of a non-resorbable material, a second surgical procedure is necessary to remove them. This procedure therefore has the disadvantage of additional trauma to the patient as well as to the healing periodontal tissues.

Clinical procedure

The area is first exposed by raising a flap developed with an intercrevicular incision to preserve keratinized gingiva. Pocket-lining epithelium is then removed from its inner aspect. All granulation tissue is removed, and the roots are thoroughly planed. A flexible Teflon (ePTFE) membrane (Gore-tex®) is carefully trimmed to cover the lesion. This consists of a narrow, open microstructure margin, which is designed to allow connective tissue penetration to produce a seal at the coronal margin of the root, as well as an occlusive membrane (*Figure 17.3*). It is adapted to fit over the intrabony defect and the root of the tooth, extending from 2–3 mm below the bone margin to just below the CEJ on the root (*Figure 17.4*). This prevents the oral epithelium and gingival connective tissue contacting the root surface during healing. It is held in place by a Teflon sling suture, which passes through both edges of the membrane upper margin and around the tooth. The flap is then sutured back with Teflon sutures to just cover the membrane. The membrane is left in place for 4–6 weeks and then removed. A further marginal incision exposes the membrane, and this is very carefully separated from the delicate healing tissue, which appears like a gelatinous red jelly. The flap is then sutured back.

It must be stressed that this technique is applicable only to the treatment of single teeth with two- or three-walled intrabony defects. At present it is still in the development stage and undergoing careful clinical assessments. As explained in the following text, GTR can be used to treat either intrabony or furcation defects.

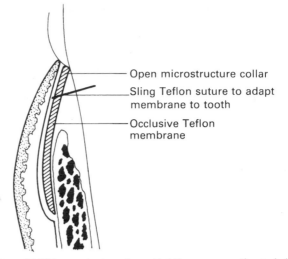

Open microstructure collar
Sling Teflon suture to adapt membrane to tooth
Occlusive Teflon membrane

Figure 17.3 Diagram to show the guided tissue regeneration technique described by Nyman *et al.* (1983). After exposure of the area by raising a flap, all granulation tissue is removed and the root surface carefully planed. A Teflon membrane is then adjusted to cover the root surface from apical to the bone margin to just below the cemento-enamel junction. It is interposed between these structures and the flap so that epithelium migrating apically over the connective tissue surface is prevented from contacting the root

Figure 17.4 An ePTFE barrier membrane secured into place with a sling suture over an intrabony defect mesial to the upper right first molar

Clinical trials of GTR using non-resorbable membranes

GTR techniques have been used for treatment of both interproximal intra-osseous defects and furcation defects in humans, and there have been many short- and long-term clinical studies of their use. Histological evaluation of the outcome of this therapy in humans has presented some difficulties due to ethical considerations. Clinical parameters are therefore used to assess the healing response in longitudinal investigations of patients undergoing this treatment. These parameters include clinical attachment level (CAL), probing pocket depth (PPD), gingival recession and bone fill, as well as bone density and height using radiographs (Garrett, 1996). The results are assessed by comparing pre- and post-treatment data over a reasonably long time scale. The response of the bone to GTR has also to be assessed by quantitative digital subtraction radiology (see Chapter 12) (Cristgau *et al.*, 1996).

Human clinical studies using non-resorbable (ePTFE) membranes have demonstrated that GTR therapy significantly improves the clinical outcome compared to conventional flap surgery. Thus, several short-term clinical studies reported significant reductions in PPD (ranging from 3.5–5.9 mm) and significant gains in CAL (ranging from 3–6 mm) and bone levels (ranging from 2.7–4.7 mm) following GTR treatment (Gottlow *et al.*, 1986; Schallhorn and McClain, 1988; Becker *et al.*, 1988; Pontoriero *et al.*, 1988, 1989; Caffesse *et al.*, 1990; Cortellini *et al.*, 1990, 1993a, 1993b, 1995b, 1996a; Gottlow, 1993; Tonetti *et al.*, 1993; Kilic *et al.*, 1997; Eickholz *et al.*, 1998). All these studies have shown that a gain in clinical attachment level may occur on teeth with a variety of intrabony and furcation defects using this technique.

Cortellini *et al.* (1993a, 1993b) treated interproximal intra-osseous defects using ePTFE membranes, and observed a significant gain in CAL, reduction in PPD and radiographic evidence of new formation of alveolar bone 1 year post-operatively, while Pontoriero *et al.* (1988) demonstrated complete resolution of more than 90% of class II furcation defects 6 months following GTR therapy.

Recently it has been also shown that these changes can be maintained over 1–5 years (Gottlow *et al.*, 1992; Weigel *et al.*, 1995; Machtei *et al.*, 1996; Cortellini *et al.*, 1996a). Gottlow *et al.* (1992) found a continuous increase in bone density in both types of defect over the 13-month test period.

When the clinical efficacy of ePTFE membranes and titanium-reinforced ePTFE membranes was compared, significant clinical improvements were obtained in both of the membrane groups, but the gain in CAL in the titanium-reinforced group was found to be greater than that in the ePTFE group (Cortellini *et al.*, 1995a).

Another recent study (Murphy, 1996) investigated the effects of prolonged placement of ePTFE membranes on the amount of regeneration. A modified surgical technique was described, which allowed substantial coverage of the barriers for a period of 4 months. Twelve intrabony defects were treated in this way, and the amount of bone fill was assessed by a re-entry procedure after 1 year. The results showed a mean bony in-fill of 95%, with three sites showing additional supracrestal bone growth. This suggests that the prolonged retention of a barrier membrane may increase the amount of regeneration. This relationship has also been found when membranes are used in connection with implants. In this situation the membrane can be completely buried and left *in situ* for 6 months (see Chapter 26).

The potential problem of prolonged retention with periodontal lesions is that of communication with the mouth via the gingival crevice, which may result in progressive bacterial contamination (see below).

There are, however, some reports that show that the results of GTR are unpredictable and on many occasions show results that have no advantage over conventional surgery (Warren and Karring, 1992; Proestakis *et al.*, 1992). In this regard, Pritlove-Carson *et al.* (1993) reported on a series of matched intrabony lesions in patients, where one lesion was treated with GTR and one with conventional surgery. They found no difference between the test and control sites in respect of probing depth, probing attachment level or recession.

With respect to the unpredictable nature of GTR treatment, it has been shown that failure to achieve the formation of new attachment can be due to a number of clinical variables. Those reported are shortcomings in the surgical technique (Caffesse and Quinones, 1992; Becker and Becker, 1990), restrictions in the size and configuration of the periodontal defect (Gottlow *et al.*, 1986) and limiting features of tooth anatomy (Lu, 1992). These studies also show that the achievement of membrane stability and total coverage of the membrane are important in achieving success.

Experimental animal studies using non-resorbable membranes

Experimental studies using prepared defects in dogs and monkeys also showed histological evidence of regenerative new cementum with embedded collagen fibres at test sites in intrabony lesions and Class II and III furcation defects (Nyman *et al.*, 1982b; Aukhil *et al.*, 1983, 1986; Gottlow *et al.*, 1984, 1990; Caffesse *et al.*, 1988, 1990; Pontoriero *et al.*, 1992). This did not occur at control sites. However, the results were variable at sites with Class III furcation involvement and extensive intrabony lesions. Thus, success was found to be partly dependent on the size, shape and apical extent of the lesion.

Bacterial contamination of membranes

The use of non-resorbable membranes has been associated with membrane contamination and/or infection when the membrane is exposed to the oral cavity (Selvig *et al.*, 1990; Tempro and Nalbandian, 1993; Grevstad and Leknes, 1993; Nowzari and Slots 1994; Nowzari *et al.*, 1996).

It has also been clearly shown that artificially buried defects in animals heal considerably better than exposed defects, and this is also found in the clinical situation (Sander and Karring, 1995a). One of the reasons for this is that exposed membranes become extensively contaminated and penetrated by bacteria from the oral and subgingival flora (Simion *et al.*, 1995) (see below), and this can significantly affect the outcome.

Several studies (Selvig *et al.*, 1992; Mombelli *et al.*, 1993; Nowzari and Slots, 1994; Simion *et al.*, 1995; De Santos *et al.*, 1996a, 1996b) have shown that the outcome of GTR procedures can be affected by bacterial contamination of the membrane. One of these studies (Nowzari and Slots, 1994) compared the bacterial contamination of 11 barrier membranes used to treat intrabony defects or furcation involvement with 16 membranes used in conjunction with dental implants with associated bony defects. The nature of bacterial contamination was determined with non-selective and selective culture and by DNA probes. All the tooth-associated membranes yielded high levels of micro-organisms. Four of the five teeth with membranes harbouring less than 10^8 micro-organisms gained 3 mm or more in probing attachment level, whereas six teeth with membranes harbouring more than 10^8 micro-organisms exhibited loss or only very small gains in attachment. In addition, three membranes with high levels of black-pigmented anaerobes lost 1–2 mm of attachment. The membranes associated with dental implants were less commonly contaminated, and when contaminated had considerably fewer bacteria present. There were 10 implant-associated membranes with no cultivable micro-organisms, and these demonstrated a mean gain of 4.9 mm of supporting bone, whilst the six implants with infected membranes only gained an average of 2 mm. The lower rate of bacterial contamination of implant-associated membranes is undoubtedly because they were buried below the surface epithelium and thus not in contact with the oral flora during the healing period. Also, the lesser effects on the outcome seen with the implant cases probably relates to the lesser degree of contamination, which occurred during placement only, and the fact that periodontal pathogens are much less likely to contaminate these membranes.

These results seem to show a direct relationship between the amount of bacterial contamination of the membrane and the formation or lack of formation of new attachment. These findings apply equally to non-absorbable and bioabsorbable membranes (De Santos *et al.*, 1996a, 1996b). Furthermore, these results would seem to indicate the importance of controlling or eliminating contamination of the membrane by periodontal pathogens with the use of careful technique and, possibly, antimicrobials.

In this last regard, it has been shown that the topical application of chlorhexidine (Simion *et al.*, 1995) or metronidazole gel (Frandsen *et al.*, 1994; Sander *et al.*, 1994) to GTR membranes during their application may reduce, but not completely prevent, bacterial contamination of the membrane. In addition, this has been reported to result in improved clinical results (Sander *et al.*, 1994). Improved clinical results of GTR treatment for furcation defects have also been reported in patients given a systemic antibiotic compared to patients given a placebo (Mombelli *et al.*, 1996). This is presumably because this reduced or delayed bacterial contamination of the membrane.

Factors affecting the success of non-resorbable membranes

The main problems associated with the use of non-resorbable ePTFE barrier membranes and those that could affect the outcome can be summarized as:

- Possible shortcomings in the surgical technique

- The configuration of the periodontal defect
- Limiting features of tooth anatomy
- Membrane contamination and/or infection whenever the membrane is exposed to the oral environment
- The need for a second surgical procedure for membrane removal.

The success of GTR procedures and the stability of the result has also been found to be detrimentally affected by poor oral hygiene, poor compliance with maintenance programmes and smoking (Cortellini *et al.*, 1996a). Patients coming into any of these categories before treatment is contemplated are best rejected for GTR.

In addition, the removal of the membrane is associated with increased morbidity for the patient, is time-consuming for the surgeon and can interfere with healing (Tonetti *et al.*, 1993; Cortellini *et al.*, 1995b). Finally, the optimal timing of membrane removal has not yet been fully determined in humans (Caton *et al.*, 1992).

These factors have led to the development of bioresorbable membranes, which are discussed below:

Bioresorbable membranes

There are basically two types of biologically resorbable membranes (Cristgau *et al.*, 1995); synthetic and natural.

1. Synthetic polymers:
   - polyurethane
   - polylactic acid
   - lactide/glycolide co-polymers, e.g. polyglactin-910
   - polylactic acid blended with citric acid ester
2. Natural biomaterials:
   - collagen.

The commonest form of synthetic bioresorbable membrane commercially available is of the lactide/glycolide co-polymer type developed by W L Gore and Associates under the trade name Resolute®, and this is supplied with a bioresorbable suture. It is a polylactate/polygalactate co-polymer, and has been used in many of the clinical trials reported below. Another commercially available synthetic bioresorbable membrane is composed of polylactic acid blended with citric acid ester, and is made by Guidor AB, Huddinge, Sweden under the trade name Guidor®. This is also supplied with a bioresorbable suture incorporated into the top margin of the membrane. It has mainly been designed for use in GTR techniques to treat gingival recession (see Chapter 18), but can also be used for intrabony and molar furcation lesions. A new polylactate based membrane, which is fabricated from a kit at the chairside, has been developed by Atrix Laboratories Inc. (Colorado, USA) under the trade name Atrisorb®.

Polylactide and polyglycoside membranes are broken down by the enzymes in the Krebs cycle, with the formation of lactic and glycolic acids (*Figure 17.5*). Whether this brings about any pH change in the tissues is uncertain, but it is unlikely to be of any significance in healing since buffering would rapidly occur.

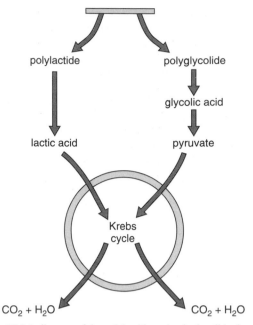

Figure 17.5 A diagram of the polylactide and polyglycolide degradation pathways in relation to resorbable membranes of these materials

Polylactic acid (PLA) degradation (*Figure 17.5*) appears to occur in two stages: first, a random non-enzymatic cleavage of the polymer, and secondly, a loss of mechanical strength and weight (Pitt *et al.*, 1981). Degradation continues to free lactic acid, which is then further metabolized in the liver to carbon dioxide and water (Bergsma *et al.*, 1995). Several studies have shown that PLA barrier membranes and sutures are safe and effective (Cutright and Hunsuck, 1971, 1972; Cutright *et al.*, 1971a, 1971b; Bergsma *et al.*, 1995).

The main difference of the Atrisorb® system is that it is fabricated from a kit at the chairside and can thus be customized for the use required. It is made by mixing polylactic acid with a solvent, N-methylpyrrodidone (NMP). This produces a flexible, semi-solid film, which can be cut to any size or shape required, and each kit contains sufficient material for the fabrication of up to 10 membranes. Excess material cannot, however, be stored for future use, and thus this results in waste. The resultant membrane can be moulded to the shape required and may be closely adapted to the shape of the defect. This obviates the need for sutures. This property is particularly useful for single surface defects on the buccal, lingual or palatal aspects of teeth, such as Class II furcation defects (see below). However, the semi-solid, flexible nature of the membrane makes it impossible to pass it through an intact contact point, and the system is therefore much less useful for interproximal intrabony defects. If used in this situation, two membranes usually have to be fabricated; the first passes under the contact to the other side to fit against the second membrane, which is applied from this side. The two are then bonded together *in situ*. This may be difficult in a surgical field contaminated by blood and saliva. If there is sufficient space it may be possible to pass a single membrane under the contact point. The membranes solidify on contact with moisture in the mouth and thus retain their shape.

There have been many attempts to make resorbable collagen membranes, and recently a number of these membranes have been produced and tested (Blumenthal, 1993; Van Swol *et al.*, 1993; Black *et al.*, 1994; Wang *et al.*, 1994). One such membrane has been produced and marketed by the German company Geistlich Biomaterials under the trade name of Bio-Gide®. The collagen is prepared from pigs which have had veterinary examination to confirm their health. The manufacture of the collagen membrane involves several technological processing steps, one of which produces a collagen bilayer. An alkaline treatment is also carried out for several hours, according to EC guidelines, to eliminate any possible viral or bacterial contamination of the material. Afterwards the structural quality of membrane is controlled by segment-by-segment analysis. Standardized processes under clean room conditions guarantee a consistently high quality biological product, which is composed of pure collagen fibres without any other organic residues or chemicals. Tests are finally carried out to confirm the biocompatibility and sterility of the end product.

It is important that a collagen membrane should be devoid of antigenicity. The locations of the collagen molecule concerned with antigenicity are the two terminal peptide regions and, during the production of Bio-Gide®, the terminal peptides are split off. Also, specific purification processes remove any fat and protein residues. In this way the immunological properties of the resultant collagen are greatly reduced and appear not to be of clinical significance. Animal experiments (Möhler, 1995) have confirmed that no inflammatory cells collect at the site of implantation of Bio-Gide®. Furthermore, no antibodies against this material were found in the implanted animals.

The resorption of collagen membranes starts with the action of collagenase, which splits the molecule at specific sites (see Chapter 1). The resultant large fragments become temperature sensitive, and are denatured at 37°C to gelatin. Gelatinases and other proteinases then degrade gelatin down to oligopeptides and amino acids (*Figure 17.6*).

Clinical trials and animal experiments with resorbable membranes

Some early trials with biodegradable membranes of polylactic acid or polyurethane failed to produce regeneration (Warren *et al.*, 1992). However, recently several human and animal studies (Caffesse *et al.*, 1994; Gottlow *et al.*, 1994; Laurell *et al.*, 1994; Lindhe *et al.*, 1995; Sander and Karring, 1995a, 1995b; Cristgau *et al.*, 1995, 1997; Becker *et al.*, 1996; Cortellini *et al.*, 1996b; Eickholz *et al.*, 1998) of improved resorbable membranes have shown that the placement of synthetic resorbable membranes in GTR procedures can result in the formation of similar amounts of new attachment to that achieved with the

Figure 17.6 The mechanism of collagen resorption in relation to resorbable membranes of this material

placement of conventional ePTFE membranes. This is the case in the treatment of both two- and three-walled intrabony defects and Class II and Class III furcation defects. The obvious advantage in using bioabsorbable membranes is the avoidance of a second surgical procedure.

Polson *et al.* (1995b) demonstrated significant reduction in PPD and gain in vertical and horizontal attachment levels in furcation defects following the use of resorbable barrier membranes. However, Cortellini *et al.* (1996b) obtained similar clinical outcomes in patients treated by GTR using either resorbable or non-resorbable membranes, whereas Hugoson *et al.* (1995) found a significant improvement in gingival recession at the sites treated with resorbable membranes compared with non-resorbable membranes at 1 year post-operatively.

A recent controlled clinical trial (Cortellini *et al.*, 1996b) compared the periodontal regeneration produced in human intrabony defects using either synthetic bioresorbable membranes (Resolute®, polylactate/polygalactate co-polymer), conventional ePTFE membranes or simple curettage of the defect. Thirty-six patients were randomly assigned to one of these three groups, and there were no significant differences in the baseline characteristics between the groups. The groups were carefully maintained for a year, and clinical attachment levels were compared with those at baseline. Significant gains in clinical attachment levels were seen in all three groups. Although there were no significant differences in the clinical attachment levels between the two membrane groups, there were significant differences between two membrane groups and the curettage-only control group. In this regard the mean gains were 2 mm greater in the two test groups. Furthermore, clinical attachment level gains of $\geqslant 4$ mm were seen in 83% of sites treated with membranes of either resorbable or non-resorbable type, whilst this was never seen in the control group. Similar results were shown in a 30-month study of paired intrabony defects (Cristgau *et al.*, 1997), and they also showed

a increase in bone density (using digital subtraction radiology) between 12 and 30 months in lesions treated with either non-resorbable or resorbable membranes. This group also reported a virtually identically structured clinical study using two types of resorbable membrane, polylactic acid or polyglactin-910, at paired intrabony sites (Cristgau *et al.*, 1998). The results were virtually the same as in their other studies, and no significant differences were seen between them.

Another study assessed the degree of bony in-fill in intrabony lesions by re-entry after 12 months in lesions treated by either non-resorbable (ePTFE) or resorbable (PLA) membranes (Weltman *et al.*, 1997). They found an average of 44% in fill for the PLA and 58% for the ePTFE membranes, with no significant difference between the two groups.

There is also a recent report of the success of GTR treatment of intrabony lesions using bioabsorbable membrane (Guidor®) carried out routinely in three specialist clinics (Falk *et al.*, 1997). They reported on the results of 203 consecutively treated intrabony defects using a bioabsorbable matrix barrier after 1 year using clinical and radiographical measurements. They found an average gain in probing attachment of 79%, and that 78% of the sites treated gained 4 mm or more. They also found an average of 3 mm bone fill measured on serial radiographs. In addition, they found that sites with membrane exposure after 2 weeks gained less clinical attachment than fully covered sites, as did sites in patients with poor plaque control. These changes in attachment were comparable to those found in clinical trials, and this shows that GTR can be successful if carefully carried out in dental practice using resorbable membranes.

There is, however, one recent study (Mayfield *et al.*, 1998) which shows that the use of bioresorbable (Guidor®) membranes did not result in any greater measurable gain in clinical attachment level than conventional flap surgery alone. Forty patients each with one suitable intrabony defect were divided into a control group receiving conventional flap surgery only and a test group treated with Guidor® membranes. They were assessed at baseline, 6 months and 12 months following surgery, by pocket probing, bone sounding and radiography. Both groups of patients showed probing depth reductions and non-significant gains in bone sounding measurements. These results were confirmed by radiography. Thus, there were no significant differences between the two groups, and this highlights the unpredictability of GTR procedures.

The bioabsorption kinetics and safety of Atrisorb® membranes have been tested in the rabbit (Coonts *et al.*, 1996) and beagle dog (Garrett *et al.*, 1997) models. In the rabbit model, test and placebo membranes were implanted subcutaneously for between 4 and 52 weeks. It showed that the Atrisorb® membranes degraded progressively with mass and molecular weight reductions, and complete degradation occurred by 13–14 months. The histopathological results showed no differences between the test and control membranes, and indicated that the Atrisorb®

membranes were biocompatible and safe. The biocompatibility of N-methylpyrrodidone (NMP) has also been shown in other studies (Bartsch *et al.*, 1976; Becci *et al.*, 1983; Ansell and Fowler, 1988). The safety and biocompatibility of Atrisorb® membranes were confirmed by histological observations around retained barrier membranes used to treat naturally occurring furcation defects in beagle dogs (Garrett *et al.*, 1996).

The clinical effectiveness of Atrisorb® membranes in treating Class II furcation lesions has been tested in beagle dogs (Polson *et al.*, 1995a; Garrett *et al.*, 1996) and humans (Polson *et al.*, 1995b, Garrett *et al.*, 1997). The beagle dog models (Garrett *et al.*, 1996; Polson *et al.*, 1995a) included treatment of both naturally occurring and surgically created Class II furcation defects. They showed 70–80% regeneration, including new bone, cementum and periodontal ligament, in both types of defect. No residual barrier was seen after 9–12 months.

The first multicentre clinical study of this membrane in humans (Polson *et al.*, 1995b) was on 29 patients with Class II furcation involvement. At 12 months, it showed a mean of 2.5 mm improvement in horizontal attachment level and 1.7 mm improvement in vertical attachment level. About half of the defects converted from Class II to Class I involvement. No adverse effects beyond those commonly associated with GTR surgery were noted. The second multicentre clinical study (Garrett *et al.*, 1997) involved 162 patients with Class II furcation involvement, and compared the use of Atrisorb® resorbable membranes with conventional Gore-tex® ePTFE membranes. Eighty-two patients were treated with resorbable membranes and 80 with ePTFE membranes. This study showed similar results for clinical improvement and tolerance between the two types of membrane, with significant improvements in both vertical and horizontal attachment levels. A majority of lesions in both groups converted from Class II to Class I involvement.

Clinical testing of bioabsorbable collagen membranes has produced results that are closely similar to those achieved with synthetic bioresorbable and non-resorbable ePTFE membranes (Blumenthal, 1993; Van Swol *et al.*, 1993; Black *et al.*, 1994; Wang *et al.*, 1994). The membrane function of Bio-Gide® has also been tested in various animal experiments. Standardized peri-implant defects in dogs were filled with a natural bone mineral (Bio-Oss®) (see below and above) and covered with Bio-Gide®. At re-entry after 4 months, histological evaluation revealed the regeneration of organized cancellous and cortical bone (Hürzeler *et al.*, 1998). In addition, the repair of prepared circumferential intrabony defects in beagle dogs has been studied comparing the results of two different cross-linked bioabsorbable collagen membranes and a non-resorbable ePTFE (Crigger *et al.*, 1996). The animals were sacrificed after 6 months and the tissues prepared for histological examination. The highly cross-linked, slowly resorbing collagen membranes did not integrate well with the tissues, and produced membrane exposure and gingival recession. In contrast, the less cross-linked, rapidly resorbing collagen membranes and

the ePTFE membranes produced good clinical results. Both these membranes also produced high levels of regeneration, with connective tissue attachment to the root surface after 6 months. The collagen membrane produced 84% and the ePTFE 53% of connective tissue attachment, but these differences were not statistically significant. Some areas of ankylosis were present with both membranes, but these were more common with the collagen membrane. The areas of ankylosis seemed to originate from the furcation. The results indicated that both types of membrane produced good levels of periodontal regeneration in these defects.

These results seem to show that clinically measurable gains in probing attachment level and histological verifiable periodontal regeneration can usually be obtained with GTR procedures using both bioresorbable or non-resorbable membranes. However, the lack of a second surgical procedure is a major advantage with bioresorbable membranes.

The clinical procedure used with bioresorbable membranes is the same as that used with non-resorbable membranes, except that they are secured with resorbable sutures. They do not, of course, need to be removed after the regenerative period.

GTR in combination with bone or bone substitute grafts

In clinical studies using GTR, some of which are cited above, there were a number of variables in the GTR technique, including the concurrent use of bone grafts, root surface conditioning and coronally positioned flaps (Schallhorn and McClain, 1988; Gantes and Garrett, 1991; Mellonig, 1991).

Combination of GTR with the use of bone grafts has been shown to have some advantages over either technique used alone (Schultz and Gager, 1990). Schallhorn and McClain (1988) reported on a clinical study combining osseous composite grafting, root conditioning and GTR. They found a significantly greater gain of mean probing attachment with the combination compared to GTR alone.

Bowers *et al.* (1989a, 1989b, 1989c) showed that periodontal regeneration could take place using human freeze-dried decalcified bone allograft (FDDBA) in intrabony defects (see previous section). They concluded that the combination of highly osteogenic material such as FDDBA with GTR might offer promise for increasing the predictability of periodontal regeneration procedures.

This combination approach was investigated by Anderegg *et al.* (1991). They compared the use of FDDBA and GTR with GTR alone on human molar furcation defects. At the 6-month re-entry, there was a distinct difference in the horizontal and vertical bone repair favouring the use of the graft. Stahl and Froume (1991) investigated the use of this combination on human intrabony defects and found gains in clinical attachment and histological evidence of new cementum, bone and periodontal ligament formation. However, the amount of new histological attachment varied from 0–1.7 mm in the four specimens studied.

Recently this combination has been investigated by Guillemin *et al.* (1993a, 1993b), using two paired sites in each of 17 patients with advanced periodontitis, one of which was treated with FDDBA and GTR and the other with GTR alone. The results were compared for the extent of bony in-fill assessed at re-entry 6 months after the procedure, and bone density was also assessed by computerized densitometric analysis. No statistically significant differences were found for either comparison between the two groups. The average bony in-fill was 58% for the GTR-alone sites and 70% for the combination sites. In addition, the combination sites showed greater mean gingival recession (0.9 mm) than the GTR-alone sites (0.4 mm).

These studies would seem to indicate that both GTR and the use of FDDBA bone graft alone can produce some periodontal regeneration. Their combined use seems to produce good results, which may be slightly better than either used alone. However, the controlled studies do not show statistically significant differences between using GTR alone or with FDDBA.

GTR in combination with hydroxyapatite-collagen grafts have also been compared with GTR alone and surgical debridement (Kilic *et al.*, 1997). GTR alone and in combination with the graft produced significantly greater gains in attachment than debridement alone. The results of GTR with the graft were slightly better than GTR alone, but these differences were not statistically significant.

The reasons for the unpredictability of GTR and bone grafting techniques may result from the cellular events leading to the formation of these tissues. These are not as simple as originally conceived, and some new views on connective tissue regeneration have a bearing on this.

GTR combined with other clinical procedures

Although histological and clinical studies on the use of barrier membranes have provided extensive evidence that some periodontal regeneration is practically feasible, the clinical results remain variable and unpredictable. In addition, studies have shown that treatment of Class III furcation defects at mandibular molars using GTR results in partial healing, whereas complete closure of the defect is obtained infrequently (Pontoriero *et al.*, 1989; Eickholz *et al.*, 1998). The biologic principles of different regenerative procedures have therefore been combined in order to attempt to achieve a greater degree of clinical success.

GTR procedures have been used in combination with root conditioning, and this has appeared to result in improved outcomes (McClain and Schallhorn, 1993; Kilic *et al.*, 1997). Antimicrobial agents have either been applied topically before membrane placement (Sander *et al.* 1994) or incorporated in the resorbable membranes (Dowell *et al.*, 1995) in order to reduce the possibility of bacterial contamination during healing. However, the addition of the antibiotic metronidazole did not appear to improve periodontal regeneration beyond that of the membrane alone (Sander *et al.*, 1994; Dowell *et al.*, 1995).

The possible use of growth factors alone or in conjunction with other procedures including GTR is discussed in the following sections.

New views on connective tissue regeneration

There have been very significant advances in this area recently (Hughes and McCulloch, 1991; Hughes, 1993, 1995). The cellular events of periodontal regeneration are not a simple race of cells, but involve the controlled integration of a number of cell signalling systems. The following factors seem, with our present knowledge, to be the most important in determining the outcome of periodontal regenerative procedures:

- Exclusion of epithelium and gingival connective tissue.
- Producing the conditions for the migration of stem and progenitor cells from the periodontal ligament and the bone marrow of the alveolar bone. This involves the integrated production of the appropriate signal molecules.
- Production of signal molecules for cementoblasts and cementum formation.
- Production of signal molecules for osteoblasts and bone formation.
- Production of signal molecules for synchronized periodontal ligament formation.

So far we have only limited means of controlling these factors, and the fine control of these systems in tissue healing almost certainly determines the type of tissue formed. Therefore, it is unlikely that periodontal regenerative procedures like GTR and bone grafting will be fully predictable until we have a better understanding of these processes and some practical means of controlling them. Some of the recent research in this area is discussed below.

Cells and extracellular matrix proteins in periodontal regeneration

The recognition that the cells involved in GTR are key factors which ultimately determine the success of periodontal regeneration has prompted a number of investigations aimed at understanding this process at the cellular and molecular levels. Morphological analysis of furcation defects treated by GTR in dogs showed that, over the first 2 weeks, the wound became occupied by granulation tissue containing numerous infiltrated inflammatory cells and blood vessels (Matsuura *et al.*, 1995). However, by 4 weeks the defect was nearly filled by new connective tissue containing many fibroblast-like cells. The cells colonizing the periodontal wound area at this stage were found to be derived from both the adjacent unwounded periodontal ligament (Gould *et al.*, 1980; Iglhaut *et al.* 1988) and the marrow spaces of adjacent alveolar bone (Iglhaut *et al.*, 1988). By 8 weeks, some new periodontal ligament associated with newly formed bone was present in the healing area (Matsuura *et al.*, 1995).

A number of recent studies have investigated the cells and tissues adherent to ePTFE membranes and samples of regenerative tissue removed from periodontal surgical sites of patients (Pritlove-Carson *et al.*, 1992, 1994; Wakabayashi *et al.*, 1996, 1997; Grosso *et al.*, 1997; Kuru *et al.*, 1997a, 1997b, 1997c, 1998a; Kuru, 1998). They showed that variable amounts of tissue were adherent to the membranes, and that the coronal part of the membrane was colonized by oral bacteria. Immunohistochemical investigations showed that vimentin-positive mesenchymal cells and keratin-positive epithelial cells were present in these tissues (Pritlove-Carson *et al.*, 1992, 1994; Kuru, 1998). Vimentin and keratin are markers of mesenchymal and epithelial cells respectively.

Recently, the cells harvested from removed ePTFE membranes and regenerated soft tissues taken from healing periodontal defects in GTR patients have been cultured and studied *in vitro* (Wakabayashi *et al.*, 1996, 1997; Grosso *et al.*, 1997; Kuru *et al.*, 1997a, 1997b, 1997c, 1998b; Kuru, 1998). These cells appeared to be fibroblast-like in morphology, and were shown to be vimentin-positive mesenchymal cells. Some of these cultured cells were also shown to express osteocalcin, osteonectin, bone sialoprotein (BSP) and high levels of alkaline phosphatase, and to form mineralized nodules *in vitro*, particularly when grown on media formulated for this purpose and stimulated by dexamethasone (Wakabayashi *et al.*, 1996, 1997; Grosso *et al.*, 1997; Kuru *et al.*, 1997b, 1997c; Kuru, 1998). Some of these cells thus appear to have osteoblast-like characteristics. Cultured cells were also found to produce extracellular matrix (ECM) proteins associated with both soft (Kuru *et al.*, 1997a) and hard connective tissues (Kuru *et al.*, 1997b), certain proteases (Wakabayashi *et al.*, 1996; Grosso *et al.*, 1997) and cytokines (Wakabayashi *et al.*, 1997). Furthermore, culture media in which these cells had been incubated *in vitro* was found to inhibit osteoclast differentiation (Rowe *et al.*, 1996).

The identification and localization of ECM proteins, which are expressed during periodontal tissue regeneration, has been studied in animals and in a few human cases. Type I collagen, along with type III, was found to be sparsely distributed and poorly organized (Pritlove-Carson *et al.*, 1994; Matsuura *et al.*, 1995). Collagen type IV was only found at basement membranes associated with blood vessels and epithelium (Pritlove-Carson *et al.*, 1994). Fibronectin was localized between the inflammatory cells in the newly formed connective tissue and at the attachment sites of the periodontal ligament to the root surface (Matsuura *et al.*, 1995). The expression of bone-associated proteins, including osteocalcin, osteonectin

and BSP, was observed in the newly formed cementum and newly formed bone, as well as in the connective tissue in close proximity to the hard tissues (Amar *et al.*, 1995, 1997; Ho *et al.*, 1995; Matsuura *et al.*, 1995).

It has also been found that samples of regenerative tissue removed from GTR surgical sites of patients had up-regulation of platelet-derived growth factor (PDGF) and transforming growth factor beta (TGFβ) receptors in comparison to those found in gingival and periodontal ligament tissue (Kuru *et al.*, 1998b; Kuru, 1998). Furthermore, PDGF and TGFβ have been detected in GCF from GTR patients, and the levels of GCF TGFβ were found to be significantly higher than in GTR patients than in GCF from conventional flap surgery patients (Kuru, 1998).

The possible use of growth factors and cell mediators to produce periodontal regeneration

The new information described above has already begun to affect clinical methods to achieve periodontal regeneration. Melcher (1976) focused on the need to stimulate the regeneration of cementum and periodontal ligament as well as bone in periodontal regeneration. He postulated that, if cells of the periodontal ligament and alveolar bone populated the healing tissue coronal to the residual alveolar bone, regeneration of new periodontium would occur.

Guided tissue regeneration seeks to produce these conditions by excluding epithelial downgrowth and thus proving an anatomical environment for the coronal migration of these cells. Bone grafts such as human freeze-dried, demineralized bone allograft seek to provide a stimulus for bone regeneration. However, it would seem likely that predictable regeneration would not occur unless cells capable of regenerating all the tissues of the periodontium, or their precursors, were stimulated by the necessary chemical messenger molecules. This would induce each cell line to differentiate and migrate into the healing area. It would also seem likely that cellular messenger molecules trigger all the stages of the complex events leading to periodontal regeneration. Recently some work has appeared in the literature, which has experimentally tested some of these events.

The control of the stem and progenitor cell in the periodontal healing process is complex and is only just beginning to be unravelled. Various locally produced growth factors seem to play a role in recruiting cells into the healing area from the bone marrow spaces and periodontal ligament, and their role has been studied in cell culture models.

Using cell culture techniques, platelet-derived growth factor (PDGF) has been found to be mitogenic and chemotactic for connective tissue cells (Ross *et al.*, 1986), and recently the role of these factors has been studied on recruitment of osteogenic cells. This was investigated by recording the behaviour cells that were enzymatically released from rat foetal calvarium cultures. It was found that both PDGF and transforming growth factor alpha (TGFα) were chemotactic for osteogenic cells (Hughes *et al.*, 1992), but the responses of different cell populations to these two factors were slightly different. The optimum concentration of PDGF was the same both for alkaline phosphatase (AlkP)-positive and -negative cells, whilst AlkP-positive cells showed two peaks of activity at different concentrations of TGFα.

Although the precise roles of different locally produced growth factors is unclear, there is evidence for the involvement of epithelial growth factor (EGF), PDGF, fibroblast growth factor (FGF), insulin-like growth factor (IGF)-I and -II and TGFα in various stages of this process (Hughes, 1995).

In addition, the systemically produced steroid hormones, glucocorticoids, are known to modulate the effects of other hormones and local mediators of cell functions. They enhance the mitogenic activity of fibroblast growth factor (Hooley and Kieran, 1974) and IGF-I (Conover *et al.*, 1986), but inhibit epidermal growth factor (Otto *et al.*, 1981). They could thus modulate the activities of growth factors in wound healing. In this regard, a potent synthetic glucocorticoid, dexamethasone, has been shown to act synergistically with cartilage-derived growth factor to produce mitogenesis in cultured mouse cells while having no effect on PDGF-produced mitogenesis (Levenson *et al.*, 1985). In contrast, it has been shown that dexamethasone acts synergistically with PDGF to induce proliferation of periodontal ligament and gingival tissue fibroblasts *in vitro* (Rutherford *et al.*, 1992). Dexamethasone has also been shown selectively to stimulate the proliferation of osteoprogenitor cells (Bellows *et al.*, 1990) and to induce adult bone marrow cells to differentiate into osteoblasts (Kasuggai *et al.*, 1991). Glucocorticoids may therefore play a role in osteogenesis.

The behaviour of three groups of cells, cementoblasts, osteoblasts and periodontal ligament fibroblasts and their stem and progenitor cells, is critical in the process of periodontal regeneration, and the factors controlling these will be discussed in turn.

Cementoblasts associated with cellular cementum from fully formed teeth appear to share most of the same phenotypical characteristics as osteoblasts. They would therefore be expected to respond to the same stimulating factors (Tenorio *et al.*, 1993, 1997; Tenorio and Hughes, 1996). However, cementoblasts from acellular cementum do not appear to share these characteristics, and may thus respond to different stimuli.

A primary requirement for periodontal regeneration is that the exposed root surface becomes populated by suitable cells from the periodontal ligament or bone marrow. Of particular importance are the cells that will develop into cementoblasts and form acellular cementum, and those which will develop into periodontal ligament fibroblasts and form the inserting collagen fibrils.

The exposed root surface in periodontal disease is pathologically altered, and this could deleteriously affect this process. In this regard it has been shown that periodontal ligament fibroblasts in culture failed to attach to or orientate to pathologically altered root surfaces (Tenorio *et al.*, 1997). It has been also shown (Hughes and Smales, 1992) that their ability to attach to normal root surfaces can be reduced but not abolished by application of bacterial lipopolysaccharide (LPS). Furthermore, it has been shown that acid conditioning of the root surface does not appear to alter this process (Tenorio *et al.*, 1997).

A number of locally produced factors have been shown to either stimulate or reduce the activity of osteogenic cells, and these include interleukin (IL)-1, IL-6, IL-11, tumour necrosis factor alpha (TNFα), interferon gamma (INFγ), bone morphogenic proteins (BMP) and the stimulation of nitrous oxide (NO) production by osteoblasts.

The role of bone morphogenic proteins (BMP) in periodontal healing seems to be considerable, since they appear to be able to regulate all stages of this process from specifying cell commitment to regulating cell function (Hughes, 1995; Hughes *et al.*, 1995). The effects of BMP-2, -4, -6 on the differentiation of osteoprogenitor cells in culture have been tested using a bone nodule formation assay system (Hughes *et al.*, 1995). All of these proteins produced differentiation of these cells right the way through to the formation of new bone, although it was found that BMP-6 appeared to act on an earlier stage of the process than the others.

It has also been shown that the expression and production of nitrous oxide (NO) by osteoblasts, as the result of appropriate signals, has an important self regulatory role on these cells and the function of osteoclasts (Hukkanen *et al.*, 1995). Certain cytokines, IL-1β, TNFα and IFNγ, either alone or in synergistic combination, stimulate the expression and production of NO by a variety of osteoblast cell lines *in vitro*. The secretion of NO by these cells significantly reduced osteoblast activity, as evidenced by reduction in DNA synthesis, cell proliferation, alkaline phosphatase activity and osteocalcin production. In addition, IL-6 is a pluripotent cytokine which is synthesized by osteoblasts, and this has also been shown to reduce osteoblast activity by inhibiting osteoblast differentiation (Hughes and Howells, 1993a). Similar effects were produced by IL-11, but the effects were more potent than those produced by IL-6 (Hughes and Howells, 1993b). Thus, there are now several known pathways that either stimulate or inhibit new bone formation.

In order for normal periodontal ligament attachment to form not only does new bone and acellular cementum need to form, but also a normal periodontal ligament space between the two has to be maintained to accommodate the inserting fibres of the periodontal ligament. This process seems to be a function of the activity of specialized periodontal ligament fibroblasts, and some knowledge of the mechanisms involved seems to be evolving. It has been shown that human periodontal ligament fibroblasts inhibit the formation of bone in rat marrow stromal cell cultures (Ogiso *et al.*, 1991). It has been further shown that these fibroblasts probably inhibit osteoblast differentiation and fulfil this function at least partially by the release of soluble factors including prostaglandins (PGs). The two most important PGs in this regard were found to be PGE2 and PGF2 alpha (Ogiso *et al.*, 1992).

The role of BMP-2 in promoting periodontal regeneration has been recently studied (King *et al.*, 1997). This was investigated using the rat buccal dehiscence model. The buccal aspect of the mandibular molars of Wistar rats was denuded of bone, periodontal ligament and some cementum, and the exposed root surfaces were acid etched. The animals were then divided into test and control groups. Human recombinant BMP-2 in a collagen gel was applied to the exposed roots of the test animals, whilst the control animals received the collagen gel alone. The flaps were sutured back into their original position and the animals were then killed either after 10 or 38 days post-operation. The mandibular tissues were then examined histologically. In the test animals of the 10-day group, there was more than twice the amount of new bone and cementum formation than was evident in the corresponding control animals. There was also no evidence of ankylosis. By 38 days there was complete periodontal regeneration of all tissues in both test and control animals, with no differences between the groups. Thus, it appears that the local application of BMP-2 in a collagen gel markedly increases the rate of periodontal regeneration in this model.

There are, however, important differences between this model and periodontal regeneration of periodontal defects, since this model would have normal, healthy root surfaces, whilst the root surfaces of the periodontal defect would be pathologically altered by the disease process. This pathological alteration of the root surface is known to affect the colonization of the root surface by progenitor cells (Hughes and Smales, 1992; Tenorio *et al.*, 1997).

Several recent experimental studies in animals have used growth factors alone, or in conjunction with either GTR or with GTR and root conditioning. The results have shown that growth factors had a significantly increased potential for inducing regenerative healing of periodontal tissues (Cho *et al.*, 1995; Park *et al.*, 1995; Sigurdsson *et al.*, 1995a, 1995b).

Platelet-derived growth factor (PDGF) in combination with insulin-like growth factor-1 (IGF-1) in a carboxymethylcellulose carrier has been tested in dogs with naturally-occurring periodontitis (Lynch *et al.*, 1991). In these experiments these factors appeared to produce regeneration of some new attachment, with formation of some new cementum, bone and periodontal ligament. This same combination has also been tested on experimental periodontitis in monkeys (Rutherford *et al.*, 1992b, 1993) with similar results.

In these experiments only the growth factors in the gel carrier separated the gingival tissue from the alveolar bone and root surface, and no attempt was made to prevent the contact of gingival connective tissue with the root surface or the carrier, as would be the case with GTR. In fact, the amount and spatial distribution of the new periodontium formed suggested that cells present in the gingival connective tissue were induced by the growth factors and contributed cells to the healing process. This possibility would seem to run contrary to all the previously held views on the role of gingival connective tissue.

A combination of dexamethasone and PDGF in a collagen carrier matrix has also been tested on local experimental periodontitis lesions in monkeys. Paired lesions with horizontal and vertical bone loss and 3–5 mm of attachment loss were used. One site received an application of PDGF and dexamethasone in the collagen-carrier, and the other the collagen-carrier only. A collagen matrix (CM) was used as the vehicle because it was thought that it might produce an environment that favoured connective tissue formation and also might act as a barrier to epithelial migration. The regeneration of some new periodontium, consisting of new cementum, bone and inserting periodontal ligament fibres coronal to the pre-treatment levels, was seen after 4 weeks in the PDGF/dexamethasone/CM sites but not in the control sites treated with CM alone. The application of PDGF/dexamethasone/CM produced five-fold more new cementum and ligament and seven-fold more supracrestal bone than the control treatments over the full time period. This included the filling of intrabony defects and increased height of alveolar bone. In these experiments, it is possible that epithelial downgrowth was prevented both by the collagen matrix acting as a barrier and as a result of the inhibition of epithelial growth factor by PDGF (Otto *et al.*, 1981).

A combination of recombinant human transforming growth factor beta-1 (TGFβ_1) and GTR with ePTFE membranes has been used on experimental periodontitis lesions in beagle dogs to evaluate bone and cementum regeneration (Wikesjö *et al.*, 1998). Supra-alveolar critical-size periodontal defects were surgically created around the third and fourth mandibular molars on both sides of the jaw in five dogs. Alternative sides in consecutive animals received either a combination of TGFβ_1 in a carrier and an ePTFE membrane (test) or an ePTFE membrane alone (control). The dogs were killed after 4 weeks and the histology of the healing lesions were assessed. Bone regeneration was seen in all animals, but was limited to the very apical aspect of the lesion. Cementum was limited, and no differences were seen between the test and control lesions. Statistical differences in favour of the test lesions were found for bone area growth and bone density. However, the amounts of bone and cementum formed were small, and would have been clinically insignificant after this time period.

Periodontal therapies using the growth factors are considered to be in the experimental stage, and therefore no growth factor therapy has received approval by the USA Food and Drug Administration to treat periodontitis in humans (The American Academy of Periodontology, 1996). Nevertheless, Howell *et al.* (1997) recently used recombinant human PDGF and insulin-like growth factor (IGF) to treat periodontal osseous defects in humans, and reported that the application of these factors significantly increased the formation of alveolar bone compared to conventional flap surgery.

Thus, there is now good evidence that specific growth factors and cell mediators may interact with competent cells in the healing periodontal wound when applied locally in a suitable vehicle. The periodontal ligament cells would seem to react by differentiating and migrating into the wound area more rapidly than the rate of epithelial downgrowth to form the tissues of some new periodontium. These factors would seem to have great potential in promoting the formation of new attachment in human periodontitis lesions, either alone in a suitable carrier or in combination with other methods, such as GTR. However, with GTR it would probably be preferable to use a resorbable membrane, such as resorbable collagen, polygalactin, polylactid or polyurethane, so that the healing process is not disturbed by membrane removal.

The diagnosis and treatment of furcation involvement

Furcation involvement is caused by bone loss between the roots of multirooted teeth, usually the molars and upper premolar teeth. There is variation in the width of the neck of these teeth, and this dictates whether furcation involvement occurs as a relatively early or late complication. The problem produced is inaccessibility to plaque control and scaling. The furcation opens buccolingually in two-rooted lower molars, buccolingually and mesiodistally in three-rooted upper molars and mesiodistally in two-rooted upper premolars. It may occasionally affect other teeth where there are aberrations in the number and shape of roots. Mesiodistal furcation involvement or the combinations that can occur with three-rooted upper molars cause the greatest access problems. Difficult and sometimes insoluble problems occur when roots lie close together or are partially fused, making the furcation extremely narrow and often totally inaccessible.

Furcation involvement results in the extraction of more molars than single-rooted teeth, and is the commonest complication of periodontitis; it often necessitates extraction because of the development of acute lateral abscesses (Hirschfeld and Wasserman, 1978).

Classification

Furcation defects are classified according to the degree of inter-radicular bone loss as Class I, II or III. This is discussed in Chapter 8.

Diagnosis

Furcation defects can be diagnosed by probing or with radiographs. Probing horizontally from within buccal or lingual pockets of lower or upper molars, as well as mesial and distal pockets of upper molars or first premolars, can detect furcation involvement hidden within the pocket. The best radiographs for confirmatory diagnosis are vertical bite wings or long cone intra-orals. They may also show on OPGs. Bisected angle periapical views are not good for this purpose, because the tube angulation has the effect of projecting marginal bone coronally. Upper molar trifurcations are more difficult to interpret on radiographs because of the superimposition of the large palatal root. Upper first premolar furcations do not appear on standard radiographs, but may show up if the tube is partly angled in a mesiodistal direction to try to project the rays between the roots.

Treatment

The aim of treatment is either to expose the furcation for access for cleaning, which is easier in a buccolingual than a mesiodistal direction, or to induce regeneration of new bone. Treatment procedures are outlined below.

Class I and II incomplete defects

Early involvement may be treated conservatively by scaling and maintenance. More definite involvement is usually treated by a gingivectomy, if the attached gingival zone is wide, or more usually an apically repositioned flap. Granulation tissue is curetted from the lesion, and the root surfaces are thoroughly scaled and planed. Minor bone reshaping may be carried out to produce a streamlined, easily cleaned contour. If a gingivectomy is used, the new gingival margin should be carefully shaped to ensure good access for cleaning after healing. Much better access is achieved with a flap, and the lesion is exposed by repositioning the flap margin next to, or even slightly apical to, the bone margin. Following healing, the furcation can be cleaned with a single tufted brush.

Guided tissue regeneration

GTR techniques have been successfully used to treat Class II furcation involvement on mandibular molars (Pontoriero *et al.*, 1988, 1989). The technique is essentially the same as that described on pp. 293. Either conventional ePTFE or bioresorbable membranes may be used with similar results. The results of clinical trials of studies using conventional ePTFE (Pontoriero *et al.*, 1988; Lekovic *et al.*, 1989; Metzler *et al.*, 1991; Yukna, 1992; Blumenthal, 1993; Black *et al.*, 1994; Demolon *et al.*, 1994; Machtei *et al.*, 1994; Mellonig *et al.*, 1994; Hugoson *et al.*, 1995; Bouchard *et al.*, 1997), synthetic bio-resorbable (Caton *et al.*, 1994; Hugoson *et al.*, 1995; Polson *et al.*, 1995b, 1995c; Bouchard *et al.*, 1997; Garrett *et al.*, 1997) and bio-resorbable collagen (Blumenthal, 1993; Van Swol *et al.*, 1993; Black *et al.*, 1994; Wang *et al.*, 1994) membranes to treat Class II furcation involvement have all produced good clinical resolution of these lesions. The results produced are broadly similar for all these types of membrane (Blumenthal, 1993; Black *et al.*, 1994; Hugoson *et al.*, 1995; Polson *et al.*, 1995b, 1995c; Bouchard *et al.*, 1997; Garrett *et al.*, 1997). In addition, other types of barrier membrane such as autogenous periosteal grafts (Lekovic *et al.*, 1989), freeze-dried allograft dura mater (Yukna, 1992) and bioabsorbable laminar bone membrane (Scott *et al.*, 1997) have also been compared with ePTFE membranes for this purpose, and have again given comparable results. All of these studies were verified by clinical and radiographical measurements, and in some cases also by surgical re-entry at 6 or 12 months. In addition, other studies have also used digital subtraction radiography for evidence of new bone formation (Eickholz and Hausemann, 1997). They have also shown comparable results for bioabsorbable and non-absorbable barrier membranes in both Class II and III defects.

In addition, the combined effects of a resorbable barrier membrane (Guidor®) and freeze-dried decalcified allograft bone (FDDBA) have been compared with the use of the same barrier membrane alone on paired Class II furcation lesions (Luepke *et al.*, 1997). The clinical parameters and bony in-fill were assessed at baseline and after 6 months, when surgical re-entry was performed. Significant gains in PAL and bony in-fill were found for both treatments, and the extent of improvement was greater but not significantly greater for the combined treatment. Similar results were seen in comparisons of combinations of bioabsorbable laminar bone or non-resorbable ePTFE membranes in combination with freeze-dried demineralized bone allograft (Scott *et al.*, 1997).

In all these clinical trials over 90% of the sites treated showed some resolution by in-filling of the defect with bone, and therefore this technique seems to produce more predicable results with furcation lesions than with other types of periodontal lesion.

Furthermore, animal studies show that a normal periodontium with new bone, cementum and periodontal ligament form in these areas, both with the use of non-resorbable ePTFE membranes (Pontoriero *et al.*, 1992) and with bioabsorbable membranes (Polson *et al.*, 1995a; Bogle *et al.*, 1997). The treated sites in the animal studies showed about 70% of regeneration with new bone, cementum and periodontal ligament.

Class III complete defects

A number of options can be considered for complete, through–through furcation defects: simple exposure, GTR, tunnel preparation, root resection, tooth division, hemisection and extraction. The choice depends on the extent and pattern of bone loss and the root anatomy.

GTR

The GTR technique may also be used to treat Class III defects, but with less predictable results (Pontoriero *et al.*, 1989; Eickholz and Hausemann, 1997). In this situation it is usually necessary to use two separate membranes on either side of the defect.

The effect of combining GTR with the application of enamel matrix derivative proteins (EMD) to the root surfaces has been investigated in five dogs (Araœjo and Lindhe, 1998). Two months prior to the start of the experiment, the mandibular first and second premolars were removed and Class III furcation defects were surgically created in mandibular third premolars. The defects were re-exposed at the start of the experiment and the root surfaces were planed. A notch was then placed in the roots at the base of the defect. On one (test) side, EMD was applied to the root surface after acid etching and a resorbable membrane was placed over the defect. On the other (control) side, only the barrier membrane was placed. The dogs were killed 4 months after the reconstructive surgery, and the tissues were examined by histology. The furcation defects on both the test and control sides were closed and harboured bone and periodontal ligament, which appeared to be in continuity with newly formed root cementum. The amounts of bone and ligament were similar in the test and control lesions. In the test lesions the cementum that formed in the apical portion of the lesion was acellular, whereas the cementum formed in the control lesions was all cellular. Thus EMD appears to be conductive to the formation of acellular cementum.

Simple exposure

If the furcation is naturally wide enough for cleaning, it can be simply exposed by the apical positioning of inverse bevel flaps; this also gains access for curettage, scaling and root planing (*Figure 17.7a*). A periodontal dressing is placed over the wound and between the roots to ensure the exposure of the furcation (*Figure 17.7b*). After healing, cleaning is carried out with a spiral interproximal brush (*Figure 17.7c*).

Tunnel preparation

This is applicable to lower molar bifurcation involvement. Exposure for curettage and scaling is gained by inverse bevel flaps buccally and lingually. The size of the furcation is then enlarged by bone contouring and sometimes by reshaping the inner root surfaces, which is only necessary if the roots are close together. If possible this should be avoided, because it can produce a high risk of root caries. The purpose of this contouring is to provide space for a spiral brush to pass freely through the furcation from the buccal to the lingual side. The flap is displaced apically to lie just below the bone margin. A periodontal pack is placed into the furcation so that the flap cannot ride up coronally. The area may need to be dressed for 2 weeks.

In some cases this procedure may be used for upper molar trifurcation involvement, but the problem is more complicated. The palatal root will usually prevent complete access from the buccal side, and additional mesial and distal approaches have to be made. These are particularly difficult for patient access using a spiral brush, and demand a high degree of manual dexterity. Patients require careful instruction in the use of spiral interproximal brushes. They must replace the heads whenever the bristles show signs of wear. Vigorous use of these brushes

(a)

(b)

(c)

Figure 17.7 The treatment of Class III furcation involvement on the 6| of a 40-year-old man. *(a)* Furcation area exposed by means of buccal and lingual inverse bevel flaps. The furcation space, the bone surface and the roots have been cleared of granulation tissue and deposits. The flap was then repositioned apically to expose the furcation area. *(b)* The postoperative result (the picture was taken 6 months after surgery). *(c)* The use of a spiral brush to clean the furcation

and allowing the metal core to contact the root will cause severe abrasion and must be avoided.

Root amputation, tooth division and hemisection (Figure 17.8)

These procedures are indicated by extensive bone

resorption around one of the roots of the affected tooth, and are only possible if the remaining roots have sufficient support to ensure function. It must be remembered that the mobility of individual roots after separation will exceed the mobility of the whole tooth. These techniques all require endodontic treatment prior to the surgery. In some cases, lack of access to narrow, curved and partially obliterated canals will preclude this treatment. Very occasionally in an emergency (e.g. when an unexpected problem is discovered during periodontal surgery) it may be necessary to amputate a root before endodontic treatment has been carried out. In this situation, one must be sure that endodontic treatment is possible and that the tooth will be functional after the procedure. The exposed pulp at the amputation site should be dressed with calcium hydroxide, and arrangements should be made for endodontic treatment soon after the surgery. In this situation it may be prudent to prescribe a course of antibiotics.

Presurgical endodontics should ensure that all of the roots to remain are filled to the apex. A small cavity is made at the entrance of the canal of the root to be removed and packed with amalgam to produce a permanent seal at the point of amputation. The floor of the pulp chamber should also be packed with amalgam for a similar purpose. In the case of tooth division or hemisection the pulpal floor will be cut through, and a permanent seal at this point is essential. The final restoration of these teeth will involve the provision of a crown(s) or a bridge.

Root amputation (Figure 17.8a)

This is particularly applicable to three-rooted upper molar teeth, when it will involve the removal of either the mesiobuccal or distobuccal root. This will allow access to the furcation area for cleaning between the remaining two roots from a buccal approach. Care should be taken to balance the occlusion on these teeth before this procedure.

Buccal and palatal inverse bevel flaps are raised to gain access. Palatal pocketing can be treated by an inverse bevel gingivectomy. Granulation tissue is curetted away to reveal the shape of the furcation and its relation to the root to be amputated. Sectioning should start in the affected furcation, and its path may be planned by passing a blunt probe through the space from the buccal to the palatal side. The cut is made with a tapered diamond bur cooled by sterile water. A wide enough space should be made to elevate the root, taking care not to remove too much substance from the part of the tooth to be retained. The base of the crown should then be shaped so that it is cleanable from a buccal approach. The remaining roots are carefully scaled and planed, and the buccal flap is placed apical to the furcation entrance between the two remaining roots. The position of the palatal gingival margin is determined by the position of the inverse bevel gingivectomy incision. A periodontal dressing is placed so that it passes between the margin of the flaps and the amputation site.

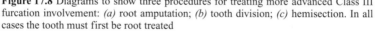

Figure 17.8 Diagrams to show three procedures for treating more advanced Class III furcation involvement: *(a)* root amputation; *(b)* tooth division; *(c)* hemisection. In all cases the tooth must first be root treated

Tooth division (Figure 17.8b)

This is carried out less frequently than the other techniques. It is indicated for extensive furcation involvement of lower molars where bone loss around both roots is similar. Buccal and lingual inverse bevel flaps are raised, and the furcation revealed by curettage. The tooth is then completely divided by extending a cut from the roof of the furcation through the crown. Each half of the tooth is reshaped into a single-rooted tooth and will be subsequently prepared to receive a crown. In this way a two-rooted molar is converted into two single-rooted teeth.

Hemisection (Figure 17.8c)

This is indicated for furcation involvement of the lower molars where there is extensive bone resorption around one of the roots. It must be ensured that adequate restoration of the remaining half of the crown is possible before embarking on this procedure.

Buccal and lingual inverse bevel flaps are raised and the area is curetted. The sectioning process is begun at the roof of the furcation, extending upwards to divide the tooth. Tooth substance is preferentially removed from the half of the tooth to be sacrificed, which is then removed with an elevator. The remaining root is scaled and planed. The remaining half of the crown is carefully contoured and smoothed, and the flaps are repositioned to eliminate any pocketing. After healing the tooth will be crowned, usually forming part of a bridge to replace the missing portion. Obviously a sufficient number of well-supported abutment teeth must be available.

Extraction

Advanced furcation involvement with extensive bone resorption around two or more roots will necessitate extraction. Teeth with uncertain prognosis may be retained on a temporary basis providing the patient is aware of the uncertainty, the teeth are symptomless and there are no signs of infection or increasing mobility. However, the effect of retaining these teeth on the prognosis of adjacent teeth should be carefully considered.

Maintenance

All teeth with furcation involvement require frequent and regular maintenance, including careful subgingival scaling. The importance of careful oral hygiene measures using spiral-tufted interproximal brushes must be stressed and taught to the patients. Care must be taken to ensure effective plaque control whilst avoiding traumatic damage to the root surface. Successful long-term maintenance of teeth with furcation involvement can be achieved in many cases (Hirschfeld and Wasserman, 1978; Knowles *et al.*, 1979).

References

Ainamo, J. (1970) Morphogenic and functional characteristics of coronal cementum on bovine molars. *Scandinavian Journal of Dental Research* **78**, 378–386

Amar, S., Petrungaro, P., Amar, A. and Van Dyke, T.E. (1995) Immunolocalization of bone matrix macromolecules in human tissues regenerated from periodontal defects treated with expanded polytetrafluoroethylene membranes. *Archives of Oral Biology* **40**, 653–661

Amar S., Chung K.M., Nam S.H. *et al.* (1997) Markers of bone and cementum formation accumulate in tissues regenerated in periodontal defects treated with expanded polytetrafluoroethylene membranes. *Journal of Periodontal Research* **32**, 148–158

American Association of Tissue Banks (1984) *Standards for Tissue Banking*. Arlington, Va: American Association of Tissue Banks

Anderegg, C.R., Martin, S.J., Gray, J.L. *et al.* (1991) Clinical evaluation of the use of decalcified freeze-dried bone allograft with guided tissue regeneration in the treatment of molar furcation invasions. *Journal of Periodontology* **62**, 264–268

Ansell, J.M. and Fowler, J.A. (1988) The acute oral toxicity and primary ocular and dermal irritation of selected N-alkyl-2 pyrrolidones. *Food and Chemical Toxicology* **26**, 475–479

Araœjo, M.G. and Lindhe, J. (1998) GTR treatment of degree III furcation defects following the application of enamel matrix proteins. An experimental study in dogs. *Journal of Clinical Periodontology* **25**, 524–530

Aukhil, I., Simpson, D.M. and Schaberg, T. (1983) An experimental study of new attachment procedure in beagle dogs. *Journal of Periodontal Research* **18**, 643–654

Aukhil, I., Petterson, E. and Suggs, G. (1986) Guided tissue regeneration. An experimental procedure in beagle dogs. *Journal of Periodontology* **57**, 727–734

Aukhil I., Petterson E., and Suggs C. (1987). Periodontal wound healing in the absence of periodontal ligament cells. *Journal of Periodontology* **58**, 71–77

Bartsch, W., Spooner, G., Dietmann, K. *et al.* (1976) Acute toxicity to various solvents in the mouse and rat. Use of ethanol, diethylacetamide, dimethylformide, dimethylsulfoxide, glycerine, N-methylpyrrolidone, polyethyleneglycol 400 and Tween 20. *Artzneimittel-Forschung* **26**, 1581–1583

Becci, P.J., Gephart, L.A., Koschier, F.J. *et al.* (1983) Subchronic feeding study in beagle dogs of N-methylpyrrolidone. *Journal of Applied Toxicology* **4**, 83–86

Becker, W. and Becker, B.E. (1990) Guided tissue regeneration for implants placed into extraction sockets and for implant dehiscences: surgical techniques and case reports. *International Journal of Periodontics and Restorative Dentistry* **10**, 377–391

Becker, W., Becker, B., Berg, L. *et al.* (1988) New attachment after treatment with root isolation procedures. Report for treated Class II and Class III furcations and vertical osseous defects. *International Journal of Clinical Periodontics and Restorative Dentistry* **3**, 9–23

Bellows, C.G., Heersche, J.N. and Aubin, J.E. (1990) Determination of the capacity for proliferation and differentiation of osteoprogenitor cells in the presence and absence of dexamethasone. *Developmental Biology* **140**, 132–138

Bergsma, J.E., Rozema, F.R., Bos, R.R. *et al.* (1995) Biocompatibility of as-polymerized poly (L-lactate) in rats using a cage implant system. *Journal of Biomedical Materials Research* **29**, 173–179

Black, B.S., Gher, M.E., Sandifer, J.B. *et al.* (1994) Comparative study of collagen and expanded polytetrafluoroethylene membranes in the treatment of human Class II furcation defects. *Journal of Periodontology* **65**, 598–604

Blumenthal, N.M. (1993) Comparison of collagen membranes with ePTFE membranes in the treatment of human Class 2 defects. *Journal of Periodontology* **64**, 925–933

Blumenthal, N.M. (1994) Future directions in periodontal regeneration therapy – a combined human collagen–bone multifunction implant. *Illinois Dental Journal* **34**, 35–38

Blumenthal, N.M., Sabet, T. and Barrington, E. (1986) Healing responses to grafting of combined collagen–decalcified bone in periodontal defects in dogs. *Journal of Periodontology* **57**, 84–90

Bogle, G., Garrett, S., Stoller, N.H. *et al.* (1997) Periodontal regeneration in naturally occurring Class II furcation defects in beagle dogs after guided tissue regeneration with bioabsorbable barriers. *Journal of Periodontology* **68**, 536–544

Bosshardt, D.D. and Schroeder, H.E. (1996) Cementogenesis reviewed. A comparison between human premolars and rodent molars. *The Anatomical Record* **245**, 267–292

Bouchard, P., Giovannoli, J.L., Mattout, C. *et al.* (1997) Clinical evaluation of a bioabsorbable regenerative material in mandibular Class II furcation therapy. *Journal of Clinical Periodontology* **24**, 511–518

Bowers, G.M., Chadroff, B., Carnevale, R. *et al.* (1989a) Histologic evaluation of new attachment apparatus formation in humans. Part I. *Journal of Periodontology* **60**, 664–674

Bowers, G.M., Chadroff, B., Carnevale, R. *et al.* (1989b) Histologic evaluation of new attachment apparatus formation in humans. Part II. *Journal of Periodontology* **60**, 675–682

Bowers, G.M., Chadroff, B., Carnevale, R. *et al.* (1989c) Histologic evaluation of new attachment apparatus formation in humans. Part III. *Journal of Periodontology* **60**, 683–693

Brookes, S.J., Robinson, C., Kirkham J. and Bownas, W.A. (1995) Biochemistry and molecular biology of amelogenin proteins of developing enamel. *Archives of Oral Biology* **40**, 1–14

Buck, B., Malinin, T. and Brown, M. (1989) Bone transplantation and human immunodeficiency virus. An estimate risk of acquired immunodeficiency syndrome (AIDS). *Clinical Orthopaedics and Related Research* **240**, 129–136

Buck, B., Resnick, L., Shah, S. and Malinin, T. (1990) Human immunodeficiency virus cultured from bone. Implications for transplantation. *Clinical Orthopaedics and Related Research* **251**, 249–253

Caffesse, R.G. and Quinones, C.R. (1992) Guided tissue regeneration: biologic rationale, surgical technique, and clinical results. *The Compendium of Continuing Education in Dentistry* **13**, 166–178

Caffesse, R.G., Smith, B.A., Castelli, W.A. and Nasjleti, C.E. (1988) New attachment achieved by guided tissue regeneration in beagle dogs. *Journal of Periodontology* **59**, 589–594

Caffesse, R.G., Dominguez, L.E., Nasjleti, C.E. *et al.* (1990) Furcation defects in dogs treated by guided tissue regeneration (GTR). *Journal of Periodontology* **61**, 45–50

Caffesse, R.G., Nasjeti, C.E., Morrison, E.C. and Sanchez, R. (1994) Guided tissue regeneration: comparison of bioabsorbable and non-bioabsorbable membranes. Histologic and histometric study in dogs. *Journal of Periodontology* **65**, 583–591

Carlisle, E. (1986) *Silicon Biochemistry*, pp. 123–136. New York: Wiley

Caton, J. and Nyman, S. (1980) Histometric evaluation of periodontal surgery. I. The modified Widman flap procedure. *Journal of Clinical Periodontology* **7**, 212–223

Caton, J. and Zander, H. (1975) Primate model for testing periodontal treatment procedures. I. Histologic investigation of localized periodontal pockets produced by orthodontic elastics. *Journal of Periodontology* **46**, 71–77

Caton, J., Nyman, S. and Zander, H. (1980) Histometric evaluation of periodontal surgery. II. Connective tissue attachment levels after four regenerative procedures. *Journal of Clinical Periodontology* **7**, 224–231

Caton, J., Wagener, C., Polson, A. *et al.* (1992) Guided tissue regeneration in interproximal defects in monkeys. *International Journal of Periodontics and Restorative Dentistry* **12**, 267–277

Caton, J., Greenstein, G. and Zappa, U. (1994) Synthetic bioabsorbable barrier for regeneration of human periodontal defects. *Journal of Periodontology* **65**, 1037–1045

Cerny, R., Slaby, I., Hammarström, L. and Wertz, T. (1996) A novel gene expressed in rat ameloblasts codes for proteins with cell binding domains. *Journal of Bone and Mineral Research* **11**, 883–891

Cho, M.I., Lin, W.L., and Genco, R.J. (1995) Platelet-derived growth factor modulated guided tissue regenerative therapy. *Journal of Periodontology* **66**, 522–530

Cristgau, M., Schmalz, G., Reich, E. and Wenzel, A. (1995) Clinical and radiographical split-mouth study on resorbable versus non-resorbable GTR membranes. *Journal of Clinical Periodontology* **22**, 306–315

Cristgau, M., Wenzel, A., Hiller, K.A. and Schmatz, G. (1996) Quantitative digital subtraction radiology for assessment of the bone density changes following periodontal guided tissue regeneration. *Dentomaxillofacial Radiology* **25**, 25–33

Cristgau, M., Schmatz, G., Wenzel, A. and Hiller, K.A. (1997) Periodontal regeneration of intrabony defects with resorbable and non-resorbable membranes: 30-month results. *Journal of Clinical Periodontology* **24**, 17–27

Cristgau, M., Bader, N., Schmatz, G. *et al.* (1998) GTR therapy of intrabony defects using two different bioresorbable membranes: 12-month results. *Journal of Clinical Periodontology* **25**, 499–509

Clergeau, L.P., Danan, M., Clergeau-Guérithault, S. and Brion, M. (1996) Healing response to anorganic bone implantation in periodontal defects in dogs. Part I. Bone regeneration. A microradiographic study. *Journal of Periodontology* **67**, 140–149

Cohen, R.E., Mullarky, R.H., Noble, B. *et al.* (1994) Phenotypic characterization of mononuclear cells following an organic bone implantation in rats. *Journal of Periodontology* **65**, 1008–1015

Conover, C.A., Rosenfeld, R.G. and Hintz, R.L. (1986) Hormonal control of the replication of human fetal fibroblasts: the role of somatomedin C/insulin-like growth factor-1. *Journal of Cellular Physiology* **128**, 47–54

Coonts, B.A., Whitman, S.L., Southard, G.L. and Polson, A.M. (1996) Biodegradation and tissue response of a polymeric barrier membrane for guided tissue regeneration (GTR). *Journal of Periodontology* **67** Abst., 65

Cortellini, P., Pini Prato, G., Baldi, C. and Clauser, C. (1990) Guided tissue regeneration with different materials. *International Journal of Clinical Periodontics and Restorative Dentistry* **10**, 137–151

Cortellini, P., Pini Prato, G. and Tonetti, M.S. (1993a) Periodontal regeneration of human infrabony defects. I. Clinical measures. *Journal of Periodontology* **64**, 254–260

Cortellini, P., Pini Prato, G. and Tonetti, M.S. (1993b) Periodontal regeneration of human infrabony defects. II. Re-entry procedures and bone measures. *Journal of Periodontology* **64**, 261–268

Cortellini, P., Pini Prato, G. and Tonetti, M.S. (1995a) Periodontal regeneration of human intrabony defects with titanium reinforced membranes. A controlled clinical trial. *Journal of Periodontology* **66**, 797–803

Cortellini, P., Pino Prato, G.P. and Tonetti, M. (1995b) Interproximal free gingival grafts after membrane removal in guided tissue regeneration treatment of intrabony defects. A randomized controlled clinical trial. *Journal of Periodontology* **66**, 488–493

Cortellini, P., Pino Prato, G.P. and Tonetti, M.S. (1996a) Long-term stability of clinical attachment following guided tissue regeneration and conventional treatment. *Journal of Clinical Periodontology* **23**, 106–111

Cortellini, P., Pino Prato, G.P. and Tonetti, M.S. (1996b). Periodontal regeneration of human intrabony defects with bioresorbable membranes. A controlled clinical trial. *Journal of Periodontology* **67**, 217–223

Crigger, M., Bogle, G.C., Garrett, S. and Gantes, B.G. (1996) Repair following treatment of circumferential periodontal defects in dogs with collagen and expanded polytetrafluoroethylene barrier membranes. *Journal of Periodontology* **67**, 403–413

Cutright, D.E. and Hunsuck, E.E. (1971) Tissue reactions to the biodegradation of polylactic acid suture. *Oral Surgery, Oral Medicine, Oral Pathology* **31**, 134–139

Cutright, D.E. and Hunsuck, E.E. (1972) The repair of fractures of the orbital floor using biodegradable polylactic acid. *Oral Surgery, Oral Medicine, Oral Pathology* **33**, 28–34

Cutright, D.E., Beasley, J.D. and Perez, B. (1971a) Histological comparison of polylactic and polyglycolic sutures. *Oral Surgery, Oral Medicine, Oral Pathology* **32**, 165–173

Cutright, D.E., Hunsuck, E.E. and Beasley, J.D. (1971b) Fracture reduction using a biodegradable material, polylactic acid. *Journal of Oral Surgery* **29**, 393–397

Demolon, I.A., Persson, G.R., Ammons, W.F. *et al.* (1994) Effects of antibiotic treatment on clinical conditions with guided tissue regeneration: 1-year results. *Journal of Periodontology* **65**, 713–717

De Santos, M., Zaccheli, G. and Clauser, C. (1996a) Bacterial contamination of barrier material and periodontal regeneration. *Journal of Clinical Periodontology* **23**, 1039–1046

De Santos, M., Zaccheli, G. and Clauser, C. (1996b) Bacterial contamination of a bioabsorbable barrier material and periodontal regeneration. *Journal of Periodontology* **67**, 1193–1200

Dowell, P., al-Arrayed, F., Adam, S. and Moran, J. (1995) A comparative clinical study: the use of human type I collagen with and without the addition of metronidazole in the GTR method of treatment of periodontal disease. *Journal of Clinical Periodontology* **22**, 543–549

Eickholz, P. and Hausemann, E. (1997) Evidence for healing of Class II and III furcations after guided tissue regeneration therapy: digital subtraction and clinical results. *Journal of Periodontology* **68**, 636–644

Eickholz, P., Kim, T.S., and Holle, R. (1998) Regenerative periodontal surgery with non-resorbable and biodegradable barriers: results after 24 months. *Journal of Clinical Periodontology* **25**, 666–676

Falk, H., Laurell, L., Ravald, N. *et al.* (1997) Guided tissue regeneration procedures of 203 consecutively treated intrabony defects using a bioabsorbable matrix barrier. Clinical and radiographic findings. *Journal of Periodontology* **68**, 571–581

Fetner, A.E., Hartigan, M.S. and Low, S.B. (1994) Periodontal repair using PerioGlas® in non-human primates: Clinical and histologic observations. *Compendium of Continuing Education in Dentistry* **15**, 932–938

Fong, C.D., Slaby, I. and Hammarström, L. (1996) Amelin, an enamel-related protein transcribed in the epithelial root sheath of rat teeth. *Journal of Bone and Mineral Research* **11**, 892–898

Frandsen, E.V.G., Sander, L., Arnbjerg, D. and Theilade, E. (1994) Effects of local metronidazole application on periodontal healing following guided tissue regeneration. Microbiological findings. *Journal of Periodontology* **65**, 921–928

Friedlaender, G. (1987) Bone banking. *Clinical Orthopaedics and Related Research* **255**, 17–21

Gantes, B.G. and Garrett, S. (1991) Coronally displaced flaps in reconstructive periodontal therapy. *Dental Clinics of North America* **35**, 495–504

Garrett, S. (1996) Periodontal regeneration around natural teeth. *Annals of Periodontology* **1**, 621–666

Garrett, S., Polson, A.M., Stoller, N.H. *et al.* (1997) Comparison of a bioabsorbable GTR barrier to a non-absorbable barrier in treating human Class II furcation defects. A multicentre, parallel design, randomized, single-blind trial. *Journal of Periodontology* **68**, 667–675

Gestrelius, S., Andersson, C., Johansson, A.-C. *et al.* (1997a) Formulation of enamel matrix derivative for surface coating. Kinetics and cell colonization. *Journal of Clinical Periodontology* **24**, 678–684

Gestrelius, S., Andersson, C., Lidström, D. *et al.* (1997b) *In vitro* studies on periodontal ligament cells and enamel matrix derivative. *Journal of Clinical Periodontology* **24**, 685–692

Gottlow, J. (1993) Guided tissue regeneration using bioresorbable and nonresorbable devices: initial healing and long-term results. *Journal of Periodontology* **64**, 1157–1165

Gottlow, J., Nyman, S., Karring, T. and Lindhe, J. (1984) New attachment formation as the result of controlled tissue regeneration. *Journal of Clinical Periodontology* **11**, 494–503

Gottlow, J., Nyman, S., Lindhe, J. *et al.* (1986) New attachment formation in the human periodontium by guided tissue regeneration. *Journal of Clinical Periodontology* **13**, 604–616

Gottlow, J., Karring, T. and Nyman, S. (1990) Guided tissue regeneration following treatment of recession-like defects in the monkey. *Journal of Periodontology* **61**, 680–685

Gottlow, J., Nyman, S. and Karring, T. (1992) Maintenance of new attachment gained through guided tissue regeneration. *Journal of Clinical Periodontology* **19**, 315–317

Gottlow, J., Laurell, L., Lundgen, D. *et al.* (1994) Periodontal tissue response to a new bioresorbable guided tissue regeneration device. A longitudinal study in monkeys. *International Journal of Periodontics and Restorative Dentistry* **14**, 437–449

Gould, T.R.L., Melcher, A.H. and Brunette, D.M. (1980) Migration and division of progenitor cell populations in periodontal ligament after wounding. *Journal of Periodontal Research* **15**, 20–42

Greenstein, G. and Caton, J. (1993) Biodegradable barriers and guided tissue regeneration. *Periodontology 2000* **1**, 36–45

Grevstad, H.J. and Leknes, K.N. (1993) Ultrastructure of plaque associated with polytetrafluoroethylene (PTFE) membranes used for guided tissue regeneration. *Journal of Clinical Periodontology* **20**, 193–198

Grosso, L.T., Iha, D.K., Niu, J. *et al.* (1997) Protease profiles of cells isolated from regenerative membranes are associated with clinical outcomes. *Journal of Periodontology* **68**, 809–818

Guillemin, M.R., Mellonig, J.T. and Brusvold, M.A. (1993a) Healing in periodontal defects treated by decalcified freeze-dried bone allografts in combination with ePTFE membranes. I. Clinical and scanning electron microscope analysis. *Journal of Clinical Periodontology* **20**, 528–536

Guillemin, M.R., Mellonig, J.T., Brusvold, M.A. and Steffensen, B.

(1993b) Healing in periodontal defects treated by decalcified freeze-dried bone allografts in combination with ePTFE membranes. Assessment by computerized densitometric analysis. *Journal of Clinical Periodontology* **20**, 520–521

Hammarström, L. (1997) Enamel matrix, cementum development and regeneration. *Journal of Clinical Periodontology* **24**, 658–668

Hammarström, L., Heijl, L. and Gestrelius, S. (1997) Periodontal regeneration in a buccal dehiscence model in monkeys after application of enamel matrix proteins. *Journal of Clinical Periodontology* **24**, 669–677

Hardwick R., Hayes, B.K., and Flynn, C. (1995) Devices for dentoalveolar regeneration: an up-to-date literature review. *Journal of Periodontology* **66**, 495–505

Hauschka, P., Mavrakos, A., Lafrati, M.D. *et al.* (1986) Growth factor in bone matrix. Isolation of multiple types by affinity chromatography on heparin sepharose. *Journal of Biological Chemistry* **261**, 12665–12674

Heijl, L. (1997) Periodontal regeneration with enamel matrix derivative in one human experimental defect. A case report. *Journal of Clinical Periodontology* **24**, 693–696

Heijl, L., Heden, G., Svördström, G. and Östgren, A. (1997) Enamel matrix derivative (Emdogain®) in the treatment of intrabony periodontal defects. *Journal of Clinical Periodontology* **24**, 705–714

Hench, L.L. (1986) Ceramic implants for humans. *Advanced Ceramic Materials* **1**, 306–310, 324

Hench, L.L. (1994) Bioceramics: theory and clinical applications. In *Bioceramics 7* (H. Andersson, R.-P. Happonen and A.Yli-Urpo, eds), pp. 3–14. Oxford: Butterworth-Heinemann

Hench, L.L. and West, J.K. (1996) Biological applications of bio-active glasses. *Life Chemistry Reports* **13**, 187–241

Hench, L.L. and Wilson, J. (1984) Surface-active biomaterials. *Science* **226**, 630–636

Hench, L.L. and Wilson, J. (1995) Bio-active glasses and glass-ceramics: a 25-year retrospective. *Ceramic Transactions* **48**, 11–21

Hench, L.L., Stanley, H.R., Clark, A.E. *et al.* (1991) Dental applications of Bioglass® implants. In *Bioceramics 4* (W. Bonfield, G.W. Hastings and K.E. Tanner, eds), pp. 231–238. Oxford: Butterworth-Heinemann

Hiatt, W. and Schallhorn, R. (1973) Intra-oral transplants of cancellous bone and marrow in periodontal lesions. *Journal of Periodontology* **44**, 194–208

Hirschfeld, L. and Wasserman, B. (1978) A long-term survey of tooth loss in 600 treated periodontal patients. *Journal of Periodontology* **49**, 225–237

Ho, S., Ivanovski, S. and Bartold, P.M. (1995) An immunohistochemical study of the extracellular matrix associated with guided tissue regeneration. *Periodontology 2000* **16**, 61–66

Hooley, R.W. and Kieran, J.A. (1974) Control of the initiation of DNA synthesis in 3T3 cells: serum factors. *Proceedings of the National Academy of Science (USA)* **71**, 2908–2911

Howell, T.H., Fiorellini, J.P., Paquette, D.W. *et al.* (1997) A phase I/II clinical trial to evaluate a combination of recombinant human platelet-derived growth factor-BB and recombinant human insulin-like growth factor-1 in patients with periodontal disease. *Journal of Periodontology* **68**, 1186–1193

Hughes, F.J. (1993) Surgical intervention: repair, guided tissue regeneration (growth factors; bone morphogenic proteins). Oral presentation at British Society of Periodontology Scientific Meeting at the Royal College of Surgery, June 5th 1993

Hughes, F.J. (1995) Cytokines and cell signalling in the periodontium. *Oral Diseases* **1**, 259–265

Hughes, F.J. and Howells, G.L. (1993a) Interleukin-6 inhibits bone formation *in vitro*. *Bone Mineralisation* **21**, 21–28

Hughes, F.J. and McCulloch, C.A. (1991) Stimulation of the differentiation of osteogenic rat bone marrow stromal cells by osteoblast cultures. *Laboratory Investigations* **64**, 617–622

Hughes, F.J. and Smales, F.C. (1992) Attachment and orientation of human periodontal ligament fibroblasts to lipopolysaccharide-coated and pathologically altered cementum *in vitro*. *European Journal of Prosthodontics and Restorative Dentistry* **1**, 63–68

Hughes, F.J., Aubin, J.E. and Heersche, J.N. (1992) Differential chemotactic responses of different populations of fetal rat calvaria cells to platelet-derived growth factor and transforming growth factor beta. *Bone Mineralisation* **19**, 63–74

Hughes, F.J., Collyer, J., Stanfield, M. and Goodman, S.A. (1995) The effects of bone morphogenic proteins 2, -4, -6 on differentiation of rat osteoblast cells *in vitro*. *Endocrinology* **136**, 2671–2677

Hugoson, A., Ravald, N., Fornell, J. *et al.* (1995) Treatment of Class II furcation involvements in humans with bioabsorbable and non-resorbable guided tissue regeneration barriers. A randomized multicentre study. *Journal of Periodontology* **66**, 624–634

Hukkanen, M., Hughes, F.J., Buttery, L.D. *et al.* (1995) Cytokine-stimulated expression of inducible nitric oxide synthase by mouse, rat and human osteoblast-like cells and its functional role in osteoblast metabolic activity. *Endocrinology* **136**, 5445–5453

Hürzeler, M.B., Kohal, R., Naghshbandi, J. *et al.* (1998) Evaluation of a new bioresorbable barrier to facilitate guided tissue regeneration around exposed implant threads. A experimental study in the monkey. *International Journal of Oral and Maxillofacial Surgery* **27**, 315–320

Iglhaut, J., Aukhil, I., Simpson, D.M. *et al.* (1988) Progenitor cell kinetics during guided tissue regeneration in experimental periodontal wounds. *Journal of Periodontal Research* **23**, 107–117

Kasuggai, S., Todescan, R., Nagata, T. *et al.* (1991) Expression of bone matrix proteins associated with mineralized tissue formation by adult marrow cells *in vitro*: inductive effects of dexamethasone on osteoblast phenotype. *Journal of Cell Physiology* **147**, 111–120

Kenney, E.B., Lekovik, V., Han, T. *et al.* (1985) The use of porous hydroxyapatite implants in periodontal defects. I. Clinical results after 6 months. *Journal of Periodontology* **56**, 82–88

Kenney, E.B., Lekovik, V., Sa Ferreira, J.C. *et al.* (1986) Bone formation within porous hydroxyapatite implants in human periodontal defects. *Journal of Periodontology* **57**, 76–83

Keeting, P.E., Oursler, M.J., Wiegand, K.E. *et al.* (1992) Zeolite A increases proliferation, differentiation, and transforming growth factor β production in normal adult human osteoblast-like cells *in vitro*. *Journal of Bone and Mineral Research* **7**, 1281–1289

King, G.N., King, N., Cruchley, A.T. *et al.* (1997) Recombinant human bone morphogenic protein-2 promotes wound healing in rat periodontal fenestration defects. *Journal of Dental Research* **76**, 1460–1470

Kilic, A.R., Efeoglu, E. and Yilmaz, S. (1997) Guided tissue regeneration in conjunction with hydroxyapatite-collagen grafts for intrabony defects. A clinical and radiological evaluation. *Journal of Clinical Periodontology* **24**, 372–383

Knowles, J.W., Burgett, F.G., Nissle, R.R. and Ramfjord, S.P. (1979) Results of periodontal treatment related to pocket depth and attachment level: 8 years. *Journal of Periodontology* **50**, 225–233

Krejci, C., Bissada, N., Farah, C. and Greenwell, G. (1987) Clinical evaluation of porous and non-porous hydroxyapatites in the treatment of human periodontal defects. *Journal of Periodontology* **58**, 521–528

Krebsbach, P.H., Lee, S.K., Matsuki, Y. *et al.* (1996) Full-length sequence, localization and chromosome mapping of ameloblastin. A novel tooth-specific gene. *Journal of Biological Chemistry* **271**, 4431–4435

Kuru, L. (1998c) Cellular and molecular basis of periodontal regeneration. PhD thesis. University of London

Kuru, L., Parkar, M.H., Griffiths, G.S. *et al.* (1997a) Extracellular matrix production by cells associated with guided tissue regeneration. *Journal of Dental Research* **76** 444 Abstr. 3447

Kuru, L., Parkar, M.H., Griffiths, G.S. *et al.* (1997b) Flow cytometry analysis of gingival and periodontal ligament fibroblasts. *Journal of Dental Research* **76** 1068 Abstr. 396

Kuru, L., Griffiths, G.S., Parkar, M.H. *et al.* (1997c) Osteoblast-like properties of regenerative periodontal cells. *Journal of Dental Research* **76** 1068 Abstr. 197

Kuru, L., Parkar, M.H., Griffiths, G.S. *et al.* (1998a) Flow cytometry analysis of gingival and periodontal ligament cells. *Journal of Dental Research* **77**, 555–564

Kuru, L., Griffiths, G.S., Parkar, M.H. *et al.* (1998b) Expression of growth factor and their receptors by regenerated periodontal tissue. *Journal of Dental Research* **77** 999 Abstr. 2942

Laurell, L., Falk, H., Fornell, J. *et al.* (1994) Clinical use of a bioabsorbable matrix barrier in guided tissue regeneration therapy. Case series. *Journal of Periodontology* **65**, 967–975

Lekovic, V., Kenney, E.B., Kovacevic, K. *et al.* (1989) Evaluation of guided tissue regeneration in Class II furcation defects. A clinical re-entry study. *Journal of Periodontology* **60**, 694–698

Leupke, P.G., Mellonig, J.T. and Brunsvold, M.A. (1997) A clinical evaluation of a bioabsorbable barrier with and without decalcified freeze-dried bone allograft in the treatment of molar furcations. *Journal of Clinical Periodontology* **24**, 440–446

Levenson, R., Iwata, K., Klagsbrun, M. and Young, D.A. (1985) Growth factor- and dexamethasone-induced proteins in Swiss 3T3 cells. *Journal of Biological Chemistry* **260**, 8056–8063

Lindhe, J., Pontoriero, R., Berglundh, T. and Araujo, M. (1995) The effect of plaque management and bioresorbable occlusive devices in GTR treatment of degree III furcation defects. An experimental study in dogs. *Journal of Clinical Periodontology* **22**, 276–283

Lindskog, S. (1982a) Formation of intermediate cementum. I. Early mineralization of aprismatic enamel and intermediate cementum. *Journal of Craniofacial Genetics and Developmental Biology* **2**, 147–160

Lindskog, S. (1982b) Formation of intermediate cementum. II. A scanning electron microscopic study of the epithelial root sheath of Hertwig. *Journal of Craniofacial Genetics and Developmental Biology* **2**, 161–169

Lindskog, S. and Hammarström, L. (1982) Formation of intermediate cementum. III. ^{3}H-proline and ^{3}H-tryptophan uptake into the epithelial root sheath of Hertwig *in vitro*. *Journal of Craniofacial Genetics and Developmental Biology* **2**, 171–177

Lu, H. (1992) Topographic characteristics of root trunk length related to guided tissue regeneration. *Journal of Periodontology* **63**, 215–219

Luo, W., Slavkin, H.C. and Snead, M.L. (1991) Cells from Hertwig's epithelial root sheath do not transcribe amelogenin. *Journal of Periodontal Research* **26**, 42–47

Lynch, S.E., Ruiz de Castilla, G., Williams, R.C. *et al.* (1991) The effects of short-term administration of a combination of platelet-derived and insulin-like growth factors on periodontal wound healing. *Journal of Periodontology* **62**, 458–467

Machtei, E.E., Cho, M.I., Dunford, R. *et al.* (1994) Clinical, microbiological and histological factors which influence the success of regenerative periodontal therapy. *Journal of Periodontology* **65**, 154–161

Machtei, E.E., Grossi, S.G., Dunford, R. *et al.* (1996) Long-term stability of Class II furcation defects treated with barrier membranes. *Journal of Periodontology* **67**, 523–527

Martin, L., McDougal, J. and Loskoski, S. (1985) Disinfection and inactivation of human T-lymphocyte virus type III/lymphadenopathy-associated virus. *Journal of Infective Disease* **152**, 400–403

Matsuura, M., Herr, Y., Han, K.Y. *et al.* (1995) Immunohistochemical expression of extracellular matrix components of normal and healing periodontal tissues in the beagle dog. *Journal of Periodontology* **66**, 579–593

Mayfeld, L., Söderholm, G., Hallström, H. *et al.* (1998) Guided tissue regeneration for the treatment of intraosseous defects using a bioabsorbable membrane. A controlled clinical study. *Journal of Clinical Periodontology* **25**, 585–595

McClain, P.K. and Schallhorn, R.G. (1993) Long-term assessment of combined osseous composite grafting, root conditioning, and guided tissue regeneration. *International Journal of Periodontics and Restorative Dentistry* **13**, 9–27

Melcher, A.H. (1976) On the repair potential of periodontal tissues. *Journal of Periodontology* **47**, 256–260

Mellonig, J.T. (1990) Regenerating bone in clinical periodontics. *Journal of the American Dental Association* **121**, 499–502

Mellonig, J.T. (1991) Freeze-dried bone allografts in periodontal reconstructive surgery. *Dental Clinics of North America* **35**, 505–518

Mellonig, J.T., Bowers, G.M., Bright, R.W. and Lawrence, J.J. (1976) Clinical evaluation of freeze-dried bone allograft in human periodontal osseous defects. *Journal of Periodontology* **47**, 125–131

Mellonig, J., Bowers, G. and Bailey, R. (1981) Comparison of bone graft materials. I. New bone formation with autografts and allografts determined by strontium-85. *Journal of Periodontology* **52**, 291–296

Mellonig, J.T., Seamons, B.C., Gray, J.L. and Towle, H.J. (1994) Clinical evaluation of guided tissue regeneration in the treatment of grade II molar furcation invasions. *International Journal of Periodontics and Restorative Dentistry* **14**, 255–271

Metzler, D.C., Seamons, B.C., Mellonig, J.T. *et al.* (1991) Clinical evaluation of guided tissue regeneration in the treatment of maxillary Class II molar furcation invasions. *Journal of Periodontology* **62**, 353–360

Möhler, H. (1995) Analysis of the immunogenicity of the collagen-membranes Bio-Gide B® and Bio-Gide®. Research report, Institute of Pharmacology, University of Zurich

Mombelli, A., Lang, N.P. and Nyman S. (1993) Isolation of periodontal species after guided tissue regeneration. *Journal of Periodontology* **64**, 1171–1175

Mombelli, A., Zappa, U., Bragger, U. and Lang, N.P. (1996) Systemic antimicrobial treatment and guided tissue regeneration. Clinical and microbiological effects in furcation defects. *Journal of Clinical Periodontology* **23**, 386–396

Murphy, K.G. (1996) Interproximal tissue maintenance in guided tissue regeneration procedures. Description of surgical technique and 1-year re-entry results. *International Journal of Periodontics and Restorative Dentistry* **16**, 463–467

Nowzari, H. and Slots, J. (1994) Micro-organisms in polytetrafluoroethylene barrier membranes for guided tissue regeneration. *Journal of Clinical Periodontology* **21**, 203–210

Nowzari, H., MacDonald, E.S., Flynn, J. *et al.* (1996) The dynamics of microbial colonization of barrier membranes for guided tissue regeneration. *Journal of Periodontology* **67**, 694–702

Nyman, S., Gottlow, J., Karring, T. and Lindhe, J. (1982a) The regenerative potential of the periodontal ligament. An experimental study in the monkey. *Journal of Clinical Periodontology* **9**, 257–265

Nyman, S., Lindhe, J., Karring, T. and Rylander, H. (1982b) New attachment following surgical treatment of human periodontal disease. *Journal of Clinical Periodontology* **9**, 290–296

Nyman, S., Lindhe, J. and Karring, T. (1983) Reattachment – new attachment. In *Textbook of Clinical Periodontology* (J. Lindhe, ed.), pp. 409–429. Copenhagen: Munksgaard

Nyman, S., Lindhe, J. and Karring, T. (1990) Reattachment – new attachment. In *Textbook of Clinical Periodontology* 2nd Edn (J. Lindhe, ed.), pp. 450–473. Copenhagen: Munksgaard

Ogiso, B., Hughes, F.J., Melcher, A.H and McCulloch, C.A. (1991a) Fibroblasts inhibit mineralized bone nodule formation by rat bone marrow stromal cells *in vitro*. *Journal of Cell Physiology* **146**, 442–450

Ogiso, B., Hughes, F.J., Davies, J.E. and McCulloch, C.A. (1992) Fibroblast regulation of osteoblast function by prostaglandins. *Cell Signalling* **4**, 627–639

Oonishi, H., Kushitani, S., Yasukawa, E. *et al.* (1994) Bone growth into spaces between 45S5 Bioglass® granules. In *Bioceramics 7* (H. Andersson, R.-P. Happonen and A.Yli-Urpo, eds), pp. 139–144. Oxford: Butterworth-Heinemann

Oonishi, H., Kushitani, S., Yasukawa, E. *et al.* (1997) Particulate bioglass compared with hydroxyapatite as a bone graft substitute. *Clinical Orthopaedics and Related Research* **334**, 316–325

Otto, A.M., Natoli, C., Richmond, K.M.V. *et al.* (1981) Glucocorticoids inhibit the stimulatory effects of epidermal growth factor on the initiation of DNA synthesis. *Journal of Cell Physiology* **107**, 155–163

Owens, P.D.A. (1978) Ultrastructure of Hertwig's epithelial root sheath during early root development in premolar teeth in dogs. *Archives of Oral Biology* **23**, 91–104

Owens, P.D.A. (1979) A light and electron microscopical study of the early stages of root surface formation in molar teeth in the rat. *Archives of Oral Biology* **24**, 901–907

Park, J.B., Matsuura, M., Han, K.Y. *et al.* (1995) Periodontal regeneration in Class III furcation defects of beagle dogs using guided tissue regenerative therapy with platelet-derived growth factor. *Journal of Periodontology* **66**, 462–477

Pitt, C.G., Gratzl, M.M., Kimmel, G.L. *et al.* (1981) Alliphatic polyesters II. The degradation of poly(DL-lactide), poly(E-caprolactone) and their copolymers *in vivo*. *Biomaterials* **2**, 215–220

Pontoriero, R., Lindhe, J., Nyman, S. *et al.* (1988) Guided tissue regeneration in degree II furcation involving mandibular molars. *Journal of Clinical Periodontology* **15**, 247–254

Pontoriero, R., Lindhe, J., Nyman, S. *et al.* (1989) Guided tissue regeneration in the treatment of furcation defects in mandibular molars. A clinical study of Class III defects. *Journal of Clinical Periodontology* **16**, 170–174

Pontoriero, R., Nyman, S., Ericsson, I. and Lindhe, J. (1992) Guided tissue regeneration in surgically produced furcation defects. An experimental study in the beagle dog. *Journal of Clinical Periodontology* **19**, 159–163

Pritlove Carson, S., Palmer, R.M., Morgan, P.R., and Floyd, P.D. (1992) Immunohistochemical analysis of cells attached to Teflon membranes following guided tissue regeneration. *Journal of Periodontology* **63**, 969–973

Pritlove-Carson, S., Palmer, R.M. and Floyd, P.D. (1993) Controlled trial of guided tissue regeneration in the treatment of periodontitis. *Journal of Dental Research* **72** 717 Abstr. 248

Pritlove-Carson S., Palmer R.M., Floyd P.D.. and Morgan, P.M. (1994) Immunohistochemical analysis of tissues regenerated from within periodontal defects treated with expanded polytetrafluoroethylene membranes. *Journal of Periodontology* **65**, 134–138

Polson, A.M., Southard, G.L., Dunn, R.L. *et al.* (1995a) Periodontal healing after guided tissue regeneration with Atrisorb® barrier in beagle dogs. *International Journal of Periodontics and Restorative Dentistry* **15**, 575–589

Polson, A.M., Garrett, S., Stoller, N.H. *et al.* (1995b) Guided tissue regeneration in human furcation defects using a biodegradable barrier. A multicentre feasibility study. *Journal of Periodontology* **66**, 377–385

Polson, A.M., Southard, G.L., Dunn, R.L. *et al.* (1995c) Initial study of guided tissue regeneration in Class II furcation involvement after use of a biodegradable barrier. *Journal of Periodontics and Restorative Dentistry* **15**, 42–55

Proestakis, G., Bratthal, G., Söderholm, G. *et al.* (1992) Guided tissue regeneration in the treatment of infrabony defects on maxillary premolars. A pilot study. *Journal of Clinical Periodontology* **19**, 766–773

Quattlebaum, J., Mellonig, J. and Hansel, N. (1988) Antigenicity of freeze-dried cortical bone allograft in human periodontal osseous defects. *Journal of Periodontology* **59**, 394–397

Quinnan, G., Wells, J. and Wittek, M. (1986) Inactivation of human T-cell lymphotropic virus type III by heat, chemicals and irradiation. *Transfusion* **26**, 481–483

Quintero, G., Mellonig, J. and Gambill, V. (1982) A 6-month clinical evaluation of decalcified freeze-dried bone allograft in human periodontal defects. *Journal of Periodontology* **53**, 726–730

Resnick, L., Veren, K., Salahuddin, S. *et al.* (1986) Stability and inactivation of HTLV-III/LAV under clinical and laboratory environments. *Journal of the American Medical Association* **255**, 1887–1891

Reynolds, M.A. and Bowers, G.M. (1996) Fate of demineralized freeze-dried bone allografts in human intrabony defects. *Journal of Periodontology* **67**, 150–157

Rosenberg, M. (1971) Free osseous tissue autografts as a predictable procedure. *Journal of Periodontology* **42**, 195–209

Ross, R., Raines, E.W. and Bowen-Pope, D. (1986) The biology of platelet-derived growth factor. *Cell* **46**, 155–169

Rowe, D.J., Leung, W.W. and Del Carlo, D.L. (1996) Osteoclast inhibition by factors from cells associated with regenerative tissue. *Journal of Periodontology* **67**, 414–421

Rummelhart, J., Mellonig, J., Gray, J. and Towle, H. (1989) Comparison of freeze-dried bone allograft in human periodontal osseous defects. *Journal of Periodontology* **60**, 655–663

Rutherford, R.B., Niekrash, C.E., Kennedy, J.E. and Charette, M.F. (1992a) Platelet-derived and insulin-like growth factors stimulate the development of periodontal attachment in monkeys. *Journal of Periodontal Research* **27**, 285–290

Rutherford, R.B., Trail-Smith, M.D., Ryan, M.E. and Charette, M.F. (1992b) Synergic effects of dexamethasone on platelet-derived growth factor mitogenesis *in vitro*. *Archives of Oral Biology* **37**, 139–145

Rutherford, R.B., Ryan, M.E., Kennedy, J.E. *et al.* (1993) Platelet-derived growth factor and dexamethasone combined with collagen matrix induce the regeneration of the periodontium in monkeys. *Journal of Clinical Periodontology* **20**, 537–544

Sampath, T.K. and Reddi, A.H. (1983) Homology of bone inductive proteins from human, monkey, bovine and rat extracellular matrix. *Proceedings of the National Academy of Sciences (USA)* **80**, 6591–6595

Sampath, T.K., Coughlin, J.E., Whetstone, R.M. *et al.* (1990) Bovine osteogenic protein is composed of dimers of OP-1 and BMP-2A, two members of the transforming growth factor-B superfamily. *Journal of Biological Chemistry* **265**, 13198–13205

Sander, L. and Karring, T. (1995a) New attachment and bone formation in periodontal defects following treatment of submerged roots with guided tissue regeneration. *Journal of Clinical Periodontology* **22**, 295–299

Sander, L. and Karring, T. (1995b) Healing of periodontal lesions in monkeys following the guided tissue regeneration procedure. A histological study. *Journal of Clinical Periodontology* **22**, 332–337

Sander, L., Frandsen, E.V.G., Arnbjerg, D. *et al.* (1994) Effect of local metronidazole application on periodontal healing following guided tissue regeneration. Clinical findings. *Journal of Periodontology* **65**, 914–920

Sanders, J., Sepe, W., Bowers, G. *et al.* (1983) Clinical evaluation of freeze-dried bone allograft in periodontal osseous defects. III. Composite freeze-dried bone allograft with and without autogenous bone grafts. *Journal of Periodontology* **54**, 1–8

Scantlebury, T.V. (1993) 1982–1992: a decade of technology development for guided tissue regeneration. *Journal of Periodontology* **64**, 1129–1137

Schallhorn, R.G. and McClain, P.K. (1988) Combined osseous grafting, root conditioning and guided tissue regeneration. *International Journal of Clinical Periodontics and Restorative Dentistry* **4**, 9–31

Schonfeld, S.E. and Slavkin, H.C. (1977) Demonstration of enamel matrix proteins on root analogue surfaces of rabbit permanent incisor teeth. *Calcified Tissue Research* **24**, 223–229

Schultz, A.J. and Gager, A.H. (1990) Guided tissue regeneration using an absorbable membrane (polygalactin 910) and osseous grafting. *International Journal of Periodontics and Restorative Dentistry* **10**, 9–17

Schwartz, K. and Milne, D.B. (1972) Growth-promoting effects of silicon in rats. *Nature* **239**, 333–334

Scott, T.A., Toule, H.J., Assad, D.D. and Nicoll, B.K. (1997) Comparison of a bioabsorbable laminar bone membrane and a non-resorbable ePTFE in mandibular furcations. *Journal of Periodontology* **68**, 678–686

Selvig, K.A., Nilveus, R.E., Fitzmorris, L. *et al.* (1990) Scanning electron microscopic observations of cell populations and bacterial contamination of membranes used for guided periodontal tissue regeneration in humans. *Journal of Periodontology* **61**, 515–520

Selvig, K., Kersten, B., Chamberlain, A. *et al.* (1992) Regenerative surgery of intrabony periodontal defects using ePTFE barrier membranes. Scanning electron microscopic evaluation of retrieved membranes versus clinical healing. *Journal of Periodontology* **63**, 974–978

Sigurdsson, T.J., Tatakis, D.N., Lee, M.B. and Wikesjö, U.M.E. (1995a) Periodontal regenerative potential of space-providing expanded polytetrafluoroethylene membranes and recombinant human bone morphogenetic proteins. *Journal of Periodontology* **66**, 511–521

Sigurdsson, T.J., Lee, M.B., Kubota, K. *et al.* (1995b) Periodontal repair in dogs: recombinant human bone morphogenetic protein-2 significantly enhances periodontal regeneration. *Journal of Periodontology* **66**, 131–138

Simion, M., Trisi, P., Maglione, M. and Piettelli, A. (1995) Bacterial penetration *in vitro* through GTAM membrane with and without topical chlorhexidine application. A light and scanning electron microscopic study. *Journal of Clinical Periodontology* **22**, 321–331

Stahl, S.S. and Froume, S. (1991) Histologic healing responses in human vertical lesions following the osseous allografts and barrier membranes. *Journal of Clinical Periodontology* **18**, 149–152

Stahl, S.S., Froum, S.J. and Tarnow, D. (1990) Human clinical and histologic responses to the placement of HTR polymer particles in 11 intrabony lesions. *Journal of Periodontology* **61**, 269–274

Stavkin, H.C. (1976) Towards a cellular and molecular understanding of periodontics. Cementogenesis revisited. *Journal of Periodontology* **47**, 249–255

Stavkin, H.C., Bringas, P., Bessem, C. *et al.* (1989a) Hertwig's root sheath differentiation and initial cementum and bone formation during long-term organ culture of mouse mandible first molars using a serumless, chemically defined medium. *Journal of Periodontal Research* **24**, 28–40

Stavkin, H.C., Bessem, C., Fincham, A.G. *et al.* (1989b) Human and mouse cementum proteins are immunologically related to enamel proteins. *Biochemica and Biophysica Acta* **991**, 12–18

Tempro, P.J. and Nalbandian, J. (1993) Colonization of retrieved polytetrafluoroethylene membranes: morphological and microbiological observations. *Journal of Periodontology* **64**, 162–168

Tenorio, D. and Hughes, F.J. (1996) An immunohistochemical investigation of the expression of parathyroid hormone receptors in rat cementoblasts. *Archives of Oral Biology* **41**, 299–305

Tenorio, D., Cruchley, A. and Hughes, F.J. (1993) An immunocytochemical investigation of the rat cementoblast phenotype. *Journal of Periodontal Research* **28**, 411–419

Tenorio, D., Foyle, D.M. and Hughes, F.J. (1997) The modulatory role of cementum matrix on osteoblastic cells *in vitro*. *Journal of Periodontal Research* **32**, 362–374

The American Academy of Periodontology (1996) The potential role of growth and differentiation factors in periodontal regeneration (Position paper). *Journal of Periodontology* **67**, 545–553

Thomas, H.F., Herold, R.C. and Kollar, E.J. (1986) Enamel proteins do not participate in murine molar cementogenesis. *Journal of Dental Research* **60**, 173. Abst. 30

Thomas, H.F. and Kollar, E.J. (1988) Tissue interactions in normal murine root development. In *Biological Mechanisms of Tooth Eruption and Root Resorption. An International Conference* (Z. Davidovich, ed.), pp. 145–151

Thomas, H.F., Herold, R.C. and Kollar, E.J. (1989) Differentiation of oclontoblasts in grafted recombinants of murine epithelial root sheath and dental mesenchyme. *Archives of Oral Biology* **34**, 27–35

Tonetti, M., Pino Prato, G. and Cortellini, P. (1993) Periodontal regeneration of human infrabony defects. IV. Determination of healing response. *Journal of Periodontology* **64**, 934–940

Turner, D. and Mellonig, J. (1981) Antigenicity of freeze-dried bone allograft in periodontal osseous defects. *Journal of Periodontal Research* **16**, 89–99

Urist, M.R. (1965) Bone formation by autoinduction. *Science* **150**, 893–899

Urist, M.R. and Strates, B. (1971) Bone morphogenic protein. *Journal of Dental Research* **60**, 1392–1406

Van Swol, R.L., Ellinger, R., Pfeifer, J. *et al.* (1993) Collagen membrane barrier therapy to guide regeneration in Class II furcations in humans. *Journal of Periodontology* **64**, 622–629

Vrouwenvelder, W.C.A., Groot, G.P. and de Groot, K. (1993) Biochemical evaluation of osteoblasts cultured in bio-active glass, hydroxyapatite, titanium alloy and stainless steel. *Journal of Biomedical Materials Research* **27**, 465–475

Wakabayashi, R.C., Wong, F., Richards, D.W. and Johnson, P.W. (1996) Protease repertoires of cells adherent to membranes recovered after guided tissue regeneration. *Journal of Periodontal Research* **31**, 171–180

Wakabayashi, R.C., Iha, D.K., Niu, J.J. and Johnson, P.W. (1997) Cytokine production by cells adherent to regenerative membranes. *Journal of Periodontal Research* **32**, 215–224

Wang, H.L., O'Neal, R.B., Thomas, C.L. *et al.* (1994) Evaluation of an absorbable collagen membrane in treating Class II furcation defects. *Journal of Periodontology* **65**, 1029–1036

Warren, K. and Karring, T. (1992) Guided tissue regeneration combined with osseous grafting in suprabony periodontal lesions. An experimental study in the dog. *Journal of Clinical Periodontology* **19**, 373–380

Warren, K., Karring, T., Nyman, S. and Gogoleweski, S. (1992) Guided tissue regeneration using biodegradable membranes of polyglactic acid or polyurethane. *Journal of Clinical Periodontology* **19**, 633–640

Watanabe, M. (1990) Implantation of hydroxyapatite granules mixed with atelocollagen and bone inductive protein in rat skull defects. In *Handbook of Bioceramics* Vol. II (T. Yamamuro, L.L. Hench and J. Wilson (eds), pp. 223–228. Boca Raton FL: CRC Press

Weigel, C., Brügger U., Hümmerle, C.H. *et al.* (1995) Maintenance of new attachment 1 and 4 years following guided tissue regeneration (GTR). *Journal of Clinical Periodontology* **22**, 661–669

Weltman, R., Trojo, P.M., Morrison, E. and Caffesse, R. (1997) Assessment of guided tissue regeneration procedures in intrabony defects with bioabsorbable and non-resorbable barriers. *Journal of Periodontology* **68**, 582–591

Wetzel, A.C., Stich, H. and Caffesse, R.G. (1995) Bone apposition onto oral implants in the sinus area filled with different grafting materials. A histological study in beagle dogs. *Clinical Oral Implant Research* **6**, 155–163

Wikesjö, U.M.E., Nilveus, R.E. and Selvig, K.A. (1992) Significance of early healing events on periodontal repair: a review. *Journal of Periodontology* **63**, 158–165

Wikesjö, U.M.E., Razi, S.S., Sigurdsson, T.J. *et al.* (1998) Periodontal repair in dogs: effect of recombinant human transforming growth factor-β_1 on guided tissue regeneration. *Journal of Clinical Periodontology* **25**, 475–481

Wilson, J. and Low, S.B. (1992) Bio-active ceramics for periodontal treatment: comparative studies in the patus monkey. *Journal of Applied Biomaterials* **3**, 123–129

Wilson, J., Low, S., Fetner, A. and Hench, L.L. (1987) Bio-active materials for periodontal treatment: a comparative study. In *Biomaterials and Clinical Applications* (A. Pizzoferrato, P.G. Marchetti, A. Ravaglioli and A.J.C. Lee, eds), pp. 223–228. Amsterdam: Elsevier Science Publishers

Wilson, J., Clark, A.E., Hall, M. and Hench, L.L. (1993) Tissue response to Bioglass® endosseous ridge maintenance implants. *Journal of Implantology* **19**, 295–302

Wilson, J., Clark, A.E., Douek, E. *et al.* (1994) Clinical applications of Bioglass® implants. In *Bioceramics 7* (H. Andersson, R.-P. Happonen and A. Yli-Urpo, eds), pp. 415–422. Oxford: Butterworth-Heinemann

Yukna, R.A. (1990) HTR-polymer grafts in human periodontal osseous defects. I. 6-month clinical results. *Journal of Periodontology* **61**, 633–642

Yukna, R.A. (1992) Clinical human comparison of expanded polytetrafluoroethylene barrier membrane and freeze-dried dura mater allografts for guided tissue regeneration of lost periodontal support. I. Mandibular molar Class II furcations. *Journal of Periodontology* **63**, 431–442

Yukna, R.A., Cassingham, R., Caudrill, R. *et al.* (1986) Six-month evaluation of calcitite (hydroxyapatite ceramic) in periodontal osseous defects. *International Journal of Periodontics and Restorative Dentistry* **6**, 34–45

Yukna, R.A., Mayer, E. and Amos, S. (1989) Five-year evaluation of Durapatite ceramic alloplastic implants in periodontal osseous defects. *Journal of Periodontology* **60**, 544–547

Zetterström, O., Andersson, C., Eriksson, L. *et al.* (1997) Clinical safety of enamel matrix derivative (Emdogain®) in the treatment of periodontal defects. *Journal of Clinical Periodontology* **24**, 697–704

18

Mucogingival problems and their treatment

As described in Chapter 1, the attached gingiva or 'functional mucosa' extends from the gingival groove to the mucogingival junction, where it meets the alveolar mucosa. At the mucogingival junction the mucoperiosteum splits so that the alveolar mucosa is separated from the periosteum by a loose, highly vascular connective tissue. The width of the attached gingiva can vary from zero to about 9 mm, widest in the incisor regions and narrowest over canines and premolars. Its boundaries are defined on the buccal side by the insertion of the buccinator, the lip muscles and the frena, as well as by the morphology of the underlying bone. On the lingual side it is bounded by the insertion of the mylohyoid muscle, the insertions of lingual frena and the bone morphology.

Reduction in width of the attached gingiva is a consequence of gingival recession produced by atrophic changes, as described in Chapter 8, and/or as the result of progressive chronic periodontal disease.

In the past it had been assumed that some width of attached gingiva is necessary to maintain gingival health by separating the stable gingival margin from the mobile alveolar mucosa. It was also assumed that the depth of the vestibular sulcus was a significant factor in gingival health. As a result of this concept, a number of surgical 'vestibular extension' procedures were devised to achieve what were considered to be adequate anatomical dimensions. There was, however, no scientific evidence for these assumptions. Fortunately for patients, notions of a normal vestibular depth were discarded and ideas about the necessary width of attached gingiva questioned. Lang and Löe (1972) reported that a narrow band of 1–2 mm attached gingiva was necessary for gingival health, but other studies indicated that this is not the case. Miyasotp et al. (1977), Wennström et al. (1982) and Salkin et al. (1987) have shown that it is possible to maintain a healthy and stable gingival margin with little or no attached gingiva, providing the individual maintains a high standard of oral hygiene. Wennström (1987) confirmed these results in a 5-year study. Addy et al. (1987) examined the relationship between frenal attachment, lip coverage and vestibular depth, and plaque and gingival bleeding scores, in 1015 schoolchildren aged 11.5–12.5 years. They found that:

1. The position of the anterior maxillary frena appeared to affect plaque retention and gingival bleeding, while the position of the mandibular labial frenum seemed to be unimportant
2. Plaque and bleeding scores in the anterior area of the mandible seemed to decrease with an increase in vestibular depth
3. Decreased upper lip coverage at rest (lack of lip-seal) was related to increased plaque and bleeding scores in both jaws.

These various findings point to the fact that variations in the width of attached gingiva are significant only when oral hygiene is poor and even then, as Addy et al. (1987) conclude, that significance is small and does not alone justify surgical interference.

However, this study on children with gingival disease is not necessarily relevant to adults with various stages of periodontal disease. The precise form of treatment necessary depends on the anatomical and pathological variables involved in the lesion and, in some cases, the views of the patient.

Mucogingival problems can arise from the effects of:

- Chronic periodontitis
- Frenal pull
- Gingival recession.

Chronic periodontitis

Chronic periodontitis may cause the following effects:

1. Periodontal pocketing extending below the mucogingival junction, where the apical limit of the pocket is:
   (a) Level with some point between the mucogingi-

val junction and the vestibular fold (*Figure 18.1*) so that, after disease has been resolved, there is enough healthy mucosa to cover the alveolar margin and produce a zone of attached mucosa and a vestibular sulcus. In this situation an apically repositioned flap may be indicated.

(b) Apical to the level of the vestibular sulcus, so that any attempt at surgery to cover the alveolar margin would obliterate the gingival sulcus. In this case the apically displaced flap procedure could be used, plus a free gingival graft if tissue destruction is great.

2. Generalized gingival recession exposing root surfaces and reducing the zone of attached gingiva. This can be treated conservatively or surgically. Several surgical procedures could be considered, including the free gingival graft combined with the coronally repositioned flap or the free connective tissue graft.

Frenal pull

Frenal pull is exerted by a frenum or muscle attachment that is inserted into an unhealthy gingival margin. This may:

1. Interfere with effective plaque removal (*Figure 18.2*) and/or
2. Pull on the wall of the pocket and thereby aggravate the lesion (*Figure 18.2*). These lesions appear rather dramatic, especially when related muscles are tensed by pulling (gently!) on the lip or cheek.

Sometimes thorough scaling, root planing and efficient home care can keep the situation stable for several years.

Figure 18.2 Gingival recession associated with soft tissue attachment

However, if gingival inflammation persists and/or there is evidence that the lesion is progressing, surgical corrective treatment is indicated.

The first situation can be corrected by a simple frenectomy; the second may require a free gingival graft.

Localized gingival recession

This may affect single or multiple teeth and may be caused by:

1. An underlying local bony dehiscence(s) with associated toothbrushing trauma
2. Direct gingival trauma from the occlusion, such as from a deep overbite associated with an Angle's Class 2, division II occlusion (*Figure 18.3*).

The first may be treated conservatively or surgically; surgical procedures include pedicle grafts and free gingival grafts and their variants (see below).

Figure 18.1 A combination of periodontal pocketing and gingival recession as a result of progressive chronic periodontitis. The pockets extend below the mucogingival junction and the gingival margin is subject to pull from muscle and frenal attachments

Figure 18.3 Destruction of gingival tissue caused by poor oral hygiene and the physical trauma of a very deep overbite, with the upper incisors impinging on the lower gingiva

The second requires orthodontic treatment for the occlusal problem plus corrective surgery where this is possible. This is dependent on the precise nature of the defect.

Surgical treatment of pocketing below the mucogingival junction

No surgical treatment should ever be contemplated unless the patient's plaque control is entirely satisfactory and all the basic treatment has been successfully completed. Surgery is also usually contraindicated in patients who smoke and refuse to give up, since their response to surgical treatment is adversely affected (Preber and Bergström, 1990; Ah *et al.*, 1994; Jones and Triplett, 1995; Miller, 1987).

A number of surgical procedures have been developed to correct mucogingival problems of this type. All have the common aims of:

- The removal of disease
- The production of a periodontal anatomy that allows effective plaque control, and therefore prevents disease recurrence.

Deep pocketing of this type may be treated by the apically repositioned flap or the apically displaced flap as appropriate. The former is described in Chapter 16.

The apically displaced flap (Figure 18.4)

The apically displaced flap technique can be used where the base of the pocket lies apical to the MGJ and the base of the vestibular sulcus and a zone of keratinized gingiva is either absent or very narrow and the vestibular depth shallow. For pocket elimination, the flap has to be moved apically by an amount equal to the depth of the pocket so that the flap margin coincides with the alveolar crest. However, where all or most of the attached gingiva has been destroyed, the flap has to be moved so that its margin is apical to the bone margin.

Procedure

If there is a usable zone of keratinized gingiva, then this is preserved by making an inverse bevel incision along the gingival margin (*Figure 18.4a*). However, if very little keratinized gingiva remains and this is grossly misshapen, than it is best discarded. In this case there is little point in making a scalloped gingival incision. A straight incision can be made, and the inflamed and frequently misshapen marginal tissue discarded. Vertical releasing incisions are made delineating the area of tissue to be moved apically, and the flap is lifted by sharp dissection through the loose connective tissue of the alveolar mucosa plus any associated muscles (*Figure 18.4b*), thus leaving the periosteum on the bone (*Figure 18.5*).

The flap is moved apical to the alveolar crest (*Figure 18.4c*) into a position that will allow the production, by secondary intention healing, of a zone of attached gingiva free of frenal and muscle attachments. After curettage and root planing of the exposed root surfaces, the flap is fixed by sutures at the releasing incisions and, if necessary, by a suture in the midline fixing the flap to the underlying mentalis muscle. The exposed alveolar margin, which is covered by periosteum, will heal by secondary intention.

A periodontal dressing is essential (*Figure 18.4d*). It is placed for 1 week and then removed; the wound is irrigated with a warm saline solution and the dressing is

(a)   (b)   (c)   (d)

Figure 18.4 The apically displaced flap technique: *(a)* an inverse bevel incision is made (where there is considerable tissue destruction and distortion a horizontal incision can be made); *(b)* the flap is dissected from the underlying periosteum; *(c)* the tissue is displaced apical to the alveolar crest; *(d)* tissue sutured to underlying muscle and held in place by periodontal dressing. Healing is by secondary intention

Figure 18.5 Apically displaced flap. A split-thickness flap has been dissected up, leaving periosteum on the bone surface

replaced for a further week. The surface of the wound becomes covered by stratified squamous epithelium over this period, but the healing period is much longer than for flap procedures that cover the bone surface. The formation of mature connective tissue and well-keratinized attached gingiva can take up to 6 weeks. During this period the patient needs to be kept on a chlorhexidine mouthwash, and should receive professional cleaning every 2 weeks.

The final result of this procedure is good, and should

Figure 18.6 Apically displaced flap. Final result 1 year after procedure. There is pocket elimination with a functional zone of attached gingiva and a good vestibular depth

produce a functional zone of attached gingiva free from muscle and frenal pull and a good vestibular depth (*Figure 18.6*).

The treatment of the effects of frenal pull

This may be treated either by a frenectomy or by a free gingival graft. The former is described below, whilst the latter is included in the section on the treatment of gingival recession.

Frenectomy

A frenectomy is indicated where the attachment of a frenum or muscle attachment is so close to the gingival margin that it interferes with efficient plaque removal and contributes to persistent gingival inflammation. This problem is most frequently found on the labial surface between the upper central incisors, but can also occur in relation to the upper canines and premolars. In the lower jaw the frena are found labial to the lower incisors and more rarely on the lingual aspect.

Procedure

1. After local anaesthesia, the lip is extended and the frenum gripped with mosquito forceps. Incisions are made with a No. 15 Swann–Morton blade on either side of the forceps through the base of the frenum. The incisions should meet at the point of the instrument. The incision on the alveolar side is made close to the alveolar bone, leaving the periosteum in place.
2. The triangle of frenal tissue should come away easily if the incisions have been made correctly.
3. The edges of the lip wound are gently undermined so that they can be approximated without tension and sutured. It is not necessary to suture the alveolar wound.
4. Swabs are placed firmly over the wound to control bleeding, and a periodontal dressing is applied. Retention of the dressing in this situation is often poor and the patient must be advised that if the dressing falls off, it is not a calamity provided that the wound is kept clean with warm saline mouthwashes and a twice-daily rinse with 0.2% chlorhexidine solution.
5. After 1 week the sutures and any dressing are removed. Usually healing is rapid and uneventful.

The treatment of gingival recession

Localized gingival recession

Localized recession of the gingival margin with considerable exposure of the root is usually associated with the presence of an underlying bony dehiscence. It is most commonly seen on the buccal surface of teeth with buccally placed roots, associated with teeth with bulbous roots, or in areas where the surface bone is naturally thin. Commonly involved teeth are the lower incisors and upper canines, premolars or first molars. Recession progresses into the attached gingival zone, decreasing this as it deepens. If it progresses into the alveolar mucosa, below the mucogingival junction, the gingival margin is no longer protected from the pull of the muscles via frenal and mucosal attachments and it may be pulled away from the root surface during facial muscle activity. This relationship also interferes with plaque removal because the gingival margin at this point is no longer accessible to clean unless the lip is physically pulled back for access. Plaque and calculus may therefore collect at the base of the lesion, producing localized gingivitis. Inflammation persists unless there is frequent professional cleaning. Lip movement also produces further tension on the gingival margin so that progressive destruction is almost inevitable.

Localized or generalized gingival recession may be managed conservatively or surgically, and these methods are described below.

Conservative management of gingival recession

Gingival recession that is not accompanied by disease, i.e. inflammation or pocketing, does not require intervention other than good plaque control and scaling when necessary unless it presents a serious cosmetic problem. The patient must be reassured that recession, especially that produced by over-enthusiastic toothbrushing, is of little significance, does not prejudice the life of the tooth and rarely justifies surgical intervention; it simply signals that a less harmful cleaning technique is needed. The main complications of gingival recession are:

- Root dentine sensitivity
- Abrasion/erosion
- Root caries.

Root dentine sensitivity

The exposed root is potentially sensitive via exposed dentinal tubules, which can transmit stimuli to the pain receptors in the pulp. When root is first exposed, the small amount of cementum covering the dentine soon wears away to uncover the dentine. This usually has open tubules containing the odontoblastic processes passing from the surface to the odontoblast cell body on the pulpal surface. This recently exposed root dentine tends to be sensitive to cold, hot and sweet stimuli, and also to drying with an air spray and the use of an ultrasonic scaler in the dental surgery. Repeated stimulation may lead to the formation of peritubular dentine, which then reduces the sensitivity; therefore, the sensitivity tends to reduce with time. The presence of fluoride ions on the surface of the root may encourage this process, and therefore gentle brushing with a fluoride-containing toothpaste helps this process. The sensitivity can return if fresh open tubules are exposed again by abrasion from toothbrushing and/or acid erosion.

Root sensitivity to cold and sweet often deters the patient from brushing properly, so that plaque accumulates on the root surface. This actually aggravates the root sensitivity, and the patient needs to be reassured that proper cleaning is necessary. Initially it may be necessary to use warm water for brushing, but in many cases adequate plaque control reduces the sensitivity. If sensitivity to cold and sweet persists, one of the toothpastes especially formulated to treat the problem (Sensodyne®, Emoform®, etc.) can be recommended. As stated earlier, sodium fluoride can be very effective as a desensitizing agent and it may be used as Lukomsky's paste (equal parts by weight of sodium fluoride, kaolin and glycerine), which is applied to the dried root on two or three occasions. An amine fluoride in a gel (Duraphat®) applied to the dried root surface is also effective and convenient to use. Another useful medicament is 1% hydrocortisone solution applied several times to dried root. Topical guanethidine (1%) has also been recommended for rapid relief from dental hypersensitivity (Hannington-Kitt and Dunne, 1993).

Generalized gingival recession resulting from periodontal disease tends to be less sensitive than single or multiple sites of localized recession from other causes. This is because the root dentine in the former situation has been irritated by the disease process over a considerable time, leading to peritubular and secondary dentine formation.

One occasionally encounters intractable root sensitivity, which does not respond to any topical applications. Usually this indicates pulp pathology, produced either by a large restoration or by a microscopic lateral pulp canal; in this situation endodontics is needed.

Abrasion/erosion

Toothbrushing using a hard brush, vigorous technique or an abrasive toothpaste can lead to surface wear, which will progressively lead to the formation of abrasion cavities. Acid erosion from acid-containing foods and drinks can lead to dissolution of the calcified content of the surface dentine. This can lead to loss of surface material *per se*, or give rise to increased rates of abrasion of the softened surface. Eventually these lesions may become large enough to require restoration.

Root caries

Food stagnation as a result of avoidance of brushing due to sensitivity or within abrasion cavities can lead to conditions that favour the development of dental caries. Root caries demands caries removal and restoration of the resulting cavity. However, root caries may cover a wide area of the exposed root and also involve some surfaces with poor access. Therefore, these lesions may be difficult to restore. Combined abrasion and carious lesions are particularly difficult to restore, because the cavities often lack mechanical retention. Furthermore, the only margin available for acid etching is the coronal enamel margin, when this is present.

The most common restorative material for these lesions is glass ionomer cement, and this produces a much better seal than composites in these situations. It also provides secondary caries protection by its ability to leach fluoride ions. However, it has low wear resistance, and patients must be warned not to use hard toothbrushes or abrasive toothpastes.

Surgical treatment of gingival recession

Contraindications to surgery for gingival recession

This form of mucogingival surgery is contraindicated if the patient's oral hygiene is unsatisfactory, if there is any gingivitis and if there is any significant periodontal attachment loss due to chronic periodontitis. It is also contraindicated in smokers, since their response to this type of surgery is poor (Miller, 1987).

Pre-operative considerations

It must be stressed that surgical intervention is required in very few cases of recession. The chief criterion for such treatment is the presence of progressive disease which is definitely associated with the recession, and which persists despite conservative measures.

Where there is inflammation and/or pocketing, i.e. the recession is involved in a progressive periodontal lesion, or where localized labial recession produces a significant cosmetic problem, intervention may be indicated.

If the recession is isolated and reflects an underlying dehiscence, a laterally repositioned graft can be an effective method of correction. If the recession is associated with a muscle attachment and a related inadequate zone of attached gingiva, a free gingival graft may be needed. These surgical techniques and some other alternatives are described in the section below.

The type of surgical treatment possible depends on the nature of the lesion(s), and these are classified below.

Classification of gingival recession

The classification of gingival recession into type defects is based upon the relationships between the base of the defect, the mucogingival junction and the height of the interdental papillae. This also gives a very reliable guide to the degree of reconstruction possible. These defects have been classified by Miller (1985a), and this is shown below, along with a summary of the clinical criteria for each group and the possible results of treatment.

Classification	*Clinical criteria*	*Possible treatment result*
Class I	Full height papillae	Recession within attached gingiva; 100% coverage possible
Class II	Full height papillae	Recession at/beyond MGJ; 100% coverage possible
Class III	Reduced papilla height	Recession at/beyond MGJ; coverage only to level related to papilla height
Class IV	Gross flattened loss of papillae	Not possible to cover

As already stated above, there are two approaches to the treatment of gingival recession:

1. *Accept and maintain*. If the degree of recession is acceptable to the patient, then a decision can be taken to try to maintain the condition. (The appropriate treatment for this has been described above.) Study models should be taken, and the condition should be reviewed at regular maintenance visits to determine whether it is stable. If the gingival recession is found to be progressing and the recession is still acceptable to the patient but is close to or beyond the mucogingival junction, then a free gingival graft can be carried out to increase the zone of attached gingiva and maintain the situation.

2. *Repair and eliminate recession*. If the recession is unacceptable to the patient and in one of the categories where successful repair is possible, then an appropriate surgical technique to repair the defect can be discussed with the patient, describing the probable outcome. The aim of these techniques is to cover the exposed root surface to the greatest degree possible and to increase and/or maintain a functional zone of attached gingiva. The possible techniques to consider are listed below.

Pedicle grafts

- Coronal repositioned flap
- Lateral repositioned flap
- Double papilla flap.

Free grafts

- Full-thickness, thick epithelial
- Connective tissue
- Connective tissue with double papilla flap.

Other regenerative techniques

- GTR with PTFE membranes
- GTR with resorbable membranes.

In reparative techniques there is still debate about the need for root surface instrumentation or conditioning.

Root surface instrumentation

Miller (1992) states that root preparation will cause a reduction in inflammation, which may result in a loss of papilla height by gingival shrinkage. This may affect the potential coverage of the exposed root surface. The reduction in vascularity may also affect the nutrient supply to the graft. However, any plaque, calculus and stain must be removed from the root surface prior to surgery, and patients undergoing these procedures must have immaculate oral hygiene.

Root surface preparation

There is still considerable debate about the need to prepare the surface and, if this is deemed necessary, about which method of preparation should be used. A number of clinical researchers have reported good results using citric acid at pH 1 for between 2–3 minutes (Register and Burdick, 1975, 1976; Crigger *et al.*, 1978; Garrett *et al.*, 1978; Nyman *et al.*, 1981; Miller, 1982). This can be applied with a brush or a cotton bud, and may either be burnished into the root surface or left alone. Tetracycline has also been used as a solution in a similar manner to citric acid, and beneficial results have been reported on its use (Terranove *et al.*, 1986; Wicksjö *et al.*, 1986; Demirel *et al.*, 1991). Terranove *et al.* (1986) showed that biochemical manipulation of the dentine surface could affect the cells attaching to it and their growth. They found that treatment of the dentine surface with tetracycline increased the binding of fibronectin to its surface, and also that the absorbed fibronectin encouraged the attachment of fibroblasts to its surface and stimulated their growth. Furthermore, they also showed that the absorbed fibronectin suppressed the attachment of epithelial cells to the dentine surface and their growth.

Pedicle grafts

Laterally repositioned flap

The laterally repositioned flap is an effective procedure for treating an isolated area of gingival recession where a suitable donor site of keratinized tissue is present. The procedure was first introduced by Grupe and Warren (1956), and has been modified in small detail by several other clinicians. The exposed root is covered by mobilizing a pedicle graft from a suitable adjacent area, which is then slid laterally to cover the defect. It is suitable for treating single tooth narrow areas of gingival recession with adequate interdental bone height and an adjacent donor area with an adequate zone of keratinized attached gingiva. This is a one-stage procedure whereby a pedicle flap is elevated by part full thickness and part split-

thickness dissection from an adjacent area of keratinized tissue. The blood supply that nourishes the flap over the avascular root surface is supplied by the wide base of the pedicle flap and from the periosteum over the bone surrounding the denuded roots. The flap is secured into position over the denuded root with interrupted silk sutures. The colour blend and root coverage are excellent in well-chosen cases. However, it is generally not suitable for treating isolated wide areas of recession or multiple recessions.

Procedure (*Figure 18.7*)

The area should receive preparatory periodontal treatment to remove all plaque and calculus from the root surface and resolve any gingival inflammation in the surrounding area and the rest of the mouth.

Preparation of the recipient area

Incisions are made down the margins of the defect to remove epithelium from its edges (*Figure 18.7a*). These incisions meet apically at the base of the defect, where the incision is carried into the vestibule. More tissue should be removed from the margin of the defect that is to receive the leading edge of the sliding pedicle graft. This is to allow bone to be uncovered at this margin so that the sutured edge of the flap will lie over bone rather than root surface. This is very important to the success of this procedure, and it dictates that the interproximal bone in this area must be at its normal height – i.e. there should be no interdental bone resorption. All the detached tissue should be carefully removed from around the exposed root surface, and the root is carefully planed clean and smooth. Some clinicians have recommended root conditioning with citric acid for this procedure. Also, if the recipient tooth has a bulky, outstanding root, this lessens the chances of success, and planing back of these prominent roots with a Kirkland No. 7 curette has been advocated. This would normally be followed by root conditioning.

Preparation of the pedicle graft

A gingival crevicular incision is then made around the next two teeth, and a releasing incision is made from the

(a)   *(b)*   *(c)*

Figure 18.7 Diagram to illustrate laterally repositioned flap technique: *(a)* incisions are made around the defect and along the gingival margin, then a releasing incision is made approximately two teeth away from the defect; *(b)* a part full-thickness and part split-thickness flap is dissected from the underlying bone and *(c)* moved laterally to cover the defect gingival incision into the vestibule (*Figure 18.7a*). This should produce a flap that is twice as wide as the gingival defect. A part split-thickness and part full-thickness flap is then carefully developed. The full thickness mucoperiosteal flap is raised from the tooth, and this will provide the part of the flap covering the exposed root so that the root is directly covered by periosteum. The part of the flap related to the adjacent tooth which when raised will expose the donor area bone should be developed as a split-thickness flap. This allows the exposed donor area of bone to retain its periosteal covering for protection and additional blood supply. This part of the flap is dissected up to separate the gingival epithelium and connective tissue from the underlying periosteum over the bone (*Figure 18.7b*). Great care should be taken with this stage of the procedure, as perforation of the flap will mean inevitable failure. However, if this technique is attempted in an area potentially involving important nerves, such as in the lower premolar area, then a total full-thickness flap should be raised to avoid nerve damage. The dissection of the flap is carried into the alveolar mucosa so that the flap can be moved laterally without any tension.

Repositioning of pedicle graft

The flap is moved across the root surface so that its leading margin approximates the receiving edge of the gingival tissue, making sure that the resulting suture line will lie over bone (*Figure 18.7c*). These margins are brought together and sutured using 4/0 or 5/0 silk sutures. Care must be taken that the flap fits tightly around the neck of the affected tooth. Three or four sutures may be needed to close the defect tightly, and one of these is placed in the vestibule so that no residual eyelet defect is produced. An interdental suture is also placed in each interproximal space covered by the flap. A denuded area of periosteum-covered bone is left distal to the flap (or mesially to the flap if it was moved distally).

A moist sterile gauze is pressed firmly over the flap to fix it in position and minimize any underlying blood clot. A periodontal dressing such as Coe-Pack is placed over the wound area.

Post-operative care

The usual post-operative instructions are given, with emphasis on the need to avoid vigorous lip movements. This procedure produces very little swelling or discomfort, and healing is usually uneventful.

The dressing and sutures are removed after 1 week, by which time the suture line should be united and the denuded area covered by healing tissue.

The wound rarely needs to be covered for more than a week. The patient is instructed to keep the area clean with a twice-daily chlorhexidine mouthwash and frequent warm saline washes. Irritation of the healing graft must be avoided. Careful toothbrushing with a soft brush can be started when the pack and sutures are removed, but this should gently clean the tooth surface down to the gingiva and not onto it.

Two weeks after surgery, the suture line should be fading and the denuded area should be covered with epithelium. One month after surgery the wound is fully healed, but it is still unwise to probe the gingival crevice over the defect. Probing is best left for about 6 months, and should be carried out with great care.

Mode of healing

The exact form of healing that takes place after the laterally repositioned flap procedure is still debated. There are two possibilities:

1. Crevicular epithelium grows down the inner surface of the flap against the root surface to form a long epithelial attachment, and the gingival fibre bundles keep the flap closely adapted to the root. It is also feasible that hemidesmosomes connect the epithelial downgrowth to the root surface so that a firm attachment is formed.
2. Epithelial downgrowth does not take place and a fibrous tissue connection forms between the flap and the root surface. This could imply the deposition of new cementum on to the root surface so that Sharpey's fibres can be formed. The differentiation of cementoblasts and formation of cementum seem unlikely without the concomitant formation of crestal bone, and so far no evidence of such repair has been produced.

Whichever form of healing actually does take place, at a clinical level the graft can remain stable for many years, providing that the gingival margin is free of plaque and therefore free of inflammation. Slight recession of the graft may take place, but the recurrence of marked recession of pocketing or the development is rare.

Modification of laterally repositioned flap

The standard laterally repositioned flap can sometimes result in some gingival recession in the donor area, and a modification that spares the marginal gingiva at the donor site has been devised (Pennel *et al.*, 1965). This is only possible if a sufficiently wide zone of attached gingiva is present in the donor area to produce the desired zone of keratinized tissue at the recipient site. It has the advantage of leaving the interdental papillae *in situ* at the recipient site, which makes it easier to secure the pedicle graft at the required height. It also leaves a much smaller exposed area at the donor site than the conventional technique.

Procedure

Recipient site

Horizontal incisions are made across the base of the two interdental papillae of the recipient tooth so that these are retained in their original positions. These will form a butt joint against which the repositioned sliding flap will lie. Two vertical incisions are then made down to the vestibule on either side of the recession area to expose bone around its margin (*Figures 18.8a* and *18.9a*). This tissue is cut off by a further horizontal incision at its base, and the tissue is removed. The root surface is carefully scaled and planed, and may be conditioned if desired.

Figure 18.8 Modified laterally repositioned flap. *(a)* Horizontal incisions below papillae of recipient teeth and below gingival margins of donor teeth. Bone is exposed around root of recipient tooth and a sloping vertical incision is made to delineate flap; *(b)* flap slid over defect and sutured in place

(a)

(b)

Figure 18.9 Clinical pictures of modified laterally repositioned flap: *(a)* incisions; *(b)* sutured into new position. (Courtesy Mr C A Waterman)

Donor site

A slightly sloping horizontal incision is then made from the tip of the distal vertical recipient site incision, and is carried below the interdental papillae and marginal gingiva of the donor site teeth. A further slightly sloping vertical incision is then made distally down into the vestibule to delineate the donor flap (*Figures 18.8a* and *18.9a*).

This flap is carefully dissected up as a split-thickness flap, leaving the periosteum in place. This flap is then fully mobilized and slid across to cover the defect where it fits into a butt joint with the recipient site papillae (*Figures 18.8b* and *18.9b*). The flap is sutured into position with resorbable 5/0 gut sutures. Two sutures join it to the retained papillae at the recipient site, and a further two or three join the vertical flap margin to the mesial edge of the recipient site. Only a small area of donor site periosteum is left uncovered with this procedure.

The area is covered with either a conventional pack, such as Coe-Pack, or a Surgicel/cyanoacrylate pack. With this latter method, Surgicel is placed over the area and held in place using cyanoacrylate glue (Superglue). This can also be covered with Vaseline® with tetracycline powder mixed into it if required (Miller, 1982, 1985b, 1992). Coe-Pack is replaced after a week for a further week if necessary. The latter pack is left until it drops off, usually after 3 weeks.

Healing of both the donor and recipient sites is usually uneventful.

Double papilla flap

This technique was introduced by Cohen and Ross (1968), and is a variant of the laterally repositioned flap. The basic technique is similar, except that the donor tissue is mobilized from the adjacent papillae rather than from an adjacent tooth. There is less exposure of donor site bone with this procedure, and less tension is placed on the donor tissue. The interdental septum at the papillary area is of greater thickness than the facial or lingual alveolar plates, and is less likely to be damaged when the overlying tissues are disturbed. A disadvantage of this technique is that the proximal papillae must be of sufficient bulk both mesio-distally and cervico-apically to cover the defect. Small papillae imply small interdental septa, and under these conditions this procedure would fail to cover the defect as well as possibly causing damage to the underlying bony septa.

Procedure (*Figure 18.10*)

This procedure is suitable for a recession defect on a tooth with bulky mesial and distal papillae. The exposed root surface is scaled and root planed. A V-shaped incision is made around the margin of the recessed gingiva to expose connective tissue at its edge (*Figure 18.10a*). The distal tissue is bevelled to expose a wider zone of connective

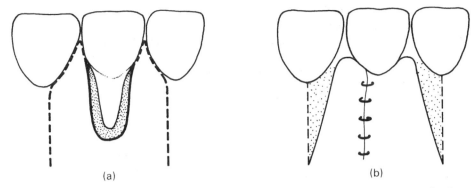

Figure 18.10 Double papilla flap. *(a)* Incisions (i) around root to expose bone with wider zone distally to provide base for suture line; (ii) delineating flap margins. *(b)* Papillae transposed to cover defect and sutured over bone exposed distal to defect

tissue to accept the mesial portion of the graft. Mesial and distal vertical incisions are made and carried into the vestibule to mobilize the two papillae (*Figure 18.10a*). The two papillary flaps are carefully raised and repositioned to cover the labial surface of the exposed root so that the join line coincides with the distal margin of the defect. The flaps are sutured together in this position with resorbable 5/0 medium gut sutures (*Figure 18.10b*). This correct positioning is very important, since placement of sutures at the midline of the exposed root will lead to inadequate co-adaptation of tissue. This will result in the creation of a dehiscence at the suture line and failure of the procedure. The most apical suture is passed through the periosteum to stabilize the position of the graft. In addition, either mesial and distal sutures or a sling suture around the tooth can be placed to stabilize the graft further. A dressing such as Coe-Pack may be carefully placed over the area for a week.

Coronally repositioned flap

The coronally repositioned flap (Harvey, 1965; Bernimoulin *et al.*, 1975) can be used on its own or in combination with other procedures to treat multiple areas of recession. It can also be used in combination with other procedures to treat localized recession. On its own it cannot increase the amount of keratinized gingiva that is already present at the site. This may however be achievable if it is combined with other procedures that can fulfil this function. An example of this is its combination with the free gingival graft to treat the combined problem of gingival recession and lack of attached gingiva.

Procedure

The free gingival graft is first carried out to increase the attached gingival zone (see full description in the following section). After complete healing, a full-thickness mucoperiosteal flap is raised and extended to the base of the vestibule. It is then moved upwards in a coronal direction to cover the exposed roots of the teeth, and

maintained in this position by interdental suturing and the placement of a periodontal dressing. In the combined procedure the free gingival graft is used to provide new keratinized attached gingiva, and the coronally repositioned flap to carry this up over the root surface.

Free grafts

Full-thickness, thick epithelial flap

The free gingival graft was introduced by Nabors (1966). It is designed to increase the width of keratinized gingiva (Sullivan and Atkins, 1968a), but can also be used to treat gingival recession (Sullivan and Atkins, 1968b, 1969; Miller, 1988). Unlike the pedicle graft, this procedure takes keratinized palatal epithelium and connective tissue from its original site and relocates it to a remote donor site. The graft is placed over a freshly prepared bed of connective tissue and sutured in place. The underlying connective tissue bed nourishes the graft until it builds its own blood supply. This occurs as the result of blood vessels growing into it from the underlying connective tissue base (see below).

As this graft retains none of its own blood supply and is totally dependent on the bed of recipient vessels, it was originally developed to increase the zone of attached gingiva and not specifically to cover denuded root. New attached gingiva is produced by grafting keratinized palatal mucosa and its inductive connective tissue over a recipient bed previously covered by non-keratinized alveolar mucosa. However, several modifications have improved this procedure's root coverage capabilities. Maynard (1977) developed two procedures: first, the placement of a free gingival graft to create a band of keratinized gingiva, and secondly, a coronally repositioned flap (see above) to pull the tissue coronally over the exposed root(s). Holbrook and Ochsenbein (1983) used thick, stretched, free gingival grafts with intricate suturing to improve the graft's adaptation to the recipient bed and limit the amount of dead space, which could hinder vascularization. Miller (1982, 1985b) emphasized root planing and citric acid treatment of the exposed roots.

All of these modifications have improved the capability of free grafts to survive over avascular root surfaces. The coverage of wide or multiple areas of recession are best treated by the double procedure of Maynard (1977) (see below), whilst the free graft alone, using the modifications of Holbrook and Ochsenbein (1983) and Miller (1982, 1985b), can be used to cover single narrow root surface defects (*Figure 18.12a*).

Procedures

The procedure differs in several details according to whether the aim is only to increase the zone of attached gingiva, leaving the existing gingiva undisturbed (procedure 1), or whether the aim is additionally to cover area(s) of root exposed by gingival recession (procedure 2).

Suitable donor and recipient sites are chosen and local analgesia given.

Preparation of recipient site

The following technique has been proposed by Miller (1982, 1985b).

For procedure 1, an incision is made along the muco-gingival junction (*Figure 18.11a, c*). For type 2 procedures, an incision is made along the gingiva of the recipient site to allow butt joining of the graft to adjacent tissue (*Figure 18.11b, c*). The apical margin of the flap is raised and dissected through the connective tissue as a split-thickness flap to delineate the connective tissue bed of the recipient site (*Figure 18.11d*). This extends into the area previously covered by non-keratinized alveolar mucosa. Bulow Dry Foil is then placed over the bed to act as a template for the graft and trimmed to size.

Root preparation

This is only necessary for type 2 procedures, and the method outlined is that proposed by Miller (1985b).

If the exposed root surface is buccally prominent, it is planed back to reduce the possibility of recurrence and to reduce localized pressures on the graft. This is done either using a Kirkland No. 12 curette or a Gracey curette. A butt joint is made at the cement enamel junction of the tooth. The root surface is then conditioned using pH 1 citric acid with cotton buds or a burnishing technique. It is left until there is a frosted finish on the root surface after profuse rinsing.

Preparation of donor site

The template is placed on the palate and the graft outlined. It is delineated with a No. 15 Swann–Morton blade, making an incision about 3 mm deep so that the graft includes an adequate thickness of connective tissue. In fact, it is this connective tissue layer which is the func-

tional part of the graft. A split-thickness graft is carefully dissected from the underlying deeper connective tissue with the No. 15 blade. The graft should be at least 2–3 mm thick, and any adipose tissue on the inner side can be left for root coverage. However, if root coverage is not being attempted, then it should be 1–2 mm thick with no adipose tissue.

Placement of graft

The graft should be placed *in situ* (*Figures 18.11e and 18.12b*) and trimmed quickly, if necessary, to help to maintain its vitality. The flap raised at the recipient site can be cut off at this point as it is no longer needed, and the graft can be sutured in place.

Three types of suture have been described for use with this procedure (Miller, 1982, 1985; Jahnke *et al.*, 1993). These are (*Figure 18.11f, g*):

1. Papillary sutures positioned interdentally (*Figure 18.11f*)
2. Apical stretching sutures (*Figure 18.11f*)
3. Vertical stabilizing sutures (*Figure 18.11g*).

The vertical stabilizing sutures (*Figure 18.11g*) criss-cross over the graft without going through it. The suture passes from the palatal aspect of the tooth through the right interdental space before passing diagonally across the surface of the graft to its base at the opposite corner. It penetrates through the periosteum at the base of the graft and then crosses diagonally in the opposite direction to the left interdental space. It finally passes through this to meet the starting end and be tied off palatally.

These sutures allow the graft to be approximated closely to the root surface, whilst still allowing flow of nutrient. Resorbable catgut sutures are used to avoid trauma to the healing area. To protect the graft, Surgicel is placed over the area and held in place using cyanoacrylate glue (Superglue). This is then covered with Vaseline into which tetracycline powder has been mixed (Miller, 1982, 1985b, 1992). This is left until it drops off, usually after 3 weeks, and cleanliness is maintained using chlorhexidine mouthwashes. The patient may be placed on tetracycline for 2 weeks.

The palate can be similarly covered or an acrylic stent may be used, although there is good healing after only 1 week.

The end result can look extremely good (*Figure 18.12c*), and this is a very predictable procedure with good long-term results. However, in some cases it can look bulky or of a different colour.

Healing of the graft

Vascularization of the gingival graft takes place from the underlying connective tissue bed. This can commence as early as the first 2–4 days post-operatively, before which nutrients to the graft are supplied by tissue fluid. Capillary buds grow from the underlying connective tissue into the graft and these vessels anastomose and mature to form a

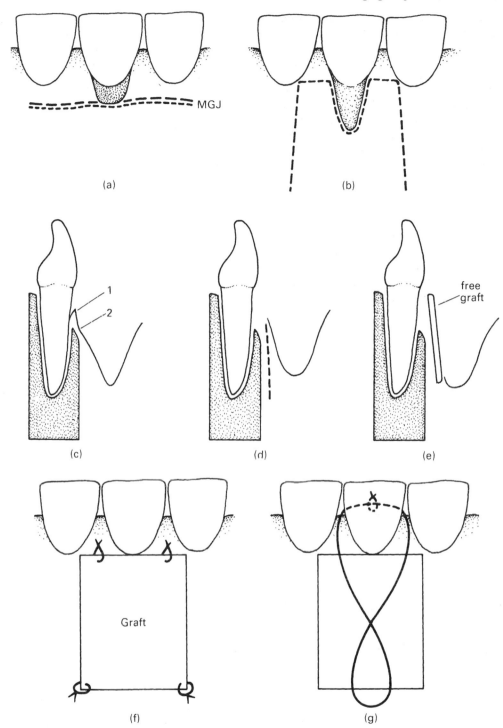

Figure 18.11 Free gingival graft. *(a)* Incision for procedure 1 at mucogingival junction. *(b)* Incisions for procedure 2 to cover exposed roots. Horizontal incision across base of papillae, which are left *in situ*. The incision carries around the recession area. Two vertical incisions delineate flap. *(c)* Incision for procedure 1(1) and 2(2) in other plane. *(d)* Dissection of split-thickness flap to leave tissue over bone to nourish free graft. *(e)* Free graft in position. *(f)* Papillary and apical stretching sutures. *(g)* Vertical stabilizing sutures

new vasculature, which is complete by about the four-teenth day. Because nutrition to the graft is minimal during the first 2–3 days, the surface layers of the epithelium degenerate, necrose and are desquamated. A layer of new epithelium is present after 4–5 days, rete pegs are formed at 7–14 days and keratinization takes about 28 days. The maturation process takes place under the inductive influence of the palatal connective tissue.

(a)

(b)

(c)

Figure 18.12 Free gingival graft to treat localized gingival recession. *(a)* Pre-operative picture showing recession of |1̄ extending to mucogingival graft; *(b)* free graft placed into position before suturing; *(c)* post-operative result after 1 year showing coverage of root and increase in attached gingival zone. (Courtesy Mr C A Waterman)

Factors affecting success

1. Incorrect choice of site for procedure, i.e. wrong class of gingival recession.
2. If the graft is too thick and this becomes vascularized, the tablet of tissue stands away from the rest of the tissue.
3. If the graft is too thin it may perforate and necrose.

4. If the underlying blood clot is too thick the graft may be discarded.

Connective tissue graft

This type of graft has a number of advantages over the free epithelial graft (Edel, 1974; Langer and Langer, 1985; Jahnke *et al.*, 1993). These include the following:

1. There is a closed palatal wound
2. The aesthetic result is claimed to be better
3. There is a better potential blood supply from the periosteum beneath and the split-thickness flap above.

This procedure was introduced by Langer and Langer (1985) as a method of gaining root coverage in cases with severe recession involving either isolated or multiple teeth. The subepithelial connective tissue graft is a combination of a pedicle graft and a free autogenous connective tissue graft performed simultaneously. In this procedure, the connective tissue receives a blood supply from the periosteum beneath and the split-thickness flap above, and this increases its chances of survival over the avascular root surface. The procedure also avoids an open palatal wound and produces a better aesthetic result because it avoids the problem of colour differentiation that occurs between a full-thickness graft and the surrounding tissues (Schluger *et al.*, 1990).

Procedure

Preparation of recipient site

A horizontal incision is made around the teeth to be treated and the area is bounded by two vertical relieving incisions, which extend well beyond the mucogingival junction to create a wide base for the flap. The horizontal incision passes along the base of each included interdental papilla and then into the gingival crevice buccally to each tooth (*Figures 18.13* and *18.14*). Great care must be taken

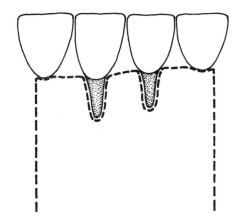

Figure 18.13 Incisions for connective tissue graft at recipient site. The incision passes across the base of the papillae to leave these *in situ* for suturing

(a)

(b)

(c)

Figure 18.14 Connective tissue graft. *(a)* Incisions: the papillae are left *in situ* for suturing; *(b)* a special scalpel handle with two blades 1.5 mm apart for taking optimum thickness connective tissue graft from palate; *(c)* the connective tissue graft in position over root surfaces and prepared bed. (Courtesy Mr C A Waterman)

not to lift the papillae. The incisions are carefully deepened and the flap is dissected from the underlying periosteum and deep connective tissue as a split-thickness flap. The edge of the flap is first raised and held under tension with fine tissue forceps to allow careful sharp dissection with a No. 15 blade. Great care must be taken not to perforate the flap as this will compromise its blood supply, which is an important source of nutrient to the connective tissue graft. The flap is freed apically so that there will be very little tension when it is ultimately

pulled coronally. The size of the connective tissue graft is determined by the size of the recipient base, and its height and length are measured. The graft must be large enough to cover the exposed roots and connective tissue bed in all directions. The connective tissue bed is the second important source of blood supply to the overlying graft.

Root preparation

Root planing of the exposed roots is carefully carried out. Additional preparation with citric acid or tetracycline may also be carried out as described in the last section. Opinion is divided as to whether this is necessary or indeed beneficial.

Preparation of donor site

The donor site is prepared palatally by making two parallel horizontal bevelled incisions 3 mm from the gingival margin using a No. 15 blade (*Figure 18.15a*). The incisions are made from the canine to the first molar area, since the connective tissue is thicker and better vascularized in this area and the rugae are of no concern because the graft is taken internally. A split-thickness flap is raised with or without mesial and distal vertical relieving incisions. A wedge of connective tissue of about 1.5 mm thickness, along with its thin border of epithelium, is carefully dissected out (*Figure 18.15b*). Care should be taken to avoid the palatine vessels, but staying anterior to the first molar should avoid this problem. The length of the flap and the depth of the dissection depend on the size of the recipient area to be covered. This procedure leaves the outer epithelialized flap to be replaced for primary intention wound closure.

A special scalpel handle (*Figure 18.14b*) has been devised to accept two blades 1.5 mm apart for use in obtaining a suitable connective tissue graft. This was designed by Harris (1992) for use in the double papilla graft/connective tissue graft (see below), but can also be used in this procedure if available.

It is advisable to suture the palatal flap back into position immediately after removing the donor tissue, as this will reduce the size of the blood clot that will form. A method of suturing that produces compression will also further this aim. Horizontal mattress sutures are used, and they begin by passing through the mesial interproximal space on the buccal surface. They then penetrate the palatal mucosa apical and distal to the base of the graft

Figure 18.15 *(a)* Incisions for connective tissue graft from palate. Two parallel incisions 1.5 mm apart are made from canine to first molar. Connective tissue graft is then dissected out. *(b)* Resultant graft with thin epithelialized upper margin

before exiting the palate mesially. They finally cross to the distal interproximal space to be tied on the buccal surface. These sutures compress the palatal flap and approximate its edges. This should bring about rapid haemostasis. A dressing is optional, and usually unnecessary. The patient reports much less discomfort and bleeding problems than with the free gingival graft because of the full coverage.

Graft placement

The connective tissue graft is carefully positioned over the denuded roots with its epithelialized border coronally (*Figure 18.14c*). It is stretched slightly to extend mesially and distally to cover the full length of the prepared bed, and should extend down apically over the full depth of the prepared bed. Some authorities advocate suturing the graft to the papillae separately using interrupted chrome gut interdental sutures and an atraumatic needle. Alternatively, the graft and the overlying flap may be secured into place together (see below). This second method does, however, depend on completely covering the connective tissue graft right up to its thin epithelial border. This thin border of epithelium is left on the graft because it helps to colour-blend it with the adjacent tissues. It must be placed coronally to the cement–enamel junction.

Replacement of the recipient overlying flap

The recipient flap is repositioned coronally to cover as much of the connective tissue graft as possible. It is sutured in place using resorbable gut sutures, either separately by interdental gut sutures, or in combination with securing the graft. In this alternative form of suturing, the gut sutures pass through the flap, the graft and, finally, the papilla. The graft is protected by using a surgical cyanoacrylate and Vaseline covering (see previous section). The patient is instructed to use chlorhexidine mouthwashes, and may be put on tetracycline for 2 weeks. The area is left until the pack comes off by itself,

usually after 2–3 weeks. The appearance of a patient before and 6 months after these procedures is shown in *Figure 18.16*.

Connective-tissue graft with double papilla flap

In both the above techniques when used separately, the graft over the root surface relies on the collateral circulation bringing nutrient from nearby areas. In this modification, proposed by Harris (1992), the graft is covered over the root surface with tissue brought together by a double papilla type flap. The graft gets its blood supply both from the underlying periosteum mesial, distal and apical to the exposed root, and from the covering double papilla pedicle flaps.

Procedure

Preparation of recipient site

The recipient site incisions are the same as those previously described for a double papilla graft coverage of a recession defect (see previous section). The tips of the papillae are left *in situ* (*Figures 18.17a and 18.18a*) to allow the graft to be sutured to them. For this combined procedure, split-thickness flaps are raised from both papillae.

Root preparation

The root surface is planed thoroughly to reduce any labial bulbosity of the affected tooth. It is then conditioned with tetracycline, using a 250 mg tetracycline capsule dissolved in 2 ml saline.

Preparation of donor site

The procedure is the same as that described for the connective tissue graft (see previous section). A special

(a)   (b)

Figure 18.16 *(a)* Gingival recession at lower incisor prior to connective tissue graft with coronally repositioned flap. *(b)* Appearance 6 months postoperatively. (Courtesy Dr A Sidi)

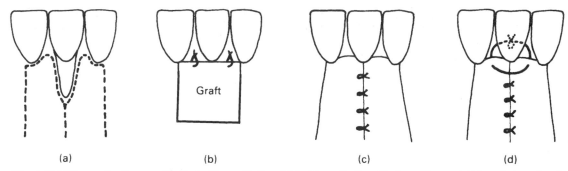

Figure 18.17 Connective tissue graft with double papilla flap. *(a)* Incisions: the tips of both papillae are left for suturing of graft. *(b)* Connective tissue graft sutured to papillae. *(c)* Double papillae flaps brought together and sutured over graft. *(d)* A sling suture tied lingually to hold flap tightly over graft

Figure 18.18 Connective tissue graft with double papilla flap. *(a)* Incisions: the tips of the papillae are left *in situ* for suturing; *(b)* double papilla flap coronally repositioned to cover graft and sutured into position. (Courtesy Mr C A Waterman)

scalpel handle (*Figure 18.14b*) has been devised to obtain an optimum thickness connective tissue graft with this procedure (Harris, 1992). It accepts two blades 1.5 mm apart, which give an ideal incision in order to remove the graft.

Placement of the graft

The graft is tried in place and its size slightly modified if necessary. It is sutured into position in three parts, using 3/0 or 4/0 catgut:

1. The connective tissue graft is sutured to the remaining interdental papillae (*Figure 18.17b*)
2. The flaps are brought together as a double papilla (*Figures 18.17c* and *18.18b*)
3. A sling suture is used to hold the flap over the graft (*Figure 18.17d*).

The area is dressed using Surgicel and cyanoacrylate, and this is covered with Vaseline and tetracycline. This last covering is made by mixing the contents of one 250 mg capsule of tetracycline into the Vaseline. Dietary restrictions are imposed, and the patient is instructed to use a

chlorhexidine mouthwash until normal oral hygiene can be carried out.

Resolution

The pack is left in position until it comes off naturally, usually after 2–3 weeks. Following this, the resolution back to health and normal oral hygiene is usually quick and uneventful.

Histological result of grafting procedures over exposed root surfaces

At best, all the grafting techniques that cover exposed root surfaces may result in a connective tissue attachment to the root surface, although this is extremely unlikely on present day knowledge of tissue relationships. Downgrowth of junctional epithelium occurs rapidly, and may act to protect the root surface from the resorptive effects of gingival connective tissue (see Chapter 17). This results in the formation of a long junction epithelium, which may be firmly adherent to the root surface. This relationship can be stable, but it is not as resistant to either inflammation or to trauma as would be the case if complete regeneration including bone had occurred. Regeneration in this context implies the restoration of the various components of the periodontium lost through disease or trauma in their appropriate locations, amounts and relationships to each other (Aukhil, 1991).

Guided tissue regeneration

To have any chance of regenerating bone, cementum and periodontal attachment in these areas, some form of guided tissue regenerative (GTR) technique needs to be performed. Standard GTR using Gore-tex® membranes always requires a secondary procedure to remove the PTFE membrane. This has the disadvantage of disturbing any newly formed osteoid material. Also, flaps replaced over Gore-tex membranes may shrink, and therefore coverage of any osteoid that might form may be difficult with this two-stage technique. However, the use of two-stage GTR techniques for buccal recession in monkeys have been shown to give rise to a reduction in gingival recession, a gain in connective tissue attachment and the formation of new bone (Gottlow *et al.*, 1990). They have also been used successfully clinically to treat buccal gingival recession, including defects in excess of 5 mm (Tinti and Vincenzi, 1990a, 1990b; Pini Prato *et al.*, 1992).

In addition, space maintenance is a problem with the use of PTFE membranes because they easily collapse and thus eradicate any space between the membrane and the root surface into which healing tissue from the periodontal ligament may grow (Nyman *et al.*, 1982). To avoid this disadvantage, techniques have evolved to help maintain this space with conventional PTFE membranes (Tinti *et al.*, 1992, 1993, 1994). These include the use of a suture to tent the membrane inwards (Pini Prato *et al.*, 1992, 1993; Tinti and Vincenzi, 1990a, 1990b), the use of a cast gold framework (Tinti and Vincenzi, 1993) and the use of a titanium-reinforced membrane, which can be curved to produce the space.

If an area of localized recession is to be treated with GTR techniques, it must have some remaining attached keratinized gingiva between the base of the defect and the mucogingival junction. This is because GTR procedures for gingival recession cannot increase the amount of keratinized gingiva already at the site, and this must be provided over the grafted area by the coronal repositioning of the flap. Thus gingival recession defects must be treated at an earlier stage in their development than in the case of lesions treated with gingival grafting techniques.

Clinical procedure using two-stage GTR with PTFE membranes

A full-thickness mucoperiosteal flap is developed from a crevicular horizontal incision, sparing the interdental papillae, and vertical relieving incisions. It is raised until freely mobile to allow subsequent coronal repositioning. A single tooth Gore-tex membrane is modified so that it can be tented out to give a space between the membrane and the root to allow tissue ingrowth. This is accomplished either by placing a suture to tent it inwards (*Figure 18.19a*) or by tying it to a suitably bent gold bar or pre-cast gold framework. Recently, Gore-tex membrane with an incorporated metal framework has been manufactured to allow the membrane to be tented to the correct shape (*Figure 18.19b*). This membrane is then placed and secured by a sling suture to cover the exposed root surface, leaving a gap for tissue ingrowth (*Figure 18.19c, d*). The flap is then coronally repositioned to cover the membrane, and sutured into place with PTFE sutures.

After 4–8 weeks, a marginal flap is gently lifted to allow the membrane to be removed. This should leave a definite soft tissue attachment against the root of the tooth. The flap is sutured back after membrane removal and the sutures are removed 1 week later. The healing is usually uneventful thereafter. It is not yet known whether new hard tissues form after this procedure. In this connection, it is also not known whether tenting of the membrane fully prevents downgrowth of gingival epithelium.

Clinical and laboratory trials of the two-stage technique

A clinical and histological investigation of the two-stage GTR techniques using ePTFE membranes for buccal recession has been carried out in monkeys (Gottlow *et al.*, 1990). It has shown that this technique can produce a reduction in gingival recession, a gain in connective tissue attachment and the formation of new bone.

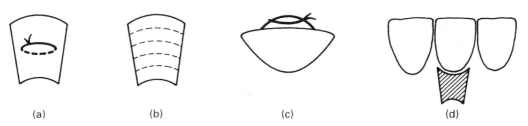

(a)   (b)   (c)   (d)

Figure 18.19 PTFE (Gore-tex™) membrane for guided tissue regeneration on localized recession. *(a)* Membrane tented with suture; *(b)* membrane with incorporated metal wires for tenting; *(c)* and *(d)* tented membrane in position over exposed root

Clinical trials of these techniques in humans have shown that they can reduce gingival recession and produce an apparent gain in clinical attachment (Pini Prato *et al.*, 1992, 1993; Tinti *et al.*, 1992, 1993; Tinti and Vincenzi, 1993, 1994). Reductions in soft tissue recession of 55–83% have been achieved by these techniques.

Resorbable membranes

Resorbable membranes do not need to be removed because they are degraded by body tissues (see Chapter 17). They may also provide the suitable conditions for bone regrowth and the formation of new attachment (Brady *et al.*, 1973; Gottlow *et al.*, 1992; Laurell *et al.*, 1992). One advantage of these techniques is that they are one-stage procedures and are thus preferred by patients. Furthermore, because of the lack of a second surgical procedure to remove the membrane, there is no interference with the healing tissue as could occur in the two-stage GTR procedure. The procedure is also considerably easier than other grafting procedures because it only involves a single surgical site and a full-thickness mucoperiosteal flap is raised.

A multilayered resorbable membrane barrier membrane (Guidor®, Guidor AB, Huddinge, Sweden) has been produced, which is designed for use in the treatment of gingival recession by producing space between the membrane and the root surface. This membrane is unidirectional, having spacer bars on the inner surface to lift it away from the root surface and create the space required for new attachment formation. The use of this membrane has been shown effectively to prevent the downgrowth of junctional epithelium and to allow integration of the flap connective tissue with new attachment on the root surface (Lundgren *et al.*, 1994; Gottelow *et al.*, 1994a, 1994b).

Clinical procedure for a one-stage procedure with a resorbable membrane

The procedure is similar to that described above for ePTFE membranes, but differs in some minor details. It involves the raising of a full-thickness mucogingival flap, which will subsequently be coronally repositioned over the membrane. The flap must include some keratinized gingiva, since this technique cannot increase this tissue (see above). A flap is outlined (*Figures 18.20a* and *18.21a*) with an inverse bevel incision, which allows partial removal over papillae tips; the remainder of these are left *in situ* to facilitate suturing. Vertical relieving incisions are made down to the vestibule to allow a full-thickness mucoperiosteal flap to be fully mobilized. The exposed root surface is cleaned and reduced in bulbosity using a Kirkland 13 and Gracey 11/12 and 13/14 curettes. The margin of a flap is slightly raised on the lingual side to accommodate the resorbable retaining suture tie submucosally. A bioresorbable membrane is placed and trimmed to cover the osseous recession defect and to cover the adjacent bone mesially, distally and apically by a few millimetres. A suitable membrane for this procedure is the Guidor polylactate membrane (Guidor®, Guidor AB, Huddinge, Sweden), which has two layers with added spacers on the underside to lift it away from the root surface and so aid the ingrowth of new cementum, bone and collagen fibre-forming cells. It may be necessary to raise the apical edge of the retained interdental papilla in order to touch the edge of the membrane beneath. The membrane adapts itself well to the shape of the root and surrounding bone (*Figure 18.21b*). It is then tied in place with resorbable sutures, using a sling suture technique to suspend the membrane from the lingual surface of the tooth (*Figure 18.20b*). It is tied off on the lingual aspect and the ends are tucked below a small lingual flap, which is raised for this purpose, taking care to avoid the lingual aspects of the papillae. The flap is sutured coronally using a minimum of four black silk sutures, two through the papilla and two in the relieving incisions (*Figures 18.20c* and *18.21c*). No packing is applied, or the space below the membrane would be eliminated and there would be no ingrowth of healing tissue. The patients are instructed not to brush the operated area for 6 weeks and to rinse daily for 2 minutes with chlorhexidine mouthwashes. This is to minimize the risk of bacterial contamination of the membrane (Nowzari and Slots, 1994). Two-weekly careful professional cleaning may also be undertaken during this period. As a further precaution against infection, tetracycline may be prescribed for 2 weeks. The external sutures are removed

(a)   (b)   (c)

Figure 18.20 Guided tissue regeneration for gingival recession using resorbable membranes. *(a)* Incisions sparing tips of papillae; *(b)* membrane held in position with sling suture; *(c)* flap coronally positioned over membrane. It is sutured to papillae and also vertically

Figure 18.21 Guided tissue regeneration using resorbable membrane to cover localized gingival recession. *(a)* Incisions; sparing tips of papillae. Full-thickness mucoperiosteal flap. *(b)* Guidor resorbable membrane in position over root surface and surrounding bone. It adapts itself well to the shape of the root and adjacent bone. *(c)* Flap coronally repositioned and sutured over membrane (Courtesy Mr C A Waterman)

after 4 weeks, and at 6 weeks the patient is instructed to start to clean this area with a careful non-traumatic brushing technique.

Clinical trials of one-stage techniques

A clinical and histological investigation of the one-stage GTR technique using bioresorbable membranes for the treatment of buccal recession has been carried out on

monkeys (Gottlow *et al.*, 1994b). It has shown that this technique can produce a reduction in gingival recession, a gain in connective tissue attachment and the formation of new bone. The amount of these tissues formed was of the same order as seen for non-resorbable membranes (Gottlow *et al.*, 1990). In addition, clinical studies in humans have shown that bioresorbable membranes produce similar reductions in recession to those seen with non-resorbable membranes (Rachlin *et al.*, 1996; Roccuzzo *et al.*, 1996; Waterman, 1997). Only these three studies of bioresorbable membranes have been reported to date, but they show 60–83% reductions in gingival recession, which are similar to or better than those seen with non-resorbable membranes. Only one clinical study of the use of Guidor® resorbable membranes for the treatment of buccal recession has used a re-entry technique 1 year after the placement of the membrane to measure new bone growth in humans (Waterman, 1997). It showed a mean increase in bone height of 1.95 ± 0.14 mm for all 17 of the sites, which included a variety of tooth sites, treated in 13 patients.

This technique therefore appears to have the potential to allow bone regeneration to occur in areas of buccal osseous defects such as those associated with localized gingival recession (Waterman, 1997). The histology of the attachment of this bone to the root surface has not been studied in humans, but results in monkeys (Gottlow *et al.*, 1994b) seem to indicate that new attachment is formed.

References

Addy, M., Dummer, P.M.H., Hunter, M.L. *et al.* (1987) A study of the association of fraenal attachment, lip coverage and vestibular depth with plaque and gingivitis. *Journal of Periodontology* **58**, 752–757

Ah, M.K.B., Johnson, G.K., Kaldahl, W.B. *et al.* (1994) The effect of smoking on the response to periodontal therapy. *Journal of Clinical Periodontology* **21**, 91–97

Aukhil, I. (1991) Biology of tooth-cell adhesion. *Dental Clinics of North America* **35**, 359–468

Brady, J.M., Cutright, D.E. and Miller, R.A. (1973) Resorption rate, route of elimination and ultra-structure of the implant site of poly-lactic acid in the abdominal wall of the rat. *Journal of Biomedical Materials Research* **7**, 155–166

Bernimoulin, J.P., Luscher, B. and Muhlemann, H.R. (1975) Coronally repositioned periodontal flap. Clinical evaluation after 1 year. *Journal of Clinical Periodontology* **2**, 1–13

Cohen, D.W. and Ross, S.E. (1968) The double papilla repositioned flap in periodontal therapy. *Journal of Periodontology* **39**, 65–70

Crigger, M., Bogle, G., Nilveus, R. *et al.* (1978) The effect of topical citric acid application on the healing of experimental furcation defects in dogs. *Journal of Periodontal Research* **13**, 538–549

Demirel, K., Baer, P.N. and McNamara, T.F. (1991) Topical application of doxycycline on periodontally involved root surfaces *in vitro*: comparative analysis of substantivity on cementum and dentin. *Journal of Periodontology* **62**, 312–316

Edel, A. (1974) Clinical evaluation of free connective tissue grafts used to increase the width of keratinized gingiva. *Journal of Clinical Periodontology* **1**, 185–196

Garrett, J.S., Crigger, M. and Egelberg, J. (1978) The effects of citric acid on diseased root surfaces. *Journal of Periodontal Research* **13**, 155–163

Gottlow, J., Karring, T. and Nyman, S. (1990) Guided tissue regeneration following treatment of recession type defects in the monkey. *Journal of Periodontology* **61**, 680–685

Gottlow, J., Lundgren, D., Nyman, S. *et al.* (1992) New attachment formation in the monkey using Guidor®, a bioabsorbable GTR device. *Journal of Dental Research* **71** 1535, Abstr.

Gottlow, J., Laurell, L., Teiwik, T. and Genon, P. (1994a) Guided tissue regeneration using a bioresorbable matrix barrier. *Practical Periodontics and Aesthetic Dentistry* **6**, 71–81

Gottlow, J., Laurell, L., Lundgren, D. *et al.* (1994b) Periodontal response to a new bioresorbable guided tissue regeneration device: A longitudinal study in monkeys. *International Journal of Periodontics and Restorative Dentistry* **14**, 437–449

Grupe, H.E. and Warren, R.F. (1956) Repair of gingival defects by a sliding flap operation. *Journal of Periodontology* **27**, 92–95

Hannington-Kitt, J.G. and Dunne, S.M. (1993) Topical guanethidine relieves dental hypersensitivity and pain. *Journal of the Royal Society of Medicine* **86**, 514–515

Harris, R.J. (1992) The connective tissue and partial thickness double pedicle graft: A predictable method of obtaining root coverage. *Journal of Periodontology* **63**, 477–486

Harvey, P.M. (1965) Management of advanced periodontitis. I. Preliminary report of a method of surgical reconstruction. *New Zealand Dental Journal* **61**, 180–187

Holbrook, T. and Ochsenbein, C. (1983) Complete coverage of denuded root surface with a one-stage gingival graft. *International Journal of Periodontics and Restorative Dentistry* **3**, 8–27

Jahnke, P.V., Sandifer, J.B., Gher, M.E. *et al.* (1993) Thick free gingival and connective tissue autografts for root coverage. *Journal of Periodontology* **64**, 315–322

Jones, J.K. and Triplett, R.G. (1992) The relationship of cigarette smoking to intra-oral wound healing: a review of evidence and implications for patient care. *Journal of Maxillofacial Surgery* **50**, 237–239

Lang, N.P. and Löe, H. (1972) The relationship between the width of keratinized gingiva and gingival health. *Journal of Periodontology* **43**, 623–627

Langer, B. and Langer, L. (1985) Subepithelial connective tissue graft technique for root coverage. *Journal of Periodontology* **60**, 715–720

Laurell, L., Gottlow, J., Nyman, S. *et al.* (1992) Gingival response to Guidor®, a bioabsorbable device in GTR therapy. *Journal of Dental Research* **71** 1536, Abstr.

Lundgren, D., Mathisen, T. and Gottlow, J. (1994) The development of a barrier for guided tissue regeneration. *Journal of Swedish Dental Association* **86**, 741–756

Maynard, J.G. Jnr (1977) Coronal positioning of a previously placed autogenous gingival graft. *Journal of Periodontology* **48**, 151–155

Miller, P.D. (1982) Root coverage using a free soft tissue autograft following citric acid application. I. Technique. *International Journal of Periodontics and Restorative Dentistry* **2**, 65–70

Miller, P.D. (1985a) A classification of marginal tissue recession. *International Journal of Periodontics and Restorative Dentistry* **5**, 9–13

Miller, P.D. (1985b) Root coverage using the free soft tissue autograft following citric acid application. III. A successful and predictable procedure in areas of deep wide recession. *International Journal of Periodontics and Restorative Dentistry* **5**, 15–37

Miller, P.D. (1988) Regenerative and reconstructive periodontal plastic surgery. Mucogingival surgery. *Dental Clinics of North America* **32**, 287–306

Miller, P.D. (1992) Personal communication

Miller, P.D. Jnr (1987) Root coverage with free gingival graft. Factors associated with incomplete coverage. *Journal of Periodontology* **58**,
674–681

Miyasoto, M., Crigger, M. and Egelberg, J. (1977) Gingival condition in areas of minimal and appreciable width of keratinized gingiva. *Journal of Clinical Periodontology* **4**, 200–209

Nabors, J. (1966) Free gingival grafts. *Periodontics* **4**, 243–245

Nowzari, H. and Slots, J. (1994) Microorganisms in polytetrafluoroethylene barrier membranes for guided tissue regeneration. *Journal of Clinical Periodontology* **21**, 203–210

Nyman, S., Lindhe, J. and Karring, T. (1981) Healing following surgical treatment and root demineralization in monkeys with periodontal disease. *Journal of Clinical Periodontology* **8**, 249–258

Nyman, S., Gottlow, J., Karring, T. and Lindhe, J. (1982) The regenerative potential of the periodontal ligament. *Journal of Clinical Periodontology* **9**, 257–265

Pennel, B.M., Higgason, J.D., Towner, J.D. *et al.* (1965) Oblique rotated flap. *Journal of Periodontology* **36**, 305–309

Pini Prato, G., Tinti, C., Vincenzi, G. *et al.* (1992) Guided tissue regeneration versus mucogingival surgery in the treatment of human buccal gingival recession. *Journal of Periodontology* **63**, 919–928

Preber, H. and Bergström, J. (1990) Effect of cigarette smoking on periodontal healing following surgical therapy. *Journal of Clinical Periodontology* **17**, 324–328

Rachlin, G., Koubi, G., Dejou, J. and Franquin, J.C. (1996) The use of resorbable membrane in mucogingival surgery. A case series. *Journal of Periodontology* **67**, 621–626

Register, A.A. and Burdick, F.A. (1975) Accelerated reattachment with cementogenesis to dentin, demineralized *in situ*. I. Optimum range. *Journal of Periodontology* **46**, 646–655

Register, A.A. and Burdick, F.A. (1976) Accelerated reattachment with cementogenesis to dentin, demineralized *in situ*. II. Defect repair. *Journal of Periodontal Research* **47**, 263–267

Roccuzzo, M., Lungo, M., Corrente, G. and Gandolofo, S. (1996) Comparative study of a bioresorbable and a non-resorbable membrane in the treatment of human buccal gingival recessions. *Journal of Periodontology* **67**, 7–14

Salkin, L.M., Freedman, A.L., Stein, M.D. and Bassiouny, M.A. (1987) A longitudinal study of mucogingival defects. *Journal of Periodontology* **58**, 164–166

Schluger, S., Youdelis, R., Page, R.C. *et al.* (eds) (1990) Mucogingival problems. In *Periodontal Diseases* (S. Schluger, R. Youdelis, R.C. Page *et al.*, eds). Philadelphia: Lea and Febiger

Sullivan, H.C. and Atkins, J.H. (1968a) Free autogenous gingival grafts. I. Principles of successful grafting. *Periodontics* **6**, 121–129

Sullivan, H.C. and Atkins, J.H. (1968b) Free autogenous gingival grafts. III. Utilization of grafts in the treatment of gingival recession. *Periodontics* **6**, 152–160

Sullivan, H.C. and Atkins, J.H. (1969) The role of free gingival grafts in periodontal therapy. *Dental Clinics of North America* **13**, 133–148

Terranove, V.P., Franzetti, L.C., Hic, S. *et al.* (1986) A biochemical approach to periodontal regeneration. Tetracycline treatment of dentin promotes fibroblast adhesion and growth. *Journal of Periodontal Research* **21**, 330–337

Tinti, C. and Vincenzi, G. (1990a) Guided tissue regeneration with Goretex: new perspectives. *Quintessence International* **6**, 45–49

Tinti, C. and Vincenzi, G. (1990b) Treatment of gingival recession with guided tissue regeneration with Gore-tex membrane: clinical variations. *Quintessence International* **6**, 465–468

Tinti, C. and Vincenzi, G. (1994) Expanded polytetrafluoroethylene titanium-reinforced membranes for regeneration of mucogingival recession defects, a 12 case report. *Journal of Periodontology* **65**, 1088–1191

Tinti, C., Vincenzi, G., Cortellini, P. *et al.* (1992) Guided tissue regeneration in the treatment of human facial recession. *Journal of Periodontology* **63**, 554–560

Tinti, C., Vincenzi, G. and Cocchetto, R. (1993) Guided tissue regeneration in mucogingival surgery. *Journal of Periodontology* **64**, 1184–1191

Trombelli, L., Schincaglia, G., Checchi, L. and Calura, G. (1994) Combined guided tissue regeneration, root conditioning, and fibrin-fibronectin system application in the treatment of gingival recession. A 15 case report. *Journal of Periodontology* **65**, 769–803

Trombelli, L., Schincaglia, G., Zangari, F. *et al.* (1995) Effects of tetracycline HCl conditioning and fibrin–fibronectin system application in the treatment of gingival recession with guided tissue regeneration. *Journal of Periodontology* **66**, 313–320

Waterman, C. (1997) A re-entry study to determine the hard and soft tissue changes following treatment of buccal defects using a bioabsorbable membrane. *Journal of Periodontology* **68**, 982–989

Wennström, J.L. (1987) Lack of association between the width of attached gingiva and the development of soft tissue recession. A 5-year longitudinal study. *Journal of Clinical Periodontology* **14**, 181–184

Wennström, J., Lindhe, J. and Nyman, S. (1982) The role of keratinized gingiva in plaque associated gingivitis in dogs. *Journal of Clinical Periodontology* **9**, 75–85

Wicksjö, U.M.E., Baker, P.J., Christersson, L.A. *et al.* (1986) A biochemical approach to periodontal regeneration: tetracycline treatment conditions dentin surfaces. *Journal of Periodontal Research* **21**, 322–369

19

The periodontal abscess

A periodontal or lateral (as opposed to apical) abscess is a localized area of inflammation in which the formation of pus has taken place in the periodontal tissues. It is produced by endogenous pyogenic micro-organisms, possibly toxic factors in the plaque and/or some reduction in host resistance caused by local or systemic factors.

A number of factors appear to provoke the formation of an abscess:

1. Obstruction of the opening to a deep pocket, frequently one which is tortuous, e.g. associated with a furcation defect.
2. Gingival injury with a foreign body, e.g. toothbrush bristle or woodstick, etc., which carries bacteria into the tissues. Careless subgingival scaling may also carry micro-organisms into damaged tissue, as can powerful irrigation of a pocket.
3. Incomplete removal of plaque and subgingival calculus from the depths of a pocket. Frequently after scaling there is tightening of the gingival cuff, which may occlude a pocket containing bacteria.
4. Infection of tissues damaged by excessive occlusal stress, which may be produced by:
    (a) A blow on a tooth.
    (b) Excessive orthodontic pressure.
    (c) Bruxism (see p. 369).
5. As a consequence of pulp disease:
    (a) Where a periapical lesion spreads up the lateral surface of a tooth.
    (b) Where lateral pulp canals link with the periodontal ligament. This is especially common in the furcation. Accessory pulp canals are extremely common, and may not be evident on the radiograph. The furcation abscess produced by pulp pathology is frequently misdiagnosed as a primary periodontal lesion.
    (c) Perforation of the lateral wall of a tooth during endodontics or post preparation.
6. Altered host response, as in diabetes. Diabetes has frequently been diagnosed following the appearance of multiple periodontal abscesses.

The main direct cause of a lateral abscess is bacterial invasion of the soft tissue wall of the pocket and multiplication therein. This leads to an acute inflammatory response with the formation of pus, which is the main feature of an abscess.

Bacterial invasion of the tissues in periodontitis has mainly been described in cases of advanced chronic periodontitis (Frank, 1980; Saglie *et al.*, 1982a, 1982b, 1985, Manor *et al.*, 1984), and an abscess is most common at this stage of the disease. Some studies have indicated that putative periodontal pathogens may penetrate epithelium, epithelial cells and connective tissue in this situation (Saglie *et al.*, 1986, 1988; Papapanou *et al.*, 1994; Sandros *et al.*, 1994) and, if the body's defence mechanisms do not control this situation quickly, could easily lead onto the formation of an abscess.

Clinical features

The onset of symptoms can be sudden, with pain on biting and a deep throbbing pain. The involved tooth may feel high and mobile. The overlying gingiva becomes red, swollen and tender, but at first there is no fluctuation or discharge of pus. There may be enlargement of the associated lymph glands.

The next stage is characterized by the presence of pus. This may discharge into a periodontal pocket when the symptoms reduce, or the pus may track through the bone to form an abscess under the alveolar mucoperiosteum. Once the pus enters the soft tissue the severe pain diminishes and the abscess appears as a red, shiny and very tender swelling over the alveolus. The abscess usually points and discharges, but if this does not happen the inflammation may spread into the surrounding connective tissue to produce a cellulitis. This occurs most commonly if the patient's resistance is low. If the abscess is in the upper jaw, depending upon the tooth involved, the lip, cheek, side of the nose or the infra-orbital area and lower eyelid may swell. Infection in the vicinity of the infra-orbital foramen is particularly dangerous. If the abscess is in the lower jaw, the lower lip, chin, cheek, angle of the mandible and neck may swell. If infection involves the lower third molar, there may also be trismus and difficulty in swallowing. At this stage the patient is obviously unwell, in pain and distressed, and the temperature may be elevated.

Differential diagnosis

These clinical features can be produced by both periapical and periodontal abscesses, and a differential diagnosis must be made because the treatments for the two forms of abscess are different. Sometimes a differential diagnosis may not be easy. A number of features must be taken into account:

1. The position of the abscess swelling. If this is over the root apex, it is likely to be periapical.
2. The presence of periodontal disease with pocketing and bone destruction. If the periodontal condition is generally quite good and pocketing is absent or shallow, the abscess is unlikely to be periodontal.
3. If the involved tooth is heavily filled it is likely that pulp pathology is present, and a history of sensitivity to hot and cold tends to confirm this. If the tooth is non-vital, the abscess could be periapical or periodontal, or both as a combined abscess. Pulp vitality tests can be extremely misleading but, if the tooth gives a normal reading, this points to periodontal infection. If the tooth is caries free and unfilled, the abscess is likely to be periodontal.
4. Pus discharging from the gingival margin is usually indicative of a lateral periodontal abscess. However, it must be remembered that about 1% of apical abscesses of palpal origin also discharge via this route by tracking up the periodontal ligament. In this latter situation rapid (within a few days) endodontic treatment is necessary to prevent the development of a perio/endo lesion as a result of the abscess tract becoming epithelialised to form a secondary periodental pocket leading to the cyrex.
5. Radiographs taken in the earliest stages provide little useful information, but once the lesion is established its position can be identified (*Figure 19.1*). However, a periodontal abscess on the facial or lingual aspect of the tooth may not be clearly discernible on the radiograph. A radiograph taken with a gutta-percha point inserted gently into the suspected pocket can help to define the origin of the abscess.

Treatment of the abscess

Treatment depends upon the stage of abscess development, the amount of bone loss and whether pulp pathol-

Figure 19.1 Radiographic appearance of a periodontal abscess that is on the palatal aspect of the central incision

ogy is also involved. The initial aims of treatment are the relief of pain and control of infection. Once these have been achieved the residual lesion must be treated; otherwise, recurrent abscess formation is inevitable.

In the first stage, infection can be controlled by an antibiotic (e.g. penicillin V 250 mg four times a day for 5 days, or erythromycin in the same dosage if the patient is sensitive to penicillin). If an anaerobic infection is suspected, then metronidazole 200 mg three times per day for 5 days, or a combination of amoxycillin 250 mg/metronidazole 200 mg three times per day for 5 days could be prescribed. The use of metronidazole is contraindicated in patients who cannot be relied upon to refrain from alcohol and during pregnancy. Grinding the opposing tooth can also help to relieve the occlusion.

Once the abscess is fluctuant and pointing, drainage is essential. The abscess is incised under local anaesthesia, but the injection must be made well away from the inflamed area. Regional anaesthesia or even general anaesthesia may be needed if the inflamed area is large. This is supplemented by regular hot salt water mouthwashes. The drainage incision should be horizontal and made through the most fluctuant site. The margins of the wound may be spread to facilitate drainage. If adequate drainage is established, an antibiotic may not be needed. Relieving the occlusion by grinding the opposing tooth should allow the patient to eat on the other side of the mouth.

If the infection has spread to produce a cellulitis or tissue space infection, an intramuscular injection of Triplopen or erythromycin should bring this under control, and drainage can then be established.

Once the acute condition is under control, treatment of the residual condition can be started. If there is considerable bone loss, extraction may be necessary. If the tooth is to be conserved, a flap can be raised and the bone defect associated with the abscess curetted. Frequently the abscess has perforated the facial or lingual plate of bone, leaving a bridge of marginal bone. If this bridge of bone is narrow, it may be cut away and the fragments of bone used as a graft in the bone defect. If the bridge is wide, it is conserved in the hope that the perforation will repair. On the first occasion of abscess formation the prognosis can be good, but if recurrent abscesses have been present the prognosis may be doubtful. If it is obvious that the tooth's prognosis is hopeless it should be immediately extracted under local anaesthia since this will produce immediate drainage and obviate the need for any antibiotics.

The combined periodontal–periapical lesion

The combined lesion can develop in a number of ways:

1. Where an apical abscess has spread laterally to create a periodontal lesion or united with a pre-existing lateral lesion.
2. Where pulp infection has spread via accessory canals into the periodontal tissues. This is most frequent in the furcation, where accessory canals are common.
3. Where a periodontal lesion extends close to the tooth apex and causes secondary pulpal infection.
4. Where a lateral canal is exposed within a pocket and infection spreads from this source into the pulp producing secondary pulpitis and apical infection.

At one time the presence of a combined periapical–periodontal lesion justified extraction, especially if occurring in a furcation. Today, endodontics has achieved a high level of success and predictability, and the prognosis for a tooth involved in a combined lesion can be good.

Treatment

Once acute inflammation has been controlled and the occlusion adjusted, root-canal treatment should be initiated. A lateral compression technique is necessary to occlude accessory canals, and when endodontics has been satisfactorily completed, periodontal surgery can be carried out.

If a multirooted tooth is involved and (i) bone destruction about one root is much more advanced than that about the other root(s), or (ii) the furcation defect is of such labyrinthine complexity that it cannot be kept clean, or (iii) the divergent roots of neighbouring teeth, usually the buccal roots of upper molars, are very close together or actually touch, then root resection is indicated (see Chapter 17).

References

Frank, R.M. (1980) Bacterial penetration in the apical pocket wall of advanced human periodontitis. *Journal of Periodontal Research* **15**, 563–573

Manor, A., Lebendiger, M., Shiffer, A. and Torvel, H. (1984) Bacterial invasion of the periodontal tissues in advanced periodontitis in humans. *Journal of Periodontology* **55**, 567–573

Papapanou, P.N., Sandros, J., Lindberg, K. *et al.* (1994) *Porphyromonas gingivalis* may multiply and advance within stratified human junctional epithelium. *Journal of Periodontal Research* **29**, 374–375

Saglie, F.R., Carranza, F.A. Jnr, Newman, M.G. *et al.* (1982a) Identification of tissue-invading bacteria in human periodontal diseases. *Journal of Periodontal Research* **17**, 452–455

Saglie, F.R., Newman, M.J., Carranza, F.A. Jnr and Pattison, G.L. (1982b) Bacterial invasion of gingiva in advanced periodontitis in humans. *Journal of Periodontology* **53**, 217–222

Saglie, F.R., Carranza, F.A. Jnr and Newman, M.J. (1985) The presence of bacteria within the oral epithelium of human periodontal disease. I. A scanning and transmission electron microscopic study. *Journal of Periodontology* **56**, 618–624

Saglie, F.R., Rezende, J.H., Pertuiset, J. *et al.* (1986) The presence of bacteria within the oral epithelium in periodontal disease. II. Immunochemical identification of bacteria. *Journal of Periodontology* **57**, 492–500

Saglie, F.R., Pertuiset, J., Rezende, J.H. *et al.* (1988) *In situ* correlative immuno-identification of mononuclear infiltrates and invasive bacteria in diseased gingiva. *Journal of Periodontology* **59**, 688–696

Sandros, J., Papapanou, P.N., Nannmark, U. and Dahlén, G. (1994) *Porphyromonas gingivalis* invades the human pocket epithelium *in vitro*. *Journal of Periodontal Research* **28**, 219–226

20

Early onset periodontitis

A variety of names have been given to a form of periodontal disease characterized by deep pockets and advanced alveolar bone loss in children, adolescents and young adults, without any associated systemic disease. Gottlieb (1923, 1928) designated the condition(s) diffuse atrophy of alveolar bone, and subsequently other names were devised: deep cementopathia, paradontosis, periodontosis, juvenile periodontitis, prepubertal periodontitis, rapidly progressive periodontitis. Page and Baab (1985) suggested that all forms of these diseases be designated early onset periodontitis (EOP).

At a population level there is direct correlation between oral hygiene status, the degree of gingival inflammation and the severity of periodontal destruction. However, at an individual level there is a great deal of variation in the way in which the tissues respond to plaque irritation. Some individuals with poor oral hygiene suffer little periodontal destruction, while others with little plaque have advanced periodontal destruction. Two hypotheses have been proposed to account for this variation:

1. Certain plaque bacteria have a greater potential for tissue destruction than others, and when they are present disease will occur
2. Host factors determine the tissue response to plaque.

Of course, both of these factors could be important in both adult periodontitis and EOP.

Early onset periodontitis can be practically divided into three groups:

1. Prepubertal periodontitis – severe gingivitis and destructive periodontitis in primary dentition
2. Juvenile periodontitis:
   • Localized – severe localized attachment loss in permanent first molars and incisors
   • Generalized – involvement of these teeth and a few or many other teeth
3 Rapidly progressive periodontitis – generalized rapid attachment loss in permanent dentition.

Prepubertal periodontitis

This is an extremely rare form of periodontal disease characterized by rapid periodontal destruction of the primary dentition (Page *et al.*, 1983a). The gingivae are grossly inflamed, and the patient commonly has other bacterial infections. In some cases the condition may affect the permanent dentition as well. In many instances there is a familial pattern to the disease, and most if not all cases are probably genetically mediated. A number of inherited conditions described in Chapter 6 also produce these effects, including hypophosphatasia, Papillon–Lefèvre syndrome, cyclic neutropenia, familial neutropenias and Chediak–Higashi syndrome.

Rapidly progressive periodontitis

Rapidly progressive periodontitis (RPP) is characterized by severe generalized periodontal destruction, and may affect any or all of the permanent dentition of patients between the ages of 20 and 35 years (Page *et al.*, 1983b). The clinical features and subgingival flora resemble active chronic periodontitis, with *Porphyromonas gingivalis*, *Prevotella intermedia*, *Eikenella corrodens* and *Actinobacillus actinomycetemcomitans* all being reported to be present. There is a lack of epidemiological evidence for this condition as a separate entity, although there is evidence of some cases having a familial tendency. On present available evidence it is difficult to justify the classification of this condition as a separate disease entity, as it could well represent a rapidly progressive chronic periodontitis in a susceptible individual.

It is also important to distinguish this condition from post-juvenile periodontitis (see below), and to remember that some conditions, such as Down's syndrome (see Chapter 6), have a high susceptibility to severe rapidly progressive periodontitis in the permanent dentition.

Juvenile periodontitis

Usually multiple names for a disease entity indicate an ill-defined knowledge of the precise aetiology and pathogenesis; indeed, it is possible for similar clinical manifestations to be produced by different causal factors and pathological processes. In this text the term juvenile periodontitis (Butler, 1969) is used because it refers to the general population affected, and does not imply any particular cause or disease process. Baer (1971) described juvenile periodontitis as a well-defined clinical entity different from adult periodontitis in that it appears to start around puberty, seems more common in girls, appears to occur in families, and is rapidly progressive.

Two forms of the disease were described; local and general. In the localized form, the tissue destruction is restricted to the first molars and incisors and is characterized by a symmetrical distribution; in the generalized form, many or all the teeth are involved. Gradations between these two extremes are often seen. The variability of these forms was recently demonstrated by Yosof (1990) in a study of 47 Malaysian children (22 boys and 25 girls) with the condition. He divided the children into four groups according to the distribution of the bone loss:

Type 1 Bone destruction limited to first molars and incisors (14.9%)

Type 2 Bone destruction involving first molars and incisors and some other teeth (25.5%)

Type 3 Generalized destruction but worse around the first molars and incisors (14.9%)

Type 4 Generalized involvement of more than 14 teeth (44.7%)

Juvenile periodontitis (JP) has distinctive clinical and bacteriological features, which justify its classification as a separate disease entity.

The main epidemiological and clinical features of this disease are described in the following section.

Prevalence

On the basis of the epidemiological studies detailed below, JP appears to occur in approximately 1 in 1000 adolescents and seems to have a racial predisposition, occurring most frequently in people of West African origin. Recent epidemiological studies using precise diagnostic criteria have reported an incidence of between 0.1 and 2.9% (Saxen, 1980a, 1980b; Saxby, 1984, 1987; Kronauer et al., 1986; Bial and Mellonig, 1987; Melvin et al., 1991; Hart et al., 1991; Papapanou, 1994). These studies all confirm that the prevalence varies amongst different ethnic groups, and a study in the UK (Saxby, 1984) showed an incidence of 0.02% for Caucasians, 0.8% for Afro-Caribbeans and 0.2% for Asians. In a later study, Saxby (1987) examined the prevalence of JP in a sample of 7266 schoolchildren in the West Midlands, UK.

The subjects were initially screened by assessments of probing depths around incisors and first molars, and positive subjects were then confirmed by full mouth clinical and radiological examination. An overall prevalence of 0.1% was found, and subjects in both sexes were affected with equal frequency. However, highly significant differences were observed between different ethnic groups, with a prevalence of 0.02% in Caucasians, 0.2% in Asians and 0.8% in Afro-Caribbeans, which was virtually identical to the earlier study. Similar findings were found by Melvin et al. (1991), who examined a racially mixed population in Florida, USA. Armed service recruits, 3158 male and 1855 female, were examined in a three-step procedure. First, panoramic radiographs of these subjects were screened, and secondly, areas suggestive of bone loss were further examined with bite wing radiographs. Finally, the recruits with radiographic evidence of bone loss were subject to careful clinical examination. Thirty cases of JP were identified, with a female : male ratio of 1.1 : 1. There were significant ethnic differences, with a prevalence of 2.9% in Blacks, 0.09% in Caucasians and 0.8% in those of Oriental and Hispanic origin. JP was more prevalent in Black males than females, with a ratio of 1 : 0.52, whilst it was more prevalent in Caucasian females than males, with a ratio of 4.3 : 1. In another recent study of the radiographs of 1038 children aged 10–12 years, Neely (1992) found a prevalence rate of 4.6 per thousand. In addition, an examination of 2500 children in Chile by Lopez et al. (1991) found a JP prevalence of 0.32%, and in Iraq Albander (1993) recorded a prevalence of 1.8%. The disease also seems more prevalent in Africa, as exemplified by Nigerian studies (Hartley and Floyd, 1988). However, too many variables, e.g. oral hygiene, nutritional status and socio-economic factors, enter into the picture to allow valid comparison, and in the Chilean study (Lopez et al., 1991) the authors state that JP was found most commonly in people from low socio-economic groups.

Age of presentation

The patient is usually an adolescent at the time of examination, but may be much younger; the onset of the disease may be several years before the time of examination. Sjobin et al. (1993) carried out a retrospective study of early radiographs of 118 young patients aged 13–19 years with JP, taken when they were 5–12 years old, and compared these with early radiographs of 168 13–19-year-olds without JP. They found that some of the individuals with JP had bone loss around primary teeth.

A similar clinical picture to JP, but with obvious signs of gingival inflammation, has been found in individuals in their 20s, and has been called post-juvenile periodontitis. It appears to result from the evolution of JP.

Sex ratios

Many of the earlier studies reported that the condition appeared more commonly in females than males, at a ratio of about 3 : 1 (Baer, 1971; Manson and Lehner, 1974). In Iraqi children Albander (1993) recorded a ratio of 3.5 : 1, and the ratio of girls to boys in the Lopez *et al.* (1991) study was 7 : 1. However, there are certain qualifications that need to be applied to all epidemiological data before such assertions can be accepted. In this regard, it has been suggested that some of the findings reflect the way in which the data were collected. In those studies based upon patients presenting at periodontal clinics, the adolescent girl (who is usually more concerned about her appearance and wellbeing than the adolescent boy) will figure more frequently. Also, the patient is more likely to be accompanied by the mother, to whom enquiries about the family are made. Fathers are often invisible, and prevalence in males may be under-estimated simply because they are not examined.

When the data are obtained from balanced epidemiological surveys (Saxby, 1987; Melvin *et al.*, 1991), an almost equal (1.1 : 1) sex prevalence is found. Furthermore, one of these studies (Melvin *et al.*, 1991) showed very different sex ratios in Black and Caucasian subjects, with a male to female ratio of 1 : 0.52 in Black subjects and 1 : 4.3 in Caucasians. They also found that there is no female preponderance of JP cases after correction has been made for selection bias. Thus, the method of collecting data must be scrutinized before conclusions can be drawn.

Clinical manifestations

The gingivae usually show few, if any, signs of clinical inflammation, and little or no supragingival plaque and calculus. Subgingival calculus deposits are usually absent from root surfaces and, because of the absence of clinical inflammation and gingival bleeding, the condition may escape detection until it becomes advanced, when mobility and drifting of teeth (usually incisors) occur. An acute periodontal abscess may develop at this stage, and the associated pain and swelling bring the patient to the dentist for examination. As stated, the condition is frequently localized to the incisors and first molars, but may affect other teeth (Astemborski *et al.,* 1989).

In regularly attending patients the disease should be diagnosed much earlier, and at this stage treatment is more successful. The early clinical signs are periodontal pocketing and attachment loss, often on the mesial surface of the first molar (*Figure 20.1*). Attachment loss may increase rapidly. Baer (1971) estimated that 50–75% of the attachment of affected teeth may be lost in 4–5 years.

Figure 20.1 Juvenile periodontitis. A periodontal probe measuring a 10 mm pocket mesial to the ⎽6 of an 18-year-old girl. Note the lack of clinical inflammation, plaque and calculus

Bone destruction

The pattern of bone destruction and distribution of the lesions represent two of the intriguing aspects of the disease. In the classic case, advanced bone destruction is localized to the incisors and first molars in a symmetrical or mirror-image distribution (*Figure 20.2*). Deep angular or crescentic bone defects around these teeth, particularly the affected molars, are characteristic, and the areas of bone resorption are sharply demarcated from the neighbouring bone, which appears completely healthy on the radiograph. Because the alveolar bone is thinner around incisors, these teeth often lose all the interdental bone and this appears on the radiographs as marked horizontal bone loss. Other teeth, in particular second premolars and second molars, may be involved.

With regular attenders, the first radiographical signs are likely to be seen on routine bite wing radiographs, usually on the mesial surface of the first molar. Any early signs of bone loss on these teeth should be taken seriously, and should lead to a detailed examination of the patient. These radiographs should always be checked for any signs of bone loss, since they clearly show the alveolar crest. They are probably the only means of early diagnosis of JP, since children and adolescents are unlikely to have a detailed periodontal examination.

In a proportion of cases, apparently random, asymmetrical involvement occurs. On rare occasions the condition may spread with time to other teeth, so that the bone around almost every tooth is involved.

Familial tendency

Many researchers have described a familial tendency in this disease. Benjamin and Baer (1967) described its occurrence in twins, siblings, cousins and other family connections. This has suggested a genetic transmission and, because of the apparently greater frequency in

Figure 20.2 Juvenile periodontitis. Classic first molar–incisor involvement in a 12-year-old boy. The orthopantogram shows advanced bone loss around the upper and lower first molars and incisors

females, an X-linked dominant inheritance has been suggested (Melnick *et al.*, 1976; Spektor *et al.*, 1985). However, reinterpretation of this evidence (Hart *et al.*, 1992) supports the notion of autosomal transmission. In this connection, some studies have suggested that it is an autosomal recessive condition (Saxen, 1980c; Long *et al.*, 1987), and still others that it is autosomal dominant (Roulston *et al.*, 1985; Boughman *et al.*, 1986). Boughman *et al.* (1986) reported one child with JP and dentinogenesis imperfecta (a genetically transmitted autosomal dominant fault), which both showed genetic markers on chromosome 4, whilst the same group also discovered a family in which five generations displayed JP and dentinogenesis imperfecta always occurring together (Roulston *et al.*, 1985). In yet another study by one of these groups (Boughman *et al.*, 1988), genetic-model testing was used on 28 families with a history of JP. They showed that an autosomal recessive mode of inheritance was most applicable to the data.

The various genetic studies showed that, if a patient has JP, there is a 50% chance that the disease will develop in a brother or sister (Saxen, 1980c; Spektor *et al.*, 1985; Van Dyke *et al.*, 1985).

It has also been shown that JP occurs frequently in blood group B (Kaslick *et al.*, 1971). Tissue typing has also been used to determine a possible predisposition to JP. The major histocompatibility complex MHC (see Chapter 3) has at least six human leucocyte antigen (HLA) types, and the composition of these is genetically determined and varies in different individuals. Available information indicates a great variation in HLA profiles amongst JP patients (Saxen, 1980c; Saxen and Koskimies, 1984), although there is an increased frequency of antigens A9, A28 and B15 in these patients (Reinholdt *et al.*, 1977). Thus, although there is much evidence to support the genetic inheritance of JP, its mode of inheritance is still unclear. It is also not known how the genes are expressed.

General health

There seems to be no relationship with any systemic condition, although a somewhat similar dental picture is found in the rare Papillon–Lefèvre syndrome but with a generalized distribution and also involving the deciduous dentition.

The role of cementum

Gottlieb (1928) first suggested that the underlying cause of periodontosis was a defect in cementum formation. This concept has been re-examined more recently (Lindstog and Blomlöf, 1983; Blomlöf *et al.*, 1986). They carried out a comparative histological study on teeth from patients with JP, adult chronic periodontitis and healthy controls. They found that the cementum on the teeth from JP subjects had extensive areas of hypoplasia in both the exposed and intra-alveolar root surfaces. This suggests that the defect is related to impaired cementum formation rather than the pathology of the pocket. This defect in cementum formation could be hereditary, and could be an important aetiological factor.

Bacteriology

The subgingival microflora of JP is scanty when compared with that associated with adult periodontitis, and its composition is very difficult. Examination with dark-ground microscopy shows that it is dominated by coccoid and straight non-motile rods (Liljenberg and Lindhe, 1980). The dominant cultivable microflora consists of Gram negative capnophilic and facultative rods, and these make up about two-thirds of the isolates (Newman and Socransky, 1977). The principal bacteria present are *Actinobacillus actinomycetemcomitans*, *Capnocytophaga* species and *Eikenella corrodens*. Some motile anaerobic rods, mainly *Campylobacter* (*Wolinella*) *recta*, may also be present in some cases (Slots, 1976; Zambon *et al.*, 1983a). Using selective media for *Actinobacillus*, *A. actinomycetemcomitans* can be isolated from nearly all JP patients (Slots *et al.*, 1980; Zambon *et al.*, 1983a). Mandell (1984) found 100-fold higher numbers of *A. actinomycetemcomitans* and 50-fold higher numbers of *E. corrodens* in active versus non-active sites.

The bacteria associated with JP may invade the periodontal connective tissue in this condition (Gillett and Johnson, 1982; Carranza *et al.*, 1983; Christersson *et al.*, 1987), and *A. actinomycetemcomitans* is the principal invading species (Saglie *et al.*, 1982).

Several bacteria associated with JP produce substances capable of damaging the host defences and tissues, and these will be described in association with each type of bacteria. By far the most important bacteria associated with this condition is *A. actinomycetemcomitans*, and this has been the subject of most of the research on this subject. This is therefore the first type described below.

Actinobacillus actinomycetemcomitans

Numerous studies have shown the association between *A. actinomycetemcomitans* and JP and have suggested that it plays an important role in its pathogenesis (Haffajee *et al.*, 1984; Zambon, 1985). *A. actinomycetemcomitans* is found in low numbers in the subgingival flora of healthy and adult chronic periodontitis sites, whereas in JP it is found in 97% of affected sites and forms up to 70% of the total flora at these sites (Zambon, 1985). Furthermore, resolution of JP coincides with a reduction or elimination of this bacteria from the subgingival flora, and recurrence of disease is associated with its recolonization of the site (Slots and Rosling, 1983).

However, there is now no doubt that a significant number of young healthy subjects also harbour *A. actinomycetemcomitans* in their oral flora. The global distribution of *A. actinomycetemcomitans* varies considerably, and in normal periodontally healthy individuals its prevalence is about 13% in Finland (Alanuusua and Asikainen, 1988), 20–25% in urban USA (Slots *et al.*, 1980) and 60% in Panama (Eisenmann *et al.*, 1983). Interestingly, this bacterial distribution seems to mirror the relative occurrence of JP in these three countries, which was lowest in Finland, intermediate in the USA and highest in Panama (Lindhe and Slots, 1989). Possibly, if there is a higher infection rate with this bacteria in the population, then there is a higher risk that susceptible individuals may acquire the bacteria and develop JP (Slots and Schonfeld, 1991). This may to some extent explain the higher prevalence of JP in black subjects in the USA and UK. It is possible that the high level of *A. actinomycetemcomitans* infection in these subjects represents a carriage of the bacteria from African populations with high prevalence of JP (Franklin, 1978). Tracing *A. actinomycetemcomitans* transmission in racial and family groups is being aided

by the development of sensitive microbial genetic methods to trace genotypes of this bacteria in various populations (Di Rienzo and Slots, 1990; Zambon *et al.*, 1990).

Similarly, familial distribution of *A. actinomycetemcomitans* may be due to transmission of bacteria between family members, and this could be particularly relevant in families with one or more members susceptible to JP. Convincing evidence of intra-familial transmission was produced by Zambon *et al.* (1983a), who found that each infected subject in the family harboured the same biotype and serotype of the bacteria. This was also shown with genetic methods using restriction fragment length polymorphism (RFLP) typing of strains (Di Rienzo and Slots, 1990). They showed at least one common RFLP type in each infected family member.

More than one serotype or genotype of *A. actinomycetemcomitans* can colonize the oral cavity of an individual. Asikainen *et al.* (1991) recovered two serotypes from 1 of 13 infected Finnish subjects, and Chung *et al.* (1989) found two serotypes in 3 of 12 infected Korean patients. In addition, Di Rienzo and Slots (1990) found two and three RFLP types in two Black families. Both the intra-familial transmission of strains of *A. actinomycetemcomitans* and the presence of uninfected members in affected families (Zambon *et al.*, 1983a) shows that close contact between individuals is necessary for transmission to occur. The apparently poor transmissibility of this organism may in part explain the low prevalence of JP.

However, as many as 25% of the adolescents in the USA harbour periodontal strains of *A. actinomycetemcomitans*, but only 0.1% of this group develop JP. This could either be because host factors determine disease development or because only certain strains of *A. actinomycetemcomitans*, alone or in combination with other bacteria, have pathogenic potential (Slots and Schonfeld, 1991).

Three serotypes of *A. actinomycetemcomitans* can be distinguished, and in a study in the USA (Zambon *et al.*, 1983c), serotype b has been detected in twice as many JP affected sites as serotypes a and c. In Finland (Asikainen *et al.*, 1991), serotype b has been mainly found in periodontitis patients and serotype c in healthy individuals.

Using restriction fragment length polymorphism (RFLP) typing of *A. actinomycetemcomitans*, different patterns were observed, and these did not correspond to serotypes of the bacteria (Di Rienzo and Slots, 1990). One of these RFLP types named RFLP B seemed particularly virulent, and was present in the flora of three subjects who converted from health to JP. This genotype was not recovered from any healthy sites.

It has also been suggested (Preus *et al.*, 1987) that genetic material acquired by phage infection could influence the virulence of *A. actinomycetemcomitans*. They found that phage infected bacteria were present in 12 sites that had experienced bone loss within the preceding year in five JP patients, whilst nine non-progressing sites infected with the bacteria had non-phage infected strains.

A. actinomycetemcomitans strains also vary in their

ability to produce the leucotoxin (see below) against human PMNs and monocytes. It has been found that sites with JP lesions are usually infected with strongly leucotoxin-producing strains, whilst the healthy sites are generally infected with non leucotoxin-producing strains (Zambon *et al.*, 1983b; Tsai and Taichman, 1986).

A. actinomycetemcomitans produces a variety of factors that could increase its virulence and potentially damage the tissues of the host. These are:

- A leucotoxin, which can destroy PMNs and monocytes
- Chemotactic inhibition factors
- Surface-associated material (SAM), which stimulates bone resorption
- A lipopolysaccharide (LPS), which can also cause bone resorption
- Proteases that degrade immunoglobulins
- Collagenase, which may degrade connective tissue collagen
- Extracellular outer membrane vesicles
- Factors affecting the immune response
- Factors damaging host cells.

Leucotoxin

It was first shown by Baehni *et al.* (1979) that *A. actinomycetemcomitans* strain Y4 isolated from a patient with JP was cytotoxic to PMNs. It was later shown that some strains of *A. actinomycetemcomitans* associated with JP produce a leucotoxin, which can kill PMNs and monocytes (Taichmann *et al.*, 1980; McArthur *et al.*, 1981; Zambon *et al.*, 1983b; Ohta and Kato, 1991). The purified leucotoxin has a mass of 115 000 Daltons, and its amino acid sequence and sequence of its coding gene has major similarities with similar toxins from other bacteria, notably *Escherichia coli* haemolysin, *Pasturella haemolytica* leucotoxin and *Pseudomonas aeruginosa* leucotoxin (Ohta and Kato, 1991). It appears to be mainly present in the outer cell membrane and in the extracellular outer membrane vesicles (Lai *et al.*, 1981; Ohta and Kato, 1991).

A. actinomycetemcomitans strains vary in their ability to produce the leucotoxin (see above), and the strains can be classified into leucotoxin-producing strains (Y4 (ATCC 43718), ATCC 29522 and 29524) and non-leucotoxin-producing strains (627, 652) (Ohta and Kato, 1991). Zambon *et al.* (1983a) found a high prevalence of leucotoxin activity in serotype b, and low or none in the other two serotypes. However, Chung *et al.* (1989) found variation in leucotoxic activity between all three strains. This is partly explained by the work of Kolodrubetz *et al.* (1989), who cloned the leucotoxin gene and showed that copies of it were present in both the leucotoxin-producing and the non-leucotoxin strains, and concluded that this was probably responsible for the strain differences in leucotoxin production.

There have been two relatively recent studies of its mechanism of leucotoxicity (Iwase *et al.*, 1990; Sakurada, 1990). These showed that it had a membranolytic activity producing pores in the target cell (Iwase *et al.*, 1990), and that phospholipid was the receptor on the cell for the toxin whose activity resulted in a rapid influx of Ca^{2+} into the cell (Sakurada, 1990). These results indicate that its mechanism of action is very similar to that of *E. coli* haemolysin and *P. aeruginosa* leucotoxin (Ohta and Kato, 1991). JP patients produce antibodies directed against this leucotoxin (Tsai *et al.*, 1981).

Lipopolysaccharide (LPS)

LPS is a major integral component of the outer membrane of Gram negative bacteria, and the LPSs of the bacteria associated with JP have been shown to stimulate bone resorption *in vitro* using the foetal mouse calvarium model. The LPS of *A. actinomycetemcomitans* has a broad spectrum of immunological and endotoxic activities, including stimulating *in vitro* bone resorption, the production of IL-1, an IL-1 inhibitor and prostaglandin (PG) E_2 from macrophages, and polyclonal activation of B-lymphocytes (Iino and Hopps, 1984; Nishihara *et al.*, 1987, 1988; Garrison *et al.*, 1988; Koga *et al.*, 1991). It seems likely that the bone resorptive activities of this LPS are the result of its stimulation of PGE_2 and IL-1 release from osteoblasts and other cells (Koga *et al.*, 1991).

The potency of these materials from different bacterial sources varies significantly and, in respect of the bacteria associated with JP, the LPSs from *A. actinomycetemcomitans*, *Capnocytophaga* and *E. corrodens* are less active in stimulating bone resorption than that from *P. gingivalis*. The LPS from *E. corrodens* releases cytokines such as IL-1 and IL-6 from osteoblasts and fibroblasts, but most other bacteria associated with JP do not produce this effect (Reddi *et al.*, 1995a; Wilson, 1995). However, all Gram negative LPSs are known to activate the complement cascade by the alternative pathway, which in turn generates prostaglandins, and this is the probable mechanism of bone resorption by these materials.

LPSs are much less potent than the corresponding surface-associated material (SAM) (see below). In this regard, SAM is 1000 times more potent than the corresponding LPS (Hopps and Sisney-Durrant, 1991).

Patients with JP have high serum antibody levels to the LPS from *A. actinomycetemcomitans* (Ebersole *et al.*, 1983).

Surface-associated material (SAM)

It has been shown during the last decade that proteins associated with the outer surfaces of some but not all putative periodontal pathogens are potent inducers of bone resorption and tissue pathology *in vitro* (Wilson *et al.*, 1985, 1993; Meghji *et al.*, 1992a, 1992b; Wilson and Henderson, 1995). This capsular or surface-associated material (SAM) has been shown to stimulate the production of prostaglandin E_2 (PGE_2) and collagenase from bone cells (Harvey *et al.*, 1987). SAMs are much more potent bone resorbing agents than lipopolysaccharide (see Chapter 5 and above).

The SAM of *A. actinomycetemcomitans* is composed of a bacterial capsule and other molecules loosely bound to the outer surface of the external membrane. It is extremely active at inducing bone resorption *in vitro* at very low concentrations (Wilson *et al.*, 1985; Kamin *et al.*, 1986), and is much more potent in stimulating bone resorption than the corresponding SAM from other putative periodontal pathogens. However, it induces bone resorption by different mechanisms to the SAMs from other bacteria (Wilson *et al.*, 1988), which do so by stimulating osteoclasts to produce bone resorption by inducing cytokines such as interleukin (IL)-1 and tumour necrosis factor (TNF) and prostaglandins (see Chapter 5).

The SAM from *A. actinomycetemcomitans* is composed of several proteins and peptides. A 64 KDa protein appears to be the factor that produces the bone resorption, and its precise mechanism of action is under investigation. There is some evidence that it could directly stimulate the proliferation and differentiation of osteoclasts, or act indirectly to do this by stimulating osteoblasts to produce signals other than the cytokines or prostaglandins mentioned above (Kamin *et al.*, 1986). In addition, the SAM contains a peptide component that stimulates fibroblasts to produce IL-6 (Reddi *et al.*, 1994, 1996b), and it appears to produce this effect by mimicking the action of IL-1 and stimulating the release of IL-6 directly. This may significantly contribute to bone resorption, because IL-6 stimulates the proliferation of osteoclast precursors (Löwick *et al.*, 1989; Roodman, 1992).

The constituents of the SAM from *A. actinomycetemcomitans* have been recently characterized (Wilson and Henderson, 1995), and it is made up of a number of proteins and peptides with potent biological actions that are relevant to the pathology of juvenile periodontitis (Wilson and Henderson, 1995). These include three main components:

1. A protein with potent osteolytic activity, which has close homology to the molecular chaperone from *Escherichia coli* known either as as chaperonin 60 or GroEL (Meghji *et al.*, 1992a; Kirby *et al.*, 1995).
2. A protein with anti-mitotic activity, which has been termed, gapstatin (White *et al.*, 1995).
3. A potent cytokine-inducing peptide, which acts by stimulating IL-6 gene transcription (Nair *et al.*, 1996). This cytokine is pro-inflammatory and plays a role in the differentiation and maturation of T- and B-lymphocytes (see Chapter 3 and Table 3.1).

The main cytokine ultimately released from connective tissue and bone cells by SAMs from Gram negative bacteria is IL-6, and it seems that this release may either be by stimulated IL-1, as with *E. corrodens*, or by direct stimulation, as with *A. actinomycetemcomitans*. This is of particular relevance because IL-6 has been shown to stimulate the formation of osteoclasts (Löwick *et al.*, 1989; Roodman, 1992).

These proteins are active in very low concentrations, and it is presumed that their actions are important in the pathogenesis of juvenile periodontitis by stimulating alveolar bone resorption (Wilson *et al.*, 1985, 1993; Kirby *et al.*, 1995; Reddi *et al.*, 1995b), inhibiting bone and periodontal ligament regeneration and repair (Kamin *et al.*, 1985; Wilson *et al.*, 1988; Meghji *et al.*, 1992a) and promoting B-lymphocyte and plasma cell proliferation (Reddi *et al.*, 1995c, 1996a, 1996b; Wilson *et al.*, 1996; Henderson *et al.*, 1996).

JP patients produce high levels of serum antibodies to SAM from *A. actinomycetemcomitans*, and serum from these patients can block the bone resorbing activity of this SAM (Meghji *et al.*, 1992b). However, it has not yet been clearly established what role these antibodies play *in vivo* in protecting against these defects.

Chemotactic inhibition factors

A. actinomycetemcomitans produces factors that inhibit the chemotaxis of PMNs (Van Dyke *et al.*, 1980, 1982; Astemborski *et al.,* 1989). These factor(s) could reduce the number of PMNs in the local lesion available to phagocytose and kill these bacteria.

Proteases that degrade immunoglobulins

A. actinomycetemcomitans produces proteolytic enzymes that degrade immunoglobulins (Killian, 1981). This could reduce the local effectiveness of antibodies produced against this bacteria.

Collagenase

A. actinomycetemcomitans produces a collagenolytic proteinase that can attack collagen (Robertson *et al.*, 1982). This could contribute to degradation of collagen and connective tissue breakdown in the periodontal tissues.

Extracellular outer membrane vesicles

A. actinomycetemcomitans produces numerous extracellular outer membrane vesicles, which are shed from the surface of the bacteria (Holt *et al.*, 1980). These vesicles contain the leucotoxin (see above) and LPS (Lai *et al.*, 1981; Nowotney *et al.*, 1982; Tervahartiala *et al.*, 1989; Koga *et al.*, 1991). Their small size could easily permit them to cross epithelial barriers such as the pocket epithelium (Maryland and Grenier, 1989).

Factors affecting the immune response

A. actinomycetemcomitans produces a potent polyclonal B-lymphocyte activating factor (Bick *et al.*, 1981), which may contribute to the pathogenesis of the condition by inducing B-lymphocytes to produce antibodies with determinants unrelated to the bacterial antigens. This may in part be due to the LPS and SAM proteins present in outer membrane vesicles (see above).

Factors damaging host cells

A. actinomycetemcomitans produces an epitheliotoxin, which can damage epithelial cells and could facilitate bacterial penetration of the junctional and pocket epithelium (Birkedal-Hansen *et al.*, 1992). It also produces a fibroblast-inhibiting factor, which may impair tissue repair (Stevens and Hammond, 1982). The surface-associated material (SAM) from this bacteria is the most potent material of this type to stimulate bone resorption *in vitro* (see above). It also has anti-mitotic activity, which could inhibit bone and periodontal ligament regeneration and repair, and also pro-inflammatory properties, which could promote B-lymphocyte and plasma cell proliferation (see above).

Factors released by the other Gram negative, capnophilic bacteria associated with JP could also contribute to the pathology of this disease. The most important of these are *Eikenella corrodens* and *Capnocytophaga* species.

Eikenella corrodens

Both the SAM and LPS from *E. corrodens* stimulate bone resorption *in vitro*. The SAM appears to do this by first releasing IL-1 and TNF from its target cells, which then stimulates the release of PGE$_2$ and collagenase (Holt and Ebersole, 1991; Henderson and Blake, 1992). It has been shown that the inhibition of bone DNA and collagen production by osteoblasts in murine calvaria produced by low titres of this SAM may be due to this mechanism because it is blocked by indomethacin, an inhibitor of prostaglandins (Meghji *et al.*, 1992b). This SAM also produces polyclonal B-lymphocyte activation (Bick *et al.*, 1981).

E. corrodens also produces factors that inhibit PMN chemotaxis (Van Dyke *et al.*, 1982).

Capnocytophaga species

The LPS of *Capnocytophaga* species produces weak bone resorption *in vitro* by the same mechanism as *E. corrodens*.

These bacteria also produce proteases, which can degrade types I and IV collagens, immunoglobulins and the glycosaminoglycan components of proteoglycans (Killian *et al.*, 1983; Seddon and Shah, 1989; Söderling *et al.*, 1991).

Finally, they produce factors that inhibit PMN chemotaxis (Van Dyke *et al.*, 1982).

Host response

Local

The primary defence of the periodontal pocket is provided by PMNs, and reduction in their function gives rise to severe disease. It has been shown that PMNs from the periodontal pockets of JP cases have reduced chemotactic activity and phagocytic function, which could in part be related to the secretion of leucotoxin by *A. actinomycetemcomitans* (Murray and Patters, 1980).

The local lesion of JP in the connective tissue adjacent to the pocket and junctional epithelium is mainly populated by plasma cells and blast cells (Liljenberg and Lindhe, 1980). Gingival explant cultures have been shown to produce immunoglobulins against the associated bacteria, and this shows that plasma cells in the local tissues are capable of local production of these immunoglobulins (Hall *et al.*, 1990).

General

The majority of patients with JP have peripheral blood PMNs with an impaired ability to react to chemotactic stimuli (Clark *et al.*, 1977; Van Dyke *et al.*, 1980). This appears to be caused by a cell-associated defect.

Patients with JP have increased levels of serum and salivary IgG, IgM and IgA (Sandholm and Gronblad, 1984; Sandholm *et al.*, 1987). Specific IgG antibodies to *A. actinomycetemcomitans* are raised in 55% of untreated and 28% of treated JP cases. In addition, specific salivary IgA antibody to this bacteria is raised in 27% of untreated and 20% of treated JP cases (Sandholm and Gronblad, 1984; Sandholm *et al.*, 1987).

It has also been shown that T-lymphocytes show an impaired blastogenic response to some Gram negative bacteria (Lehner *et al.*, 1974). More recently it has been shown that a considerable number of JP cases have overall raised antibody titres to *A. actinomycetemcomitans* (Ebersole *et al.*, 1982; Ranney *et al.*, 1982), and over 90% develop neutralizing antibodies against its leucotoxin (Tsai *et al.*, 1981), its LPS (Ebersole *et al.*, 1983) and the bone resorbing activity of its SAM (Meghji *et al.*, 1992b).

Aetiology

From these findings it appears that JP is a distinct bacterial disease from adult chronic periodontitis. It seems that the susceptibility to infection by certain Gram negative, facultative bacteria is mainly the result of impaired PMN function, which may be inherited. The impaired lymphocytic blastogenic response to certain

Gram negative bacteria may also play a part, as may the inherited cementum hypoplasia. These impairments may be further compromised by infection with a suitable strain of *A. actinomycetemcomitans* and its production of leucotoxin and chemotactic inhibitor, which could allow the bacteria to invade the tissues. Its production of SAM with its potential to stimulate bone resorption may also be a key factor.

The tendency of the disease to stabilize in early adult life may well be associated with the production of neutralizing antibodies against the leucotoxin, SAM and LPS.

None of these findings fully explain the condition. The bacterial theory may explain the classic incisor–first molar syndrome, as these teeth erupt first and are exposed to the oral flora for longer. However, it does not explain classic distributions where some teeth are spared, e.g. upper incisors involved and lower incisors spared, or the cases with a random or asymmetrical distribution of lesions.

Post-juvenile periodontitis

Post-juvenile periodontitis is seen in patients over 20 years of age, and shows some of the features of localized JP. The main differences are that the gingival condition and bacterial flora resemble chronic periodontitis. The gingival tissues show clinically obvious inflammation associated with supra- and subgingival plaque and calculus. It would seem that the marked attachment loss seen in this condition mainly results from the active phase of JP. It seems likely that when JP comes under control by the development of effective immunity the pockets become colonized by the usual indigenous bacteria associated with chronic periodontitis, which produce clinically obvious inflammation. Further progression of the condition then becomes related to the same factors which operate in chronic periodontitis.

Diagnosis of juvenile periodontitis

The early diagnosis of JP depends on careful and regular periodontal examinations of children and young adolescents from the time of eruption of the permanent teeth. This needs to include careful periodontal probing around the first molars and incisors. It should, of course, be remembered that deep false pocketing is a feature around erupting teeth. JP usually starts on the first molar, and early signs of bone loss may be noticed on routine bite wing radiographs. Full-mouth radiographs may be necessary for comprehensive diagnosis. As the condition has a familial tendency, siblings and offspring of JP patients should always be carefully examined.

Treatment of juvenile periodontitis

Early diagnosis on this condition is very important because the chances of saving affected teeth are only good if treatment is given before significant attachment is lost.

JP is mainly associated with *A. actinomycetemcomitans* infection, and elimination of this bacteria with antibiotics is the mainstay of the primary treatment of this disease. *A. actinomycetemcomitans* is susceptible to tetracycline, a bacteriostatic, protein synthesis-inhibiting antibiotic *in vitro*. Following systemic administration of tetracycline, the serum and crevicular fluid concentrations are high enough to suppress the bacteria *in vivo*. A combination of systemic tetracycline and scaling and root planing has been shown to suppress *A. actinomycetemcomitans* much better than scaling alone (Slots and Rosling, 1983), and this has been shown to be an effective treatment for JP. This has therefore become the mainstay of the primary treatment of this disease. However, recently it has been shown that tetracycline often fails to eliminate *A. actinomycetemcomitans* completely from the subgingival flora (Mandell *et al.*, 1986).

Topical application of tetracycline into the pocket produces much higher local concentrations in the pocket than systemic administration. However, in spite of this, topical application only reduces the numbers of *A. actinomycetemcomitans* to a very limited extent (Nakagawa *et al.*, 1991), and this suggests that its *in vivo* susceptibility is much less than *in vitro*. It is also probable that local tetracycline fails to inhibit *A. actinomycetemcomitans* within the periodontal lesion or at other sites in the mouth, and may thus allow a more rapid recolonization of the site.

A. actinomycetemcomitans is only moderately susceptible to metronidazole, but is 2–4 times more susceptible to its hydroxy-metabolite (Pavicic *et al.*, 1991). The combination of metronidazole and amoxycillin has been found to be very effective in eliminating *A. actinomycetemcomitans* from the subgingival flora (Van Winkelhoff *et al.*, 1989). Complete elimination of *A. actinomycetemcomitans* was found in 97% of all the patients treated with this combination of scaling and root planing (Van Winkelhoff *et al.*, 1992), and two out of four patients who were still positive for this bacteria were colonized by metronidazole resistant stains. After 2 years of follow-up, recolonization by *A. actinomycetemcomitans* was found in only one out of 48 patients (Pavicic *et al.*, 1994). This highly predictable therapy may be explained by the synergism found between metronidazole and amoxycillin (Pavicic *et al.*, 1991), and this also occurs between the hydroxy-metabolite of metronidazole and amoxycillin. Thus, on present evidence, metronidazole and amoxycillin would seem to be the antibiotics of choice for the elimination of *A. actinomycetemcomitans* from the subgingival flora (Pavicic *et al.*, 1992).

In addition, Saxen and Asikainen (1993) compared the systemic administration of metronidazole and tetracycline as adjuvants in the treatment of juvenile periodontitis in 27 patients who were all positive for *A. actinomycetemcomitans* at the affected sites. At baseline they were divided into three groups. One group received metronidazole (200 mg tds for 10 days), one group received tetracycline (250 mg tds for 10 days), and the final control group received no antibiotics. All groups received full periodontal treatment consisting of scaling and root planing, maintenance, and periodontal surgery when indicated. The clinical parameters were measured at 6 and 18 months after treatment, and bacterial samples were also taken for *A. actinomycetemcomitans* culture at the same time intervals. The clinical condition markedly improved in all groups. *A. actinomycetemcomitans* was eliminated from all the test sites in the metronidazole group, 17 out of 26 sites in the tetracycline group and 19 out of 26 sites in the control group. They therefore concluded that metronidazole was more effective than tetracycline in eliminating *A. actinomycetemcomitans* from infected juvenile periodontitis pocket sites. Therefore, there is evidence that the adjuvant administration of metronidazole alone is effective treatment for the complete elimination of *A. actinomycetemcomitans* in juvenile periodontitis.

Thus, providing sufficient support is remaining on the affected teeth, the aim of the primary treatment is elimination of *A. actinomycetemcomitans* from the pockets by a combination of antibiotics, oral hygiene instruction and scaling and root planing. This should be followed by regular 3-monthly maintenance scaling to prevent recolonization.

If *A. actinomycetemcomitans* reinfects a site(s), the patient should be retreated with the appropriate antibiotic(s) based on the results of microbiological sensitivity tests. Regular microbiological monitoring of *A. actinomycetemcomitans* in the subgingival flora should be carried out if such facilities are available. Practitioners should refer patients to a dental hospital if oral microbiological facilities are not available to them locally.

Where appropriate, periodontal surgery may be considered for the treatment of residual deep pockets. Where there is insufficient support remaining, extractions and prosthetic replacement need to be considered. A plan for such treatment follows.

1. *Microbiology.* Samples of subgingival flora of affected sites should be taken for microbiological investigation, and in particular to monitor *A. actinomycetemcomitans* and its antibiotic sensitivity. A suitable collection and transport system using an appropriate medium must be worked out with the microbiology laboratory.
2. *Oral hygiene instruction and counselling.* This should be given to the patient, with emphasis laid on the special nature of the condition and therefore the special responsibility of the patient in maintaining a high level of home care.
3. *Antibiotics.* These should be administered: either metronidazole 200 mg and amoxycillin 375 mg three times daily for 7 days, or metronidazole 200 mg three times daily for 10 days, or tetracycline 250 mg four times daily for 14 days.

4. *Scaling and root planing of affected sites.* Subgingival calculus deposits are usually absent. However, debridement and root planing help to create conditions unfavourable to the microflora.
5. *Extraction.* This may be necessary, with immediate replacement of anterior teeth or teeth with a hopeless prognosis due to excessive bone loss and drifting.
6. *Periodontal surgery.* Localized inverse bevel periodontal surgery should only be carried out if the patient's co-operation is good, and is best done with pre-operative and post-operative antibiotic administration. Any suprabony pockets in posterior teeth can be eliminated by apical positioning, but with anterior teeth replaced flaps are necessary because of aesthetic considerations. A majority of teeth with this condition will have deep intrabony pocketing with associated angular bony defects. These lesions should be curetted with the aim of producing bony in-fill with or without the placement of a bone or bone substitute graft. Certain isolated intrabony lesions with suitable morphology can be treated with guided tissue regenerating and/or bone grafting techniques (see Chapter 14). The tissues heal rapidly after surgery, and often show evidence of in-fill of bone defects. In some cases, advanced bone loss around one of the roots of a first molar may be treated by root amputation or hemisection.
7. *Occlusal adjustment.* Migration of incisors is a late characteristic of JP, but orthodontic treatment of these cases is usually contraindicated. If teeth that are to remain have drifted into premature contact, these should be treated by selective grinding. In a few cases, after successful periodontal treatment and after the condition has become fully stable, gentle orthodontic retraction of labially drifted upper incisors might be considered if they can be stabilized behind the lower lip or splinted in a stable position.
8. *Prosthetics.* Any necessary partial dentures must be carefully designed so that gingival irritation is avoided and abutment teeth loaded as near axially as possible. Chrome cobalt skeleton dentures are usually indicated, and acrylic dentures should only be used in the immediate replacement phase.
9. *Maintenance.* The observation by Waerhaug (1977) that successfully treated cases can subsequently show signs of relapse indicates that long-term maintenance is essential. These patients should be recalled every 3 months for oral hygiene reinforcement and scaling. The affected sites should be monitored, and if any deterioration occurs, samples of subgingival flora be taken for microbiological investigation in order to monitor possible recurrence of *A. actinomycetemcomitans*. If this bacteria is found by the microbiologists, its antibiotic sensitivity should be determined. Appropriate antibiotic treatment can then be given to eliminate this bacteria from the flora. For these reasons it is usually appropriate to refer these cases to a dental hospital, where microbiological facilities are available.

Evaluation of treatment procedures for JP

Antibiotics and scaling and root planing

It has been shown by Christersson *et al.* (1985) that scaling and root planing alone may improve the clinical condition somewhat, but it fails to reduce significantly the number of *A. actinomycetemcomitans* in the subgingival flora. However, a number of studies have shown that a 2-week course of tetracycline or related drugs brought about clinical improvement and significantly reduced the numbers of *A. actinomycetemcomitans* (Slots and Rosling, 1983; Christersson *et al.*, 1985; Novak *et al.*, 1991). However, tetracycline often fails to eliminate *A. Actinomycetemcomitans* from the subgingival flora (Mandell *et al.*, 1986). Penicillin and metronidazole used separately have been reported to be ineffective in treating JP (Mitchell, 1984; Kunihira *et al.*, 1985), but in contrast, metronidazole and amoxycillin used in combination have been found to be very effective (Van Winkelhoff *et al.*, 1989, 1992). In a 2-year follow-up study (Pavicic *et al.*, 1994), this combination of drugs with scaling and root planing (see above) has been shown to eliminate *A. actinomycetemcomitans* totally from the subgingival flora for 2 years. Recently, however, the administration of metronidazole alone has been shown to be effective in eliminating *A. actinomycetemcomitans* from the flora (Saxen and Asikainen, 1993).

Antibiotics and surgery

A combination of antibiotics and surgery seems to be very effective in controlling JP. A 2-week course of tetracycline plus replaced flap surgery (Lindhe and Liljenberg, 1984) controlled the progress of the disease in 16 study patients, although two patients had recurrence and needed retreatment. After 5 years of follow-up, there was improvement in all clinical measurements and evidence of bony in-fill of bone defects. Bacterial monitoring of this combination of treatment (Kornmann and Robertson, 1985) showed that sites with high levels of *Actinobacillus actinomycetemcomitans* showed a better response to surgery plus tetracycline than to scaling plus tetracycline. It has also been shown that surgery plus tetracycline can completely eliminate *A. actinomycetemcomitans* from the subgingival flora for up to 12 months (Mandell and Socransky, 1988). However, it has now been shown (Pavicic *et al.*, 1994) that this can be achieved for 2 years with metronidazole and amoxycillin plus scaling and root planing (see above). There are as yet no reported studies of these antibiotics in combination with surgery.

References

Alanuusua, S. and Asikainen, S. (1988) Detection and distribution of *Actinobacillus actinomycetemcomitans* in the primary dentition. *Journal of Periodontology* **59**, 504–507

Albander, J.M. (1993) Juvenile periodontitis – pattern of progression in relationship to clinical periodontal parameters. *Community Dentistry and Oral Epidemiology* **21**, 185–189

Asikainen, S., Lai, C.-H., Alanuusua, S. and Slots, J. (1991) Distribution of *Actinobacillus actinomycetemcomitans* serotypes in periodontal health and disease. *Oral Microbiology and Immunology* **6**, 115–118

Astemborski, J.A., Boughman, J.A., Myrick, P.O. *et al.* (1989) Clinical and laboratory characteristics of early onset periodontitis. *Journal of Periodontology* **60**, 557–563

Baehni, P.C., Tsai, C.-C., McArthur, W.P. *et al.* (1979) Interactions of inflammatory cells and oral micro-organisms. VII. Detection of leucotoxic activity of plaque-derived Gram negative micro-organisms. *Infection and Immunity* **24**, 233–243

Baer, P.N. (1971) The case for periodontitis as a clinical entity. *Journal of Periodontology* **42**, 516–519

Benjamin, S.D. and Baer, P.N. (1967) Familial patterns of advanced alveolar bone loss in adolescence (periodontitis). *Periodontics* **5**, 82–88

Bial, J.J. and Mellonig, J.T. (1987) Radiographical evidence of juvenile periodontitis (periodontosis). *Journal of Periodontology* **58**, 321–326

Bick, P.H., Betts-Carpenter, A., Holdman, L.V. *et al.* (1981) Polyclonal B-cell activation induced by extracts of Gram negative bacteria isolated from periodontally diseased sites. *Infection and Immunity* **34**, 43–49

Birkedal-Hansen, H., Caulfield, P.W., Wannameumier, Y. and Pierce, R. (1992) A sensitive screening assay for epitheliotoxins produced by oral organisms. *Journal of Dental Research* **61**, 192 Abstr. 125

Blomlöf, L., Hammerström, L. and Linskog, S. (1986) Occurrence and appearance of cementum hypoplasias in localized and generalized juvenile periodontitis. *Acta Odontologica Scandinavica* **44**, 313–320

Boughman, J.A., Halloran, S.L. and Roulston, D. (1986) An autosomal dominant form of juvenile periodontitis (JP): its localization to chromosome No. 4 and linking to dentinogenesis imperfecta. *Journal of Craniofacial and Genetic Development Biology* **6**, 341–350

Boughman, J.A., Beaty, T.H., Yang, P. *et al.* (1988) Problem of genetic model testing in early onset periodontitis. *Journal of Periodontology* **59**, 332–337

Butler, J.H. (1969) A familial pattern of juvenile periodontitis (periodontosis). *Journal of Periodontology* **40**, 115–118

Carranza, F.A., Saglie, F.R., Newman, M.G. and Valentin, P.L. (1983) Scanning and transmission electron microscopic study of tissue-invading micro-organisms in localized juvenile periodontitis. *Journal of Periodontology* **54**, 598–617

Christersson, L., Slots, J., Rosling, B. and Genco, R.J. (1985) Microbiological and clinical effects of surgery treatment of localized juvenile periodontitis. *Journal of Clinical Periodontology* **12**, 465–476

Christersson, L.A., Wikesjö, U.M.A., Albini, B. *et al.* (1987) Tissue localization of *Actinobacillus actinomycetemcomitans* in human periodontitis. I. Light, immunofluorescent and electron microscopic studies. *Journal of Periodontology* **58**, 529–539

Chung, H.-J., Chung, C.-P., Son, S.-H. and Nisengard, R.J. (1989) *Actinobacillus actinomycetemcomitans* serotypes and leukotoxicity in Korean localized juvenile periodontitis. *Journal of Periodontology* **60**, 509–511

Clark, R.A., Page, R.C. and Wilde, G. (1977) Defective neutrophil chemotaxis in juvenile periodontitis. *Infection and Immunity* **18**, 694–700

Di Rienzo, J.M. and Slots, J. (1990) Genetic approach to the study of epidemiology and pathogenesis of *Actinobacillus actinomycetemcomitans* in localized juvenile periodontitis. *Archives of Oral Biology* **35**, 79S–84S

Ebersole, J.L., Taubman, M.A., Smith, D.C. and Socransky, S.S. (1982) Humoral immune responses and the diagnosis of human periodontal disease. *Journal of Periodontal Research* **17**, 478–480

Ebersole, J.L., Taubman, M.A., Smith, D.J. *et al.* (1983) Human immune responses to oral micro-organisms. II. Serum antibody responses to antigens from *Actinobacillus actinomycetemcomitans* and correlation with localized juvenile periodontitis. *Journal of Clinical Immunology* **3**, 321–331

Eisenmann, A.A.C., Eisenmann, R., Sousa, O. and Slots, J. (1983) Microbiological study of localized juvenile periodontitis in Panama. *Journal of Periodontology* **54**, 712–713

Franklin, E.R. (1978) Periodontal diseases, a socio-economic problem in Black Africa. *Odonto-Stomatologie Tropicale* **6**, 16–28

Garrison, S.W., Holt, S.C. and Nichols, F.C. (1988) Lipopolysaccharide-stimulated PGE$_2$ release from human monocytes. Comparison of lipopolysaccharide prepared from suspected periodontal pathogens. *Journal of Periodontology* **59**, 684–687

Gillett, R. and Johnson, N.W. (1982) Bacterial invasion of the periodontium in a case of juvenile periodontitis. *Journal of Clinical Periodontology* **9**, 93–100

Gottlieb, B. (1923) Die diffuse Atrophie des Alveolarknochens Weitere Beitrage zur Kenntnis des Alveolarschwandes und dwssen Wiedergutmachung durch Zementwachstum. *Zeitschrift für Stomatologie* **21**, 195–262

Gottlieb, B. (1928) The formation of the pocket: diffuse atrophy of alveolar bone. *Journal of the American Dental Association* **15**, 462–476

Haffajee, A.D., Socransky, S.S., Ebersole, J.L. and Smith, D.J. (1984) Clinical, microbiological and immunological features associated with treatment of active periodontal lesions. *Journal of Clinical Periodontology* **11**, 600–618

Hall, F.P., Falkler, W.A. and Suzuki, J.B. (1990) Production of immunoglobulins in gingival tissue explant cultures from juvenile periodontitis patients. *Journal of Periodontology* **61**, 603–608

Hart, T.C., Marazita, M.L., Schenkein, H.A. *et al.* (1991) No female preponderance for juvenile periodontitis after correction for ascertainment bias. *Journal of Periodontology* **62**, 745–749

Hart, T.C., Marazita, M.L., Schenkein, H.A. and Diehl, S.R. (1992) Reinterpretation of the evidence for X-linked dominant inheritance of juvenile periodontitis. *Journal of Periodontology* **63**, 169–173

Hartley, A.F. and Floyd, P.D. (1988) Prevalence of juvenile periodontitis in school children in Lagos, Nigeria. *Community Dentistry and Oral Epidemiology* **16**, 299–301

Harvey, W., Kamin, S., Meghji, S. and Wilson, M. (1987) Interleukin 1-like activity in capsular material from *Haemophilus actinomycetemcomitans*. *Immunology* **60**, 415–418

Henderson, B. and Blake, S. (1992) Therapeutic potential of cytokine manipulation. *Trends in Pharmacological Science* **13**, 145–152

Henderson, D., Poole, S and Wilson, M. (1996) Bacterial modulins: a novel class of virulence factors which cause host tissue pathology by inducing cytokine synthesis. *Microbiological Reviews* **60**, 316–341

Holt, S.C. and Ebersole, J.L. (1991) The surface of selected periodontopathic bacteria: possible role in virulence. In *Periodontal Disease Pathogens and Host Immune Response* (S. Hamada, S.C. Holt and J.R. McGhee, eds), pp. 79–96. Tokyo: Quintessence Publishing Co. Ltd

Holt, S.C., Tanner, A.C.R. and Socransky, S.S. (1980) Morphology and ultrastructure of oral strains of *Actinobacillus actinomycetemcomitans* and *Haemophilus aphrophilus*. *Infection and Immunity* **30**, 588–600

Hopps, R.M. and Sisney-Durrant, H.J. (1991) Mechanisms of alveolar bone loss in periodontal disease. In *Periodontal Disease Pathogens and Host Immune Response* (S. Hamada, S.C. Holt and J.R. McGhee, eds), pp. 307–320. Tokyo: Quintessence Publishing Co. Ltd

Iino, Y. and Hopps, R.M. (1984) The bone resorbing activities of lipopolysaccharides from the bacteria *Actinobacillus actinomycetemcomitans*, *Bacteroides gingivalis* and *Capnocytophaga ochracia* isolated from human mouths. *Archives of Oral Biology* **29**, 59–63

Iwase, M., Lalley, E.T., Berthold, P. *et al.* (1990) Effects of cations and osmotic protectants on cytolytic activity of *Actinobacillus actinomycetemcomitans* leukotoxin. *Infection and Immunity* **58**, 1783–1788

Kamin, S., Harvey, W., Wilson, M. and Scutt, A. (1986) Inhibition of fibroblast proliferation and collagen synthesis by capsular material from *Actinobacillus actinomycetemcomitans*. *Journal of Medical Microbiology* **22**, 245–249

Kaslick, R.S., Chasens, A.I., Tuckman, M.A. and Kaufman, B. (1971) Investigation of periodontosis with periodontitis: literature survey and findings based on ABO blood groups. *Journal of Periodontology* **42**, 420–427

Killian, M. (1981) Degradation of immunoglobulins A1, A2, and G by suspected principal periodontal pathogens. *Infection and Immunity* **34**, 757–765

Killian, M., Thompson, B., Petersen, P.E. and Bleeg, H.S. (1983) Occurrence and nature of bacterial IgA proteases. *Annals of the New York Academy of Science* **409**, 612–624

Kirby, A.C., Meghji, S., Nair, S.P. *et al.* (1995) The potent bone-resorbing mediator of *Actinobacillus actinomycetemcomitans* is homologous to the molecular chaperone GroEL. *Journal of Clinical Investigation* **96**, 1185–1194

Koga, T., Nishihara, T., Amano, K. *et al.* (1991) Chemical and biochemical properties of cell-surface components of *Actinobacillus actinomycetemcomitans*. In *Periodontal Disease Pathogens and Host Immune Response* (S. Hamada, S.C. Holt and J.R. McGhee, eds), pp. 117–127. Tokyo: Quintessence Publishing Co. Ltd

Kolodrubetz, D., Dailey, T., Ebersole, J. and Kraig, E. (1989) Cloning and expression of leukotoxin gene from *Actinobacillus actinomycetemcomitans*. *Infection and Immunity* **57**, 1465–1469

Kornmann, K.S. and Robertson, P.B. (1985) Clinical and microbiological evaluation of juvenile periodontitis. *Journal of Periodontology* **56**, 443–446

Kronauer, E., Borsa, G. and Lang, N.P. (1986) Prevalence of incipient juvenile periodontitis at age 16 in Switzerland. *Journal of Clinical Periodontology* **13**, 103–108

Kunihira, D., Caine, F. and Palicanis, K. (1985) A clinical trial of phenoxymethyl penicillin for adjunctive treatment of juvenile periodontitis. *Journal of Periodontology* **56**, 352–360

Lai, C.-H., Listgarten, M.A. and Hammond, B.F. (1981) Comparative ultrastructure of leukotoxic and non-leukotoxic strain of *Actinobacillus actinomycetemcomitans*. *Journal of Periodontal Research* **16**, 379–389

Lehner, T., Wilton, J.M.A., Ivanyi, L. and Manson, J.D. (1974) Immunological aspects of juvenile periodontitis (periodontosis). *Journal of Periodontal Research* **9**, 261–272

Liljenberg, B. and Lindhe, J. (1980) Juvenile periodontitis. Some microbiological, histopathological and clinical characteristics of juvenile periodontitis. *Journal of Clinical Periodontology* **7**, 48–61

Lindhe, J. and Liljenberg, B. (1984) Treatment of localized juvenile periodontitis results after 5 years. *Journal of Clinical Periodontology* **11**, 399–410

Lindhe, J. and Slots, J. (1989) Periodontal disease in children and young adults. In *Textbook of Clinical Periodontology* (J. Lindhe, ed.), pp. 193–220. Copenhagen: Munksgaard

Lindstog, S. and Blomlöf, L. (1983) Cementum hypoplasia in teeth affected by juvenile periodontitis. *Journal of Clinical Periodontology* **10**, 443–451

Long, J.C., Nance, W.E. and Waring, P. (1987) Early onset periodontitis: a comparison and evaluation of two proposed modes of inheritance. *Genetics and Epidemiology* **4**, 13–24

Lopez, N.J., Rios, V., Pareja, M.A. and Fernandez, O. (1991) Prevalence of juvenile periodontitis in Chile. *Journal of Clinical Periodontology* **18**, 529–533

Löwick, C.W.G.M., van der Pluijm, G., Bloys, H. *et al.* (1989) Parathyroid hormone (PTH) and PTH-like protein (PLP) stimulate interleukin-

6 production by osteogenic cells: a possible role of interleukin-6 in osteoclastogenesis. *Biochemical and Biophysical Research Communications* **162**, 1546–1552

Mandell, R.L. (1984) A longitudinal microbiological investigation of *Actinobacillus actinomycetemcomitans* and *Eikenella corrodens* in juvenile periodontitis. *Infection and Immunity* **45**, 778–780

Mandell, R.L. and Socransky, S.S. (1988) Microbiological and clinical effects surgery plus doxycycline on juvenile periodontitis. *Journal of Periodontology* **59**, 373–379

Mandell, R.L., Tripodi, L.S., Savitt, E. *et al.* (1986) The effect of treatment on *Actinobacillus actinomycetemcomitans* in localized juvenile periodontitis. *Journal of Periodontology* **57**, 94–99

Manson, J.D. and Lehner, T. (1974) Clinical features of juvenile periodontitis (periodontosis). *Journal of Periodontology* **45**, 636–640

Maryland, D. and Grenier, D. (1989) Biological activities of outer membrane vesicles. *Canadian Journal of Microbiology* **35**, 607–613

McArthur, W.P., Tsai, C.-C., Baehni, P.C. *et al.* (1981) Leucotoxic effects of *Actinobacillus actinomycetemcomitans*. *Journal of Periodontal Research* **16**, 159–170

Meghji, S., Henderson, B., Nair, S. and Wilson, M. (1992a) Inhibition of bone DNA and collagen production by surface-associated material from bacteria implicated in the pathology of periodontal disease. *Journal of Periodontology* **63**, 736–742

Meghji, S., Wilson, M., Henderson, B. and Kinane, D. (1992b) Antiproliferative and cytotoxic activity of surface associated material from periodontopathic bacteria. *Archives of Oral Biology* **37**, 637–644

Meghji, S., Henderson, B. and Wilson, M. (1993) High titre antisera from patients with periodontal disease inhibit bacterial-capsule-induced bone breakdown. *Journal of Periodontal Research* **28**, 115–121

Meghji, S., Barber, P., Wilson, M. and Henderson, B. (1994) Bone resorbing activity of surface-associated material from *Actinobacillus actinomycetemcomitans* and *Eikenella corrodens*. *Journal of Medical Microbiology* **41**, 197–203

Melnick, M., Shields, E.D. and Bixler, D. (1976) Periodontitis: a phenotypic and genetic analysis. *Oral Surgery, Oral Medicine, Oral Pathology* **42**, 32–41

Melvin, W.L., Sandifer, J.B. and Grey, J.L. (1991) The prevalence and sex ratio of juvenile periodontitis in a young racially mixed population. *Journal of Periodontology* **62**, 330–334

Mitchell, D. (1984) Metronidazole: its use in clinical dentistry. *Journal of Clinical Periodontology* **11**, 145–158

Murray, P. and Patters, M. (1980) Gingival crevice neutrophil function in periodontal lesions. *Journal of Periodontal Research* **15**, 463–469

Nair, S.P., Meghji, S., Wilson, M. *et al.* (1996) Bacterially induced bone destruction: mechanisms and misconceptions. *Infection and Immunity* **64**, 2371–2380

Nakagawa, T., Yamada, S., Oosuka, Y. *et al.* (1991) Clinical and microbiological study of local minocycline delivery (Periocline) following scaling and root planing in recurrent periodontal pockets. *Bulletin of Tokyo Dental College* **32**, 63–70

Neely, A.L. (1992) Prevalence of juvenile periodontitis in a circumpubertal population. *Journal of Clinical Periodontology* **19**, 367–372

Newman, M.G. and Socransky, S.S. (1977) Predominant cultivatable microbiota in periodontitis. *Journal of Periodontal Research* **12**, 120–128

Nishihara, T., Koga, T. and Hamada, S. (1987) Extracellular proteinous substances from *Haemophilus actinomycetemcomitans* induce mitogenic responses in murine lymphocytes. *Oral Microbiology and Immunology* **2**, 48–52

Nishihara, T., Koga, T. and Hamada, S. (1988) Suppression of murine macrophage interleukin-1 release by the polysaccharide portion of the lipopolysaccharide of *Haemophilus actinomycetemcomitans*. *Infection and Immunity* **56**, 619–625

Novak, M.J., Stamatelakys, C. and Adair, S.M. (1991) Resolution of early lesions of juvenile periodontitis with tetracycline therapy alone: long term observations in four cases. *Journal of Periodontology* **62**, 628–633

Nowotney, A., Behling, U.H., Hammond, B. *et al.* (1982) The release of toxic microvesicles by *Actinobacillus actinomycetemcomitans*. *Infection and Immunity* **37**, 151–154

Ohta, H. and Koga, K. (1991) Leucotoxic activity of *Actinobacillus actinomycetemcomitans*. In *Periodontal Disease Pathogens and Host Immune Response* (S. Hamada, S.C. Holt and J.R. McGhee, eds), pp. 143–154. Tokyo: Quintessence Publishing Co. Ltd

Page, R.C., Altman, L.C., Ebersole, J.L. *et al.* (1983b) Rapidly progressive periodontitis, a distinct clinical condition. *Journal of Periodontology* **54**, 197–209

Page, R.C. and Baab, D.A. (1985) A new look at the etiology and pathogenesis of early onset periodontitis. *Journal of Periodontology* **56**, 748–751

Page, R.C., Bowen, T., Altman, L. *et al.* (1983a) Prepubertal periodontitis. I. Definition of a clinical disease entity. *Journal of Periodontology* **54**, 257–271

Papapanou, P.N. (1994) Epidemiology and natural history of periodontal disease. In *Proceedings of the 1st European Workshop on Periodontology* (N.P. Lang and T. Karring, eds), pp. 23–41. London: Quintessence Publishing Co. Ltd

Pavicic, M.J.A.M.P., Van Winkelhoff, A.J. and de Graaff, J. (1991) Synergistic effects between amoxycillin, metronidazole and its hydroxy-metabolite against *Actinobacillus actinomycetemcomitans*. *Antimicrobial Agents and Chemotherapy* **35**, 961–966

Pavicic, M.J.A.M.P., Van Winkelhoff, A.J. and de Graaff, J. (1992) Susceptibilities of *Actinobacillus actinomycetemcomitans* to a number of antimicrobial combinations. *Antimicrobial Agents and Chemotherapy* **36**, 2634–2638

Pavicic, M.J.A.M.P., Van Winkelhoff, A.J., Douqué, N.H. *et al.*, (1994) Microbiological and clinical effects of metronidazole and amoxycillin in *Actinobacillus actinomycetemcomitans* associated periodontitis: a 2-year evaluation. *Journal of Clinical Periodontology* **21**, 107–112

Preus, H.R., Olsen, I. and Namork, E. (1987) The presence of phage-infected *Actinobacillus actinomycetemcomitans* in localized juvenile periodontitis. *Journal of Clinical Periodontology* **14**, 605–609

Ranney, R.R., Yanni, N.R., Burmeister, J.A. and Tew, J.G. (1982) Relationship between attachment loss and precipitating antibody to *Actinobacillus actinomycetemcomitans* in adolescents and young adults having severe periodontal destruction. *Journal of Periodontology* **53**, 1–7

Reddi, K., Poole, S., Nair, S. *et al.* (1994) Comparison of the IL-6 inducing activity of periodontopathic bacterial surface-associated proteins. *Journal of Dental Research* **73**, 816 Abstr. 237

Reddi, K., Henderson, B., Meghji, S. *et al.* (1995a) Interleukin-6 production by lipopolysaccharide-stimulated fibroblasts is potentially inhibited by napthoquinone (vitamin K) components. *Cytokine* **7**, 287–290

Reddi, K., Meghji, S., Wilson, M. and Henderson, B. (1995b) Comparison of the osteolytic activity of surface-associated proteins of bacteria implicated in periodontal disease. *Oral Diseases* **1**, 26–31

Reddi, K., Wilson, M., Poole, S. *et al.* (1995c) Relative cytokine stimulating activities of surface components of the oral periodontopathic bacterium, *Actinobacillus actinomycetemcomitans*. *Cytokine* **7**, 534–541

Reddi, K., Wilson, M., Nair, S. *et al.* (1996a) Comparison of the pro-inflammatory cytokine-stimulating activity of surface-associated proteins of periodontopathic bacteria. *Journal of Periodontal Research* **31**, 120–130

Reddi, K., Nair, S., White, P.A. *et al.* (1996b) Surface-associated material from the bacterium, *Actinobacillus actinomycetemcomitans*, contains a peptide which in contrast to lipopolysaccharide, directly stimulates interleukin-6 gene transcription. *European Journal of Biochemistry* **236**, 871–876

Reinholdt, J., Bay, I. and Svjgaard, A. (1977) Association between HLA antigens and periodontal disease. *Journal of Dental Research* **56**, 1261–1263

Robertson, P.B., Lantz, M., Marucha, P.T. *et al.* (1982) Collagenolytic activity associated with *Bacteroides* species and *Actinobacillus actinomycetemcomitans*. *Journal of Periodontal Research* **17**, 275–283

Roodman, G.D. (1992) Interleukin-6: An osteotropic factor? *Journal of Bone and Mineralisation Research* **7**, 475–478

Roulston, D., Schwartz, S., Cogan, M.M. *et al.* (1985) Linkage analysis of dentinogenesis imperfecta and juvenile periodontitis: creating a 5 point map of 4q. *American Journal of Human Genetics* **37**, 206 Abstr.

Saglie, F.R., Carranza, F.A. Jnr, Newman, M.G. *et al.* (1982) Identification of tissue-invading bacteria in human periodontal disease. *Journal of Periodontal Research* **17**, 452–455

Sakurada, S. (1990) Leucotoxic mechanism of *Actinobacillus (Haemophilus) actinomycetemcomitans* leukotoxin on human neutrophils. *Japanese Journal of Oral Biology* **32**, 103–114

Sandholm, L. and Gronblad, E. (1984) Salivary immunoglobulins in patients with juvenile periodontitis and their healthy siblings. *Journal of Periodontology* **55**, 9–12

Sandholm, L., Tolo, K. and Olsen, I. (1987) Salivary IgG, a parameter of periodontal disease activity? High responder to *Actinobacillus actinomycetemcomitans* Y4 in juvenile and adult periodontitis. *Journal of Clinical Periodontology* **14**, 289–294

Saxby, M. (1984) Prevalence of juvenile periodontitis in a British school population. *Community Dentistry and Oral Epidemiology* **12**, 185–187

Saxby, M. (1987) Juvenile periodontitis. An epidemiological study in the West Midlands of the United Kingdom. *Journal of Clinical Periodontology* **14**, 594–598

Saxen, L. (1980a) Prevalence of juvenile periodontitis in Finland. *Journal of Clinical Periodontology* **7**, 177–186

Saxen, L. (1980b) Juvenile periodontitis. *Journal of Clinical Periodontology* **7**, 1–19

Saxen, L. (1980c) Heredity of juvenile periodontitis. *Journal of Clinical Periodontology* **7**, 276–288

Saxen, L. and Asikainen, S. (1993) Metronidazole in the treatment of juvenile periodontitis. *Journal of Clinical Periodontology* **20**, 166–171

Saxen, L. and Koskimies, S. (1984) Juvenile periodontitis – no linkage with HLA-antigens. *Journal of Periodontal Research* **19**, 441–444

Seddon, S.V. and Shah, H.N. (1989) The distribution of hydrolytic enzymes among Gram negative bacteria associated with periodontitis. *Microbial Ecology in Health and Disease* **2**, 181–190

Sjobin, B., Mattson, L., Unell, L. and Egelberg, J. (1993) Marginal bone loss in the primary dentition of patients with juvenile periodontitis. *Journal of Clinical Periodontology* **20**, 32–36

Slots, J. (1976) The predominant cultivatable organisms in juvenile periodontitis. *Scandinavian Journal of Dental Research* **49**, 248–255

Slots, J. and Rosling, B. (1983) Suppression of periodontopathic microflora in localized juvenile periodontitis by systemic tetracycline. *Journal of Clinical Periodontology* **10**, 465–486

Slots, J. and Schonfeld, S.E. (1991) *Actinobacillus actinomycetemcomitans* in localized juvenile periodontitis. In *Periodontal Disease Pathogens and Host Immune Response* (S. Hamada, S.C. Holt and J.R. McGhee, eds), pp. 53–64. Tokyo: Quintessence Publishing Co. Ltd

Slots, J., Reynolds, H.S. and Genco, R.J. (1980) *Actinobacillus actinomycetemcomitans* in human periodontal disease: a cross-sectional microbiological investigation. *Infection and Immunity* **29**, 1013–1020

Söderling, E., Mäkinen, P.L., Syed, S.A. and Mäkinen, K.K. (1991) Biochemical comparison of proteolytic enzymes present in rough- and smooth-surfaced *Capnocytophaga* isolated from the subgingival plaque of periodontitis patients. *Journal of Periodontal Research* **26**, 17–23

Spektor, M.D., Vandersteen, G.E. and Page, R.C. (1985) Clinical studies of one family manifesting rapidly progressing juvenile periodontitis and prepubertal periodontosis. *Journal of Periodontology* **56**, 93–101

Stevens, R.H. and Hammond, B.F. (1982) Inhibition of fibroblast proliferation by extracts of *Capnocytophaga* spp. and *Actinobacillus actinomycetemcomitans*. *Journal of Dental Research* **61**, 347 Abstr. 1515

Taichmann, N.S., Dean, R.T. and Sanderson, C.J. (1980) Biochemical and morphological characterization of the killing of human monocytes by leukotoxin derived from *Actinobacillus actinomycetemcomitans*. *Infection and Immunity* **28**, 258–268

Tervahartiala, B., Uitto, V.-J., Kari, K. and Laako, T. (1989) Outer membrane vesicles and leukotoxic activity of *Actinobacillus actinomycetemcomitans* from subjects with different periodontal status. *Scandinavian Journal of Dental Research* **97**, 33–42

Tsai, C.-C. and Taichmann, N.S. (1986) Dynamics of infection by leukotoxic strain of *Actinobacillus actinomycetemcomitans* in juvenile periodontitis. *Journal of Clinical Periodontology* **13**, 330–331

Tsai, C.-C., McArthur, W.P., Bachni, P.C. *et al.* (1981) Serum neutralizing activity against *Actinobacillus actinomycetemcomitans* leukotoxin in juvenile periodontitis. *Journal of Clinical Periodontology* **8**, 338–348

Van Dyke, T.E., Horoszewicz, H.O., Cianciola, L.J. and Genco, R.J. (1980) Neutrophil chemotactic dysfunction in human periodontitis. *Infection and Immunity* **27**, 124–132

Van Dyke, T.E., Bartholomew, E., Genco, R.J. *et al.* (1982) Inhibition of neutrophil chemotaxis by soluble bacterial products. *Journal of Periodontology* **53**, 502–508

Van Dyke, T.E., Schweinebraten, M., Cianciola, L.J. *et al.* (1985) Neutrophil chemotaxis in families with juvenile periodontitis. *Journal of Periodontal Research* **20**, 503–514

Van Winkelhoff, A.J., Rodenberg, A.J., Goené, R.J. *et al.* (1989) Metronidazole plus amoxycillin in the treatment of *Actinobacillus actinomycetemcomitans* associated periodontitis. *Journal of Clinical Periodontology* **16**, 128–131

Van Winkelhoff, A.J., Tijhof, C.J. and de Graaff, J. (1992) Microbiological and clinical results of metronidazole plus amoxycillin therapy in *Actinobacillus actinomycetemcomitans*-associated periodontitis. *Journal of Periodontology* **63**, 52–57

Waerhaug, J. (1977) Plaque control in the treatment of juvenile periodontitis. *Journal of Clinical Periodontology* **4**, 29–40

White, P.A., Wilson, M., Nair, S.P. *et al.* (1995) Characterization of an anti-proliferative surface-associated protein from *Actinobacillus actinomycetemcomitans* which can be neutralized by sera from a portion of patients with localized juvenile periodontitis. *Infection and Immunity* **63**, 2612–2618

Wilson, M. (1995) Bacterial activities of lipopolysaccharides from oral bacteria and their relevance to the pathogenesis of chronic periodontitis. *Scientific Progress* **78**, 19–34

Wilson, M. and Henderson, B. (1995) Virulence factors of *Actinobacillus actinomycetemcomitans* relevant to the pathogenesis of inflammatory periodontal diseases. *FEMS Microbiological Reviews* **17**, 365–379

Wilson, M., Kamin, S. and Harvey, W. (1985) Bone resorbing activity from purified capsular material from *Actinobacillus actinomycetemcomitans*. *Journal of Periodontal Research* **20**, 484–491

Wilson, M., Meghji, S. and Harvey, W. (1988) Effect of capsular material from *Haemophilus actinomycetemcomitans* on bone collagen synthesis *in vitro*. *Microbios* **54**, 181–185

Wilson, M., Meghji, S., Barber, P. and Henderson, B. (1993) Biological activities of surface associated material from *Porphyromonas gingivalis*. *FEMS Immunology and Medical Microbiology* **6**, 147–155

Wilson, M., Reddi, K. and Henderson, D. (1996) Cytokine-inducing components of periodontopathic bacteria. *Journal of Periodontal Research* **31**, 393–407

Yosof, Z.A. (1990) Early-onset periodontitis: radiographic patterns of alveolar bone loss in 55 cases from a selected Malaysian population. *Journal of Periodontology* **61**, 751–754

Zambon, J.J. (1985) *Actinobacillus actinomycetemcomitans* in human periodontal disease. *Journal of Clinical Periodontology* **12**, 1–20

Zambon, J.J., Christersson, L.A. and Slots, J. (1983a) *Actinobacillus actinomycetemcomitans* in human periodontal disease. Prevalence in patient groups and distribution of biotypes and serotypes within families. *Journal of Periodontology* **54**, 707–711

Zambon, J.J., de Louca, C., Slots, J. and Genco, R.C. (1983b) Studies of leukotoxin from *Actinobacillus actinomycetemcomitans* using the promyelocytic HL-60 cell line. *Infection and Immunity* **40**, 205–212

Zambon, J.J., Slots, J. and Genco, R.C. (1983c) Serology of oral *Actinobacillus actinomycetemcomitans* and serotype distribution in human periodontal disease. *Infection and Immunity* **41**, 19–27

Zambon, J.J., Gregory, G.J. and Smutko, J.S. (1990) Molecular genetic analysis of *Actinobacillus actinomycetemcomitans* epidemiology. *Journal of Periodontology* **61**, 75–80

21

Acute and infectious lesions of the gingiva

Introduction

Acute lesions are, by definition, of sudden onset, limited duration and with well-defined clinical features; by contrast with chronic gingivitis, which is frequently not obvious, acute gingival lesions are usually easier to diagnose.

There are some pathological conditions that can affect other parts of the oral mucosa as well as the gingivae that are impossible to classify because their aetiology is uncertain, e.g. erythema multiforme, or because they may be chronic with acute episodes, e.g. the fungal disease candidiasis. Syphilis, tuberculosis and other bacterial and viral infections may occasionally involve the gingiva, but the lesions are widespread, involving many parts of the mouth as well as other parts of the body.

The gingival lesions to be described include:

1. Traumatic lesions, both physical and chemical
2. Viral infections
   - Acute herpetic gingivostomatitis
   - Herpangina
   - Hand, foot and mouth disease
   - Measles
   - Herpes varicella/zoster virus infections
   - Glandular fever
   - HIV infection and AIDS (see Chapter 7)
3. Bacterial infections
   - Acute ulcerative necrotizing gingivitis (see Chapter 22)
   - Tuberculosis
   - Syphilis
4. Fungal infections
   - Candidiasis
5. Gingival abscess
6. Aphthous ulceration
7. Erythema multiforme
8. Drug allergy and contact hypersensitivity.

Traumatic lesions

Physical injury can be mechanical or thermal. A carelessly wielded toothbrush or woodstick, a sharp piece of food such as a fish-bone, hot food and drink are the most common causes of injury. Occasionally the cause is rather more bizarre; a cigarette burn, a pencil pushed into the mouth, a hair-grip, a musical instrument – the range of human oral activity is extensive.

Chemical causes of damage include aspirin placed against the gum to alleviate toothache, escharotics such as silver nitrate, even hydrogen peroxide solution used too strong and too frequently. Careless use of a caustic by the dentist, e.g. phenol, trichloracetic acid, can cause considerable tissue damage.

Usually there is little doubt about the diagnosis. The patient is aware of the accident and may suffer immediate and fairly severe pain. The acute symptoms may last for a day or so, and be followed by several days of soreness and sensitivity to further irritation. A localized area of inflammation and ulceration may form. In the case of a burn, there may be vesicle formation followed by ulceration. The wound is seen as a bright red area denuded of epithelium and with a ragged edge of necrotic tissue, which can be felt by the tongue (*Figure 21.1*). The healing wound is quickly covered by epithelium unless secondary infection takes place, as it might do in the debilitated individual. In this case pain persists, the wound may suppurate and this may be accompanied by lymph gland enlargement and malaise. Abscess formation may follow damage by a piece of woodstick or bone if the foreign object is not removed.

Treatment

Frequently the wound heals without any active intervention. The patient should and probably will avoid irritant foods or hot drinks. Rinsing with cold water or a very dilute saline solution might soothe. Strong antiseptics should be avoided. Troches containing a topical anaes-

Figure 21.1 Traumatic ulcer caused by a burn. (Courtesy Professor C Scully)

(a)

(b)

Figure 21.2 *(a)* Acute herpetic gingivostomatitis. The grey membrane of sloughing epithelium is in contrast to the underlying gingival inflammation. *(b)* Herpetic lesions in the cheek. (Courtesy Professor F Nally)

thetic, e.g. benzocaine lozenge, can be recommended, and some analgesic such as aspirin or paracetamol prescribed.

If the cause of the injury is still there, e.g. a fish-bone, it should be removed as gently as possible.

If there is secondary infection, an antibiotic may need to be prescribed.

It can be helpful to protect the wound with a bland dressing such as carboxymethylcellulose gelatin paste (Orabase), which is spread gently over the wound several times a day. However, this is rarely necessary since the usual cause of secondary infection is the persistance of the traumatic object. Its removal will bring about resolution.

Viral infections

Acute herpetic gingivostomatitis

Primary infection by the herpes simplex virus (HSV) type I usually occurs in children (1–10 years), but may affect older children or adults. The virus is transmitted by infected saliva or skin lesion contact. Infection in neonates can produce encephalitis or meningitis, but in children or adults it produces either a febrile illness or subclinical infection. The incubation period is about 5 days. Symptoms appear abruptly, with mild to severe fever. Temperature may be raised as high as 39.4°C. There is lymph gland enlargement and malaise, and the mouth and throat may be very painful. In young children there is irritability, profuse salivation and refusal to eat, even before the oral lesions become apparent. Small vesicles form on the gingivae, the tongue, buccal mucosa and lips, in fact anywhere in the mouth (*Figure 21.2b*). Usually the vesicles burst before they are seen, and the resultant round or irregular ulcers form a grey membrane surrounded by bright red mucosa. There is an acute gingivitis with redness, swelling and bleeding (*Figure 21.2a*). Symptoms subside in 10–21 days as the titre of protective antibodies rises.

A large proportion (30%) of patients who have had a primary herpetic infection early in life develop recurrent infection years later. The commonest recurrent lesion is on the lip (herpes labialis or cold sore). The lesion develops at the mucocutaneous junction of the upper lip and on the skin up to the nostril, although it can occur on the lower lip, and rarely on the gingiva or palate. An itching or burning sensation precedes the appearance of the lesion and a blister or cluster of blisters form, which burst, crust and heal after about 10 days. The blisters occur as a result of reactivation of latent virus in the trigeminal ganglion. This can occur as a result of any infection that lowers the resistance or dries the skin, or as a result of excessive exposure to sunlight.

Laboratory diagnosis may be made by direct smear to show characteristic giant cells, or by staining with specific fluorescent antisera to HSV. The virus can be isolated in tissue culture. A considerably raised antibody titre indicates recent infection.

Treatment

Treatment of the oral infection is largely symptomatic and supportive, i.e. bed rest, cool, soft food and plenty of fluid. In the infant, milk of magnesia or 55% Dequadin paint may be gently applied on cotton wool to the lesions. Benzocaine lozenges are useful in the older child or adult.

Aspirin or paracetamol will help to reduce pain and temperature. Phenergan is a useful sedative in the child.

In severe cases, acyclovir (Zovirax®) tablets (200 mg five times daily for 5 days) or suspension (5 ml of suspension five times daily for 5 days) may be prescribed. Acyclovir cream (apply five times daily for 5 days) may also be used as a preventive measure for herpes labialis.

Herpangina

This is an acute febrile illness caused by infection with Coxsackie A types 1–6, 8, 10, 16 or 22. It occurs in sporadic outbreaks, mainly in children. The patient complains of a sore throat, due partly to oral ulceration. Small ulcers appear mainly on the anterior faucial walls but also on the hard and soft palate, posterior pharyngeal wall, buccal mucosa and tongue. They heal in a few days and recovery is uneventful in 7–10 days.

Hand, foot and mouth disease

This is an acute febrile illness caused by infection with Coxsackie A type 16 or, occasionally, 5 or 6. It occurs in sporadic outbreaks, affecting mainly young children. Maculopapular and vesicular lesions appear on the skin and oral mucosa. The skin lesions mainly affect the hands, arms and feet. The oral vesicles break down into small ulcers. Recovery is uneventful in 10–14 days.

Measles

Measles is a severe febrile illness affecting mainly children, and protective vaccination is available against it. There is fever, malaise, cough, conjunctivitis, photophobia and lacrimation. There is a typical blotchy macular rash. Oral lesions known as Koplik's spots precede the skin lesions by a number of days. These are bluish-white specks surrounded by a bright red margin, and they occur mainly on the buccal mucosa.

Recovery takes place in 2–3 weeks in otherwise healthy, fit and well-fed children, but the infection can be serious in previously unexposed populations, particularly when poor and malnourished. Vaccination against measles is available for all children as part of their vaccination programme.

Herpes varicella/zoster virus infections

Varicella or chickenpox is an acute febrile illness, mainly of children. It produces a widespread maculopapular or vesicular eruption on the skin. Small vesicles also form on the oral mucosa, including the tongue and gingiva. Recovery is uneventful in 2–3 weeks.

Herpes zoster or shingles is caused by reactivation of latent varicella virus or re-infection of a person who has previously had chickenpox. It is commonest in middle-aged to older adults and affects sensory nerves, producing a severe neuralgia. A vesicular eruption occurs on the skin or mucosa innervated by the affected sensory nerve. If the trigeminal nerve or sensory portion of the facial nerve is affected, the vesicles can affect the skin of the face and oral mucosa.

Glandular fever

Glandular fever is caused by infection with the Epstein–Barr virus (EBV), which is a herpes-like virus. It is thought to be spread in infected saliva, and is most common in children, adolescents and young adults. The infection may be prolonged, and this particularly occurs in adults. It is characterized by fever, malaise, sore throat, headache, chills, cough and widespread lymphadenopathy. The liver and spleen may also be enlarged. There is oral involvement with a pharyngitis and oral lesions, which take the form of palatal petechiae. There is also an acute gingivitis and stomatitis.

Good oral hygiene and regular professional cleaning are important to treat the gingivitis. Sometimes acute necrotizing ulcerative gingivitis (ANUG) may occur and require treatment.

HIV infection and AIDS

The oral features and other aspects of this infection are fully discussed in Chapter 7.

Bacterial infections

The commonest acute gingival bacterial infection, ANUG, is described separately in Chapter 22. Other bacterial infections affecting the oral mucosa are described below.

Tuberculosis

Oral lesions are rare, and are usually secondary to sputum infection from open pulmonary tuberculosis. Deep ulcers may occur on any part of the oral mucosa, and a tuberculous gingivitis has been reported (Shafer *et al.*, 1983).

Tuberculosis is once again on the increase in immigrant, immunosuppressed and poor groups.

Syphilis

Secondary syphilis occurs about 6 weeks after primary infection, and it produces a widespread skin rash and oral eruption. In the mouth ulcers known as mucous patches form, and also irregular, long, winding ulcers known as snail track ulcers. These lesions are teeming with spirochaetes, and are highly infectious. The ternary lesions are rarely seen today but gumma can occur in the mouth, usually affecting the palate.

Figure 21.3 Thrush (acute pseudomembranous candidiasis). Creamy white particles are present on the attached gingiva over the right upper incisors and premolars. (Courtesy Professor C Scully)

Fungal infections

Candidiasis

The fungus *Candida albicans* is normally found in the mouth as a saprophyte until some changes in the balance of the oral flora or alteration in the local and systemic defence mechanisms occur, producing lowered resistance. The fungus then proliferates and infects the tissues. It is the most common fungal infection of the mouth. Factors that predispose to infection include prolonged use of antibiotics, steroids, and immunosuppressive drugs. It is also associated with diabetes, leukaemia and conditions of the gastrointestinal tract that promote malabsorption and malnutrition. Vaginal candidiasis is common in pregnancy, and the newborn infant may be infected from the vagina. It is also a very common feature of HIV infection, and its presence in a severe form should alert one to the possibility of this infection.

Candidiasis occurs in many forms. Three forms tend to be confined to the mouth; fortunately, these are usually transient and easy to treat.

Acute pseudomembranous candidiasis (thrush)

Thrush is found in infants, debilitated older adults and patients with HIV infection. Lesions occur in the gingivae, tongue, cheeks and throat. They are creamy white, elevated patches, which can be wiped away to leave a raw red base (*Figure 21.3*). The patient complains of a sore dry mouth or throat. Diagnosis can be made by demonstrating the yeasts in scrapings from the lesion.

In infants, a suspension of nystatin (100 000 iu/ml) can be painted on the lesions two or three times a day. In adults, amphotericin B lozenges BP (10 mg) or nystatin pastilles DPF (100 000 iu) are sucked three or four times a day. In severe cases, miconazole oral gel DPF can be used.

Acute atrophic candidiasis

This form is usually associated with an upset in balance between tissues and oral flora, which follows the prolonged use of steroids or antibiotics. The mucosa is thin, fiery red and painful.

Nystatin or amphotericin B reduces the symptoms.

Chronic atrophic candidiasis (denture sore mouth)

This condition is produced by *Candida* infection of tissue that is being irritated by a denture, often one that is worn day and night. The most usual site is the palate, where the tissue is bright red and spongy. The condition is often accompanied by an angular cheilitis, which is produced by overclosure following alveolar resorption under the denture. The corners of the mouth become folded and wet and subsequently infected by *Candida albicans*.

Treatment consists of leaving the denture out as much as possible; coating the lesions and the denture, when worn, with nystatin or amphotericin B; and remodelling the dentures and remaking them when the infection is controlled.

Gingival abscess

The term 'gingival abscess' should be used for abscesses confined to the gingivae. These abscesses are often associated with physical damage to the gingival margin by a woodstick, fish-bone, etc. with subsequent infection of the wound, but they can also arise within the wall of a gingival pocket where drainage has been impeded.

The abscess appears as a localized, shiny, painful, red swelling (*Figure 21.4*); associated teeth are sensitive to percussion. The abscess may discharge spontaneously or spread into the underlying tissue to form a periodontal abscess.

Figure 21.4 Gingival abscess caused by injury from a carelessly used dental woodstick

Figure 21.5 Aphthous ulceration. (Courtesy Dr F Nally and Editor of *Dental Update*)

Treatment

If the cause of the abscess is still present, it should be carefully removed. Drainage can be established by hot salt water mouthwashes used every 2 hours. If the lesion persists, it can be curetted under local anaesthesia or incised if it is pointing. If persistent and severe, a systemic antibiotic may very occassionally be needed. Any residual pocketing can be removed by thorough subgingival curettage or localized gingivectomy.

Aphthous ulceration

Recurrent mouth ulcers are the most common lesions of the oral mucosa. There are three types of ulcer: minor aphthous ulcers, major aphthous ulcers and herpetiform ulcers. Their common characteristics are that they are painful lesions, which appear without any reason, last for several days or weeks, heal and then, after a variable interval, recur. The cause is as yet unknown, but it is thought that the ulcers may be a manifestation of auto-immunity to a component of the oral mucosa. Several related factors have been suggested, such as emotional stress and hormonal change. In a number of patients the ulcers appear to be related to the menstrual cycle, the peak incidence being found in the post-ovulation period. There may be ional stress and hormonal change. In a number of patients the ulcers appear to be related to the menstrual cycle, the peak incidence being found in the post-ovulation period. There may be a relationship between ulceration and iron-deficiency anaemia, deficiency of folic acid and vitamin B12.

Minor aphthous ulcers (Mikulicz's aphthae)

These are the most common type. One or several small ulcers occur on non-keratinized oral mucosa, especially the lips, cheeks, vestibule and margins of the tongue (*Figure 21.5*). They are shallow ulcers less than 10 mm in length, with a surrounding zone of inflammation and slight swelling. They may be very painful or scarcely noticed by the patient unless traumatized. Sometimes tissue breakdown is heralded by localized paraesthesia. The ulcer(s) may last for 4–14 days, heal without scarring and recur after weeks or months. They are found in the age group 10–40 years, slightly more frequently in females than males.

Major aphthous ulcers (periadenitis mucosa necrotica recurrens)

These are much less common than the minor variety. They are larger (up to 30 mm), last as long as 40 days and are much more painful. Sometimes they recur so rapidly that involvement seems continuous. They can be found anywhere on the oral mucosa. They start as a submucosal nodule, which breaks down to form a deep crater-like ulcer with considerable tissue destruction. This heals with a scar.

Herpetiform ulcers

Despite their name, these ulcers are not related to herpes. They are most frequent in females and occur as a group of pin-head ulcers, which may coalesce to form a large, painful ulcer. They can occur on any part of the oral mucosa, including the tongue, palate and oropharynx, in which case they cause dysphagia (discomfort or pain on swallowing).

Treatment

Treatment for all aphthous ulceration is symptomatic, and depends on the frequency and severity of the ulceration. The patient needs to be reassured that the ulcer is not malignant. In the case of minor ulcers treatment may be unnecessary, but if they are painful, topical anaesthetics or applications of Bonjela can be useful. Where the ulcer is more painful and persistent, the application of topical corticosteroid preparations, such as 0.1% triamcinolone (Adcortyl A in Orabase), may be beneficial. Tablets of hydrocortisone hemisuccinate (2.5 mg, Corlan) can be used four times a day, allowing the tablet to dissolve next to the ulcer.

Very rarely, systemic corticosteroids may be needed in severe cases, but in these patients it is essential to have comprehensive blood tests and assessment of iron, folic acid and vitamin B12 levels.

If the patient has a problem keeping the mouth clean, a 0.2% chlorhexidine mouthwash is useful and can speed up the rate of healing.

Erythema multiforme

This is a syndrome of multiple aetiology with a wide spectrum of clinical features. The oral and cutaneous lesions may occur separately or together. In about a third of cases the condition is recurrent.

The aetiology of the syndrome may involve several underlying mechanisms. Drug allergy can cause the condition, especially to long-acting sulphonamides, penicillin and barbiturates. Several cases have also been associated with *Mycoplasma pneumoniae* infection, which causes primary atypical pneumonia. In many cases no cause can be found.

The major form of the disease produces systemic involvement, whilst the minor form produces local manifestations only. The patient is usually a child or young adult. In the major form there is a skin eruption with conjunctivitis and lesions of the mouth and upper respiratory tract. The patient becomes progressively ill over 7–14 days with fever and malaise.

In the mouth there is diffuse inflammation of the oral mucosa and gingivae. There are widespread erosions on the mucosa, and these have a red, velvety base and bleed freely. Some vesicles also form. The lips are severely involved with extensive crusting, and they may crust together at night. Eating, talking and oral examination are painful.

On the skin there is an extensive erythematous and macular rash. Iris target lesions with a central bulla that breaks down to crust may be seen. The hands, feet and flexural surfaces are most involved.

There is a diffuse conjunctivitis, which can become secondarily infected to produce corneal ulceration. The upper respiratory tract is often involved, with epistaxis, dysphagia and tracheitis. Pneumonia, urinogenital involvement, nephritis and myocarditis can occur in severe cases.

In the minor form there are local manifestations in the mouth or the skin or both, and no fever or prostration.

The patient should be referred to a physician. In the minor form, topical corticosteroids may be used in the mouth. In the major form systemic steroids and supportive treatment are necessary. If *Mycoplasma pneumoniae* infection is present, a course of tetracycline is given.

Drug allergy and contact hypersensitivity

As the number and variety of drugs and chemicals used as food additives increase, oral manifestations of hypersensitivity become more common.

Adverse reactions are basically of two types:

1. Those following systemic administration of a drug or chemical
2. Those following direct contact with the oral mucosa.

Drug allergy

These reactions can be provoked by penicillin, diazepam, local anaesthetics, codeine, tetracycline, barbiturates and many other drugs in common use.

Manifestations depend on the type of allergic response provoked, ranging from simple drying of the mouth to the most severe response, anaphylactic shock, which is potentially fatal. A severe reaction is angioneurotic oedema, in which there is swelling of the face, eyelids, lips, tongue and even pharynx. A fairly common response, especially to penicillin, is urticaria, skin rash, pains in the joints and fever. In the mouth, patches of inflammation, vesicles and ulcers may appear. Hypersensitivity to drugs may involve type I, II, III or IV mechanisms.

Contact hypersensitivity

Reactions of the oral mucosa have been reported to chewing gum, mouthwashes, toothpaste, sweets, cosmetics, topical antibiotics, periodontal dressings, etc. Often flavouring agents, such as peppermint, menthol, cinnamon and eugenol, are implicated.

Symptoms start with a burning sensation of the oral mucosa and swelling and redness of the tongue, lips and gingivae. The epithelium may peel off to leave very sore ulcerated areas. The gingivae are characteristically bright red and sensitive, and because the patient cannot clean the mouth it can become very dirty.

Management

The drug or chemical suspected must be immediately withdrawn. Antihistamines such as Piriton are useful where symptoms are mild, but more severe reactions, e.g. angioneurotic oedema, may require injection of hydrocortisone hemisuccinate.

In anaphylactic shock, intramuscular injection of 0.5 ml of 1 : 1000 adrenaline is necessary.

The mouth can be kept clean by frequent warm water or weak saline mouthwashes.

Reference

Shafer, W.G., Hine, M.K. and Levy, B.M. (1983) *A Textbook of Oral Pathology*, 4th Edn. Philadelphia: Saunders

22

Acute necrotizing ulcerative gingivitis

This condition has many synonyms, including acute ulcerative gingivitis (AUG), acute necrotizing gingivitis (ANG), Vincent's disease, trench mouth and fuso-spiro-chaetal gingivitis. Acute necrotizing ulcerative gingivitis (ANUG) is an acute necrotizing inflammatory disease produced by endogenous infection where systemic changes, as yet not precisely defined, predispose the gingiva to invasion by some bacteria in the oral flora, in particular spirochaetes and fusiform bacteria.

In Western countries, ANUG is usually seen in the 16–30 years age group. Epidemiological studies from 1950–1960 reported a 5% incidence of this condition in young adults, particularly in large groups living in cramped conditions, such as military recruits and college students. However, the prevalence of the disease has reduced markedly over the past 20 years, and this may reflect improved general health and nutrition and better standards of plaque control. More recently the disease has been seen in patients with HIV infection and AIDS (see Chapter 7), and this now needs to be considered in the diagnosis of this condition.

In some developing countries, such as Africa, ANUG is often seen in children and is frequently associated with malnutrition and infectious disease such as measles and herpes simplex infections (Osuji, 1990). Environmental factors are entirely responsible for this situation, because it occurs in the poor, malnourished children and not in those children from rich families who are of the same race and tribe. In a few of these affected children with severe malnutrition and recent infections the infection may spread from the gingiva to involve the oral and facial tissues, producing a condition known as cancrum oris or noma. This may result in massive oro-facial necrosis and is life-threatening. If the child recovers from the infection, gross facial deformity results.

In a study of 58 Nigerian children with ANUG, Osuji (1990) found five cases of cancrum oris. These children all had a recent history of febrile illness. Predisposing factors for cancrum oris are severe malnutrition, infectious childhood diseases, HIV infection and any disease in which the immune system is compromised, as well as poor oral hygiene.

Clinical features of ANUG

In developed countries the condition is a disease of young adults, and occurs equally in both sexes. It appears to be seasonal, occurring most frequently in autumn and winter months. The condition rarely occurs in a clean mouth, and then only if there is a major predisposing factor.

The condition is very painful, and plaque accumulates around the affected areas. Patients complain of gingival soreness, which is sometimes severe, and eating becomes difficult. There may be spontaneous gingival bleeding, an objectionable taste and a powerful halitosis.

ANUG is characterized by necrotic ulceration of the affected gingival margins (*Figure 22.1*). In the early stages of the disease, the gingival papillae become red and swollen and the tips of the papillae become ulcerated (*Figure 22.1a*). Necrotic ulceration of the papillae increases, and the ulcers may spread laterally along the gingival margins. The ulcers are painful to touch and are covered by a yellowish-grey slough. They have a characteristic 'punched out' appearance (*Figure 22.1b*), and if the 'false membrane' of sloughing tissue is removed a raw and bleeding surface is exposed.

The ulceration may be localized to one area or involve the whole mouth. Localized infections are most often seen around the lower anterior teeth. They may also be related to sites of bacterial stagnation, such as a partially erupted lower third molar.

There are frequently no systemic symptoms, although cervical or submandibular lymphadenopathy is commonly present. In some severe cases there may be mild to moderate fever and malaise and more marked lymphadenopathy. In a study of 35 ANUG patients presenting at an urban USA dental school, Falker *et al.* (1987) found lymphadenopathy in 61% and fever in 39% of their cases.

(a)

(b)

Figure 22.1 *(a)* Early papillary lesions of acute necrotizing ulcerative gingivitis. *(b)* Acute ulcerative gingivitis (involving gingivae in the lower jaw). (Courtesy Dr F Nally and Editor of *General Practitioner*)

Ulceration can also rarely occur on the contacting surface of the tongue or cheek, the palate and the fauces (Vincent's angina), but only when there is very severe debilitation. When ANUG occurs in association with HIV infection, the lesion may spread more deeply and lead to exposure and infection of the underlying bone (Chapter 7).

Even without active intervention, the acute symptoms will subside and the ulcers heal in 10–14 days. However, the normal gingival form does not return; the gingival margin becomes thickened by fibrous repair tissue and the papillae retain the concave shape of the healed ulcer. This saucer-shaped deformity of the gingiva is so characteristic of ANUG that an episode of previous infection can be diagnosed years later.

Once an episode of ANUG has occurred there is a tendency for recurrence, and in a susceptible individual this can occur more than once a year. This can result in progressive destruction of the periodontal tissues, with typical loss of the interdental papillae and the formation of characteristic gingival craters. The additional stagnation produced by this tissue deformity also encourages the progression of any underlying chronic periodontitis.

Predisposing factors

The main predisposing factors in most cases are poor oral hygiene, smoking and emotional stress. However, it can be precipitated by malnutrition, blood dyscrasias such as acute leukaemia, infections such as AIDS and glandular fever, malignant neoplasms and chemotherapy. Probably any condition in which the immune and defence systems are compromised would act in the same way.

The reduction in this condition in recent times probably reflects better standards of oral hygiene and improved health and nutrition. The name 'trench mouth' derives from the high prevalence of ANUG in soldiers suffering the appalling conditions of trench warfare in the First World War. The disease occurred in groups living together in these grossly unhygienic conditions and under immense stress.

Microbiology

ANUG is a mixed bacterial infection caused by a group of anaerobes consisting of spirochaetes and fusiform bacteria, which is often termed a fuso-spirochaetal complex. These bacteria include *Treponema vincentii, T. denticola, T. macrodentium, Fusobacterium nucleatum, Prevotella intermedia* and *Porphyromonas gingivalis* (Loesche *et al.*, 1982). These bacteria are all found in large numbers in the slough and necrotic tissue at the surface of the ulcer, and also invade a small distance into the underlying intact tissue at the base of the ulcer (Courtois *et al.*, 1983). Spirochaetes can be seen under electron microscopy to invade the greatest distance into the tissue. The aetiological role of these bacteria is suggested by the fact that ANUG resolves rapidly following short-term treatment with metronidazole.

Other bacterial species commonly found in the subgingival flora are also present on the surface of the lesion in lesser numbers.

There are many reports of ANUG in closely confined groups of young adults (see above). However, there is no evidence that the condition is transmissible. This view is supported by experiments in which the inoculation of micro-organisms from affected to healthy animals did not result in development of ANUG, except when the recipients were severely immunosuppressed. It is therefore thought that the reported group outbreaks of ANUG are due to common exposure to stressful conditions and poor oral hygiene rather than direct transmission of an infecting agent. This view is supported by the fact that all of the bacteria infecting the tissues in ANUG are the same as those found in the subgingival flora of patients with chronic gingivitis and periodontitis who do not develop ANUG.

Smoking

A clear association between smoking and the prevalence of ANUG was demonstrated over 40 years ago (Stammers, 1944; Pindborg, 1947, 1949). A number of more recent studies (MacGregor, 1992) have also indicated that smoking is an important predisposing factor in ANUG (see also Chapter 4). Stammers (1944) examined over 1000 cases of ANUG, and found that nearly all of them were smokers. More recently, in a study in Edinburgh, Kowalik and Nisbet (1983) found that 98 out of 100 cases of ANUG were smokers. Similarly, Falker *et al.* (1987), in a study of 35 ANUG patients in an urban dental school, found that 83% of them were smokers.

Smokers tend to have poorer levels of oral hygiene and greater deposits of calculus than non-smokers, but this is not sufficient to explain the association. Smoking may cause vasoconstriction of gingival blood vessels (Bergström and Floderus-Myrhed, 1983) and in this way favour the colonization of an anaerobic bacterial flora. Of more possible relevance would seem to be the effects of smoking on serum IgG antibodies to subgingival bacteria (Haber, 1994), on the numbers of T-helper lymphocytes (Ginns *et al.*, 1982; Costabel *et al.*, 1986) and neutrophil function (Eichel and Shahrik, 1969; Armitage *et al.*, 1975; Bridges *et al.*, 1977; Kenny *et al.*, 1977; Codd *et al.*, 1987; Nowak *et al.*, 1990; Kalra *et al.*, 1991; Lannon *et al.*, 1992; Selby *et al.*, 1992; MacFarlane *et al.*, 1992; Totti *et al.*, 1994; Ryder *et al.*, 1994) (See Chapter 4).

Host responses

The exact way in which the predisposing factors trigger the infection is not clear. However, the fact that ANUG occurs in AIDS and in severely immunosuppressed animals suggests that immunosuppression might be an important factor.

ANUG usually develops when there is poor oral hygiene and pre-existing gingivitis. However, it will rarely occur in a clean mouth when a severe debilitating factor is present, e.g. acute leukaemia.

Emotional stress as a predisposing factor in ANUG has long been recognized by clinicians. However, there are only a few well-controlled studies that demonstrate the association between ANUG and stress. Stress may alter behaviour (such as decreasing oral hygiene) and reduce salivary and local blood flow, and probably affects immune function. Despite some knowledge of these effects, it is not entirely clear how they operate to predispose to this condition.

There is a clear relationship between nutritional deficiency and ANUG in developing countries. This may operate by compromising the defence mechanisms to such a degree that the disease spreads more easily.

Histopathology

The histopathological changes of ANUG are largely non-specific. The surface epithelium and adjacent connective tissue on the surface of the lesion is necrotic. There is a dense acute inflammatory infiltration of the underlying tissues, with large numbers of polymorphonuclear neutrophil leucocytes (PMNs) in the tissues. Bacteria can be seen invading this area, with the spirochaetes spreading deepest. Below this area is viable tissue infiltrated with plasma cells, lymphocytes and some macrophages.

Diagnosis

The diagnosis is easily made on clinical grounds without the need to take a bacterial smear to show the fuso-spirochaetal flora. Nevertheless, it is important to take a very careful history to determine the underlying predisposing factors in each individual case.

Treatment

Treatment is divided into two stages:

1. Control of the acute phase
2. Management of the residual condition.

Control of the acute phase

This is achieved by cleaning the wound and using an antibacterial agent. The lesion is irrigated with warm water or 5-vol hydrogen peroxide solution, gently cleaned and the teeth lightly scaled. The patient is prescribed an oxygen-releasing mouthwash, such as hydrogen peroxide DPF or sodium perborate (Bocasan) DPF, to be used three times daily. The scaling of the affected teeth is completed over the next few days. This may suffice in very mild cases, but most cases requires an antibiotic in addition. ANUG is an anaerobic infection, thus oral metronidazole (200 g three times daily for 3–5 days) is the first choice (Shinn, 1962; Shinn *et al.*, 1965). It gives rapid relief of symptoms and is not prone to produce hypersensitivity reactions. Side effects may include nausea, headaches, a metallic taste and tachycardia. It should not be prescribed in early pregnancy, if there is blood dyscrasia, or in patients who drink alcohol heavily; alcohol must be totally avoided when taking metronidazole, since it precipitates nausea and vomiting. In these cases, phenoxy-methyl penicillin (250 mg four times daily for 5 days) is an effective alternative. Erythromycin or tetracycline may be used if both metronidazole and penicillin are contra-indicated. A 2% chlorhexidine mouthwash might also be helpful in some cases, but should only be used during the short period in which mechanical oral hygiene is compromised.

It is also vital to determine the predisposing factors in each individual case and to counsel the patient on controlling these when appropriate.

Management of the residual condition

This is essential if recurrence is to be avoided. Meticulous supra- and subgingival scaling is carried out together with the removal of all predisposing local factors, such as overhanging filling margins, partially erupted teeth and food impaction.

Residual gingival deformity needs to be corrected by gingivoplasty in early cases, and by inverse bevel flap procedures in all other cases. Any underlying chronic periodontitis lesion, e.g. pocketing, can be dealt with at the same time.

The maintenance of a high standard of oral hygiene is essential, therefore regular inspection and scaling should be organized.

Patients suffering unexplained recurrence should undergo medical examination and blood screening for major predisposing factors.

References

Armitage, A.K., Dollery, C.T., George, C.F. *et al.* (1975) Absorption and metabolism of nicotine from cigarettes. *British Medical Journal* **4**, 313–316

Bergström, J. and Floderus-Myrhed, B. (1983) Co-twin study of the relationship between smoking and some periodontal disease factors. *Community Dentistry and Oral Epidemiology* **11**, 113–116

Bridges, R.B., Kraal, J.H., Huang, L.J.T. and Chancellor, M.B. (1977) The effects of tobacco smoke on chemotaxis and glucose metabolism of polymorphonuclear leucocytes. *Infection and Immunology* **15**, 115–123

Codd, E.E., Swim, A.T. and Bridges, R.B. (1987) Tobacco smokers neutrophils are desensitized to chemotactic peptide-stimulated oxygen uptake. *Journal of Laboratory and Clinical Medicine* **110**, 648–652

Costabel, U., Bross, K.J., Reuter, C. *et al.* (1986) Alterations in immunoregulatory T-cell subsets in cigarette smokers. A phenotypic analysis of bronchoalveolar and blood lymphocytes. *Chest* **90**, 39–44

Courtois, G., Cobb, C. and Killoy, W. (1983) Acute necrotizing ulcerative gingivitis. A transmission electron microscope study. *Journal of Periodontology* **54**, 671–679

Eichel, G. and Shahrick, H.A. (1969) Tobacco smoke toxicity: loss of human oral leucocyte function and fluid cell metabolism. *Science* **166**, 1424–1428

Falker, W.A. Jnr, Martin, S.A., Vincent, J.W. *et al.* (1987) A clinical and demographic and microbiologic study of ANUG patients in an urban dental school. *Journal of Clinical Periodontology* **14**, 307–314

Ginns, L.C., Goldenheim, P.D. and Miller, L.G. (1982) T-lymphocyte subsets in smoking and lung cancer. Analysis of monoclonal antibodies and flow cytometry. *American Review of Respiratory Disease* **126**, 265–269

Haber, J. (1994) Cigarette smoking: a major risk factor for periodontitis. *Compendium of Continuous Education in Dentistry* **15**, 1002–1014

Kalra, J., Chandhary, A.K. and Prasad, K. (1991) Increased production of oxygen free radicals in cigarette smokers. *International Journal of Experimental Pathology* **72**, 1–7

Kenny, E.B., Kraal, J.H., Saxe, S.R. and Jones, J. (1977) The effects of cigarette smoke on human polymorphonuclear leukocytes. *Journal of Periodontal Research* **12**, 227–234

Kowolik, M.J. and Nisbet, T. (1983) Smoking and acute ulcerative gingivitis. *British Dental Journal* **154**, 241–242

Lannan, S., McLean, A., Drost, E. *et al.* (1992) Changes in neutrophil morphology and morphometry following exposure to cigarette smoke. *International Journal of Experimental Pathology* **73**, 183–191

Loesche, W.J., Syed, S.A., Laughton, B.E. and Stoll, J. (1982) The bacteriology of acute necrotizing ulcerative gingivitis. *Journal of Periodontology* **53**, 223–230

MacFarlane, G.D., Herzberg, M.C., Wolff, L.F. and Hardie, N.A. (1992) Refractory periodontitis associated with abnormal polymorphonuclear leucocyte phagocytosis and cigarette smoking. *Journal of Periodontology* **63**, 908–913

MacGregor, I.D.M. (1992) Smoking and periodontal disease. In *Drugs, Diseases and the Periodontium* (R.A. Seymour and P.A. Heasman, eds), pp. 118–119. Oxford: Oxford University Press

Nowak, D., Ruta, U. and Piasecka, G. (1990) Nicotine increases human polymorphonuclear leukocytes' chemotactic response – possible additional mechanism of lung injury in cigarette smokers. *Experimental Pathology* **39**, 37–43

Osuji, O.O. (1990) Necrotizing ulcerative gingivitis and cancrum oris in Ibadan, Nigeria. *Journal of Periodontology* **61**, 769–772

Pindborg, J.J. (1947) Tobacco and gingivitis. I. Statistical examination of the significance of tobacco in the development of acute ulceromembranous gingivitis and in the formation of calculus. *Journal of Dental Research* **26**, 261–264

Pindborg, J.J. (1949) Tobacco and gingivitis. II. Correlation between consumption of tobacco, acute ulceromembranous gingivitis and calculus. *Journal of Dental Research* **28**, 460–463

Ryder, M.I. (1994) Nicotine effects on neutrophil F-actin formation and calcium release: implications for tobacco use and respiratory disease. *Experimental Lung Research* **20**, 283–296

Selby, C., Drost, E., Brown, D. *et al.* (1992) Inhibition of neutrophil adherence and movement by acute cigarette smoke exposure. *Experimental Lung Research* **18**, 813–827

Shinn, D.L. (1962) Metronidazole in acute ulcerative gingivitis. *Lancet* **1**, 1191

Shinn, D.L., Squires, S. and McFadzean, J.A. (1965) The treatment of Vincent's disease with metronidazole. *Dental Practitioner* **15**, 275–280

Stammers, A. (1944) Vincent's infection: observations and conclusions regarding the aetiology and treatment of 1017 civilian cases. *British Dental Journal* **76**, 147–155

Totti, N., McCuster, K.T., Campbell, E.J. *et al.* (1994) Nicotine is chemotactic for neutrophils and enhances neutrophil responsiveness to chemotactic peptides. *Science* **227**, 169–171

23

Epulides and tumours of the gingiva

Epulides

The term 'epulis' means a 'lump on the gum', and these lesions are the commonest localized enlargements of the gingiva. They are best described as chronic inflammatory hyperplasias. These can be fibrous epulides, pyogenic granulomata or giant-cell granulomata, the first two being much more common than the third.

Fibrous epulis (fibro-epithelial polyp)

This usually arises from an interdental papilla and is a firm, pink nodule of varying shape (*Figure 23.1*). Fibrous epulides usually associate with a source of chronic irritation such as calculus or the rough edge of a restoration. Similar lesions can occur on the cheek as the result of

cheek biting, or related to the margin of an ill-fitting denture (denture granuloma).

Histologically the lesion consists of hyperplastic connective tissue covered by stratified squamous epithelium.

These lesions should be treated by excision with care to remove any irritating factor. The whole lesion should be placed in formal saline fixative and sent for histological confirmation of the diagnosis.

Pyogenic granuloma

The pyogenic granuloma usually arises from the interdental papilla. It appears as an elevated, pedunculated or sessile mass with a smooth or lobulated surface (*Figure 23.2*). It is deep red or reddish-purple in colour, and the surface may be ulcerated. It also has a tendency to bleed, either spontaneously or on provocation with slight trauma. It may develop rapidly to a variable size and then remain stable for an indefinite period.

Figure 23.1 A fibrous epulis arising from the interdental papilla between $\overline{32|}$ of a 35-year-old woman

Figure 23.2 A pyogenic granuloma arising from the interdental papilla between $|45$ of a 15-year-old boy

The lesion appears to result from local irritation, but in some cases there may be a hormonal conditioning factor, such as in the lesions occurring in pregnancy (pyogenic granulomata of pregnancy) and at puberty (Chapter 6).

Histologically, the overlying stratified squamous epithelium is usually thin and atrophic but may show signs of hyperplasia in some parts of the lesion. The connective tissue contains vast numbers of endothelium-lined vascular spaces and proliferation of endothelial cells and fibroblasts. There is a moderately intense infiltration of polymorphonuclear neutrophil leucocytes (PMNs), lymphocytes and plasma cells, with high numbers of PMNs at the surface of the lesion particularly when ulceration is present.

The lesion should be carefully excised with care to remove all affected tissue and any local irritating factor. Lack of care in these respects can lead to recurrence of the lesion. The whole lesion should be placed in formal saline fixative and sent for histological confirmation of the diagnosis.

Giant-cell epulis

The giant-cell epulis or granuloma is usually found growing from the gingival margin between teeth anterior to the permanent molars, and its development may be related to the resorption of the deciduous molars (*Figure 23.3*). The lesion is rounded, soft and purplish-red in colour. It may grow rapidly in its early stages, and tends to bleed easily.

Histologically, the connective tissue consists of numerous multinucleated giant cells (macrophage polykaryons) and plump spindle-shaped cells in a loose fibrous stroma. It is covered by stratified squamous epithelium.

A giant-cell granuloma of the jaw may erode through the outer alveolar plate and appear as a gingival swelling. This should be distinguished from the epulis by radiological investigation.

The treatment is total excision of the lesion, along with the basal tissue from which it arose. The alveolar bone at the base of the lesion should also be curetted thoroughly. Histological confirmation of the diagnosis is essential, and the lesion must be immediately placed in formal saline fixative for this purpose.

Neoplasms of the gingiva

True benign or, occasionally, malignant neoplasms may arise from the gingival or periodontal tissue, and may sometimes resemble an epulis.

Epithelial neoplasms

Squamous-cell papilloma

The squamous-cell papilloma usually appears as a warty nodule with a white surface if keratinized and a pink one if not (*Figure 23.4*). It may be related to the common wart of the skin and be due to infection with human papilloma virus (HPV).

The whole lesion should be excised and submitted for histological examination to confirm the diagnosis.

Figure 23.3 A giant-cell epulis arising from the interdental and buccal gingiva between |45 of a 15-year-old boy

Figure 23.4 A squamous cell papilloma on the gingiva between |23 in a 40-year-old woman

Squamous-cell carcinoma

These tumours may occasionally occur on the gingiva but are more common on other parts of the oral mucosa, such as the tongue, lips, buccal mucosa, floor of the mouth or alveolar mucosa. Carcinoma of the gingiva usually presents as an ulcerated lesion with rolled edges, but it may sometimes have an exophytic or verrucous type of growth. Any fast growing lesion or ulcer that fails to heal should be regarded with suspicion; 95% of oral cancer occurs after the age of 40 years, and it becomes more common with increasing age. Gingival carcinomas are closely related to the underlying bone and rapidly invade the periosteum and bone. Metastasis is common, and early diagnosis is essential if treatment is to have any chance of success. Suspicious lesions should be quickly referred to a specialist maxillofacial surgeon and oral pathologist to confirm the diagnosis by biopsy and institute treatment.

Figure 23.5 A benign true fibroma beneath the gingival and alveolar mucosa related to |1 in a 25-year-old woman. The tumour has caused displacement at |1

Figure 23.6 A benign osteoma in the maxilla producing swelling of the overlying gingiva (Courtesy Professor C Scully)

Connective-tissue neoplasms

Benign and, occasionally, malignant neoplasms arising in the connective tissue can sometimes involve the gingival tissues. They may present as firm masses that stretch the overlying mucosa, and may displace adjacent teeth. They may also sometimes resemble epulides. Suspicious lesions should be referred to a specialist maxillofacial surgeon and oral pathologist for definitive diagnosis.

(a)

(b)

Figure 23.7 *(a)* A tumour of dental tissue origin, resembling an epulis, arising from the mesial interdental and buccal gingiva related to |1 in a 16-year-old girl. *(b)* Photomicrograph of a low-power view of a histological section of the above lesion. It shows the features of an adenomatoid odontogenic tumour

These neoplasms may include benign fibromas (*Figure 23.5*) and myxomas, and their equivalent malignant sarcomas. It should also be borne in mind that benign and malignant bone tumours may also produce gingival swelling (*Figure 23.6*).

Lymphoid neoplasms

Lymphomas such as Hodgkin's and non-Hodgkin's lymphomas may produce deposits beneath the oral mucosa including the gingiva. In addition, deposits from a leukaemia may seed in the gingiva and multiply (see Chapter 6). All such cases should be quickly referred to specialists in these conditions.

Dental tissue neoplasms

Tumours of odontogenic origin may be found in the jaws and occasionally arise from dental epithelial remnants in the periodontium, such as the epithelial rests of Malassez, and occur in the periodontium or gingiva. Those in the gingiva may resemble epulides, and those within the bone may expand the alveolar plate and produce a gingival swelling. They include adenomatoid odontogenic tumours, squamous odontogenic tumours and calcifying epithelial odontogenic tumours. Careful radiographic examination is necessary in these cases, and they should be referred to a specialist maxillofacial surgeon and oral pathologist for definitive diagnosis and treatment. The clinical appearance and histology of an adenomatoid odontogenic tumour of the gingiva are shown in *Figure 23.7a, b*.

24

Occlusion

The term 'occlusion' applies to any contact between the mandibular and maxillary teeth in any position of the mandible. The occlusion is therefore of importance to restorative and prosthetic dentistry as well as to orthodontics and periodontics. Unfortunately, each of these specialties has been concerned with a particular aspect of occlusion and has developed its own beliefs and vocabulary, leading to confusion. Many of the concepts valuable to prosthetics or orthodontics may be irrelevant or even contrary to an understanding of the role of occlusal relationships and occlusal stresses in periodontics. Many of the ideas still in current use were developed before knowledge of the neurophysiology of the masticatory system had been acquired, and therefore represent a static view of occlusion in which anatomical stereotypes are important. The idea of malocclusion as expressed by Angle's classification is of this generation. The concept of 'balanced occlusion', in which bilateral cuspal contacts are made in lateral excursions, may well be important in prosthetics, but under certain circumstances can be contrary to periodontal health. Health of the tooth-supporting tissues does not depend primarily on the conformity of the occlusion to any particular anatomical stereotype. However, occlusal stresses can play a role in periodontal pathology (Chapter 8).

Three important aspects of masticatory function need to be considered:

1. During normal mastication, teeth are separated by the food bolus and make contact at the end of the chewing cycle and during swallowing. It has been estimated that the total duration of tooth contact in a 24-hour period is 17.5 minutes, made up of 9 minutes chewing contact and 8.5 minutes swallowing contact. Therefore, normal functional tooth-to-tooth contact is occasional and transient, and by itself is unlikely to cause damage.
2. The activity of the masticatory system is largely under the control of the trigeminal nerve nucleus, which, subject to the control of the higher centres, operates various forms of reflex activity. These constitute a feedback mechanism, which protects the various tissues of the masticatory system, including the periodontium. For example, the presence of a hard object such as a piece of bone or nut in the bolus of soft food stimulates proprioceptors in the periodontal ligament, which by reflex activity causes the jaw to open. In this way, stress on the teeth and supporting tissues is controlled, unless the higher centres dictate that a conscious effort be made to crack the nut.
3. All the tissues of the masticatory system except the teeth have considerable powers of adaptation, and bone, connective tissue and epithelium are in a state of constant activity and renewal. The masticatory system is not a rigid system; like other vital tissues, it is immensely flexible and allows a range of environmental changes to be absorbed without damage.

Excessive occlusal stress

Attempts to define the word 'excessive' in most situations tend to beg the question. Excessive occlusal stresses are those that exceed the limits of tissue adaptation and therefore cause pathology. Occlusal trauma pathology is the damage to the supporting tissues when subject to excessive occlusal stresses. Forces generated during mastication depend largely on the consistency of the food. Peak pressures on an adult molar have been estimated at 0.4–1.8 g, but because of the powers of adaptation of the periodontal tissues it is impossible to define excessive occlusal stress in precise numerical terms.

Excessive stresses appear to be engendered by:

1. Abnormal or parafunctional activity
2. Dental treatment
3. Occlusal disharmony

4.   Destruction of the periodontal tissues by disease, i.e. chronic periodontitis.

These factors are frequently inter-related.

Parafunction

Parafunctional activity is outside the range of functional activity. It is usually habitual and the patient is often unaware of such habits, during which contact may be made between the upper and lower teeth (as in clenching and grinding), between the teeth and the soft tissues (cheeks, lips and tongue) or between the teeth and some foreign body (e.g. pencil, pipe, etc.). These habits may be associated with psychological factors, e.g. anxiety, anger, frustration, or with occupational or recreational activity.

Bruxism

The most common tooth-to-tooth habits are clenching and grinding, i.e. bruxism. A large proportion of patients with periodontal disease indulge in this habit. Many patients are aware of clenching their teeth when under stress during the day, but few people are aware of a night grinding habit unless complained of by someone else. It has been estimated that during clenching or grinding the individual might impose a load of over 20 g on a tooth over periods of 2.5 seconds at a time. This is far in excess of normal functional stresses and causes 'flow' within the visco-elastic periodontal ligament and distortion of the alveolar bone, from which the tissues are slow to recover. Furthermore, the excessive load tends to affect the proprioceptive nerve endings, which are either overridden or set at a higher tolerance level, thereby impairing the protective reflex mechanism. Muscle activity becomes abnormal and the habit is perpetuated. Such disturbed muscle activity may also interfere with temporomandibular joint function. Bruxism is the most usual cause of advanced attrition in the Western world.

Night grinding occurs during the rapid eye movement (REM) periods of sleep when dreaming activity takes place. The grinding does not occur in the intercuspal position but rather in the retruded position of the mandible.

In the absence of gingival inflammation or periodontal destruction, the supporting tissues may adapt to the load of primary occlusal trauma. Where there is pre-existing inflammatory periodontal disease, the tissues usually similarly adapt. In early to moderate periodontitis the adaptive response is the same, but in advanced periodontitis the rate of disease progress may be accelerated by the fusion of the marginal inflammatory and the intra-alveolar 'trauma' lesions (Chapter 8).

There are two causes of bruxism – nervous tension and occlusal interference. These two factors often act together so that an occlusal interference in an anxious person may provoke bruxism, whereas a relaxed individual may adapt to it.

Diagnosis of bruxism

There may be a definite history of bruxism but, as stated, many patients are unaware of parafunction. A number of signs help in its detection:

1.   Advanced attrition is the most obvious clue; also wear facets that could be produced only in extreme positions of mandibular movements
2.   Increased tooth mobility patterns, which are not commensurate with the amount of attachment loss or degree of gingival inflammation
3.   The presence of widened periodontal ligament spaces seen in radiographs
4.   Hypertonicity of the muscles of mastication
5.   Temporomandibular joint discomfort.

Dental treatment

One of the most common causes of excessive occlusal stress in the partially dentate patient is the badly designed partial denture. Many abutment teeth suffer abnormal loading because the stress is either greater than normal, or is applied in an abnormal direction. The tooth used as an abutment for a free-end saddle denture is particularly vulnerable, especially when clasps without occlusal rests are used. As the denture sinks into the soft tissues, lateral and distal forces are imposed on the abutment teeth. In most cases oral hygiene is poor, and the combined effect of gingival inflammation under the denture and excessive occlusal loads make loss of abutment teeth more than likely. In denture design axial loading of abutment teeth is imperative, and where soft-tissue support is necessary this should be spread over as large an area as possible.

Orthodontic treatment can cause excessive occlusal stress in two ways. Large forces can cause rapid tooth movement and damage to the supporting tissues. If the alveolar plates of bone are thin they may be perforated; thus, tipping a lower incisor forward against a thin labial plate may produce a dehiscence. Slow orthodontic movement allows tissue adaptation and less likelihood of trauma. Tooth movement can also produce occlusal disharmonies, with harmful results.

Failure to contour the cusps of restorations or to check the occlusion in both intercuspal and functional positions can produce cuspal interference. Unfortunately modern dental amalgams set rapidly and leave little time for careful occlusal adjustment, which is very important if the restoration is to have correct occlusion relationships. Occlusal composite restorations need careful occlusal adjustment after the restoration has set.

Failure to occlusally balance cast restorations such as

crowns and bridges can produce more serious occlusal disharmony.

Failure to replace a lost tooth can result in drifting of other teeth, with resultant disharmonies.

Occlusal disharmony

Functional harmony is a very important attribute of the healthy masticatory system, with all parts of the unit – muscles, ligaments, temporomandibular joints – working smoothly together. Occlusal disharmonies are tooth contacts that interfere with smooth closing movement along any pathway into intercuspal position. A common mistake is to assume that malocclusions are always associated with occlusal disharmonies. So flexible is the tooth eruption mechanism that even gross tooth malalignment does not necessarily produce cuspal interference; rather, it is external interference with the fully erupted dentition which produces disharmony. Badly executed dentistry can create interferences, but the most common cause is tooth loss. After tooth extraction, neighbouring teeth may tip and drift and opposing teeth overerupt until a new position of stability is reached. Thus after extraction of the lower first molar the second and third molars tip mesially and lingually, and the distal cusps of these teeth come into interfering contact with upper molar cusps. Moreover, because of the tilt, plaque may be allowed to collect on the mesial and lingual aspects of these teeth, producing gingival inflammation and pocketing.

Effects of occlusal interference

1. The path of closure of the mandible may alter to avoid the interference. This may put an excessive load on other teeth, e.g. occlusal interference between molar cusps may produce a path of closure forward of the normal pathway and forward posturing of the mandible so that the upper incisors become overloaded (*Figure 24.1b*). This may result in drifting of the incisors, which is more likely when there is already loss of tooth support caused by periodontal disease.

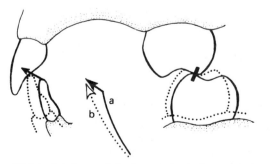

Figure 24.1 An interference between posterior teeth may produce *(a)* a slide from the initial contact into the intercuspal position, or *(b)* forward posturing of the mandible so that it closes through a forward path

2. If there is no adaptation to the interference, the involved teeth make contact in what is called an initial or premature contact, from which a slide carries the mandible into the position of maximum intercuspation (*Figure 24.1a*). This may produce excessive stress on those teeth involved directly, as well as on those teeth indirectly stressed at the end of the slide. Drifting and occlusal trauma may result.
3. The interference may also initiate parafunctional habits.

The diagnosis of occlusal trauma

A number of clinical features point to the presence of occlusal trauma, and a diagnosis should be based on the presence of several features together, rather than only one.

1. Tooth mobility is affected by the load on the tooth and its duration, by the proportion of tooth invested in supporting tissue and by the morphology of the root(s). It is also affected by inflammation of the attachment apparatus. Increased tooth mobility may be a sign of occlusal trauma or of hyperfunction, i.e. increased loading of the tooth without evidence of tissue breakdown. Assessment of mobility (outside the laboratory) is entirely subjective, teeth being given a score from 0 to 3 (Chapter 11). It can be detected by having the patient grind the teeth from side to side while the operator rests the fingers on the facial surfaces of the teeth. It is more usually tested for by pressing the blunt end of an instrument against one side of the tooth while a finger rests on the tooth under examination and a neighbouring tooth which acts as a fixed point.
2. The presence of tooth wear that appears to be greater than one might expect in a patient of that age and which cannot be attributed to any special diet or deficiency in tooth mineralization.
3. The migration of one or more teeth. This is usually seen in the anterior segment, often related to (i) loss of posterior support and/or (ii) an abnormal path of closure due to tooth interference between posterior teeth (*Figure 24.1*). Where bone loss due to periodontal disease has taken place, tooth migration can be rapid and a common cause of patient alarm. Food impaction may occur following tooth drifting and breaking of interproximal contacts.
4. Operators with a sensitive ear may be able to detect that the percussion note of an affected tooth is dull rather than resonant.
5. There may be hypertrophy and hypertonicity of the muscles of mastication, most obviously of the masseters. This is detected by palpation but sometimes can actually be seen, especially in the bruxist patient.
6. Signs of temporomandibular pain dysfunction syndrome with jaw deviation, joint clicking, discomfort and even pain due to muscle spasm.

7. Radiographic evidence, together with mobility, offers evidence of occlusal trauma. The signs are:
   (a) Widening of the periodontal space
   (b) Funnel-like or crescentic resorption of the alveolar crest around a tooth
   (c) Loss of definition of the lamina dura; this is an unreliable sign as other factors, including root morphology, affect the radiographic appearance of the socket wall.
8. Tooth sensitivity may be associated with both occlusal trauma and pulp pathology brought about by excessive loading. Sometimes patients have an awareness of a discrepancy in their occlusion, a positive occlusal sense, and a patient may be able to point to the tooth involved.

Occlusal analysis

This is an analysis of static jaw relationships as well as of the relationships of the teeth during mandibular movements. A large number of articulators have been designed to replicate jaw movement but each of them has its limitations, and the almost inevitable errors in bite registration and model mounting frequently nullify the accuracy of the articulator. A more fundamental criticism of mechanical aids is that they simply cannot reproduce the flexibility of vital tissues. However, fully adjustable articulators are necessary in carrying out complex restorative procedures. In a periodontal analysis study models are useful, but careful oral examination is essential.

The examination of static jaw relations should include a record of the teeth in the arch, tooth alignment and such tooth deviations as tilting, overeruption and plunger cusps. Inter-arch examination records the Angle's classification, overbite, overjet, gross malocclusions such as crossbite, and any details of cusp to fossa relationships which appear abnormal.

The examination of functional relationships is a great deal more difficult, and can be carried out properly only with experience and great attention to detail. The starting point for this examination has been the subject of much debate. The intercuspal position (ICP) as the end point of functional movement would appear to be the natural starting point for analysis, but it is not a fixed position and may well be the end point of a habitual mandibular closing path that compensates for and therefore masks the disharmonies we are trying to detect. The only fixed and reproducible position is the retruded contact position (RCP), where the jaw rotates around its hinge axis. Although some people swallow in RCP, it is an abnormal and strained position in the majority. However, it is useful because of its reproducibility.

The essential requirement for recording RCP is to have the patient sitting in a relaxed position. Some operators even go as far as hypnotizing the patient! With the dental chair slightly reclined and the patient sitting comfortably, the operator puts one hand on the patient's chin, with the thumb resting on the incisal edge of the lower incisors.

The patient is instructed to relax the jaw and allow the operator to move it freely up and down. When the muscles relax the mandible can be rotated around its hinge axis without discomfort, and when the thumb is removed the jaw can come together in RCP. Once the patient has learned the feel of this position, he or she can reproduce it at will and allow the operator to register a number of contact relations using coloured bite papers or soft occlusal indicator wax. Sometimes muscle tension is so great that closing pathways cannot be altered in this way, and a bite-guard may be needed as an aid to overcome abnormal muscle patterns of activity.

An initial cusp contact in centric relation can be detected by placing coloured paper or indicator wax over the upper posterior teeth, guiding the patient into tooth contact in RCP and then sliding from there into complete closure (ICP). The direction of the slide can be observed, and the point of initial contact will be marked on the teeth or seen by perforations in the indicator wax. Similarly, tooth contacts in working and non-working sides during lateral excursions and tooth contacts in protrusive movement can be defined. These techniques can be learned only by practical experience.

It should be possible to link signs of occlusal disharmony, such as drifting, mobility and faceting, with the site of an occlusal disharmony and an associated slide. Thus a premature contact in RCP between the distal slope of an upper molar cusp will produce a forward slide so that the lower incisors come forward against the upper incisors.

Occlusal adjustment

Adjustment can be carried out by selective grinding, restorative dentistry or orthodontics. Whatever technique is used, the objectives remain the same:

1. To direct occlusal forces along the long axis of the tooth and as far as possible reduce lateral components of force
2. To distribute forces over as many teeth as possible in maximum intercuspation and to establish 'group function' during lateral and protrusive movements by creating simultaneous gliding contacts between working teeth
3. To establish bilateral contact between posterior teeth in RCP and a sagittal movement of no more than 1 mm between RCP and ICP
4. Thereby, to eliminate the signs and symptoms of occlusal disharmony.

Selective grinding (Schuyler, 1935)

The greatest danger of selective grinding is that it can be indiscriminate. One is faced with a bewildering array of coloured dots and smudges and multiple perforations in the occlusal wax. Before any tooth grinding is carried out, the consequences of any adjustment must be determined. Central to this analysis is the location of cuspal inclines,

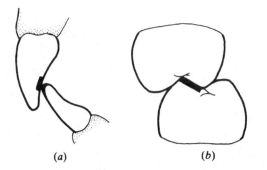

Figure 24.2 Centric stops *(a)* on incisors and *(b)* on posterior teeth

which act as centric stops or supporting cusps in maximum interdigitation and thus maintain the vertical dimension of the face (*Figure 24.2*). Selective grinding is carried out with a handpiece and diamond stones, and should proceed in a methodical manner as follows:

1. Elimination of gross occlusal disharmonies that are obvious to the eye, such as plunger cusps, malposed and extruded teeth, and discrepancies in marginal ridge height. Where there is a widened buccolingual diameter caused by attrition, the diameter can be reduced. Keeping the positions of supporting cusps in mind, these obvious sources of occlusal disharmony can be corrected to a considerable degree as a first step. In severe cases this stage may have to involve extraction of grossly over-erupted teeth or the restora-

tive treatment of these teeth with cast crowns to reduce the occlussal height.
2. Correction of prematurities in RCP. These may be divided into two groups, with or without prematurities in lateral excursions. These situations and their corrections are shown in *Figure 24.3*.
3. Correction of protrusive disharmonies. The contact between incisors and canines should be a smooth glide into the edge-to-edge position, with as many anterior teeth as possible in contact. In adjustment of protrusive contact, it is essential to remember that the incisal edge (or close to it) of the lower incisors is a centric stop (*Figure 24.4*). One of the most common mistakes is the reduction of an incisal edge obviously above the line of the rest of the incisors in order to achieve an improved appearance. The almost inevitable result is overeruption of the reduced tooth, with recreation of the interference and consequent aggravation of the problem.
4. Correction of disharmonies in lateral excursions (*Figures 24.5* and *24.6*). The objective of this adjust-

(a)

(b)

Figure 24.3 Correction of interferences between posterior teeth in RCP. If there is no interference in lateral excursions, the fossa is ground as in *(a)*. If there is interference in lateral excursions, the cusp is ground as in *(b)*

Figure 24.4 Correction of interference between incisors in protrusive movements. The adjustment should not disturb the centric stop

Figure 24.5 Correction of working side interference according to the BULL rule

(a)

(b)

Figure 24.6 The correction of a lateral movement in the non-working side depends upon the relationships of the interfering cuspal inclines in other excursions. In *(a)* the buccal cusp of the lower tooth is in interfering contact in two positions, while in *(b)* the palatal cusp of the upper tooth is in interfering contact in two positions and is therefore the one to be corrected ment is group function on the working side and disarticulation of the non-working side. Non-working side contacts (called balancing contacts in prosthetics) are frequently associated with advanced periodontal destruction and TMJ dysfunction. A premature contact between buccal cusps in working movement and position is corrected by grinding the buccal cusp of the upper tooth, while a lingual cusp contact is corrected by grinding the lingual cusp of the lower tooth. This is the so-called BULL rule (*Figure 24.5*).

Correcting a non-working side contact can be a problem, as the contact is frequently between the buccal incline of the palatal cusp of the upper tooth and the lingual incline of the lower buccal cusp – i.e. supporting cusps. It is almost impossible to avoid cutting these surfaces, and the adjustment will depend upon the form of contact made by these surfaces in other positions (*Figure 24.6*). If a cuspal incline is in premature contact in both working and non-working positions, this can be adjusted. On other occasions, very precise adjustment of the cuspal incline is needed so that the cusp tip, as the centric stop, is retained, thus avoiding overeruption. If grinding a centric stop is unavoidable, the occlusion will need to be supervised in case there is resultant tipping of involved teeth, which would create a further interference.

Finally, the adjusted surfaces are polished smooth. Not infrequently the patient remarks on an improvement in the feel of the occlusion. After some weeks mobility and other features of occlusal disharmony should reduce if the adjustment has been carried out correctly.

Treatment of bruxism

The first step in the control of any parafunctional habit must be discussion with the patient. Frequently once the individual becomes aware of a habit and the damage that it can do, he or she can bring it under some degree of daytime control.

If occlusal disharmonies play a role in provoking or aggravating a clenching or grinding habit, selective grinding should help to relieve the parafunction. However, the psychological substrate of stress will remain and, apart from reassuring the patient that the dental problems can be controlled, attempts to alleviate psychological problems have no place in dental treatment. Further dental treatment involves the use of bite-guards aimed at limiting the effects of excessive occlusal stress.

There are basically two forms of bite-guard, both of which are made in acrylic:

1. The occlusal shield, which fits over the occlusal surfaces, incisal edges and facial and lingual tooth convexities (*Figure 24.7*)
2. The anterior bite plate (*Figure 24.8*).

Where attrition is severe or where there has been collapse of the posterior segments so that the freeway space is increased, the occlusal shield can be useful, especially in cases where there has been considerable periodontal

Figure 24.7 Bite-guard with occlusal coverage

Figure 24.8 Bite-guard with anterior bite plate

destruction. Usually it is fitted over the teeth of the jaw in which there is most periodontal destruction. The occlusal surface must be flat and highly polished so that the teeth in the opposing jaw can skid across the surface without impedance. The thickness of the bite-guard must be adjusted so that the freeway space is not encroached upon, otherwise muscle tension will be intensified rather than diminished. 'Opening the bite' can be a dangerous procedure, which may accelerate periodontal destruction. Sheikholeslam *et al.* (1993) have shown that where there are signs of craniomandibular disorders, i.e. headaches, neck or TMJ pain, in patients with nocturnal bruxism, full arch maxillary plane occlusal splints remove or relieve the symptoms. Alas, symptoms often recur on discontinuing the use of the splint.

Where there is an obvious bruxism habit with symptoms of muscle spasm and where the lower anterior teeth are well supported by bone, a bite-guard with an anterior bite plate is extremely useful. This disengages the posterior teeth, thus eliminating any cuspal interference and interrupting the reflex activity that causes muscle spasm. It is also useful where the freeway space is small. The anterior bite plate may be used as an initial form of control of bruxism in the appropriate case and then, if necessary, the occlusal shield can be used for long-term control, in which case it can also be used as a splint. Depending on the habit pattern, the bite-guard is worn at night or during the day, and any necessary adjustments are made until the minimal thickness compatible with comfort and efficiency is obtained. Patients with bite-guards must adhere to a strict oral hygiene regime and avoid sugar between meals.

References

Schuyler, C.H. (1935) Fundamentals in the correction of occlusal disharmony, natural and artificial. *Journal of the American Dental Association* **22**, 1193–1202

Sheikholeslam, A., Holmgren, K. and Rise, C. (1993) Therapeutic effects of the maxillary plane occlusal splint in signs and symptoms of craniomandibular disorders in patients with nocturnal bruxism. *Journal of Oral Rehabilitation* **20**, 473–482

25

Splinting

When the periodontal tissues are no longer capable of withstanding the stresses of function, teeth become mobile. This mobility can interfere with function. In many cases, treatment of the periodontal lesion and occlusal adjustment, if necessary, is all that is required to strengthen the supporting tissues, reduce mobility and re-establish function. When such local treatment fails to achieve these ends and chewing is uncomfortable, and/or where periodontal support is so reduced that increasing mobility is inevitable, further tooth support is needed (Lindhe and Nyman, 1977).

A splint is a device for supporting weakened tissues. It serves two purposes:

1. It provides rest where wound healing is in process
2. It permits function where the tooth or teeth and periodontium alone cannot perform adequately.

There has been a great deal of debate about the role of splinting in periodontal treatment, largely because the role of the splint has been misunderstood. A splint does not make loose teeth tight. A splint controls mobility when the splint is in place, and when the splint is removed the tooth mobility becomes manifest again. Only the removal of disease and subsequent healing can achieve a real reduction in tooth mobility.

The aims of splinting teeth are:

- To protect the tooth-supporting tissues during the healing period after an accident or following surgery
- To bring into function teeth that cannot be used to eat efficiently or in comfort without artificial support.

If splinting is carried out incorrectly it may make firm teeth loose, as, for example, when a loose first premolar is linked to a stable second premolar, overloading the latter tooth and thus producing two loose teeth.

There are many types of splint, temporary and permanent, fixed and removable, but every splint should meet certain requirements:

1. It should incorporate as many firm teeth as is neces-

sary to reduce the extra load on individual teeth to a minimum.
2. It should hold the teeth rigid and not impose torsional stresses on any incorporated teeth.
3. It should extend around the arch so that anteroposterior forces and faciolingual forces are counteracted.
4. It should not interfere with the occlusion. If possible, gross tooth disharmonies should be eliminated before the application of the splint.
5. It should not irritate the pulp.
6. It should not irritate the soft tissues, gingivae, cheeks, lips or tongue.
7. It should be designed so that it can be kept clean. Interdental embrasure spaces should not be blocked by the splint.

Temporary and provisional splints

Temporary splints are used to assist healing after injury or after surgical treatment. They should be reasonably easy to apply to mobile teeth, and also easy to remove after healing has taken place. They should not be left in place for longer than 2 months. If adequate stabilization has not taken place in that time, a more permanent form of splinting is necessary. Most temporary splints do not involve destroying tooth tissue.

Composite filling materials can be acid-etched to the surface of mobile teeth and linked together. This is the simplest form of temporary splinting, and one that is especially useful in emergencies (*Figure 25.1*).

The *wire and acrylic splint* (*Figure 25.2*) is also fairly easy to apply, and is frequently used for the stabilization of incisors. It is stronger and more reliable than the composite-filling splint. Usually the teeth from canine to canine, or first premolar to first premolar, are included in the splint. A length of 0.05 mm (0.002 inch) stainless-steel wire is looped around the teeth, with the lingual arch wire just incisal to the cingula. The ends of the wire are

Figure 25.1 Emergency splint made with composite filling material

Figure 25.2 Wire splint placed prior to covering with acrylic resin

twisted together distal to the last tooth included. The interdental wires are looped around both lingual and facial arch wires and twisted tight so that the arch wire is pulled tight around the teeth just apical to the contact point. After any necessary adjustment in position, the arch wire and interdental wires are finally tightened, their ends trimmed and tucked out of the way into embrasure spaces. A thin mix of quick-set acrylic is run over the wire, care being taken to avoid blocking out embrasure spaces. When set, the acrylic is trimmed smooth and polished so that it is comfortable to the soft tissues.

Orthodontic bands may also be used, especially in posterior segments where they are not obvious; 0.12 mm (0.005 inch) stainless-steel bands are fitted to the teeth to be splinted and welded together. Alternatively, the splint can be fabricated on a model and cemented into position. The edges of the bands must be contoured and polished to reduce plaque retention and avoid soft-tissue irritation.

Acrylic bite-guards, already described for the treatment of bruxism, may also be used as splints. The splint should cover the occlusal surface of the teeth and extend 1–2 mm over the facial surfaces of the teeth. In order to obtain adequate stability and rigidity in the upper jaw

considerable palatal coverage is needed, and in the lower jaw the lingual acrylic needs to be brought well down in the lingual vestibule without impeding muscle activity. The occlusal surface must be designed to allow free excursion of the mandible, with no greater than 1 mm increase in vertical dimension in the molar regions. Very careful adjustment of the occlusion in the mouth is essential, otherwise opposing teeth will be subject to excessive stress.

The *intracoronal splint* can be regarded as a semi-permanent rather than temporary splint, and many consist of a continuous intracoronal bar or of sections of wire in the so-called A-splint. These are described below.

1. *The continuous intracoronal bar.* A transverse groove, 2–3 mm wide, is cut in the lingual surface of anterior teeth coronal to the cingulum, or in the occlusal surface of posterior teeth. The groove is made about 1.5 mm deep and slightly undercut. A stainless-steel wire is bent to fit the groove, which is filled with self-curing acrylic, and the wire quickly pressed home. After the acrylic has set it is shaped and polished.

Alternatively, a gold bar may be cast to fit the preparation and cemented in place. As occlusal pressures may push anterior teeth away from the bar, it is advisable to improve retention by making pin-hole preparations in the base of the groove, but even with this added retention it is not advisable to splint upper anterior teeth in this way. The horizontal-pin splint represents a variation of the continuous intracoronal bar. It is strong and well retained, but can be used only where some pulp recession has taken place.

A form of continuous intracoronal bar, used to stabilize a posterior segment, consists of MOD amalgam fillings placed in the teeth to be stabilized and then subsequently linked by a bar cemented with acrylic into a channel cut through the amalgams.

2. *The Rochette splint.* Acid-etch composite materials provide an opportunity for splinting without radical tooth preparation. An impression of the teeth to be splinted is taken, and a chrome-cobalt splint, fitting the lingual surface of these teeth, is constructed. The lingual tooth surfaces are dried and etched and the splint is glued into position with the composite material.

If carefully prepared and in good occlusal balance, this form of splinting provides excellent stability and may be regarded as a semi-permanent splint.

Permanent splints

Permanent splints may be fixed or removable.

Fixed splints

Fixed splints provide the most reliable form of immobilization, but do require considerable tooth preparation, skill and time. They consist of linked inlays or crowns.

Linked inlays are self-descriptive. Inlays that fit into dovetail preparations in the lingual surfaces of anterior teeth may be displaced if an excessive anterior force is exerted on any individual tooth. In the posterior region, a series of linked MOD inlays with occlusal coverage can make a satisfactory and permanent splint.

Linked crowns provide the most reliable form of immobilization and support (Lindhe and Nyman, 1979; Nyman and Ericsson, 1982). The splint is extremely strong, holds the teeth rigidly, and is the most aesthetically satisfying and unobtrusive type of splint. If teeth are missing, the multiple abutment fixed bridge may be used to replace these teeth and to stabilize a segment or a complete arch. This type of splint allows modification of the form of the teeth and in fact provides one of the most satisfactory methods of occlusal rehabilitation. This splint is difficult to make and requires a great deal of chairside time and skill. Considerable tooth preparation is necessary, and there is often the possibility of pulpal involvement. Alternatively, telescope crowns soldered together may be used. These are fitted over gold copings, which are cemented onto the teeth. The telescope superstructure may be fixed with temporary cement so that it may be removed periodically for inspection and cleaning.

One modification of the linked crown splint is the multiple pinlay splint, which reduces tooth-tissue loss to a minimum. Three parallel pin-holes are made in each tooth to be splinted. Usually six teeth are incorporated into the splint, and paralleling eighteen pin-holes presents some difficulty. Pin retention is not as good as that provided by inlays or crowns; therefore, this appliance can only be used with success where functional forces are not acting to separate the appliance from the tooth, as they might be where upper incisors are under some occlusal stress. This factor restricts the application of the pinlay splint to the lower incisors.

Removable splints

The removable splint does not involve cutting tooth tissue, it is easier to construct than a fixed splint and it can be altered or discarded at will. Like all removable appliances, the splint may act as a plaque-retention factor and source of gingival irritation unless oral hygiene is good.

Figure 25.3 Removable splint in chrome-cobalt with lingual coverage for incisor teeth

The most common type of splint is the lingual coverage splint, which is essentially a partial denture in chrome-cobalt with extensions covering the lingual surfaces of the teeth to be protected (*Figure 25.3*). The continuous clasp splint is a variation in which support is reinforced by a labial arch bar. However, removable splints have been largely superseded by fixed acid-etched splints.

Designing splints provides the opportunity for considerable ingenuity, but the choice of splint should reflect patient need rather than the artistic aspirations of the operator. Many forms of splint are complex, difficult to execute and costly, and are justified only when a good prognosis is likely. Where the prognosis is doubtful, a simple form of splint is indicated. If the prognosis is poor, the removable chrome-cobalt lingual coverage splint allows for the addition of teeth as weaker ones are lost.

References

Lindhe, J. and Nyman, S. (1977) The role of occlusion in periodontal disease and the biological rationale for splinting in the treatment of periodontitis. *Oral Science Reviews* **10**, 11–43

Lindhe, J. and Nyman, S. (1979) A longitudinal study of combined periodontal and prosthetic treatment of patients with advanced periodontal disease. *Journal of Periodontology* **50**, 163–169

Nyman, S. and Ericsson, I. (1982) The capacity of reduced periodontal tissues to support fixed bridgework. *Journal of Clinical Periodontology* **9**, 409–414

26

Dental implants and peri-implantology

This account is merely meant to be an introduction to this subject from the periodontal standpoint and not to be a comprehensive account, which can be obtained from a specialist text devoted to this subject.

Development of osseointegrated dental implants

The successful development of titanium endosseous implants over the last two decades has made it possible to place these with a degree of predictability not previously attainable (Lang and Wilson, 1992). It was first shown that titanium implants could achieve a bone-to-implant contact (Brånemark et al., 1969), and this was demonstrated in undecalcified ground sections by Schroeder et al. (1976). They referred to this contact as functional ankylosis, but Brånemark et al. (1977) later created the term 'osseointegration', which they referred to as a direct structural and functional connection between the bone and the surface of a load bearing implant.

Titanium is a highly reactive metal that spontaneously forms an oxide layer in contact with air, and this layer is resistant to further corrosion. This protects it against chemical attacks in biological tissues, and gives it excellent biocompatible properties. Also, functional loading of implants transfers masticatory forces to the jawbone, and for this reason the stiffness of the implant should be similar to that of bone. Titanium approaches this more closely than other materials (Brånemark et al., 1969). The implant requires retention to achieve ankylotic anchorage, and this is usually in the form of screw threads (Brånemark et al., 1985) and perforations (Sutter et al., 1988) and also micro-retentions in the form of plasma coatings (Schroeder et al., 1976). This provides resistance to shearing forces essential to successful osseointegration (Carlsson et al., 1988).

Clinical factors related to osseointegration

Successful osseointegration appears to require 3–6 months of quiescence after placement before any post-operational loading is applied (Brunski, 1988). Osseointegration has been shown to be achievable with either two-stage or one-stage techniques. In the two-stage technique (Brånemark et al., 1977) the implant fixtures are submerged under the mucosal tissues at the time of the installation, and this has been claimed to be necessary for success by the advocates of this technique. More recently, however, it has been shown that the non-submerged implants using a one-stage technique integrate equally well provided that they are not subjected to any loading during the osseointegration period (Albrektsson et al., 1986; Lang and Wilson, 1992).

Probably the most critical aspect in achieving success is the preparation of the implant bed. Drilling in bone generates considerable heat, which can result in bone necrosis. Therefore it is essential to use low drilling speeds (i.e. under 800 rpm) (Schroeder et al., 1988) and abundant irrigation with chilled sterile saline to minimize injury. The sequential use of drills of increasing diameter also helps to minimize thermal trauma. There must be a minimal gap between the prepared site and the implant, which is achieved by the careful use of matched precision drills in the chosen implant system.

If stability is achieved new bone will grow and replace damaged bone, resulting in an intimate bone-to-implant contact with a gap of about 20 μm or less (Schenk and Willenegger, 1977; Carlsson et al., 1988). If an implant lacks primary stability, healing will occur by fibrous replacement of the damaged bone, preventing osseointegration.

The histology of the peri-implant tissues

The head of the implant fixture penetrates through the crest of the alveolar bone and relates to the gingival or alveolar mucosa. Once the implant head penetrates the mucosa, at the second operation in the two-stage technique or at the first operation in the one-stage technique, a tight soft tissue collar will form around it. This consists of fibrous tissue with fibres running parallel to the long axis of the implant (Listgarten and Lai, 1975) and an epithelial cuff. The junctional epithelium attaches to the implant surface by hemidesmosomes and a basal lamina similar to that seen with natural teeth (Gould *et al.*, 1981).

In a series of experimental studies on the beagle dog model, aspects of the histology and pathology of the gingival and periodontal tissues around normal teeth and the peri-implant mucosa around osseointegrated implants were studied (Berglundh *et al.*, 1991, 1992, 1994; Ericsson *et al.*, 1992; Lindhe *et al.*, 1992). In this work they used specially designed light and electron-microscopical techniques that enabled them to examine the tissues adjacent to the implant (Thomsen and Ericson, 1985).

It was shown that the gingival and peri-implant mucosal tissues had several features in common (Berglundh *et al.*, 1991). In this regard, both tissues exhibited a junctional epithelium adjacent to their respective surfaces of about 2 mm in length. Apical to the junctional epithelium they found a zone of connective tissue forming a barrier between the epithelium and the bone. However, the gingiva and peri-implant mucosa also differed in several important respects. The implant surface, as expected, was devoid of cementum, and this prevented the collagen fibres in this area from inserting into its surface. The collagen fibres in the area of peri-implant mucosa between the apical end of the junctional epithelium and the bone surface seemed to originate from the crestal bone surface, and appeared to run a course parallel to the implant surface. The collagen content of this area of the peri-implant mucosa was much higher than in the corresponding area of gingiva, and the number of fibroblasts was much lower. In most respects this area of the peri-implant mucosa resembled scar tissue. However, this tissue is very important in protecting osseointegration, since it is the barrier that prevents the junctional epithelium from migrating apically.

The blood supply of the peri-implant mucosa has also been studied using the same beagle dog model, and compared with that in the gingiva adjacent to natural teeth. The supply of the peri-implant mucosa differs from that of the gingiva in important respects (Berglundh *et al.*, 1994). The gingiva receives a copious blood supply (see Chapter 1) from two major sources, namely the supra-periosteal vessels lateral to the alveolar process, and the vessels of the periodontal ligament, which anastomose freely with the alveolar bone supply. In contrast, the blood vessels of the peri-implant mucosa were found to be terminal branches of the larger vessels of the periosteum of the bone. In addition, the blood vessels lateral to the junctional epithelium in both the peri-implant mucosa and gingiva formed a characteristic crevicular plexus. However, whilst the supra-alveolar mucosa of the gingiva is richly vascularized, the corresponding area of the peri-implant mucosa was almost devoid of blood supply. Thus, the scar-like nature of this area of the peri-implant mucosa may be a reflection of its poor blood supply.

The dimensions of the peri-implant mucosa have also been studied in the beagle dog model (Berglundh and Lindhe, 1996). The width of the peri-implant mucosa between the crest of the bone and apex of the junctional epithelium was compared with the pre-operative alveolar mucosal width. This was compared at contralateral sites in each dog's jaw. On one side (control sites) the alveolar mucosal width was normal, whilst on the other side (test sites) it was reduced to 2 mm or less prior to abutment connection. It was found that the length of the junctional epithelium and peri-implant mucosa was similar on test and control sides. However, on the test side, with reduced alveolar mucosal width, this had been achieved by alveolar bone resorption and the establishment of an angular bone defect at the crestal bone margin. This implies that a certain minimal width of peri-implant mucosa is required for normal implant function, and if this is not present bone resorption will take place to re-establish this width. This finding may in part explain the marginal bone loss that has been reported to occur during the first year following abutment connection and subsequent loading of the implant system (Adell *et al.*, 1981; Pilliar *et al.*, 1991).

It is probable that once the implant system is exposed to the oral environment and is in function, a barrier mucosa of a certain minimum dimension is required to protect osseointegration (Berglundh and Lindhe, 1996; Abrahamsson *et al.*, 1996). This relationship between the alveolar bone margin and the base of the junctional epithelium appear to be closely similar for all osseointegrated implant systems, including 1- and 2-stage implant systems (Abrahamsson *et al.*, 1996).

Clinical indications for dental implants

Only a few total edentulous and partially edentulous patients will benefit from dental implants, and these must be carefully selected both on clinical grounds and the patients' wishes after they have been fully acquainted with the details and are able to make an informed judgment. Successful implants may need a team approach with co-operation between oral surgeons, periodontologists, restorative and prosthetic dentists (Lang and Wilson, 1992). Any dentist or dental specialist carrying out any part of this work needs to have undergone a lengthy course of postgraduate academic and practical training in the subject. Oral surgeons or periodontologists will easily be able to acquire the necessary surgical skills, but will need to acquire considerable restorative and prosthetic knowledge, skills and experience if they wish to carry out the full treatment.

Implants can be considered for stabilizing a full lower or upper denture. The use of anterior mandibular implants is probably the commonest use (Lang and Wilson, 1992).

They can also be used in the partially edentulous mouth to act as abutments for bridgework (*Figure 26.1*) or as single tooth replacements (*Figure 26.2*). A very careful clinical assessment has to be made to plan any of these procedures (Bahat and Handelsman, 1992).

Clinical considerations

Careful evaluation of the prognosis of the existing dentition must precede any decisions on partial cases. If implants are clinically indicated, regardless of the implant system used, success mainly depends on the patients' health and co-operation, the design of the prosthesis and the amount and quality of the bone at the implant site. All of these factors need very careful assessment, and this involves comprehensive clinical and radiographical examinations of the soft tissue and bony anatomy. Relationships of the proposed implants with vital structures such as the inferior dental canal, maxillary sinus and floor of the nose must be carefully assessed. Adequate radiographs are necessary to assess these relations as well as to assess the amount and quality of the supporting bone (Iacono and Livers, 1992). These may include panoral, lateral and occlusal views. Manual examination also is necessary in conjunction with this to assess the width of the available bone and the presence of undercuts and exostoses.

Since the long-term future of remaining natural teeth must be assured, there should not be any caries or periodontal activity on any of the remaining teeth and the patient must be willing to carry out all the necessary preventive measures to avoid this in the future. All necessary periodontal and restorative treatment must have been successfully completed on the remaining natural teeth. Periodontal stability is of critical importance because the bacterial flora associated with active periodontal disease can spread from adjacent natural teeth to the implant, resulting in peri-implant infections (see below).

(a)

(b)

(c)

Figure 26.2 A Calcitek hydroxyapatite coated osseointegrated dental implant used as the support to replace missing 1|. *(a)* A radiograph of the implant in position in the alveolar bone following stage 1. The 1| was lost due to trauma. Root resorption can be seen on 2|; *(b)* the superstructure in position (stage 2); *(c)* jacket crown tried in prior to glazing and placement. (Courtesy Professor R Watson)

Figure 26.1 Two Brånemark osseointegrated implants in the position of 64| acting as two of the abutments of a full arch bridge. (Courtesy Mr C Waterman)

It is extremely important to relate the final position of the artificial teeth of a full denture in edentulous cases, or the abutment teeth of a bridge in a partially edentulous case, to the position of the implant fixtures before these are decided upon. The final occlusion is of critical importance and this is best determined by making up a planning appliance, which acts as a stent for determining the eventual positions of the implant fixtures. The occlusion of the natural teeth must be in balance in all functional positions before any implant work is planned, and any necessary occlusal equilibration must be undertaken prior to implant planning.

No details will be given here of the basic techniques since these are best obtained from books solely devoted to this subject or books where specialist authors write separate chapters on this subject. A good detailed account from a periodontal standpoint can be found in the implant section of Wilson *et al.* (1992).

Use of guided tissue regeneration (GTR)

The biological principles of GTR (see Chapter 17) have been applied to the treatment of osseous defects in the alveolar ridge and around endosseous dental implants (Dahlin *et al.*, 1988; Buser *et al.*, 1990; Nyman *et al.*, 1990; Seibert and Nyman, 1990). The barrier membrane is adapted over the bony defect to allow cells of osseous origin to populate the area to form new bone (Dahlin *et al.*, 1989, 1991; Lazzara, 1989; Becker and Becker, 1990). This procedure has been shown to be capable of forming new bone to increase the alveolar bone height or to increase bone support around the implant at the time of installation. Either non-resorbable ePTFE or bioresorbable membranes can be used for this purpose (see Chapter 17).

The membrane function of a resorbable collagen membrane (Bio-Gide®) has also been tested in animal experiments. Peri-implant defects in dogs were filled with a bovine bone mineral (Bio-Oss®, see Chapter 17) and covered with Bio-Gide®. Histological evaluation after 4 months showed the regeneration of organized cancellous and cortical bone (Hürzeler *et al.*, 1997).

It is also very important to avoid bacterial contamination of the membrane (Becker *et al.*, 1990a), since this can seriously affect the success of the procedure (see Chapter 17). In this regard, one study has investigated the effect of bacterial contamination of 16 membranes used in conjunction with dental implants with associated bony defects (Nowzari and Slots, 1994). The nature of bacterial contamination was determined with non-selective and selective culture and by DNA probes. The 10 implant-associated membranes with no cultivable micro-organisms demonstrated a mean gain of 4.9 mm of supporting bone, whilst the six implants with infected membranes only gained an average of 2 mm. This seems to show a direct relationship between bacterial contamination of the membrane and the extent of new bone formation. Furthermore, these results would seem to indicate the importance of controlling or eliminating contamination of the membrane by periodontal pathogens, in some cases by the use of antibiotics (Sander *et al.*, 1994).

These results seems to show that clinically significant gains in bone formation on the alveolar ridge and around implants can be obtained with GTR procedures using both bioresorbable or non-resorbable membranes. The lack of a second surgical procedure is a major advantage with bioresorbable membranes.

Use of bone or bone-substitute grafts

Allograft and xenograft bone (Becker *et al.*, 1990b; Wetzel *et al.*, 1995) and synthetic bone substitutes such as hydroxyapatite (Seibert and Nyman, 1990; Wetzel *et al.*, 1995) and bioceramics and glasses (Hench, 1994) have all been used to enhance the bone support around implants, either alone or in conjunction with barrier membranes (see Chapter 17). This can be in the form of ridge augmentation via advanced flaps with autogenous and alloplastic grafting material or the placement of grafting materials into extraction sockets to preserve ridge height or to build support for a subsequent implant (Wilson *et al.*, 1993; Hench, 1994).

The osteoconductive potential of bovine anorganic cancellous bone (BACB) (Bio-Oss®), human freeze-dried demineralized bone allograft (FDDBA) and resorbable hydroxyapatite (Osteogen®) have been compared in beagle dogs receiving dental implants (Wetzel *et al.*, 1995). Titanium dental implants (ITI®) (see below) were placed into prepared edentulous sites, which were extended into the maxillary sinus by elevating the sinus floor. The area below the raised sinus floor contained the protruding implant tip and was packed with one of these materials. The implanted material was placed so that it surrounded the implant tip and extended to the bone margin below. Sites implanted with human FDDBA showed no signs of new bone formation, whereas those implanted with BACB (Bio-Oss®) or resorbable hydroxyapatite (Osteogen®) did show significant new bone formation in this area. The use of bone markers (tetracycline or calcein green) revealed rapid bone formation and remodelling, especially around the BACB particles. Thus, both BACB and resorbable hydroxyapatite were shown to be osteoconductive in this situation. However, the lack of response to FDDBA and the good response to resorbable hydroxyapatite seems to run contrary to most other research group findings (see Chapter 17).

Bioglass particulate (Bioglass®) has also been used to stimulate bone formation in extraction sockets and to thus maintain the alveolar ridge height (Hench *et al.*, 1991; Wilson *et al.*, 1993; Hench and Wilson, 1995).

Implant systems

Numerous implant systems are available, but most clinicians in this field limit themselves to one or two systems. They include the Brånemark (Nobel Pharma), Astra (Astratec) and IMZ (General Medica) systems, which are all two-stage, and the Bonefit and ITI (Straumann Institute), which are one-stage.

The response of the peri-implant mucosal tissues to plaque

The response of the gingiva adjacent to normal teeth and of the peri-implant mucosa adjacent to the suprabony surface of the implant have been compared in the beagle dog model (Berglundh *et al.*, 1992; Ericsson *et al.*, 1992; Lindhe *et al.*, 1992). Both tissues responded to *de novo* plaque formation with an increased migration of leucocytes through the junctional epithelium and the establishment of an inflammatory cell infiltrate in the adjacent connective tissue (Berglundh *et al.*, 1992). The location and composition of these lesions were similar in both situations, but the lesions in the peri-implant mucosa tended to be larger.

Two studies (Ericsson *et al.*, 1992; Lindhe *et al.*, 1992) compared the responses of these tissues to long-standing plaque irritation. In this situation, the peri-implant mucosa was much less effective than the gingiva in preventing apical proliferation of the bacterial plaque. As a consequence, with increasing exposure times, the lesion in the peri-implant mucosa became larger and extended apically to become closer to the bone margin than in the corresponding gingiva. This much poorer response to plaque on the part of the peri-implant mucosa may be partly explained by the structural differences between peri-implant mucosa and gingiva (see above). It indicates a susceptibility of the peri-implant tissues to plaque-mediated damage and, if allowed to proceed unchecked, can result in peri-implant infections.

Peri-implant infections

Since the superstructure of dental implants share the same environment as the teeth and are surrounded like them by a gingival cuff, it is to be expected that bacterial plaque will form on their surfaces. In edentulous mouths the flora associated with the natural teeth is absent, and therefore they appear to accumulate plaque less readily than implants in dentate mouths. This suggests that the presence of natural teeth may influence the composition of the subgingival flora around implants (Apse *et al.*, 1989). It seems likely that the early colonization of implants by putative periodontal pathogens could be more frequent in patients with poorly controlled periodontal disease on adjacent teeth. These teeth may therefore serve as a reservoir for potentially pathogenic bacteria to colonize adjacent implant surfaces.

The development of the bacterial flora of implants in edentulous mouths has been studied for up to 180 days after placement (Mombelli *et al.*, 1988). They showed that 80% of the cultivable bacteria were Gram positive

cocci in all sites but one. In this one site, which did show signs of clinical failure at day 120, including bleeding on probing, increased probing depth and pus formation, there was a decrease in the number of cocci, an increase in the number of rods and an appearance of spirochaetes. These changes were never seen in healthy sites. Further studies over 5 years (Mombelli and Mericske-Sterne, 1990) in 18 edentulous implant patients have shown that a predominantly Gram positive coccal flora persisted around healthy implant sites over this period. Gram negative rods such as *Fusobacterium nucleatum* and *Prevotella intermedia* were found in 9% of the samples, but *Porphyromonas gingivalis* and spirochaetes were never seen at the healthy sites. Most other studies of successful implants over recent years have shown a similar pattern (Rams *et al.*, 1984; Lekholm *et al.*, 1986; Mombelli *et al.*, 1987; Apse *et al.*, 1989; Bower *et al.*, 1989; Quirynen and Listgarten, 1990). However, one recent study (Mombelli *et al.*, 1987) compared samples from five patients with successful implants supporting overdentures for more than a year with those from seven patients with clinically failing implants who had probing depths exceeding 5 mm, suppuration and radiological loss of alveolar bone. *P. gingivalis*, *P. intermedia*, *F. nucleatum* and other putative periodontal pathogens were cultured, and spirochaetes, fusiform bacteria, motile and curved rods were commonly seen by dark field microscopy in samples from failing sites. In contrast, the healthy sites maintained a predominantly Gram positive coccal flora. There was also a 20-fold lower bacterial count in the healthy as compared with the failing sites.

In animals, ligature-induced disease has been produced around dental implants and has been shown to be clinically, radiologically and microbiologically similar to ligature-induced periodontitis (Brandes *et al.*, 1988). All of these studies would seem to indicate that implant failures after osseointegration has taken place (i.e. after 4–6 months) are probably due to bacterial infection rather than an effect of occlusal overload.

Monitoring of implant sites and diagnosis of possible implant failure

Dental implants should be regularly monitored by careful clinical and radiological measurements for signs of possible implant failure (Bahat and Handelsman, 1992; Iacono and Livers, 1992). Probing depths are best measured from a fixed reference point such as the occlusal surface or incisal edge of implant-retained crowns, or the occlusal edge of the implant head in implants retaining dentures. They may be more accurately measured with constant pressure electronic probes such as the Florida disc probe (see Chapter 12). However, this must be carried out very gently to avoid damage to the delicate junctional epithelium. Some workers have even suggested that probing around implant sites with periodontal probes always causes damage to the junctional epithelium and should not be performed (Berglundh *et al.*, 1992). Certainly, any pain elicited during probing is indicative of tissue damage and should warn the operator to stop. Thus, there is some evidence to indicate that probing should not be used around healthy implants. If this advice is adhered to, then implant failure can only be detected by radiographical evidence of bone loss, clinical signs of soft tissue inflammation or infection or a novel method based on examination of a peri-implant sulcus fluid component (see below).

Radiographs should be very carefully localized so that a constant bite block, film position and tube angulation is achieved (see Chapter 12). Only in this way can serial radiographs be compared and measured (Hollender and Rockler, 1980). Comparability of serial radiographs can also be checked by measuring the distance between the implant screw threads on each radiograph. Careful measurements can then be made of the distance from an identifiable and reproducible point on the neck of the implant to the crest of the alveolar bone. Any change in attachment level in sequential clinical measurements should be verified and, if confirmed, should be regarded as possible evidence of loss of implant support. Any measurable change in the position of the alveolar bone level in respect to the implant on radiographs should be regarded as stronger evidence of loss of implant support. Gingival inflammation, bleeding on gentle probing and the presence of calculus should also be noted.

In addition, paper point samples of the bacterial flora in the peri-implant sulcus may be taken and placed into anaerobic transport medium for anaerobic bacterial culture. Samples could also be taken for dark ground microscopy (see Chapter 13). The presence of or an increase in the numbers of black-pigmented anaerobes or spirochaetes could be taken as a possible indication of impending peri-implant infection (Mombelli *et al.*, 1987).

Finally, in the future the measurement of proteolytic enzymes in peri-implant sulcus fluid (PISF) may be of possible diagnostic value. In this regard, the total enzyme activity and enzyme concentration of several host derived proteinases, cathepsin B, elastase and dipeptidyl peptidase (DPP) IV and a bacterial protease, trypsin-like protease, in 30-second paper strip PISF samples have been shown to significantly correlate with increased attachment and bone loss around osseointegrated dental implants (Eley *et al.*, 1991). PISF samples are very easy to obtain, and if these relationships were shown to be predictive in a longitudinal study of dental implants, then one or more of these proteases could be used as a diagnostic test of possible impending implant failure as described in Chapter 13. This would, of course need confirmation from the other clinical and radiological measurements described above.

Treatment of implant sites

In many ways the treatment of dental implant sites is similar to that of natural teeth, since the aim is to prevent the development of a pathogenic bacterial flora which would lead to resorption of supporting bone. Careful oral hygiene with soft toothbrushes and dental floss should be carefully taught. Specially designed interproximal brushes that can penetrate into the peri-implant crevice can also be used.

Metallic scalers cannot be used with dental implants because they would damage the titanium surfaces of the implant, and for this reason good plaque control is also necessary to prevent calculus formation. Specially designed plastic scalers can be used to remove soft deposits, but these are ineffective for calculus removal. Recently, plastic tips have also been produced for ultrasonic scalers for use with implants. However, if calculus does form it is usually impossible to remove with these instruments. In this case the calculus should be very carefully chipped away with curettes, taking extreme care not to damage the surface. During maintenance visits the implants can be polished with a rubber cup and non-abrasive polishing paste. Regular applications of antiseptic agents such as 0.2% aqueous chlorhexidine have also been shown to be beneficial in addition to mechanical oral hygiene in some cases.

If peri-implant infections do occur then these need to be treated with the appropriate systemic antimicrobials, such as metronidazole with or without adjuvant amoxycillin (Van Winkelhoff *et al.*, 1989), and this treatment has been shown to be effective in most cases. It has also been shown to eradicate black-pigmenting Gram negative anaerobic rods and spirochaetes from subgingival implant sites (Duckworth *et al.*, 1987). Local applications of local deposit metronidazole or minocycline into the peri-implant pocket would produce a very high local concentration of these drugs, and could be used as an alternative treatment. However, there are no studies at present to indicate whether local application is as effective as systemic administration in this situation.

The failure rate of osseointegrated oral implants

A recent review (Esposito *et al.*, 1998) analysed 73 published papers on this subject, and estimated a total 5-year biological failure rate of 7.7%. The review covered all types of implant systems, but the majority were of the Brånemark type. One hundred and fifty-nine follow-up studies, up to early 1997, were initially considered in this review, but 86 of these were excluded either because they included inadequate data or because they related to extreme situations.

For the edentulous patient, fixed prostheses had a 5.8% implant failure rate whereas those supporting overdentures had a rate of 12.8%. In partially dentate patients, implants partially supporting fixed bridges failed in 4% of cases, and single tooth implants in 2.4%. In cases where bone grafts were used the failure rate increased to

14.9%, and to 7.3% when other types of adjunctive oral surgery were used.

The causes of failure were not always clear, but the higher maxillary failure rate was confirmed in these studies. About half the early failures appeared to be due to surgical technique or host-related factors. Ten% of the failures were attributed to perio-implantitis, but this cause was rare for implants of the Brånemark type. The remainder of the failures appeared to be due to overloading.

References

Abrahamsson, I., Berglundh, T., Wennström, J. and Lindhe, J. (1996) The peri-implant hard and soft tissues at different implant systems. A comparative study in the dog. *Clinical Oral Implant Research* 7, 212–219

Adell, R., Lekholm, U., Rockler, B. and Brånemark, P.I. (1981) A 15-year study of osseointegrated implants in the treatment of the edentulous jaw. *International Journal of Surgery* 10, 387–416

Albrektsson, T., Zarb, G., Worthington, P. and Eriksson, A.R. (1986) The long-term efficacy of currently used dental implants: A review and proposed criteria of success. *International Journal of Oral Maxillofacial Implants* 1, 11–25

Apse, P., Ellen, R.P., Overall, C.M. and Zarb, G.A. (1989) Microbiota and crevicular fluid collagenase activity in the osseointegrated dental implant sulcus. A comparison of sites in edentulous and partially edentulous patients. *Journal of Periodontal Research* 24, 96–105

Bahat, O. and Handelsman, M. (1992) Presurgical treatment planning and surgical guidelines for dental implants. In *Advances in Periodontics. Part IV. Implant Dentistry* (T.G. Wilson Jr, K.S. Kornman and M.G. Newman, eds), pp. 323–340. Chicago, London: Quintessence Publishing Co. Ltd

Becker, W. and Becker, B.E. (1990) Guided tissue regeneration for implants placed into extraction sockets and for implant dehiscences: surgical techniques and case reports. *The International Journal of Periodontics and Restorative Dentistry* 10, 377–391

Becker, W., Becker, B.E., Newman, M.G. and Nyman, S. (1990a) Clinical and microbiological findings that may contribute to implant failure. *International Journal of Oral Maxillofacial Implants* 5, 31–38

Becker, W., Becker, B., Handselsman, M. *et al.* (1990b) Bone formation at dehisced dental implants sites treated with implant augmentation material: a pilot study in dogs. *International Journal of Periodontics and Restorative Dentistry* 10, 93–102

Berglundh, T. and Lindhe, J. (1996) Dimension of the periimplant mucosa. Biological width revisited. *Journal of Clinical Periodontology* 14, 189–193

Berglundh, T., Lindhe, J., Ericsson, I. *et al.* (1991) The soft tissue barrier at implants and teeth. *Clinical Oral Implant Research* 2, 81–90

Berglundh, T., Lindhe, J., Marinello, C.P. *et al.* (1992) Soft tissue reactions to *de novo* plaque formation at implant and teeth. *Clinical Oral Implant Research* 3, 1–8

Berglundh, T., Lindhe, J., Jonsson, K. and Ericsson, I. (1994) The topography of the vascular systems in the periodontal and peri-implant tissues in the dog. *Journal of Clinical Periodontology* 14, 189–193

Bower, R.C., Radney, N.R., Wall, C.S. and Henry, P.J. (1989) Clinical and microscopic findings in edentulous patients 3 years after incorporation of osseointegrated implant-supported bridgework. *Journal of Clinical Periodontology* 16, 580–587

Brandes, R., Beamer, B., Holt, S.C. *et al.* (1988) Clinical microscopic observations of ligature-induced 'peri-implantitis' around osseointegrated implants. *Journal of Dental Research* 67, 287

Brånemark, T.-I., Breine, U., Adell, R. *et al.* (1969) Intraosseous anchorage of dental prostheses. Experimental studies. *Scandinavian Journal of Plastic Reconstructional Surgery* 3, 81–100

Brånemark, T.-I., Breine, U., Adell, R. *et al.* (1977) Osseointegrated implants in the treatment of the edentulous jaw. Experience from a 10 year period. *Scandinavian Journal of Plastic Reconstructional Surgery* 11(16), 1–132

Brånemark, P.I., Zarb, G.A. and Albrektsson, T. (1985) *Tissue-integrated Prostheses: Osseointegration in Clinical Dentistry.* Chicago: Quintessence

Brunski, J.B. (1988) The influence of force, motion and related quantities on the response of bone to implants. In *Non-Cemented Total Hip Arthroplasty* (R. Fitzgerald Jr, ed.), pp. 7–21. New York: Raven Press

Buser, D., Bragger, U., Lang, N.P. and Nyman, S. (1990) Regeneration and enlargement of jaw bone using guided tissue regeneration. *Clinical Oral Implants Research* 1, 22–32

Carlsson, L., Röstlund, T., Albrektsson, B. and Albrektsson, T. (1988) Removal torques for polished and rough titanium implants. *International Journal of Oral Maxillofacial Implants* 3, 21–24

Dahlin, C., Linde, A., Gottlow, J. and Nyman, S. (1988) Healing of bone defects by guided tissue regeneration. *Journal of Plastic Reconstructive Surgery* 81, 672–676

Dahlin, C., Sennerby, L., Lekholm, U. *et al.* (1989) Generation of new bone around titanium implants using a membrane technique: an experimental study in rabbits. *International Journal of Oral and Maxillofacial Implants* 4, 19–25

Dahlin, C., Andersson, L. and Linde, A. (1991) Bone augmentation at fenestrated implants by an osseopromotive membrane technique. A controlled clinical study. *Clinical Oral Implant Research* 2, 159–165

Duckworth, J., Brose, M., Avers, R. *et al.* (1987) Therapeutic implications of the bacterial pathogens associated with dental implants. *Journal of Dental Research* 66, 114

Eley, B.M., Cox, S.W. and Watson, R.M. (1991) Protease activities in peri-implant sulcus fluid from patients with permucosal osseointegrated dental implants. Correlation with clinical parameters. *Clinical Oral Implant Research* 2, 62–70

Ericsson, I., Berglundh, T., Marinello, C.P. *et al.* (1992) Long-standing plaque and gingivitis at implants and teeth in the dog. *Clinical Oral Implant Research* 3, 99–103

Esposito, M., Hirsch, J.M., Lekholm, U. and Thopsen, P. (1998) Biological factors contributing to failures of osseointegrated oral implants. I. Success criteria and epidemiology. *European Journal of Oral Science* 106, 527–551

Gould, T.R.L., Brunette, D.M. and Westbury, L. (1981) The attachment mechanism of epithelial cells to titanium *in vivo*. *Journal of Periodontal Research* 16, 611–616

Hench, L.L. (1994) Bioceramics: theory and clinical applications. *Bioceramics* 7 (In H. Andersson, R.-P. Happonen and A. Yli-Urpo, eds), pp. 3–14. Oxford: Butterworth-Heinemann

Hench, L.L. and Wilson, J. (1995) Bioactive glasses and glass-ceramics: a 25-year retrospective. *Ceramic Transactions* 48, 11–21

Hench, L.L., Stanley, H.R., Clark, A.E. *et al.* (1991) Dental applications of Bioglass® implants. In *Bioceramics 4* (W. Bonfield, G.W. Hastings and K.E. Tanner, eds), pp. 231–238. Oxford: Butterworth-Heinemann

Hollender, L. and Rockler, B. (1980) Radiographic evaluation of osseointegrated implants of the jaws. *Dentomaxillofacial Radiology* 9, 91–95

Hürzeler, M.B., Quinones, C.R., Schupback, P. *et al.* (1997) Treatment of peri-implantitis using guided bone regeneration and bone grafts, alone or in combination in beagle dogs. Part 2: histologic findings. *Journal of Oral Maxillofacial Implants* 12, 168–175

Iacono, V.J. and Livers, H.N. (1992) Special radiographic techniques for implant dentistry. In *Advances in Periodontics. Part IV. Implant Dentistry* (T.G. Wilson Jr, K.S. Kornman and M.G. Newman, eds), pp. 341–345. Chicago, London: Quintessence Publishing Co. Ltd

Lang, N.P. and Wilson, T.G. Jr (1992) Choice of implant systems and clinical management. In *Advances in Periodontics. Part IV. Implant Dentistry* (T.G. Wilson Jr, K.S. Kornman and M.G. Newman, eds), pp. 346–376. Chicago, London: Quintessence Publishing Co. Ltd

Lazzara, R. (1989) Immediate implant placement into extraction sites: surgical and restorative advantages. *The International Journal of Periodontics and Restorative Dentistry* **9**, 333–344

Lekholm, U., Ericsson, I., Adell, R. and Slots, J. (1986) The condition of the soft tissues at tooth and fixative abutments supporting fixed bridges. *Journal of Clinical Periodontology* **13**, 588–562

Lindhe, J., Berglundh, T., Ericsson, I. *et al.* (1992) Experimental breakdown of peri-implant and periodontal tissues. A study in the beagle dog. *Clinical Oral Implant Research* **3**, 9–16

Listgarten, M.M. and Lai, C.H. (1975) Ultrastructure of the intact interface between an endosseous epoxy resin dental implant and the host tissues. *Journal Biologie Buccale* **3**, 13–28

Mombelli, A. and Mericske-Sterne, R. (1990) Microbiological features of stable osseointegrated implants used as abutments for overdentures. *Clinical and Oral Implant Research* **1**, 1–7

Mombelli, A., Van Oosten, M.A., Schürch, E. Jr and Lang, N.P. (1987) The microbiota associated with successful or failing osseointegrated titanium implants. *Oral and Microbiological Immunology* **2**, 145–151

Mombelli, A., Buser, D. and Lang, N.P. (1988) Colonization of osseointegrated titanium implants in edentulous patients. *Oral and Microbiological Immunology* **3**, 113–120

Nowzari, H. and Slots, J. (1994) Microorganisms in polytetrafluoroethylene barrier membranes for guided tissue regeneration. *Journal of Clinical Periodontology* **21**, 203–210

Nyman, S., Lang, N.P., Buser, D. and Bragger, U. (1990) Bone regeneration adjacent to titanium implants using guided tissue regeneration, A report of two cases. *International Journal of Oral Maxillofacial Implants* **5**, 9–14

Pilliar, R.M., Deporter, D.A., Watson, P.A. and Valiquette, N. (1991) Dental implant design – effect on bone remodelling. *Journal of Biomedical Research* **25**, 467–483

Quirynen, M. and Listgarten, M.M. (1990) The distribution of bacterial morphotypes around natural teeth and titanium implants. *Clinical and Oral Research* **1**, 8–12

Rams, T.E., Roberts, T.W., Tatum, H. and Keyes, P.H. (1984) Subgingival bacteriology of periodontally healthy and diseased human dental implants. *Journal of Dental Research* **63**, 200

Sander, L., Frandsen, E.V.G., Arnbjerg, D. *et al.* (1994) Effect of local metronidazole application on periodontal healing following guided tissue regeneration. Clinical findings. *Journal of Periodontology* **65**, 914–920

Schenk, R. and Willenegger, H. (1977) Zur Histologie der primären Knochenheilung. Modifikationen und grenzen der Spaltheilung in Abhängigkeit von der Defektgrösse. *Unfallheilk* **80**, 155–160

Schroeder, A., Pohler, O. and Sutter, F. (1976) Gewebsreaktion auf ein Titan-Hohlzylinderimplantat mit Titan-Spritzchichtoberfläche. *Schweizerische Monatsschrift für Zahnheilkunde* **86**, 713–727

Schroeder, A., Sutter, F. and Krekeler, G. (1988) *Orale Implantogie. Allgemeine Grundlagen unt ITI-Hohlzylindersystem*. Stuttgart, New York: Georg Thieme

Seibert, J. and Nyman, S. (1990) Localized ridge augmentation in dogs. A pilot study using membranes and hydroxyapatite. *Journal of Periodontology* **61**, 157–165

Sutter, F., Schroeder, A. and Buser, D. (1988) The new concept of ITI hollow-cylinder and hollow-screw implants: Part 1. Engineering and design. *International Journal of Oral Maxillofacial Implants* **3**, 161–172

Thomsen, P., Ericson, L.E. (1985) Light and transmission electron microscopy used to study the tissue morphology close to implants. *Biomaterials* **6**, 421–424

Van Winkelhoff, A.B., Rodenburg, J.P., Goené, R.J. *et al.* (1989) Metronidazole plus amoxycillin in the treatment of *Actinobacillus actinomycetemcomitans* associated periodontitis. *Journal of Clinical Periodontology* **16**, 128–131

Wetzel, A.C., Stich, H. and Caffesse, R.G. (1995) Bone apposition onto oral implants in the sinus area filled with different grafting materials. A histological study in beagle dogs. *Clinical Oral Implant Research* **6**, 155–163

Wilson, T.G. Jr, Kornman, K.S. and Newman, M.G. (eds) (1992) *Advances in Periodontics. Part IV. Implant Dentistry*. Chicago, London: Quintessence Publishing Co. Ltd

Wilson, J., Clark, A.E., Hall, M. and Hench, L.L. (1993) Tissue response to Bioglass® endosseous ridge maintenance implants. *Journal of Implantology* **19**, 295–302

27

The relationship between periodontal and restorative treatment

Dental restorations should be designed both to minimize plaque accumulation at the gingival margin and to avoid physical injury to the periodontal tissues. The main areas where restorative dentistry and periodontics inter-relate are as follows:

- The relationship between dental restorations and gingival margins
- The occlusal relations of dental restorations
- The support from the periodontium for partial dentures or fixed bridgework
- The consequences of gingival recession
- Crown lengthening for cast restorations
- Periodontal/pulpal infections
- Dental implants.

These will be discussed below.

The relationship between dental restorations and gingival margins

Dental caries usually attacks smooth enamel surfaces, interproximally and buccal or lingual cervically, immediately coronally to the gingival margin. The enamel carious lesion tapers towards the amelodentinal junction and then spreads laterally along the junction. In this way it involves a greater area of dentine and may result in it progressing subgingivally towards the alveolar crest (*Figure 27.1*). Breakdown of the unsupported enamel may then result in damage to the attached junctional epithelium.

When the tooth is restored, the margin of the restoration often has to extend slightly subgingivally in order to eliminate the caries and unsupported enamel (*Figure 27.1*). Whatever restorative material is used – amalgam, composite, glass ionomer, gold or porcelain – the junctional epithelium fails to adhere to its surface and a pocket results. A further important factor in this process is the restorative margin itself, since even apparently

Figure 27.1 Restoration of interproximal caries. Caries below contact area extending into dentine and spreading along amelodentinal junction. The resultant restoration extends subgingivally with pocket formation

perfect margins accumulate plaque at this site. The lack of protective seal from the junctional epithelium results in the pocket becoming colonized by the bacteria found in subgingival plaque. Thus all subgingival restorations, even those judged clinically sound, will cause gingivitis of some degree, extending at least to the margin of the restoration (*Figure 27.2a*). This situation could eventually promote the development of chronic periodontitis. However, if a restoration such as an anterior crown is very carefully prepared so that the resulting margins can be cleaned by the patient, then the surrounding gingival margin will remain healthy (*Figure 27.2b*)

(a)

(b)

Figure 27.2 *(a)* Carefully prepared crown |1 with healthy surrounding gingivae (Courtesy Mr B Parkins). *(b)* Porcelain jacket crown on 1| extending subgingivally. Severe localized gingivitis is present associated with this restoration

Obviously, if the restorative margin is poor then much more damage may result. Deficient or overhanging margins become completely covered with plaque over their whole complex surface and are impossible to clean (*Figure 27.3*). Therefore, they are a potent source of gingival irritation and result in severe gingivitis and, frequently, progression to periodontitis (see Chapter 4).

Clinical considerations

In view of these problems, a cavity margin should not extend subgingivally except when absolutely necessary for caries removal (Reeves, 1991). Major precautions should also be taken to avoid deficient or overhanging cervical margins. Furthermore, all restorations with deficient or overhanging cervical margins should be removed and replaced by satisfactory ones.

Figure 27.3 A paralleling technique intra oral radiograph showing grossly overhanging amalgam restorations associated with severe gingivitis. There is also evidence of horizontal bone loss between 76| and the retained root of 8|

Amalgam restorations

Careful cavity preparation should avoid any unnecessary cervical extension. Class II preparations should be fitted with a tightly fitting and appropriately adapted matrix band, and this should be firmly wedged cervically. If the cervical floor of the restoration is at or below the cement–enamel junction, the proximal surface will be concave. In this situation a conventionally shaped wedge will fail to adapt the matrix to the cervical floor (*Figure 27.4*). A carefully contoured wedge should be used to adapt the matrix (Eli *et al.*, 1991). The cervical margin should be carefully checked with a fine explorer immediately the matrix is removed so that any small excesses can be trimmed with a fine instrument.

Figure 27.4 Section through a Class II cavity at the level of the cervical floor. It shows how a conventional wedge may fail to adapt the matrix to a proximal furrow on the tooth

Composite and glass ionomer restorations

A wide range of composite filling and veneering materials is now available for anterior and posterior teeth. In posterior teeth they should only be used for small restorations. Glass ionomers are used to restore buccal and lingual cervical cavities, and as a secondary base material for composite restorations. Both types of restoration should ideally be placed using a rubber dam, since they are very moisture sensitive.

Careful cavity preparation should avoid any unnecessary cervical extension. Matrices should be very carefully adapted, placed and wedged to avoid cervical excess. Any thin excess should be carefully fractured away after the material has fully set to leave a good tooth–restoration junction. When necessary, composites can be carefully contoured and trimmed with fine diamond stones and abrasive discs specially made for this purpose. The cervical margin should be carefully assessed with a probe and dental floss before accepting the restoration as satisfactory. Excesses with this material will not adhere to the tooth, and plaque will rapidly form between its inner surface and the tooth. This actively promotes the development of secondary caries, gingivitis and periodontitis.

Very great care indeed should be taken with the use of composite as a veneer material on anterior teeth for aesthetic purposes. Its use must be fully justified, since the potential for gingival damage is great. If it is decided appropriate to use this technique, then sufficient tooth substance must be removed labially to accommodate the veneer without over-contouring. The use of a rubber dam is mandatory. The cervical margin should be placed level with the gingival margin, and the material must be very carefully contoured to avoid it acting as a plaque trap. It must be possible to clean the margin effectively with a toothbrush.

Gold and porcelain restorations

Careful cavity preparation should avoid any unnecessary cervical extension. The margins must be very precise, and a very accurate full arch master impression should be taken, along with a full arch impression of the opposing arch and appropriate bite registration. Supragingival placement of margins makes it much easier to take an accurate impression. The restoration must precisely fit the margins without any deficiency or excess. This depends on the skills of both the dentist and the dental technician.

Periodontal care of teeth with subgingival restorations

There will be a tendency for buccal or lingual subgingival restorations to stimulate gingival recession, which may expose their cervical margin. Perhaps in this instance the gingiva knows what is good for it! The effects on the gingiva can be reduced interproximally by the regular use of floss, taking it down to just below the margin of the restoration. Obviously, any excess material at the margin will prevent this procedure. Buccally and lingually, the use of Bass technique brushing will be effective providing the bristles of the brush can reach the cervical margin of the restoration. Regular subgingival scaling should also

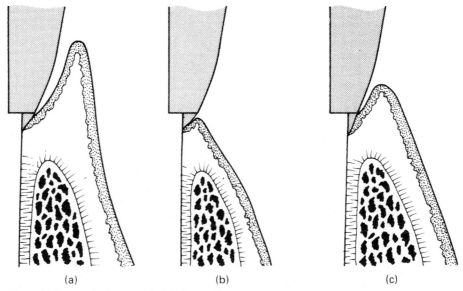

(a)   (b)   (c)

Figure 27.5 An apically repositioned flap used to expose margin of subgingival restoration with a restoration-to-bone distance less than 4 mm: *(a)* before surgery; *(b)* after healing of surgery; *(c)* months later when gingival regeneration is complete. The gingival margin has migrated coronally to cover the restorative margin again be carried out. These areas should be regularly checked by periodontal probing and, when appropriate, radiographs to watch for any loss of attachment.

Ideally, surgical pocket elimination should be carried out to expose the margin and produce a physiological sulcus. However, this is only possible if a sufficiently deep periodontal pocket is present with the alveolar bone margin 4 mm apical to the restorative margin. If this is attempted for situations with a lesser distance, the procedure is only temporarily successful in exposing the margin (Van der Velden, 1982). This is because during repair, following the surgery, the gingiva will gradually reform its physiological form and relationships and will extend coronally so that its margin is 4 mm above the bone margin (*Figure 27.5*). If a deeper pocket is present then pocket elimination surgery using gingivectomy or an apically repositioned flap, as appropriate, will be successful in exposing the margin.

Crown margins

There is a strong case for supragingival margins on crowns, provided the crown length is sufficient for retention. If not, a crown lengthening procedure should be considered (see below). Supragingival margins greatly simplify impression taking, provision of temporary crowns, the inspection of the final restoration and its cementation. Most importantly, the crown margins are accessible for cleaning.

The only possible exception to this rule is the buccal aspects of visible anterior teeth for aesthetic purposes. In this situation, the labial margin only of the crown is extended to a maximum of 0.5 mm (i.e. just) into the gingival crevice (*Figure 27.6*). Obviously, there must be

Figure 27.6 Section through an anterior crown preparation for a bonded porcelain—metal crown. The palatal finishing line is located supragingivally. The buccal finishing line is located just within the gingival crevice for aesthetic reasons. The interdental finishing line joins these two points

complete gingival health before the provision of any crown is considered. Provided the labial surface consists of highly glazed porcelain, has a precise fit and is reachable by Bass technique toothbrushing, then little harm should result. Good plaque control is essential to maintain this situation, and it should be remembered that gingivitis in this area is very unsightly.

The occlusal relations of dental restorations

All dental restorations should be in a balanced occlusion in the functional intercuspal, protrusive, retruded and lateral positions. If this is not achieved, occlusal trauma lesions may result (Chapter 24). In addition, the contact areas should be correctly restored to avoid food impaction and drifting of adjacent teeth.

With plastic restorations such as amalgam, these relationships must be checked and corrected by carving before the material reaches its final set. Composites in posterior teeth are more difficult to deal with, and this is one of their disadvantages. The intercuspal occlusion can be roughly produced by placing a cling-film membrane over the occlusal surface so that the patient can bite on this. Since this impedes light curing, the patient can only close on this material and grind immediately after placement of the composite and then open again to allow curing. This is also difficult with a rubber dam in position, which is essential to avoid moisture contamination. Therefore, composites involving the occlusal surface are usually only roughly shaped before curing and then need grinding into shape and occlusion using occlusal registering paper or wax. This is far from ideal, since it destroys the original surface of the composite and makes it impossible to achieve good occlusal contouring. These problems can be overcome by using composite inlays, which are fabricated on models outside the mouth. Their initial fit and occlusion depend on the accuracy of the impressions and bites, but their marginal seal is no better than that of conventional composites because they are luted in with composite acid etched to the enamel surface. Their life is therefore similar to conventional composites.

With cast gold or fused porcelain or bonded metal—porcelain restorations, the correct occlusion depends on the accuracy of the models and bite registration and the skill of the dental technician. If all these functions are carried out correctly, then no adjustments should be necessary at the fitting stage and the restoration(s) should be in balance in the intercuspal and functional lateral, protrusive and retruded positions (Chapter 24). Great care should also be taken to restore the correct contact area(s) with adjacent teeth. This requires accurate impressions of the arch with the restoration(s) and the opposing arch, accurate bite registration using a face bow when necessary, and functional wax bites in order to place the models correctly on an articulator.

The support from the periodontium for partial dentures or fixed bridgework

When teeth are lost and replaced by dentures or bridges, the occlusal forces applied to the prosthesis are transmitted to the remaining supporting teeth. Obviously, the greater number of teeth lost, the larger are the forces applied to the remaining teeth. In addition, chronic periodontitis can significantly reduce the support of teeth, which are therefore less able to resist occlusal forces placed upon them and, more particularly, additional forces placed upon them by prostheses.

It is essential that all periodontal disease is successfully treated before any prosthetic work, fixed or removable, is undertaken. If periodontal health cannot be achieved and advanced periodontitis persists, then the prognosis for the remaining dentition and any prosthesis will be extremely poor. In some situations with advanced chronic periodontitis, transitional dentures may have to be provided as part of a planned transition to a full denture. However, these dentures are never stable and always, to some extent, reduce the life of the remaining dentition.

The aim of any prosthesis is to spread the occlusal load of missing teeth to as many remaining teeth as possible and to avoid overloading any supporting teeth. In periodontally controlled mouths, the choice usually lies between a tooth supported, skeleton, chrome-cobalt partial denture and a fixed bridge. The tendency is to restrict the use of bridgework to short edentulous spans, where the abutment teeth have good periodontal support and health, and to use dentures for patients with greater numbers of missing teeth and consequently fewer abutment teeth. The design of a chrome-cobalt denture aims to distribute the occlusal load to as many supporting teeth as possible using occlusal rests. It also aims to minimize the stress on abutment teeth by reciprocating the forces placed upon them by retention clasps. In addition, it aims by its skeleton design, where possible, to leave uncovered the gingival margins of supporting teeth and thus to reduce its plaque retentiveness and avoid gingival trauma. However, chrome-cobalt dentures can still overstress abutment teeth if the edentulous span is long, and particularly where there is a free end saddle. In these situations, tilting and rocking of abutment teeth can occur and this can reduce their functional life. In addition, the movements of a free end saddle may cause gingival and mucosal trauma. These tendencies can be minimized by a wide distribution of occlusal loads and careful reciprocation of clasps.

These forces are much more damaging with poorly designed acrylic partial dentures. Teeth with reduced periodontal support may be rocked by ill-fitting clasps and denture components, and considerable gingival trauma may be caused by tissue coverage and denture movement. These dentures are also plaque retentive, and will cause gingival irritation if not kept scrupulously clean.

A period of periodontal adaption will follow the placement of a new partial denture, and the result will greatly depend on its design.

The problems described above may be overcome by the provision of bridgework. This is, however, extremely expensive and very demanding on clinical and technical expertise.

A 15-year longitudinal study of 108 bridges made for 102 patients by senior students in a Norwegian dental school was carried out by Valderhaug *et al.* (1993). They found that the amount of plaque was similar on crowned and control teeth, but marked gingivitis was seen more frequently in crowned teeth with subgingival margins. A slight increase in mean pocket depth was seen with crowned teeth but not in control teeth, although no differences could be detected in bone levels. There was also a steady increase in secondary caries around the abutment teeth from 3.3% at the fifth year to 12% at the fifteenth year. These findings make it clear that abutment crowns should have supragingival margins wherever possible; oral hygiene and diet should be continually monitored, as should periodontal and caries status.

The amount of support provided by abutment teeth is crucial in the success of a bridge. This is usually based on Ante's law, which proposes that in a fixed bridge the attached root surface area of the abutment teeth should be equal to or greater than the equivalent root surface area of the teeth to be replaced. The blanket application of this 'law' places great restraint on the use of bridges in subjects with reduced periodontal support. However, provided that periodontally healthy conditions are first produced and then maintained, it has been shown that satisfactory function can be achieved with bridges of a cross-arch design supported by teeth with markedly reduced periodontal support (Nyman and Lindhe, 1979; Nyman and Ericsson, 1982). In many of these cases, successful bridges were produced with the support of as little as 16% of the presumed root area of the teeth replaced. However, these bridges involved the whole arch and took maximum advantage of cross-arch support. Such bridges can also take advantage of the increased clinical crown length of treated periodontally involved teeth with attachment loss. This allows the preparation of abutments with good retention form and also for the provision of supragingival margins when aesthetics allow.

These sorts of bridges are probably preferable to partial dentures in cases with reduced periodontal attachment, especially where there is tooth mobility. This is because the full arch fixed bridge has greater rigidity and provides a more favourable distribution of function to the remaining teeth. Moreover, the mechanoreceptors within the periodontal ligament restrict by feedback the force generated by the muscles of mastication, and thereby limit the occlusal forces on the bridge.

However, as already stated, there are three important constraints on this sort of work. First, it is extremely expensive, which puts it out of reach of most patients in this category. Secondly, and most importantly, it will only be successful if existing periodontal disease is first effectively treated and then maintained, both by immaculate oral hygiene and regular 3-monthly subgingival scaling. Thirdly, this work is extremely demanding on the clinical expertise of the dentist and the technical expertise of the dental technician. This is because all of the abutment crowns must fit perfectly with superb leak-free margins which are easy to clean, and the whole occlusion must be in balance in the functional intercuspal, retrusive, lateral and protrusive positions.

Pontic design

Pontics should be designed so that the interproximal cleaning of the abutment teeth can be effectively carried out. This means that it must be possible to thread dental floss through the interproximal space between the abutments and the pontic(s). It should also be possible to pass floss under the inner surface of the pontic to clean the surface adjacent to the bridge mucosa. If such a design is provided, then floss can be threaded through using a floss threader or by using superfloss with its stiffened end. It can then reach the proximal surfaces of both abutments and the undersurface of the pontic.

The ideal design for a posterior pontic is the so-called bullet-shaped pontic (*Figure 27.7a*). This has a point contact with the ridge mucosa, and is shaped to produce wide interproximal spaces to allow floss access. Its occlusal surface is also somewhat narrowed in comparison to a corresponding natural tooth in order to reduce the occlusal loads placed upon it. This design is not possible for anterior pontics because of aesthetic considerations. These usually have a single ridge-lap design, slightly lapping over the labial aspect of the ridge (*Figure 27.7b*).

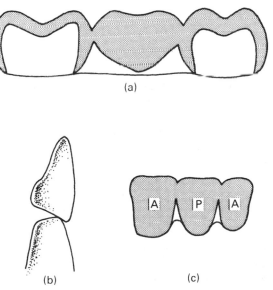

(a)

(b)   (c)

Figure 27.7 *(a)* A 'bullet-shaped' posterior pontic. This has wide interproximal spaces to allow easy passage of floss and a point contact with the ridge. *(b)* An anterior single ridge lap pontic (buccolingual view). It laps the labial ridge but remains clear palatally. *(c)* Labial view of diagram of anterior supporting crowns and pontic. The pontic (P) has wide interproximal spaces to allow the easy passage of floss to clean the proximal surface to the abutments (A) and the undersurface of the pontic

However, the undersurface should slope upwards from the labial edge so that it passes clear of the ridge surface palatally. The undersurface should be smooth and slightly convex for easy cleaning. The anterior–posterior dimensions of the labial aspect should resemble the tooth it is replacing, but should also have wide enough interproximal spaces to allow good floss access (*Figure 27.7c*).

The consequences of gingival recession

Gingival recession resulting from developmental bony dehiscences, periodontal disease or periodontal surgery exposes the root surface (Chapters 8 and 18). Trauma from toothbrushing can result in abrasion, and acids from foods and drinks can cause erosion. These processes may quickly remove the surface cementum and, progressively, the root dentine to produce abrasion/erosion cavities. This can occur on buccal and lingual surfaces, but is much more common buccally.

These cavities are often periodically sensitive to hot and cold stimuli and become retentive of food debris. The cavities or unaffected exposed root surfaces may also become carious if conditions for this are present, and this will necessitate restorative treatment. Abrasion cavities also need restoring if progressive loss of dentine is taking place or if there is persistent sensitivity.

The cavities are usually restored with glass ionomer materials using the newer dentine bonding agents. These materials are moisture sensitive, and the work is best carried out using a rubber dam. Restorations need to be very carefully placed if a good marginal seal and smooth, edge-free margins are to be achieved. Failure to do this will lead to restoration failure and gingival irritation. Obviously, further trauma and erosion need to be avoided by correct oral hygiene training and dietary advice.

Crown lengthening for cast restorations

Since the subgingival placement of restorative margins is undesirable, crown lengthening will have to be considered if the clinical crown is too short to achieve a retentive preparation (Allen, 1993). This is usually a problem with full crown preparations on molar teeth, but can also affect other teeth. Crown lengthening would usually need to be carried out with an apically repositioned flap, as it is extremely important to preserve the full amount of keratinized attached gingiva. The only possible exception to this would be where the problem is caused by gingival hyperplasia, when a gingivectomy could be considered. Soft tissue surgery alone will not achieve the objective unless there is sufficient periodontal pocketing and/or gingival hyperplasia to expose the desired amount of clinical crown. Furthermore, tooth exposure will only be permanent if the bone–gingival margin distance is kept to approximately 4 mm. Therefore, in all other cases marginal bone will also have to be reduced, usually by 1–2 mm, to achieve the desired length of clinical crown.

Where these procedures are carried out, crown preparation should be delayed for at least 20 weeks until the position of the gingival margin is stable (Wise, 1985). This is particularly important with anterior crowns, where aesthetics are important.

Periodontal/pulpal infections

There may be communication between the pulp and periodontal ligament (*Figure 27.8*) via:

- Dentinal tubules
- Lateral and accessory root canals
- The apical foramen
- Cracks and fracture lines
- Iatrogenic perforations.

These may sometimes give rise to:

- Pulpal disease with secondary periodontal involvement
- Periodontal disease with secondary pulpal involvement
- Combined lesions where coincidental periodontal and pulpal origin lesions have merged.

Pulpal disease with secondary periodontal involvement

Infection from the pulp may pass into the periodontal ligament space through the apical foramen or through lateral canals (Hiatt, 1977). Lateral canals are most common in the apical third of the root, but may also occur less commonly in the middle and coronal thirds. In addition, lateral canals are relatively common in the furcation areas of multirooted teeth (*Figure 27.8*).

Infection passing from the pulp into the apical periodontium via the apical foramen or lateral canals in the apical third usually produces an apical granuloma or abscess. Infection usually tracks through the bone to form a subperiosteal abscess, which drains into the vestibule. A very small percentage of apical abscesses, less than 1%, drain via the periodontal ligament to discharge from the gingival margin. This route is, however, more likely if infection passes via a lateral canal in the coronal or middle third of the root. This is also very likely if the infection passes via a lateral canal in the furcation area of a molar tooth (*Figure 27.8*), and in this situation it may simulate periodontal furcation infection (*Figure 27.9*). Fortunately, this is most likely to occur in a young patient with no signs of periodontal disease elsewhere in the mouth, and is therefore less likely to deceive.

Infection may also pass from the pulp to the periodontal ligament space via a fracture line due to trauma or

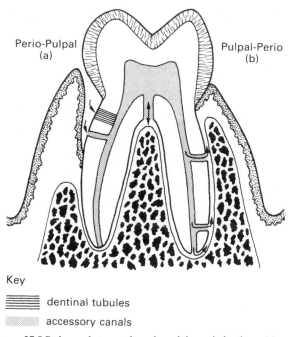

Perio-Pulpal (a)   Pulpal-Perio (b)

Key

▦ dentinal tubules

▨ accessory canals

Figure 27.8 Pathways between the pulp and the periodontium: *(a)* perio-pulpal via dentinal tubules and accessory canals; *(b)* pulpal-perio via accessory canals and apical foramen

Figure 27.9 An abscess in the furcation area of the lower molar with pus discharging from the gingival margin in a 19-year-old girl. The condition was associated with a primary pulpal infection and drained into the periodontium via accessory furcation canals. The condition resolved following successful endodontic treatment

iatrogenic perforations, which may occur during endodontic treatment or post-preparation (Tidmarsh, 1979). This also may lead to discharge of pus from the gingival margin, and could lead to misdiagnosis of a lesion of periodontal origin.

Periodontal disease with secondary pulpal involvement

Gingival recession may expose dentinal tubules to irritation from the oral involvement and lead to hypersensitivity. It can also lead to abrasion and erosion. However, secondary and peritubular dentine formation in these instances usually minimizes pulpal irritation.

Within periodontal pockets, the root surface is exposed to bacteria and their products. Scaling and root planing will remove diseased cementum and expose the dentine tubules, which may transmit irritants (*Figure 27.8*). However, secondary dentine formation usually protects the pulp from irreversible damage.

Periodontal pockets may also involve lateral canals in the coronal and middle thirds of the root and the furcation area, and infection could pass via these communications into the pulp (*Figure 27.8*). Finally, teeth with advanced chronic periodontitis could pass secondary infection from the pocket to the pulp via lateral canals in the apical third or the apical foramen.

Combined lesions

In these cases there is no clear indication from the history or examination of a primary causal link with chronic periodontitis or pulpal disease. A true combined lesion is the result of the fusion of two separate lesions, one marginal periodontal and the other pulpal. The pulpal lesion spreads to the periodontium via the apical foramen or lateral canals, and both lesions enlarge and merge together.

Diagnosis

The correct diagnosis of these conditions involves a detailed history of the onset and development of the symptoms and signs, followed by a careful clinical examination. This should be backed up by the appropriate radiographs and vitality tests. It is much more difficult to get a clear history from a chronic periodontal–pulpal lesion than immediately after an acute episode.

Clinical examination

One should be alerted to the possibility of a periodontal–pulpal lesion by discoloured clinical crowns, pus discharge from the gingival margin buccally or palatally or from the furcation area between the molar roots, and by deep localized pocketing uncharacteristic of the mouth as a whole.

When a primary pulpal lesion spreads to the periodontal ligament and thence to the previously healthy marginal periodontium, it usually spreads along a narrow pathway. When this area is carefully probed it reveals a localized narrow pocket in an otherwise healthy mouth. The pocket contains pus, but no plaque or calculus. The age of the patient may also give a clue to its origin, since pulpal disease is more common in the young than periodontitis. In particular, the discharge of pus from the furcation area of a single molar in a young patient with an otherwise healthy mouth is very suggestive of a primary pulpal lesion (*Figure 27.9*).

Vitality testing

The response of the pulp to vitality testing depends on an intact nerve supply, whereas pulpal vitality may be maintained with an intact blood supply alone. Testing may be carried out electrically, thermally or by using a bur in a cavity within a non-anaesthetized tooth. None of these tests are infallible, and both false-positives and false-negatives may occur. They are particularly likely in heavily filled, multirooted molar teeth.

Radiography

Careful long-cone paralleling radiographs should be taken of the suspected tooth. Where appropriate, radiographs of the rest of the mouth may also be needed. The radiographs of the suspected tooth should show an undistorted view of both the apical and marginal periodontium. The radiographs should be checked for widening of the apical periodontal space, apical or lateral areas of radiolucency, furcation radiolucency and the presence, extent and pattern of marginal bone loss. It should be remembered that the furcation radiolucency can be either pulpal or periodontal in origin.

Treatment

Pulpal disease with secondary periodontal involvement

The pulpal disease will have progressed to partial or total necrosis, and endodontic treatment should be commenced immediately. If drainage of pus from the gingival margin is not rapidly controlled by mechanical cleaning of the pulp chamber and root canals, a course of an appropriate antibiotic should be given. This is best based on a sample of pus, which is sent to a microbiology laboratory for antibiotic sensitivity testing. However, as speed is the essence in these cases, treatment can usually be started with amoxycillin provided that the patient is not hypersensitive to penicillin. If the infection is rapidly controlled by these measures, then the involved marginal periodontium may regenerate and successful endodontic treatment will lead to a return to full periodontal health. However, if the infection is allowed to become chronic, the healing is much less predictable. This is because the chronic infection can cause pathological changes to occur on the root surface, with the cementum becoming infected and necrotic. This leads to a downgrowth of junctional epithelium along the changed root surface, which in turn leads to the establishment of a deep chronic periodontal pocket. For this reason, rapid diagnosis and treatment of the primary pulpal disease is essential for a successful outcome. Chronic lesions will need both endodontic and periodontal treatment, including periodontal surgery. The outcome of the periodontal treatment of such lesions is doubtful.

Periodontal disease with secondary pulpal involvement

An assessment of the prognosis of the tooth in terms of its remaining alveolar bone support should be made before further treatment is planned and instituted.

Lesions of periodontal origin are invariably chronic. An assessment should first be made of the state of the pulp, and it should be ascertained whether the pulpal disease is reversible or irreversible, i.e. whether the pulp is hyperaemic or necrotic. If the pulp is necrotic, endodontic treatment should be carried out first. If, on the other hand, the pulp appears to be still vital but hypersensitive, then periodontal treatment should be carried out first to see whether the reduction in the source of irritation will lead to pulpal recovery.

The periodontal lesion should first be treated by careful, meticulous subgingival scaling and root planing. The condition of the rest of the mouth should be taken into account in the overall treatment plan. Meticulous oral hygiene must be established. The periodontal lesion will invariably require periodontal surgery, and the precise technique employed will depend upon the depth of the pocket and pattern of bone resorption (Chapters 16 and 17).

The outcome can be difficult to determine in cases associated with advanced periodontitis, and all cases should receive regular maintenance treatment.

Combined lesions

If the prognosis is reasonable, both periodontal and endodontic treatment is carried out as outlined above. The endodontic treatment should be carried out first. The periodontal treatment invariably includes periodontal surgery in these cases. The outcome of treatment is uncertain in cases associated with advanced periodontitis.

Dental implants

Osseointegrated dental implants and their clinical implications have been discussed in Chapter 26. They require very careful design, and great clinical and technical expertise. They also require careful maintenance to prevent peri-implant disease. All of this is covered in Chapter 26.

References

Allen, E.P. (1993) Surgical crown lengthening for function and aesthetics. *Dental Clinics of North America* **37**, 163–180

Eli, I., Weiss, E., Kozlovsky, A. and Levi, N. (1991) Wedges in restorative dentistry: principles and applications. *Journal of Oral Rehabilitation* **18**, 257–264

Hiatt, W.H. (1977) Pulpal periodontal disease. *Journal of Periodontology* **48**, 598–609

Nyman, S. and Ericsson, I. (1982) The capacity of reduced periodontal tissues to support fixed bridgework. *Journal of Clinical Periodontology* **9**, 409–414

Nyman, S. and Lindhe, J. (1979) A longitudinal study of combined periodontal and prosthetic treatment for patients with advanced periodontitis. *Journal of Periodontology* **50**, 163–169

Reeves, W.G. (1991) Restorative margin placement and periodontal health. *Journal of Prosthetic Dentistry* **66**, 733–736

Tidmarsh, B.G. (1979) Accidental perforation of the roots of teeth. *Journal of Oral Rehabilitation* **6**, 235–240

Valderhaug, J., Ellingsen, J.E. and Jokstad, A. (1993) Oral hygiene, periodontal condition and carious lesions in patients treated with dental bridges. A 15-year clinical and radiographic follow-up study. *Journal of Clinical Periodontology* **20**, 482–489

Van der Velden, U. (1982) Regeneration of the interdental soft tissue following denudation procedures. *Journal of Clinical Periodontology* **9**, 455–459

Wise, W.D. (1985) Stability of the gingival crest after surgery and before anterior crown placement. *Journal of Prosthetic Dentistry* **53**, 20–23

Further reading

Nevins, M. (1993) Periodontal considerations in prosthodontic treatment. In *Current Opinion in Periodontology* (R.A. Yukna, M.G. Newman and R.C. Williams, eds), pp. 151–156. Philadelphia: Current Science

Wilson, R.D. (1992) Restorative dentistry. In *Advances in Periodontics* (T. Wilson, K. Kornman and M. Newman, eds), pp. 226–244. Chicago: Quintessence Publishing Co. Ltd

Index